MYOCARDIAL AND SKELETAL MUSCLE BIOENERGETICS

ADVANCES IN EXPERIMENTAL MEDICINE AND BIOLOGY

Recent Volumes in this Series

A Continuation Order Plan is available for this series. A continuation order will bring delivery of each new volume immediately upon publication. Volumes are billed only upon actual shipment. For further information please contact the publisher.

MYOCARDIAL AND SKELETAL MUSCLE BIOENERGETICS

Edited by

Nachman Brautbar

University of Southern California School of Medicine
and Hollywood Presbyterian Medical Center
Los Angeles, California

PLENUM PRESS • NEW YORK AND LONDON

Library of Congress Cataloging in Publication Data

International Congress on Myocardial and Cellular Bioenergetics and Compartmentation (2nd: 1984: University of Southern California)
  Myocardial and skeletal muscle bioenergetics.

  (Advances in experimental medicine and biology; v. 194)
  "Proceedings of the Second International Congress on Myocardial and Cellular
Bioenergetics and Compartmentation, held February 16–18, 1984 at the University of
Southern California, Los Angeles, California"—T.p. verso.
  Includes bibliographies and index.
  1. Muscles—Congresses. 2. Heart—Muscle—Congresses. 3. Bioenergetics. 4. Cell
compartmentation. 5. Tissue respiration. I. Brautbar, Nachman. II. Title: III. Series.
[DNLM: 1. Cell Compartmentation—congresses. 2. Energy Metabolism—congresses.
3. Energy Transfer—drug effects—congresses. 4. Myocardium—metabolism—con-
gresses. W1 AD559 v.194/WG 280 I594 1984m]
QP321.I525   1984   599′.01852   86-4883
ISBN 0-306-42237-9

Proceedings of the Second International Congress on Myocardial and Cellular
Bioenergetics and Compartmentation, held February 16–18, 1984,
at the University of Southern California, Los Angeles, California

© 1986 Plenum Press, New York
A Division of Plenum Publishing Corporation
233 Spring Street, New York, N.Y. 10013

Printed in the United States of America

To my parents, wife, and children who supported me and stood
behind me at all times

PREFACE

I am pleased to present to the readers the Proceedings of the Second International Congress on Myocardial and Cellular Bioenergetics and Compartmentation which was held in Los Angeles during February 16-18, 1984.

I would like to express my deep appreciation to all those who have encouraged us to hold the Second International Congress. This endeavor could not have been possible without the generous financial support of the following: The American Society for Magnesium Research, The University of Southern California Department of Continuing Medical Education, Alpha Therapeutics, ALSEB Scientific Products, The American Physiological Society, Ciba-Geigy Corporation, Victor Gura, M.D., Merck Sharp and Dohme, Phosphoenergetics, Stuart Pharmaceuticals, and the Upjohn Company.

A note of special thanks goes to Samuel Bessman, M.D., who has been a source of constant support and encouragement for this Congress and for my research endeavors.

Nachman Brautbar

CONTENTS

I. MICROCOMPARTMENTATION AND ENERGY TRANSPORT:

III. MYOCARDIAL PRESERVATION, ISCHEMIA: CELLULAR MECHANISMS

IV. PATHOPHYSIOLOGY OF ENERGY COMPARTMENTATION:

VI. 31-P NMR:

THE PHYSIOLOGICAL SIGNIFICANCE OF THE CREATINE PHOSPHATE SHUTTLE

Samuel P. Bessman

Department of Pharmacology and Nutrition
University of Southern California School of Medicine
2025 Zonal Avenue, Los Angeles, California 90033

The creatine phosphate shuttle[1] is a mechanism found in highly developed cells which carries out an intercommunication process to signal the demand for energy and to transport the energy produced in response to the signal to those sites where energy is being utilized.

Such a system requires three discrete parts, each with a highly specific function (Fig. 1.). First, the energy utilizing function which can be called the peripheral terminus of the shuttle. Here the transport form of energy, in this case creatine phosphate, is fed into the final endergonic process, e.g., muscle contraction, by means of a transducer, an isozyme of creatine phosphokinase.

Muscle contraction is energized by ATP, by a mechanism (ATPase) which splits ATP to ADP, using the energy of the anhydride bond to cause the muscle fiber to contract. The ADP liberated by this reaction is bound by enzymes in its immediate environment, the predominant one of which is creatine phosphokinase. This enzyme catalyzes the following reaction:

(1)   Creatine PO_4 + ADP $\longrightarrow$ ATP + Creatine

Thus, creatine phosphate, the transport form of energy is transduced to ATP, the utilizable form of energy, as need arises (e.g., muscle contraction) and the chemical signal that the muscle has contracted is the liberation of free creatine at, or in the immediate vicinity of, the contractile site.

This signal then enters the intervening space (Fig. 1.) in which creatine and creatine phosphate are diffusing in opposite directions.

1

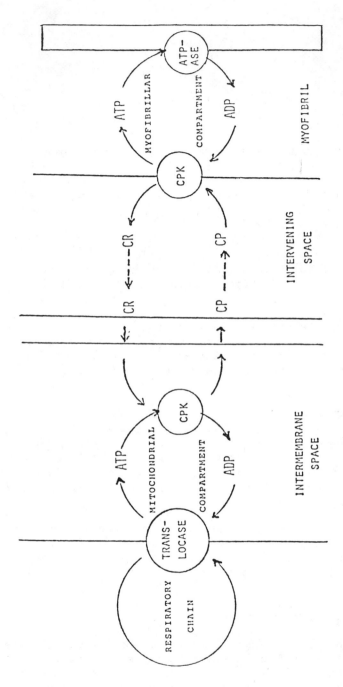

MITOCHONDRION

Legend, Figure 1. The creatine phosphate shuttle showing at the left the location within the inner membrane and the intermembrane space of the mitochondrion. The intervening space between the mitochondrion and the myofibril with the CPK attached to it. The mitochondrial compartment of the shuttle lies within the intermembrane space and the myofibril compartment lies within the myofibril. It includes the ATPase of the light chains and the CPK which is associated with the A-band [38]. The transport of energy between the myofibril and the mitochondrion therefore takes place in the form of the creatine-creatine phosphate shuttle.

When creatine arrives at the mitochondrion, the energy generating terminus, it encounters the mitochondrial isozyme of creatine kinase. Here conditions are favorable for the conversion of creatine to creatine phosphate, according to the right to left direction of reaction 1.

The ATP comes from the translocase system of the mitochondrion, donates its gamma phosphate group to creatine and produces ADP which is the immediate respiratory control stimulus for formation of more ATP. The creatine phosphate formed enters the intervening space, diffusing in the direction of the peripheral terminus, the contracting myofibril.

Thus creatine behaves as the carrier vehicle by literally transporting the energy to the energy-using system. It does this because at each end of the "track" there is a special transducer, an isozyme of creatine phosphokinase, to convert the signal, creatine, to the substrate for energy generation, ADP, at one end, and another transducer which converts creatine phosphate to immediately useful energy at the peripheral end. In communication terms, energy supply at least in heart, brain and skeletal muscle, can be regarded as a "dialogue" between two isozymes of creatine kinase.

It would seem that the most efficient process would be to generate and transmit ATP, to utilize ATP peripherally, and to return the energy generation signal, ADP to the mitochondrion. This was, and still is, the conventional view. Would any advantage accrue to the cell to convert ATP and ADP to their shuttle transport counterparts, creatine phosphate and creatine?

In any transmission system efficiency is _inter alia_ proportional to the integrity of the signal. A signal may be lost through friction, dissipation as of light, or be caught in intervening traps or barriers. In the living cell almost every endergonic reaction is energized by ATP or a direct product of ATP. There are thousands of enzymes in the cell which could trap and bind ATP in the course of its traverse. This is even more true of ADP, which has a true concentration (activity) about two orders of magnitude smaller than its nominal concentration[2].

On the other hand, creatine phosphate and creatine take part in no reactions other than the equilibrium with ATP and ADP, catalyzed by only one enzyme, creatine phosphokinase. Even though creatine phosphate may be broadcast throughout the cell, and creatine may be sent out undirected, the energy and signal can only be utilized or "interpreted" at those sites where the several isoenzymes of creatine kinase are located.

3

The binding of various isozymes of creatine kinase to specific sites in the cell of the heart, skeletal muscle, or brain focuses the energetics of that cell on those sites, perhaps not to the exclusion of others, but certainly preferentially. The first prediction of this distribution of signal and energy product organized through creatine turnover[3] did not come from muscle physiology, however, it came from a metabolic imperative related to the mechanism of insulin action.

It has been postulated[4] that insulin acts to connect hexokinase to mitochondria. This would explain the generally anabolic effects of insulin as an increase in the delivery of energy to all anabolic processes, such as membrane transport, and protein, fat and carbohydrate synthesis[5,6]. The close similarity between the energy stimulating effect of the attachment of hexokinase to mitochondria as the mechanism of insulin action and the fact that exercise causes insulin-like effects on blood glucose and anabolic processes[7] in the diabetic demanded some similar "acceptor" mechanism involving muscle contraction. Since it had been shown by Lipmann and Meyerhoff[8] that muscle exercise liberated free creatine, and Belitzer and Tsybakova[9] had demonstrated oxidative phosphorylation of creatine it was postulated that exercise sent free creatine to the mitochondrion, thereby causing accelerated respiratory control.

It has been dogma in muscle physiology that the creatine-creatine phosphate system is simply an energy buffer to maintain equilibrium ATP potential. Such a buffer should receive ATP from the mitochondrion and liberate ATP into the myofibrils, receive ADP from the contracted myofibrils and emit it into the mitochondria, causing respiratory control. This view is contradicted by both anatomical and functional evidence which is reviewed in extenso[1]. The anatomical evidence shows that specific isozymes of creatine kinase are bound to mitochondria and to myofibrils or other peripheral termini, they do not float free in the postulated buffer pool. The functional evidence shows that energy is preferentially emitted by the mitochondrion as creatine phosphate and preferentially utilized by the myofibril in the same form. The evidence also shows that creatine, not ADP, is emitted by the myofibril and received by the mitochondrion.

The first anatomical data showing a non-homogenous distribution of creatine kinase was reported by Jacobs, Heldt and Klingenberg[10], who discovered the mitochondrial bound isozyme. This finding led to the demonstration of Bessman and Fonyo[11], of respiratory control in pigeon breast mitochondria by creatine, extended by Jacobs and Lehninger[12] to heart sarcosomes. The discovery of the binding of creatine kinase to the M-line[13,14] of the myofibril and to the entire A-band[15,16] furnished an anatomical basis for the creatine phosphate shuttle.

Chemical evidence for the functional compartmentation of creatine phosphate in mitochondria was first produced by Yang et al[17], who showed, by use of ^{32}P labeled nucleotides, that the changes in specific activity of creatine phosphate over short time intervals were compatible only with the conclusion that, functionally, creatine phosphate was formed from creatine by recently synthesized ATP, which must have had special access to the mitochondrial CPK. Not only was there CPK bound to the mitochondrion, it was bound in such a way that nascent ATP was utilized preferentially over the ATP in the medium.

This was followed by the demonstration by Viitanen et al[18] that the mitochondrial CPK compartment is apparently bounded by the mitochondrial outer membrane. This was done by subjecting mitochondria to controlled membranolysis with digitonin in such a way that there was only trivial loss of CPK and of respiratory function. These mitochondria no longer exhibited the functional compartmentation of the untreated mitochondria, Figure 2. It is biochemical dogma that the outer mitochondrial membrane is permeable to nucleotides, but the absolute degree of this permeability has never been considered. Since it is a structure interposed between the cytosol and the inner membrane of the mitochondrion it appears reasonable that there should be some functional barrier. These experiments support the inference that qualitatively "permeable" membranes may not be absolutely permeable, and that some compartmentation and functional "advantage" may be effected by the intermembrane space of the intact mitochondrion. Elegant kinetic experiments from Saks' group[19,20,21] gave strong support to the concept of a mitochondrial compartment sensitive to creatine as the respiratory control signal.

Evidence for the myofibrillar end of the shuttle was first obtained by Perry[22] who showed that in the presence of trace amounts of ATP creatine phosphate could supply energy for muscle contraction. The important contribution made by these experiments was that ATP qua ATP could be regenerated and cause contraction at extremely small concentrations if there was creatine phosphate available. Since all of the experiments were conducted with creatine phosphokinase added to the medium it was not possible to postulate compartmentation of CPK with ATPase. Evidence such as this together with the experiments by Mommaerts[23] and others which showed that ATP did not break down during muscle contraction, nor did ADP rise, but that creatine phosphate breakdown did parallel muscle contraction, served to cause Hill[24] to throw down his famous "Challenge to Biochemists." There was no relation between muscle contraction and ATP and ADP economy yet biochemists insisted that nucleotides fueled muscle contraction. Experiments by Cain and Davies[25] who used fluorodinitrobenzene (FDNB) to inhibit CPK showed contractions continuing for a short time after poisoning so that there was no change in CP while ATP fell. This convinced the biochemists and the physiologists, who abandoned attempts to understand the role of creatine phosphate in muscle contraction.

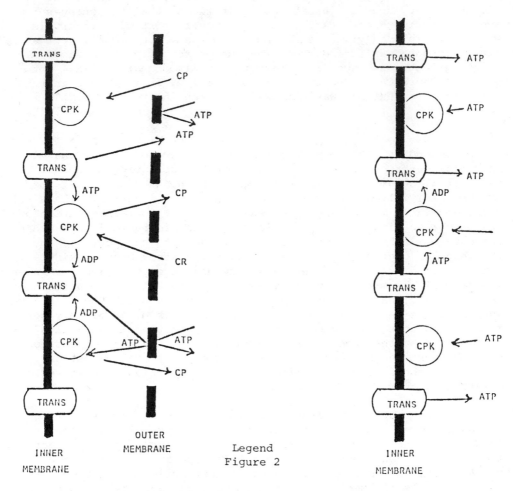

INNER MEMBRANE

OUTER MEMBRANE

Legend
Figure 2

INNER MEMBRANE

A.   Complete mitochondrial membrane system with outer and inner membranes intact. ATP generated through the translocase can be deflected if it does not hit a pool in the outer membrane and ATP from the cytosol can be deflected as well. This gives a partial separation between the larger outer pool of ATP and the intermembrane pool which has closer access to CPK.

B.   The outer membrane having been removed by detergent action permits equal access of ATP generated throughout the translocase and ATP from the cytosol to the CPK system. Therefore, there is no longer any evidence of compartmentation.

It now appears that both sides were correct and both were somewhat in error. Contraction was not normal by any stretch of the imagination when CPK was inactivated, so an intact nucleotide system, ATP and ADP, although necessary was not sufficient to support normal muscular work. It was not proper even at that juncture to relegate the CP-CPK-creatine system to the role of a simple energy buffer. It was clearly a necessary part of the energy transport system.

As frequently happens at such junctures, however, the conventional wisdom in physiology adopted the nucleotide philosophy to the exclusion of further consideration of creatine phosphate even though Perry[22] had shown that stoichiometric amounts of ATP were not necessary for myosin ATPase activity and Cain and Davies had shown that the ATP system was not sufficient to maintain contraction.

Although Perry[22] had made the seminal discovery that creatine phosphate could support myofibrillar contraction in the presence of amounts of ATP insufficient to cause any contraction at all, all of the experiments were done with added soluble creatine kinase, so no conclusions could be drawn about the role of creatine phosphate in vivo.

The first chemical evidence for a functional myofibrillar compartment was obtained by Viitanen et al[26] who showed that myofibrillar ATPase utilized creatine phosphate phosphorus preferentially by studying the time course of ^{32}P labeling of nucleotide, creatine, and inorganic phosphates. Direct evidence obtained by Savabi et al[27,28] showed that creatine phosphate produced faster and stronger contraction of glycerinated fibers than did ATP at equivalent concentrations. It was possible to cause contraction with amounts of ATP too low to cause any contraction at all if creatine phosphate was added. This was done with glycerinated fibers which still had about 25% of the original creatine kinase.

Gudbjarnason et al[29] extended Mommaerts' observations to beating mammalian hearts, showing that contraction stopped when creatine phosphate was depleted even though 80% of the ATP remained. This confirmed the existence of peripheral compartments for ATP. The role of creatine as the respiratory control stimulus was not considered even though it had been reported previously[11] however, so the complete shuttle system could not be predicted from these observations.

The creatine phosphate shuttle concept has explained why exercise in diabetics seems metabolically equivalent to dosage with insulin. It would appear, however, that exercise is not really equivalent for it can only be effective in muscle and heart. It does explain why the heart can carry on well in the absence of insulin for it is continually contracting, therefore sending itself a creatine stimulus for respiration not requiring the insulin-hexokinase effect. The effect of exercise, if it is based on the insulin principle of respiratory control (see above) should not affect the metabolism of liver, kidney or any organ which has significant concentrations either of CPK or of creatine phosphate, nor do these organs exercise.

The major effects of exercise are on muscle uptake of glucose, muscle protein synthesis, and utilization of ketones to a small extent. The true physiological significance of exercise in a diabetic is not yet completely clear, but one could predict that except for muscle and its role in utilization of blood glucose there is really little lasting beneficial effect.

Carpenter et al documented the dependence of muscle protein synthesis on the creatine shuttle[30,31,32] and Pal[33,34] has developed evidence that brain protein synthesis may be even more dependent on the shuttle than that of muscle.

Other specific termini for the shuttle have been discovered, and at each one there is found bound creatine kinase. Saks' group[35,36,37] found that membrane NaK ATPase depended upon creatine phosphate primarily for energy with plasma membrane bound CPK transducing it to ATP functionally adjacent to the ADPase.

In regard to the peculiar resistance of the heart to the skeletal muscle wastage caused by prolonged bed rest, paralysis, or the unbridled catabolism of diabetic failure, it must be recalled that the anabolic effect of insulin is mimicked by exercise. The heart is continually contracting, thereby maintaining its own respiratory control and energy economy. It never rests. It is the resting muscle which suffers the greatest damage in diabetes.

REFERENCES

1. S.P. Bessman and C.L. Carpenter, The Creatine Phosphate Energy Shuttle, in: Vol.54, "Annual Review of Biochemistry," Annual Reviews, Palo Alto, CA (1985).
2. R.L. Veech, J.W.R. Lawson, N.W. Cornell, and H.A. Krebs, Cytosolic Phosphorylation Potential, J. Biol. Chem. 254:6538 (1979).
3. S.P. Bessman, Diabetes Mellitus: Observations, Theoretical and Practical, J. Pediatr. 56:191 (1960).
4. S.P. Bessman, Fat Metabolism, A Contribution to the Mechanism of Diabetes Mellitus, in: "Fat Metabolism," V.A. Najjar, ed., The Johns Hopkins Press, Baltimore, MD (1966).
5. S.P. Bessman, A Molecular Basis for the Mechanism of Insulin Action, Amer. J. Med. 40:740 (1966).
6. S.P. Bessman, The Hexokinase-Mitochondrial Binding Theory of Insulin Action, in: "Energy, Biosynthesis and Regulation in Molecular Biology," D. Richter, ed., Walter de Gruyter Verlag, Berlin, New York (1974).

7. S.P. Bessman, B. Borrebaek, P.J. Geiger, and S. Ben-Or, Mito-
    chondrial Creatine Kinase and Hexokinase - Two Examples
    of Compartmentation Predicted by the Hexokinase Mitochond-
    rial Binding Theory of Insulin Action, in: "Microenviron-
    ments and Cellular Compartmentation," P. Srere and R.W.
    Estabrook, eds., Academic Press, Inc., New York (1978).

8. F. Lipmann and O. Meyerhof, Über die Reaktionsänderung des
    tätigen Muskels, Biochem. Z. 227:84 (1930)

9. V.A. Belitzer and E.T. Tsbakova, Phosphorylation as Related to
    Respiration, Biokhimiya 4:516 (1939).

10. H. Jacobs, H.W. Heldt, and M. Klingenberg, High Activity of
    Creatine Kinase in Mitochondria from Muscle and Brain and
    Evidence for a Separate Mitochondrial Isoenzyme of Creatine
    Kinase, Biochem. Biophys. Res. Commun. 16:516 (1964).

11. S.P. Bessman and A. Fonyo, The Possible Role of the Mitochondrial
    Bound Creatine Kinase in Regulation of Mitochondrial Respi-
    ration, Biochem. Biophys. Res. Commun. 22:597 (1966).

12. W.E. Jacobus and A.L. Lehninger, Creatine Kinase of Rat Heart
    Mitochondria: Coupling of Creatine Phosphorylation to
    Electron Transport, J. Biol. Chem. 248:4803 (1973).

13. D.C. Turner, T. Wallimann, and H.M. Eppenberger, A Protein That
    Binds Specifically to the M-line of Skeletal Muscle is
    Identified as the Muscle Form of Creatine Kinase, Proc.
    Natl. Acad Sci. (USA) 70:702 (1973).

14. T. Wallimann, D.C. Turner, and H.M. Eppenberger, Localization
    of Creatine Kinase Isoenzymes in Myofibrils, J. Cell Biol.
    75:297 (1977).

15. O.S. Herasymowych, R.S. Mani, C.M. Kay, R.D. Bradley, and D.G.
    Scraba, Ultrastructure Studies on the Binding of Creatine
    Kinase and the 165,000 Molecular Weight Component to the
    M-band of Muscle, J. Mol. Biol. 136:193 (1980).

16. J. Botts, D.B. Stone, A.T.L. Wang, and R.A. Mendelson, Electron
    Paramagnetic Resonance and Nanosecond Fluorescence Depolari-
    zation Studies on Creatine-phosphokinase Interaction with
    Myosin and Its Fragments, J. Supramol. Struct. 3:141 (1975).

17. W.C.T. Yang, P.J. Geiger, S.P. Bessman, and B. Borrebaek, Forma-
    tion of Creatine Phosphate from Creatine and ^{32}P-labeled ATP
    by Isolated Rabbit Heart Mitochondria, Biochem. Biophys.
    Res. Commun. 76:882 (1977).

18. S. Erickson-Viitanen, P. Viitanen, P.J. Geiger, W.C.T. Yang, and
    S.P. Bessman, Compartmentation of Mitochondrial Creatine
    Phosphokinase. I. Direct Demonstration of Compartmentation
    with the Use of Labeled Precursors, JBC 257:14395 (1982).

19. V.A. Saks, G.B. Chernousova, I. Voronokov, V.N. Smirnov, and
    E.I. Chazov, Energy Transport Mechanism in myocardial cells.
    Circ. Res. Supl. III, 34, 35; III-138, III-148 (1974).

20. V.A. Saks, G.B. Chernousova, D.E. Gukovsky, V.N. Smirnov, and
    E.I. Chazov, Energy Transport in Heart Cells. Mitochondrial
    isoenzyme of creatine phosphokinase. Kinetic Properties and
    Regulatory Action of Magnesium (2+) Ions, Eur. J. Biochem.
    57:273 (1975).

21. V.A. Saks, V.V. Kupriyanov, G. Elizarova, and W.E. Jacobus, Studies of Energy Transport in Heart Cells, the Importance of Creatine Kinase Localization for the Coupling of Mitochondrial Phosphorylcreatine Production to Oxidative Phosphorylation, J. Biol. Chem. 255:755 (1980).

22. S.V. Perry, Creatine Phosphokinase and the Enzymic and Contractile Properties of the Isolated Myofibril, Biochem. J. 57: 427 (1954).

23. W.F.H.M. Mommaerts, Is Adenosine Triphosphate Broken Down During a Single Muscle Twitch?, Nature 174:1083 (1954).

24. D.K. Hill, Preferred Sites of Adenine Nucleotide in Frog's Striated Muscle, J. Physiol. (London) 153:433 (1960).

25. D.F. Cain and R.E. Davies, Breakdown of Adenosine Triphosphate During a Single Contraction of Working Muscle, Biochem. Biophys. Res. Commun. 8:361 (1962).

26. S. Erickson-Viitanen, P.J. Geiger, P. Viitanen, and S.P. Bessman, Compartmentation of Mitochondrial Creatine Phosphokinase. II. The Importance of the Outer Mitochondrial Membrane for Mitochondrial Compartmentation, JBC 257:14405 (1982).

27. F. Savabi, P.J. Geiger, and S.P. Bessman, Kinetic Properties and Functional State of Creatine Phosphokinase in Glycerinated Muscle Fibers - Further Evidence for Compartmentation, Biochem. Biophys. Res. Commun. 114:785 (1983).

28. F. Savabi, P.J. Geiger, and S.P. Bessman, Myofibrillar End of the Creatine Phosphate Energy Shuttle, Amer. J. Physiol. 247:C424 (1984).

29. S. Gudbjarnason, P. Mathes, and K.A. Ravens, Functional Compartmentation of ATP and Creatine Phosphate in Heart Muscle, J. Mol. Cell. Cardiol. 1:325 (1970).

30. C.L. Carpenter, C. Mohan, and S.P. Bessman, Inhibition of Protein and Lipid Synthesis in Muscle, by 2,4-Dinitrofluorobenzene, an Inhibitor of Creatine Phosphokinase, Biochem. Biophys. Res. Commun. 111:884 (1983).

31. C.L. Carpenter, C. Mohan, and S.P. Bessman, Necessity of the Creatine Phosphate Shuttle for Muscle Protein Synthesis (Submitted for publication, 1984).

32. C.L. Carpenter, F. Savabi, and S.P. Bessman, Protein Synthesis by Isolated Skeletal Muscle Polysomes: A Terminal for the Creatine Phosphate Shuttle (Submitted for publication, 1984).

33. S.P. Bessman and N. Pal, The Krebs Cycle Depletion Theory of Hepatic Coma, in "The Urea Cycle," S. Grisolia, R. Baguena and F. Mayor, eds., John Wiley & Sons, Inc., New York (1976).

34. S.P. Bessman and N. Pal, Ammonia Intoxication: Energy Metabolism and Brain Protein Synthesis, Isr. J. Med. Sci. 18:171 (1982).

35. V.G. Sharov, V.A. Saks, V.N. Smirov, and E.I. Chazov, An Electron Microscopic Histochemical Investigation of the Localization of Creatine Phosphokinase in Heart Muscle, Biochim. Biophys. Acta 468:495 (1977).

36. D.O. Levitsky, T.S. Levchenko, V.A. Saks, V.G. Sharov, and V.N.
       Smirov, The Role of Creatine Phosphokianse in Supplying
       Energy for the Calcium Pump System of Heart Sarcoplasmic
       Reticulum, Membr. Biochem. 2:81 (1978).
37. V.A. Saks, N.V. Lipina, V.G. Sharov, V.N. Smirnov, E. Chazov,
       and R. Grosse, The Localization of the MM Isoenzyme of
       Creatine Phosphokinase on the Surface Membrane of Myocardial
       Cells and its Functional Coupling to Ouabain-inhibited
       (sodium—potassium) Ion-dependent ATPase, Biochim. Biophys.
       Acta 465:550 (1977).
38. S.P. Bessman and P.J. Geiger, The Transport of Energy in Muscle
       - The Phosphorylcreatine Shuttle, Science 211:448 (1981).

ORGANIZATION OF THE MITOCHONDRIAL MATRIX

Paul A. Srere and Balazs Sumegi

Veterans Administration Medical Center, 4500 South Lancaster Road and Department of Biochemistry, Univ. of Texas Health Science Center, Dallas, TX

Heart tissue has a high oxidative capacity due to its high content of mitochondria. In addition it is known that the oxidative capacity of mitochondria is correlated to their cristal content and heart mitochondria are known to contain many closely packed cristae. Measures of the inner membrane content (surface area) of heart mitochondria have been made by a number of groups of electron microscopists using stereomorphology (see 1 for review). Their data indicate that a rat heart mitochondrion contains about 60 μm^2 of inner membrane surface area for each μm^3 of mitochondrial volume. I have shown that these figures are consistent with an average spacing of cristae within a heart mitochondrion of about 150 A^2. One can calculate a diameter of 60 A for a spherical protein molecule with a molecular weight of about 80,000. Therefore, it is readily seen that a theoretical construct of a heart mitochondrion would place almost all of the matrix proteins next to the inner membranes.

Further insight as to the nature of the matrix space of mitochondria is obtained from the protein content of this compartment which has been determined to be greater than 300 mg per ml[3,4]. For a cubical packing configuration of spherical protein molecules one cannot expect a concentration higher than 59%. This then indicates that the milieu of the mitochondrial matrix is quite different from that used to study enzymes in vitro. For example, under these conditions of high protein concentration the exclusion of solvent from a significant portion of the total volume creates a condition referred to by Minton[5] as macromolecular crowding. He has shown both theoretically and experimentally that under these conditions the apparent equilibrium constants of monomer-protomer equilibria of proteins change due to a change in activity coefficients. An example of this effect has been demonstrated by the conversion of active dimers of the enzyme triose phosphate dehydrogenase to its inactive tetramers in the presence a 30% protein solution[6]. A recent report showed that a nucleic ligase could exhibit a "blunt-end" ligase activity only in the presence of a high concentration of polyethylene glycol[7]. The change in specificity of the ligase was attributed to crowding effect brought about by the volume exclusion of polyethylene glycol.

Another consequence of the high protein concentration becomes apparent if we compare the mitochondrial matrix to protein crystals whose protein concentration is also in the range of 30–70%[8]. Bishop and Richards[9] have shown that small molecules can diffuse unhindered through the bulk water of crystals but larger molecules show decreased diffusion rates. I have calculated that molecules of the size of NAD and CoA (20 A) would have difficulty passing through the pores of a dense protein solution.

A number of workers who have studied metabolite pools in the mitochondrion have reported the existence of two pools of acetyl CoA[10] and of some amino acids[11]. These apparent anomalous results might be explained by the physical nature of the matrix, i.e., small pores, ion-exchange like conditions and small amounts of bulk water.

Just these few considerations of the composition of the mitochondrial matrix indicates that models for metabolism within it based on results in dilute solutions are probably far from the mark.

Organizational Aspects. The notion of organized enzyme systems is an old one[12–14] but data supporting the notion has always been suspect. Those of us who were raised in the "grind and find" tradition of biochemistry found that fractionations which yielded the desired enzyme with a difficult-to-remove other enzyme a nuisance. Such contaminations were considered artifacts and seldom was it considered that these interactions were meaningful associations indicative of large enzyme complexes within the cell.

It is now clear that the sequential enzymes of many metabolic pathways are organized to some extent. This may be a common location on membranes or a structural component of the cell or by interactions of sequential enzymes. Evidence has been presented for organization of glycolysis, protein synthesis, pyrimidine synthesis, ureogenesis, and nucleic acid synthesis[15]. I will present here a summary of the evidence for interactions of

the Krebs tricarboxylic acid (TCA) cycle enzymes with each other
and with mitochondrial membranes. In addition, I will present
some recent data we have obtained on the organization of fatty
acid oxidation enzymes in the mitochondrial matrix.

We showed a number of years ago that when citrate synthase
and malate dehydrogenase were coimmobilized we could show a kinetic rate enhancement over the free enzymes[16]. Later we were able
to show that in the presence of 14% polyethylene glycol citrate
synthase and mitochondrial malate dehydrogenase (MDH) would specifically co-precipitate[17]. The cytosolic isozyme of MDH did not
interact with citrate synthase nor did at least six other metabolically unrelated proteins or enzymes. Fahien and Kmiotek[18]
were able to reproduce these results and were able to show that
the enzymes could be crosslinked in the presence of polyethylene
glycol. Similar results had been reported by Mosbach's group[19].
In a different type of experiment Beeckman and Kanarek[20] showed
that immobilized MDH could bind both fumarase and citrate synthase and the stoichiometry of these interactions were reported.

The interaction of pyruvate dehydrogenase complex (PDC) and
citrate synthase has been reported by Sumegi et al[21]. This
interaction has been characterized in several ways including
chromatography, centrifugation, and kinetic studies[21,22]. As
with the other interactions discussed the binding was shown to be
specific in that among other controls MDH could not replace
citrate synthase nor could α keto glutarate dehydrogenase complex
(KGDC) replace PDC. Porpaczy et al[23] were able to demonstrate by
similar techniques that a specific binding between succinate
thiokinase (STK) and α KGDC existed.

A total of nine specific interactions can be visualized for
the enzymes of the TCA cycle (including PDC) and thus far four of
them have been demonstrated. We have not studied the others as
yet. It is interesting to note that the interactions do not seem
to exhibit a species specificity. Enzymes that interact have
been derived from beef, pig, chicken, and rat, and even though
immunological differences can be detected between the same enzyme
from different species, no differences in specific enzyme bin-
dings have been reported. It would appear that the binding sites
have been evolutionarily conserved.

In a study of the locational interactions between Krebs cycle
enzymes and membranes we have reported that a number of Krebs
cycle enzymes, citrate synthase, malate dehydrogenase, and
fumarase can bind to the inner surface of the inner mitochondrial
membrane. The cytosolic isozyme of MDH did not bind nor was
binding seen to the outer membrane or to the outer surface of the

inner membrane. We have since that time extended the study to include the enzymes isocitrate dehydrogenase (NAD), PDC, and KGDC. No binding has been observed with ICDH (NADP) or with STK. In addition, inner membrane fractions from rat, rabbit, pig, beef, lemon, fruit, and yeast tissues will bind these enzymes (pig, rat, and beef sources). For citrate synthase we have observed that low concentrations of substrates can inhibit binding. The most effective inhibitor of binding of citrate synthase is oxalacetate which at 5 μM releases all the bound citrate synthase from the membranes.

Since the major metabolic fuel of heart tissue is fatty acids we extended our studies to include some mitochondrial enzymes of fat metabolism. Several authors consider the enzymes of fatty acid β-oxidation as soluble matrix enzymes since they appear in the supernatant fraction of disrupted mitochondria[24-26]. In spite of the fact that the acyl-CoA dehydrogenase transfers hydrogen atoms from the substrate to the enzymes of terminal oxidation (these enzymes are components of the inner membrane) some consider it to be a soluble matrix enzyme.

On the other hand, others claim that enzymes of fatty acid β-oxidation are membrane bound[27-30]. These contradictory reports are mainly obtained from studies on the fractionation of mitochondria by different techniques under different conditions, and until now reconstitution binding experiments have not been reported.

The contradiction in the localization of the enzymes of fatty acid β-oxidation and our results with the Krebs cycle enzymes prompted us to look for specific interaction between the enzymes of fatty acid β-oxidation and the inner mitochondrial membrane.

The experiments were made, if not otherwise stated, in 50 mM HEPES buffer, pH 7.0 containing 1 mM β-mercaptoethanol. Membrane fractions and protein were incubated for 30 min at 0-4°C in 100 l volume. This mixture was centrifuged for 30 min at 40,000 g. The sedimented pellet was resuspended in the original buffer solution and the activities were determined both in the resuspended pellet and the supernatant solution. The volume of pellet was determined by using inulin [^{14}C] carboxylic acid assuming a homogeneous distribution in the water of each fraction. The recovery of enzymatic activities was between 95-105%. In the case of crotonase the reaction rate was not directly proportional to the enzyme concentration. Therefore, the amount of enzyme was determined with the aid of a calibration curve.

Table I   Binding of the Enzymes of Fatty Acid
β-Oxidation and Some Related Enzymes to the
Inner Mitochondrial Membrane

Enzyme	Enzyme Activity Added	Enzyme Activity Bound
	units	
Crotonase	1.6 ± 0.1	0.32 ± 0.03(20)
β-Hydroxyacyl CoA dehydro-genase	0.75 ± 0.08	0.54 ± 0.045(72)
Thiolase	0.12 ± 0.01	0.095 ± 0.007(83)
Succinyl-CoA transferase	0.07 ± 0.01	0.0022 ± 0.0007(3)
Carnitine acetyl transferase	0.40 ± 0.03	0.34 ± 0.03(86)

Pig heart mitochondrial inner membranes (1.4 mg) and
thiolase (5 µg), β-hydoxyacyl CoA dehydrogenase (5 µg),
carnitine acetyl transferase (5 µg), crotonase (4.1
µg), or succinyl CoA transferase (20 µg) in 100 µl of
50 mM Hepes pH 7.0 were incubated at 0-4°C for 30 min.
The membranes were reisolated by centrifugation and the
enzyme activities were estimated. Over 95% of added
enzyme activities were recovered. The values represent mean ± S.E. for all experiments shown in this
Table and as controls in Tables III and IV. Hence,
they are the averages of six experiments. The percent
bound is shown in parantheses.

Binding of the so called soluble matrix enzymes of the fatty
acid β-oxidation and some selected enzymes to the inner
mitochondrial membrane was measured (Table I). It can be seen
that the thiolase, β-hydroxylacyl-CoA dehydrogenase, and carnitine acetyl transferase bind very well to the inner membrane.
The binding of crotonase is smaller but significant while the

succinyl-CoA transferase does not bind to the membrane under our experimental conditions. Saturation binding was observed for thiolase, β-hydroxylacyl-CoA dehydrogenase and crotonase, but for carnitine acetyl transferase the amount of bound protein was directly proportional to the added enzyme in the 0.05-3 mg/ml concentration range.

The binding of crotonase and carnitine acetyl transferase is largely independent of pH in the pH 6.5-8 range while the binding of thiolase and β-hydroxyacyl CoA dehydrogenase is markedly inhibited by increasing pH.

Increase of ionic strength up to 0.5 M inhibits the binding of all studied proteins. However, the binding of carnitine-acetyl transferase and crotonase are less sensitive to an increase of ionic strength than the thiolase and β-hydroxyacylCoA dehydrogenase (Table II).

Table II   Effect of Ionic Strength on the Binding of the Enzymes of Fatty Acid β-Oxidation to the Inner Mitochondrial Membrane

Enzyme	2 mM HEPES	50 mM HEPES	100 mM HEPES	200 mM HEPES
	Bound Enzymes % of Total			
Carnitine acetyl transferase	92 ± 3	93 ± 3	90 ± 3	79 ± 3
Thiolase	92 ± 3	83 ± 3	48 ± 2	9 ± 1
Crotonase	21 ± 1	20 ± 1	20 ± 1	19 ± 1
β-hydroxyacyl-CoA dehydrogenase	86 ± 3	72 ± 3	14 ± 2	7 ± 1

The experimental conditions were the same as in Table I except that the ionic strength was changed as shown in the Table.

Different treatments of the membrane were performed to be able to characterize the membrane component responsible for the binding of the above mentioned enzymes. Trypsin treatment and heat denaturation markedly decreased binding of enzymes of fatty acid β-oxidation to the mitochondrial inner membrane, but only slightly affected the binding of carnitine acetyl transferase (Table III).

Table III   Effect of Different Treatments of Inner Membrane on the Binding of the Enzymes of Fatty Acid β-Oxidation and Carnitine Acetyl Transferase

Enzyme	Boiled[b] % inhibitor	Trypsin treated[a] % inhibitor
Crotonase	84	44
β-hydroxyacyl CoA dehydrogenase	85	28
Thiolase	68	39
Carnitine acetyl transferase	40	5

In all cases the treated membranes were reisolated by centrifugation and washed extensively with 50 mM HEPES, pH 7.0.   1.4 mg of treated or untreated membranes were used for binding studies.   All other conditions were the same as described in Table I.   The values represent mean of three experiments.   The numbers indicate percent inhibition compared to untreated membranes.

[a]Pig heart inner membranes (10 mg) were incubated in 1 ml of 50 mM HEPES, pH 7.0 containing 200 µg trypsin for 15 min at room temperature.   The proteolysis was stopped by the addition of trypsin inhibitor.

[b]Pig heart inner membranes (10 mg) were placed in a boiling bath for 5 min and after reisolation were used for binding studies.

The carnitine acetyl transferase (CAT) binds to phosphatidyl choline liposomes showing that the CAT is able to incorporate into a pure lipid bilayer without the presence of a binding protein. In the case of the enzymes of β-oxidation the substitution of the inner mitochondrial membrane by mitoplasts, whole mitochondria, erythrocytes (not shown), or liposomes resulted in a substantial decrease in the binding of these enzymes (Table IV). These data indicate the importance of the protein composition and orientation of inner membrane in the binding process.

The data presented here show that the studied enzymes of fatty acid β-oxidation bind to the matrix surface of mitochondrial inner membrane. However, the binding is inhibited by increasing of ionic strength. Experiments with different membranes, trypsin treated and heat denaturated inner membranes, show that a protein component of the inner membrane is responsible for the binding. It is also known that carnitine palmityl transferase which is involved in the transport of acyl groups through the membrane is bound to the inner membrane. In spite of the contradictory results about the localization of acyl CoA dehydrogenase it seems to be probable that it should interact with the membrane to be able to transfer the hydrogen atoms from the substrate to the enzymes of terminal oxidation.

These data suggest that all enzymes of fatty acid β-oxidation are organized on the inner surface of inner mitochondrial membrane so that the intermediates can get from one enzyme to another without dissolving into the bulk water solution of the matrix. Therefore, the long chain acyl-CoA intermediates that are poorly water soluble can remain in the hydrophobic environment of the lipid membrane while they are catabolized to smaller hydrophilic molecules.

The oxidation of fatty acid was studied in broken mitochondria, soluble mitochondrial extract, and detergent treated mitochondria[31-33]. In these cases, the time course of the end product accumulation showed a lag phase and the intermediates of β-oxidation were detectable showing the properties of a non-organized enzyme system without channelling.

In contrast with this, in an intact system[34-36] the time course of end-product accumulation did not show a lag phase, and the intermediates of β-oxidation were either nondetectable or detectable only with extremely sensitive techniques in extremely small amounts. These data indicate that there is a channelling of intermediates among the enzyme components of fatty acid β-oxidation in intact system.

Table IV   Binding of the Enzymes of Fatty Acid
            β-Oxidation and Carnitine Acetyl
            Transferase to Different Membranes

Enzymes	Inner Membranes[+] % Bound Enzyme	Mitoplasts[*] % Bound Enzyme	Liposomes % Bound Enzyme
Crotonase	20	7	2.0
β-hydroxyl-acyl CoA dehydrogenase	72	28	2.3
Thiolase	83	9.1	4.3
Carnitine acetyl transferase	86	83	59

Pig heart mitochondrial inner membranes (1.4 mg/ml), mitoplasts (2.8 mg/ml), or liposomes (30 mg phosphatidylcholine per 1 ml 50 mM Hepes, pH 7.0) was incubated with thiolase (5 µg), β-hydroxylacyl CoA dehydrogenase (5 µg), carnitine acetyl transferase (5 µg) or crotonase (4.1 µg) in 50 mM Hepes, pH 7.0 for 30 min at 0-4°C. The mixture was centrifuged and the enzyme activities were determined in the supernatant fluid and in the resuspended pellet. The values represent mean of three experiments.

[*]In these experiments the enzyme content of mitoplast was determined and used as a blank value.

[+]The values in this column represent the average values for all these experiments in Tables I, III, and IV.

The ratio of acetyl CoA/CoA can be an important regulatory factor of the β-oxidation[37]. Therefore, it was important to check whether carnitine acetyl transferase binds to the inner membrane. The data presented above show that CAT binds to all membranes, including phosphatidyl choline liposomes. That is, in contrast to the enzymes of fatty acid β-oxidation, which bind to a protein component of the inner membrane, the CAT bind to the membrane lipids. As for the physiological importance of this phenomenon, the simultaneous binding of CAT and thiolase to the membrane may be advantageous because CAT can recover the CoA (whose concentration is very low in muscle tissue) from acetyl-CoA from the last enzyme (thiolase) of fatty acid β-oxidation.

Binding of the succinyl-CoA transferase to the inner membrane that initiates the muscle ketone body catabolism was also tested, but no binding was detected. So, our data do not support the idea of an organization of the enzymes of ketone body catabolism on the surface of the inner membrane.

Conclusion. We have presented evidence which shows that some enzymes of fatty acid oxidation can bind to a protein component of the matrix side of the inner membrane of heart mitochondria. This observation along with our previous studies on the nature of the mitochondrial matrix and the binding of tricarboxylic acid cycle enzymes indicates that the mitochondrial matrix is a highly organized system.

Acknowledgements. Supported by the Veterans Administration, USPHS Grant No. 2-R01-AM11313-16, NSF Grant No. PCM-8204114, and Welch Grant No. I-975. We are indebted to our colleagues for unpublished data and to Ms. Penny Perkins for manuscript preparation. Thiolase was a gift of Dr. Gilbert (Baylor).

References

1. Reith, A. Barnard, T., and Rohr, H.-P. Stereology of Cellular Reaction Patterns, CRC Critical Reviews in Toxicology, 4:219-269 (1976).

2. Srere, P. A. The Structure of the Mitochondrial Inner Membrane-Matrix Compartment, Trends Biochem. Sci., 7: 375-378 (1982).

3. Srere, P. A. The Infrastructure of the Mitochondrial Matrix, Trends Biochem. Sci., 5:120-121 (1980).

4. Hackenbrock, C. R. Chemical and Physical Fixation of Isolated Mitochodnria in Low-Energy and High-Energy States, Proc. Natl. Acad. Sci. 61:598-605 (1968).

5. Minton, A. P. Excluded Volume as a Determinant of Macro-molecular Structure and Reactivity, Biopolymers, 20:2093-2120 (1981).

6. Minton, A. P. and Wilf, J. Effect of Macromolecular Crowding upon the Structure and Function of an Enzyme: Glyceralde-hyde-3-phosphate Dehydrogenase, Biochemistry, 20:4821-4826 (1981).

7. Zimmerman, S. B. and Pheiffer, B. H. Macromolecular Crowding Allows Blunt-end Ligation by DNA Ligases from Rat Liver or Escherichia coli, Proc. Natl. Acad. Sci. USA, 80:5852-5856 (1983).

8. Srere, P. A. Protein Crystals as a Model for Mitochondrial Matrix Proteins, Trends Biochem. Sci., 6:4-6 (1981).

9. Bishop, W. H. and Richards, F. M. Properties of Liquids in Small Pores, J. Mol. Biol. 38:315-328 (1968).

10. Fritz, I. B. "Cellular Compartmentalization and Control of Fatty Acid Metabolism", Academic Press, New York (1968).

11. Schoolwerth, A. C. and LaNoue, K. F. The Role of Micro-compartmentation in the Regulation of Glutamate Metabolism by Rat Kidney Mitochondria, J. Biol. Chem. 255:3403-3411 (1980).

12. Loeb, J. "The Organism as a Whole from a Physicochemical Viewpoint", Knickerbocker Press, New York (1916).

13. Srere, P. A. and Mosbach, K. Metabolic Compartmentation: Symbiotic, Organnelar, Multienzymic, and Microenvironmental. Ann. Rev. Microbiol. 28:61-83 (1974).

14. Welch, G. On the Role of Organized Multienzyme Systems in Cellular Metabolism: A General Synthesis, Prog. Biophys. Molec. Biol. 32:103-191 (1977).

15. Srere, P. A. and Estabrook, R. "Editors of Microenvironments and Metabolic Compartmentation", Academic Press, New York (1978).

16. Srere, P. A., Mattiasson, B., and Mosbach, K. An Immobilized Three-Enzyme System: A Model for Microenvironmental Compartmentation in Mitochondria. Proc. Natl. Acad. Sci. USA 70:2534-2538 (1973).

17. Halper, L. A. and Srere, P. A. Interaction between Citrate Synthase and Mitochondrial Malate Dehydrogenase in the Presence of Polyethylene Glycol. Arch. Biochem. Biophys. 184:529-534.

18. Fahien, L. A. and Kmiotek, E. Complexes between Mitochondrial Enzymes and Either Citrate Synthase or Glutamate Dehydrogenase, J. Biol. Chem. 254:5983-5990 (1979).

19. Koch-Schmidt, A., Mattiasson, B., and Mosbach, K. Aspects on Microenvironmental Compartmentation, Eur. J. Biochem. 81: 71-78 (1977).

20. Beeckmans, S. and Kanarek, L. Demonstration of Physical Interactions between Consecutive Enzymes of the Citric Acid Cycle and of the Aspartate-Malate Shuttle, Eur. J. Biochem. 117:527-535 (1981).

21. Sumegi, B., Gyocsi, L., and Alkonyi, I. Interaction between the Pyruvate Dehydrogenase Complex and Citrate Synthase, Biochim. Biophys. Acta 616:158-166.

22. Sumegi, B. and Alkonyi, I. A Study on the Physical Interaction between the Pyruvate Dehydrogenase Complex and Citrate Synthase, Biochim. Biophys. Acta 749:163-171 (1983).

23. Porpaczy, Z., Sumegi, B., and Alkonyi, I. Association between the α-Ketoglutarate Dehydrogenase Complex and Succinate Thiokinase, Biochim. Biophys. Acta 749:172-179 (1983).

24. Chapman, M. F., Miller, L. R., and Ontko, J. A. Localization of the Enzymes of Ketogenesis in Rat Liver Mitochondria, J. Cell. Biol. 58:284-306 (1973).

25. Brdiczka, D., Pette, D., Brunner, G., and Miller F. Kompartimentierte Verteilung von Enzymen in Rattenlebermitochondrien, Eur. J. Biochem. 5:294-304 (1968).

26. Haddock, B. A., Yates, D. W., and Garland, P. B. The Localization of Some Coenzyme A-Dependent Enzymes in Rat Liver Mitochondria, Biochem. J. 119:565-573 (1970).

27. Landriscina, C., Papa, S., Coratelli, P., Mazzarella, L., and Quagliariello, E. Enzymatic Activities of the Matrix and Inner Membrane of Pigeon-Liver Mitochondria, Biochim. Biophys. Acta 205:136-141 (1970).

28. Allmann, D. W., Galzigna, L., McCaman, R. E., and Green, D.E. The Membrane Systems of the Mitochondrion, Arch. Biochem. Biophys. 117:413-419 (1966).

29. Wit-Peeters, E. M., Scholte, H. R., Van Den Akker, F., and DeNie, I. Intramitochondrial Localization of Palmityl-CoA Dehydrogenase, β-Hydroxyacyl-CoA Dehydrogenase and Enoyl-CoA Hydratase in Guinea-Pig Heart, Biochim. Biophys. Acta 231:23-31 (1971).

30. Beattie, D. S.   The Submitochondrial Distribution of the Fatty Acid Oxidizing System in Rat Liver Mitochondria, Biochem. Biophys. Res. Commun. 30:57-62 (1968).

31. Blank, M. L., Cress, E. A., Stephens, N., and Snyder, F. On the Analysis of Long Chain Alkane Diols and Glycerol Ethers in Biochemical Studies, J. Lipid Res. 12:638-640 (1971).

32. Davidoff, F. and Korn, E. D.   The Reactions of trans-α, β-Hexadecenoyl Coenzyme A and cis- and trans-β, γ-Hexadecenoyl Coenzyme A Catalyzed by Enzymes from Guinea Pig Liver Mitochondria, J. Biol. Chem. 240:1549-1558 (1965).

33. Fleming, P. J. and Hajra, A. K.   Biosynthesis and Characterization of a Phosphatidic Acid Analog Containing β-Hydroxy Fatty Acid, Biochem. Biophys. Res. Commun. 55:743-751.

34. Garland, P. B., Shepherd, D., and Yates, D. W.   Steady-State Concentrations of Coenzyme A, Acetyl-Coenzyme A and Long-Chain Fatty Acyl-Coenzyme A in Rat-Liver Mitochondria Oxidizing Palmitate, Biochem. J. 97:587-594 (1965).

35. Rabinowitz, J. L. and Hercker, E. S.   Incomplete Oxidation of Palmitate and Leakage of Intermediary Products during Anoxia, Arch. Biochem. Biophys. 161:621-627 (1974).

36. Stanley, K. K. and Tubbs, P. K.   The Role of Intermediates in Mitochondrial Fatty Acid Oxidation, Biochem. J. 150:77-88 (1975).

37. Olowe, Y. and Schulz, H.   Regulation of Thiolases from Pig Heart - Control of Fatty Acid Oxidation in Heart, Eur. J. Biochem. 109:425-429 (1980).

THE TIME COURSE OF ATP CLEAVAGE BY CONTRACTING AMPHIBIAN AND MAMMALIAN SKELETAL MUSCLES

Earl Homsher

Dept. of Physiology, School of Medicine, UCLA, Los Angeles, Ca.

INTRODUCTION

The purpose of this paper is to describe our current under-standing of the factors affecting the rate of energy utilitiza-tion, or ATP hydrolysis, by contracting muscles. While there are a variety of ways in which this question might be approached, historically the most productive methods have been the measurement of the enthalpy (heat+work) production and the measurement of changes in the high energy phosphate content of contracting muscles. The former technique involves the recording of heat and work production by thermopiles and work by force and displacement transducers. This technique has the advantage that it has a good frequency response (resolving changes in the rate of energy liberation in 10 msec) is quantitatively very accurate (to a fraction of a mW/g), and is non-destructive. Its primary disadvantage is its non-specificity; i.e., the myothermal recording represents the sum of all the rections taking place. The latter technique involves the measurement of the change in chemical content of acid extracts of paired whole muscles (one a control and the other an experimental muscle) which are rapidly frozen at specific times during a contraction. This technique has the advantage that it is specific for those metabolites assayed (usually ATP, ADP, AMP, creatine, creatine phosphate, and phosphate). The disavantages are that it is inherently destructive, can not resolve time points much better than ca. 50 ms in whole muscles, and it requires a large number of replications (and thus much time) to obtain the desired accuracy. The technique also measures only total amounts and says nothing about compartmentation. Recently, in collaboration with Drs. Michael Ferenczi and David Trentham, we have developed a variation of the rapid freezing technique which can be applied to single muscle fibers, can be used to resolve changes in the 10 ms range, and can be used to examine the reaction kinetics of ATP hydrolysis by mechanically and chemically skinned single muscle fibers. This paper will contain a brief description of the technique and results obtained using glycerinated rabbit psoas fibers.

In the studies using unpoisoned and oxygenated frog skeletal muscles described below, there are rarely any changes in the muscles' nucleotide content which exceed 40 nmol nucleotide/g of muscle (even when as much as 5 umol creatine phosphate/g of muscle has been consumed). This is because under the aegis of creatine kinase in the muscle, any ADP formed is rapidly rephosphorylated to ATP. Therefore in the discussion below we will use the term "high-energy phosphate" (abbreviated by ~ P) hydrolysis rather than "ATP" hydrolysis.

ISOMETRIC TETANIC CONTRACTIONS

A frog sartorius muscle at rest at 0 C consumes about 0.8nmol ~ P/g s, and when the muscle is stimulated the rate ~P hydrolysis increases about 500 fold to 0.35 umol/g s (Kushmerick and Paul, 1976; Curtin and Woledge, 1978; Homsher and Kean, 1978). Figure 1 shows the time course of tension, enthalpy production, and enthalpy derived from ~ P hydrolysis during an isometric tetanus of a frog sartorius muscle. Notewothy is the fact that the enthalpy production begins at a high rate and then over the course of ca. 2-5 seconds declines to a steady rate called the stable maintenance heat rate (Aubert, 1956) while the rate of ~ P hydrolysis is linear from the start of the tetanus. With the cessation of stimulation the rate of enthalpy production and ~ P hydrolysis fall to low values. It was once accepted that the enthalpy production during the contraction, called the initial heat, was directly associated with processes using energy, while the heat produced above the basal rate after the muscle relaxed, the recovery heat, was associated with the processes of ATP resynthesis (glycolysis and oxidative phosphorylation). Results of studies like that shown in Fig. 1 have caused this concept to be discarded. During the early part of the tetanus, heat in excess of that generated by the measured ~ P hydrolysis is produced and this can amount to 30-40 mJ/g, the isometric unexplained heat. This is an amount of energy equivalent to about 1 umol ATP hydrolyzed/g. Furthermore, during recovery more oxygen is consumed than is necessary to resynthesize the amount of ~ P hydrolyzed during the tetanus (Kushmerick and Paul, 1976; Paul 1982). Studies of the behavior of the enthalpy liberation and ~ P hydrolysis rate as a function of initial sarcomere length have been most useful in understanding the isometric behavior of the

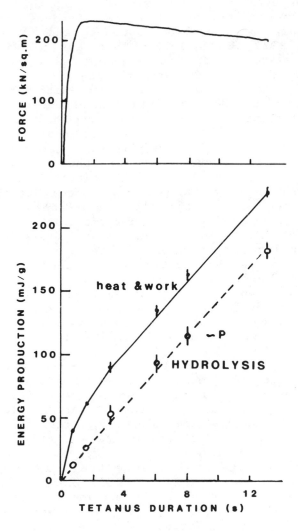

Figure 1.   The time course of force production (upper panel), and energy liberation (lower panel) during an isometric tetanus of frog skeletal muscle at 0°C.   The solid line in the lower panel is the energy liberated as heat+work while the dashed line is the amount of enthalpy which should have been liberated as judged by the measured amount of ~P hydrolysis.   Data is from Homsher, et al. (1979).

muscle.   At sarcomere lengths greater than 2.2µm the stable
maintenance heat rate and   ~ P hydrolysis rate decline linearly
with decreasing overlap and at a sarcomere length near 3.65 um,
both reach values which are 30% of the value observed at full
overlap (Infante, et al., 1964; Sandberg and Carlson, 1966;
Homsher et al, 1972; Smith, 1972).   This result indicates that
about 1/3 of the steady state rate of energy liberationin tetanus
is associated with the calcium release and sequestration
mechanism while the remainder is associated with thick and thin
filament interaction.   Measurement of the amount of unexplained
enthalpy at different sarcomere lengths have shown it to be only
slightly reduced at zero thick and thin filment overlap which
tends to indicate that it is primarily a consequence of a reaction involving calcium cycling within the cell (Curtin and
Woledge, 1981; Homsher and Kean, 1982).   Finally the unexplained
enthalpy is produced only during the intial part of the tetanus
(the first 2-5 sec); thereafter, the energy liberation is fully
accounted for by the measured ~ P hydrolysis (Curtin and Woledge,
1979; Homsher et al., 1979). Such results are consistent with the
notion that during the early part of the tetanus a reaction
occurs which produces heat but does not involve high energy
phosphate hydrolysis.   During recovery, after the muscle has
relaxed, this reaction is reversed at the expense of ATP hydrolysis.   A likely candidate for this reaction is calcium binding to
the intracellular calcium binding protein, parvalbumin.   In frog
muscles there are about 0.8 umol of parvalbumin   calcium binding
sites per gram muscle (Gosselin-Rey and Gerday,1977), and given
the enthalpy change accompanying calcium binding to parvalbumin
(Curtin and Woledge, 1978) most of the unexplained enthalpy could
explained if, during the maintained tetanus the parvalbumin calcium binding sites were being saturated.   After relaxation the
calcium would be gradually returned to the sarcoplasmic reticulum
at a rate limited by the dissociation rate of calcium from the
calcium-parvalbumin complex.

In mammalian skeletal muscle there is very little
parvalbumin (Robertson et al., 1981) and, perhaps as a
consequence, both the rate of heat production and ATP proceed at
a linear rate (Gibbs and Gibson, 1972; Wendt and Gibbs, 1973;
Crow and Kushmerick, 1982). Furthermore in both fast and slow leg
muscles of the mouse, there does not appear to be an energy
imbalance of the type seen in amphibian skeletal muscle.   The
basal rate of ~ P hydrolysis of resting mouse skeletal muscle is
about 0.02 µmol/g s   (at 20°C) and during a tetanus it can rise
to 1 µmole/g s and 3 umol/g s in the slow and fast muscle respectively.   Assuming that there are 0.3 µmol myosin ATPase sites per
gram of muscle(Ebashi et al., 1969) and that the 2/3 of the ~ P
is consumed by actomyosin, the catalytic site activity of whole
slow and fast muscle myosin is respectively 2 s^{-1} and 6 s^{-1}.

SHORTENING CONTRACTIONS

When a tetanically stimulated muscle is allowed to shorten, the rate of energy liberation increases markedly over the isometric rate of energy liberation. In two very important papers, Hill (1938, 1964) showed that during shortening not only does the rate of work production increase in a fashion dicatated by the force velocity curve, but the rate of heat production also increases over the isometric rate. Figure 2 shows a plot of the

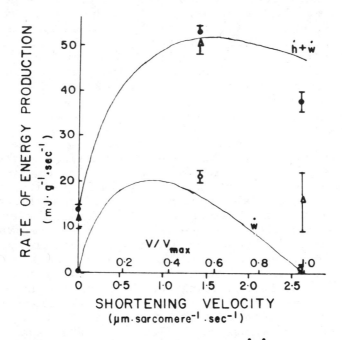

Figure 2. The rate of energy liberation (ḣ+ẇ) and work production (ẇ) during shortening at various velocities. Solid lines are from work of Hill (1964); the filled circles are (ḣ+ẇ) measurments from Homsher et al (1981, 1982); open circles are work rates (ẇ) based on measurements from Homsher et al (1981, 1982); open triangles represent the amount of enthalpy produced by the measured ~P hydrolysis (Homsher et al [1981,1982]).

rate of energy liberation as a function of shortening velocity and shows that at shortening velocities near one-half maximal, the rate of energy liberation is 4-5 times that seen under isometric circumstances. Both the increased rate of work production and heat production are derived from the interaction of the thick and thin filaments and the increased rate of heat production as shown by their dependence on the amount of thick and thin filament overlap (Gordon, et al, 1966; Homsher, et al, 1983). The most obvious interpretation of this result is that the increased rate of energy liberation is a consequence of an increased rate of ATP hydrolysis attendant to an increased rate of crossbridge cycling. Tests of this idea (Kushmerick and Davies, 1969; Curtin et al, 1974; Rall et al 1976; Homsher et al, 1981; Homsher et al, 1982) have shown that the rate of ~P hydrolysis at first increases as the shortening velocity increases and as shortening velocity approaches maximal values, the ~P hydrolysis rate declines so that at the maximal shortening velocity, it is little different from the isometric rate. In experiments designed to measure the extent to which the energy liberation during shortening could be explained by the measured high energy phosphate splitting during shortening , it was found that the rate of ~P hydrolysis could completely account for the rate of energy liberation at velocities of shortening up to half maximal (were force exerted during shortening is 25% of the isometric tetanic force). However, at higher velocities, near the V_{max} for example, (during which maintained force was about 2% of the isometric force, only about half of the energy liberated during shortening is explained·by ~P hydrolysis. When the muscles ceased shortening, the rate of enthalpy production returns to the isometric rate consistent with the new muscle length. In muscles which had shortening at one-half the maximal velocity, the rate of ~P hydrolysis also falls to a rate similar to that seen in an isometric contraction. However in muscles which had shortened at near maximum velocities, there is, prior to the return to the isometric rate, a burst of ~P hydrolysis, not accompanied by enthalpy production, occurs so that, over the total period of shortening and tension redevelopment all the energy liberated can be explained as ultimately being derived from ~P hydrolysis. To explain these results, one might argue that as filaments slide past one another more rapidly, the rate of attachment and detachment of crossbridges must also increase and thus increase the rate of energy liberation. Further at really high velocities of shortening, the time during which a given actin remains in the poisition necessary for a crossbridge to attach may be so short as to effectively reduce the rate of crossbridges attachment and thereby reduce the rate of crossbridge cycling. Huxley (1973) has shown that such a hypothesis can account for the rate of energy liberation by shortening muscles. However, this simple hypothesis requires that the time course of ~P hydrolysis paral-

lel the rate of energy liberation. The failure to observe such a
parallelism at high shortening velocities must therefore imply
that each crossbridge attachment does not obligate the concomitant hydrolysis of an ATP molecules and there is not a tight
temporal coupling between ATP hydrolysis and the liberation of
energy. While it is not difficult to imagine possible
crossbridge mechanisms to account for the above results, little
definitive data exists to constrain such hypotheses.

At the present no data is available which describes how that
rate of enthalpy production and ~P hydrolysis change during
shortening of mammalian muscle.

ATP HYDROLYSIS BY ISOLATED MUSCLE PROTEINS

Using the techniques of transient kinetic analysis (see
Taylor 1979 for a review of this subject) the hydrolysis of ATP
by acto-myosin subfragment 1 has been analyzed and a reaction
mechanism has been has been developed as shown below:

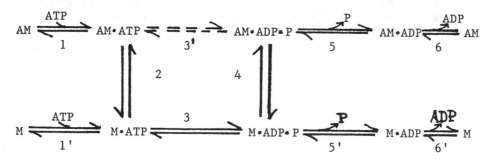

Lymn-Taylor Mechanism

In this mechanism A represents actin, M a myosin subfragment 1
head, P inorganic phosphate, and ATP and ADP their usual designa-
tion. M•ATP and M•ADP•P are detached cross bridge states. Each
step is labled with a number. The normal pathway for a
crossbridge involved in ATP hydrolysis (Lymn and Taylor, 1971)
would be through steps 1,2,3,4,5, and 6. Recent data however has
shown that another hydrolysis pathway could occur via steps
1,3',5,and 6 (Stein et al., 1979). Crossbridge detachment could
occur by a rapid equilibrium at steps 2 and 4 and could therefore
act to remove force on a crossbridge. The in vitro work on
rabbit proteins indicates that reactions 1 and 2 are very rapid
(> 1000 s^{-1} at physiological ATP levels) and that steps 3 and 3'
occur at a rates of ca. 100 s^{-1} with an equilibrium constant for
step 3 of about 10. Step 5 may be the rate limiting step for the
acto-subfragment 1 system having a rate of $10-20$ s^{-1}. In the
absence of calcium ATP is hydrolyzed via steps 1',3,5', and 6,'

in which the rate limiting step is 5 which has a value of about 0.05 s^{-1}. While this reaction scheme accounts for the behavior of isolated proteins, one could ask whether a similar mechanism occurs in the intact muscle filament lattice. If it does, how how do force and shortening affect the rate constants for the various steps? To answer such questions it would be necessary to perform transient kinetic analyses of ATP hydrolysis in an intact fiber lattice; i.e., to suddenly increase the ATP concentration from zero to some known value and to monitor the time course of ATP hydrolysis and the mechanical behavior of the fiber. However, because the rate of diffusion of ATP into the skinned muscle fiber lattice is slow compared to the rates of the reactions of interest, there was no method available to perform transient kinetic analyses on the mechanically constrained fiber lattice.

STUDIES USING "CAGED ATP"

Recently Kaplan et al (1978) synthesized P^3-1-(2-nitro)-phenylethyl-adenosine 5'-triphosphate, more simply known as caged-ATP. The structure of caged ATP is shown in Fig. 3. The

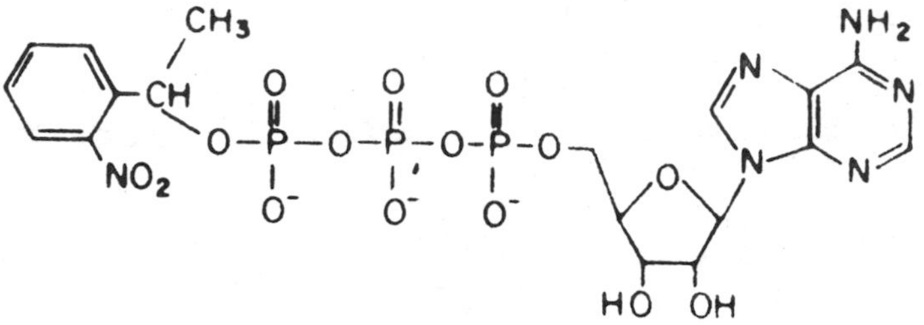

Figure 3. Caged ATP

presence of the 1-(2)-nitrophenylethanol group on the terminal phosphate prevents muscle ATPases from hydrolyzing the ATP even though it can easily diffuse into the filament lattice of chemically skinned muscle fibers. Kaplan et al (1978) synthesized the compound because it can, upon exposure to light at wave lengths near 350 nm, be photolyzed to ATP (as well as a proton, and 2-nitrosoacetophenone) so that transient kinetic studies could be performed on structured systems. McCray et al (1980) further showed that by the use of laser flash photolysis, ATP can be released from caged ATP at a rate of ca. 100 s^{-1}. Goldman et al (1982) have used caged ATP photolysis to study tension transients in skinned muscle fibers. In collaboration with Drs. M.A. Ferenczi and D.R. Trentham (Ferenczi, et al., 1983), we developed a technique to monitor transient kinetics of ATP hydrolysis in single chemically skinned muscle fibers. To do this [2-^{3}H] caged ATP was synthesized and diffused into glycerinated rabbit psoas

fibers which had earlier been put into rigor by exposing them to
several salt solutions lacking ATP. After several minutes of
equilbration with the caged-ATP solution, the chamber in which
the fiber was bathed was rapidly removed from about the fiber.
The fiber, whose force output was constantly monitored, was then
exposed to a 50 ns pulse of focused laser light at 347 nm to
release tritiated ATP. At times ranging from 50 ms to 8 s, after
the laser flash, the fiber was frozen (and the chemical reactions
halted) by squeezing it between two copper blocks at liquid
nitrogen temperature. The frozen fiber was then extracted in in
acidic methanol at -20 for 24 hr during which time more than 98%
of the labelled nucleotide was removed from the fiber. The fiber
itself was then collected and assayed for total protein while the
fiber extract was lyophilized and the residue dissolved in water.
The nucleotides in the fiber extract (i.e., tritiated caged ATP,
ATP, ADP, and AMP) were isolated by ion-pair reverse phase HPLC
and the amount of each assayed by liquid scintillation counting.
With this information and the knowledge of the specific activity
of the caged ATP incubation solution, one can calculate the fluid
volume occupied by the fiber, the concentration of ATP released
by the flash photolysis, and the amount of ADP and AMP formed by
the enzymatic action of the fiber.

The results of two types of flash photolysis experiments
(i.e., ATP release in the absence of calcium [$<1x10^{-8}$M] and in
the presence of calcium [$2x10^{-5}$ M] are shown in Figs. 4 and 5.
Figure 4 shows the effects of photolytic release of ATP on force
production in the absence(A) and presence (B) of calcium. In
the absence of calcium there is a biphasic response in which a
first phase lasting about 40 ms (during which tension changes
very little) is followed by an exponential decline in force
whose rate constant is 11 s^{-1}. In the presence of calcium the
force response is also biphasic in which there is first a period
(lasting about 13 ms) during which tension changes very little
followed by a rise in force with a rate constant of 28 s^{-1}.
These results are similar to the tension responses reported by
Goldman et al (1982). Figure 5 is a plot of the time course of
ATP hydrolysis by fibers in the absence (A) and presence (B) of
calcium (due to a technical limitation, data points earlier than
50 ms after the laser pulse were not obtained). In both cases
the time course of ATP hydrolysis is biphasic and consists of a
rapid initial burst of ADP formation, complete within 50 ms,fol-
lowed by a slower steady-state rate of ATP cleavage. Based on
protein assays of the rabbit muscle it is estimated that the
concentration of myosin subfragment 1 heads in the fiber is
about 0.180 mM (Yates and Greaser,1983), and therefore the magnitude of the burst of ATP cleavage corresponds to about molecule
of ATP cleaved per subfragment 1 head. Further, since the
earliest data point is at 50 ms, we can provide only a lower
limit for the rate of the phosphate burst; i.e., it is greater
than 35 s^{-1}.

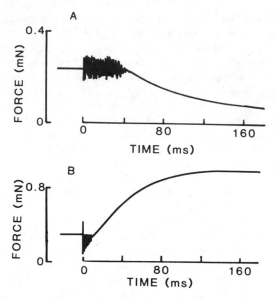

Figure 4. The time course of tension changes in glycerinated
fibers in response to the release of ATP from caged ATP provoked
by pulse of laser light at time zero. The fibers had been first
relaxed in a solution containing 6mM ATP, 7.3 mM MgCl$_2$, 100 mM
TES buffer (pH was 7.1) 10 mM glutathione, calcium buffered with
25 mM EGTA. The fiber was then transferred though several washes
of the same buffer, but containing no ATP, and allowed to go into
rigor. The fibers wee then placed in a similar buffer containing
2-3 mM caged ATP. The noise in the tension records after the
laser pulse is an artifact caused by the laser pulse.

   Both of these results are in good accord with the Lymn-Taylor
mechanism. In the presence of calcium ions the steady state rate
of ATP hydrolysis corresponds to about 2 moles MgATP cleaved per
mole of myosin subfragment 1 head per second, while in the
absence of calcium the steady state rate of MgATP cleavage is at
least 10 fold smaller. Both results are in accord with the rate
limiting step of the crossbridge mechanism being associated with
the release of products and are similar to those obtained in
purified protein systems. This technique should be of use in
elucidating the chemical kinetics of crossbridge behavior.

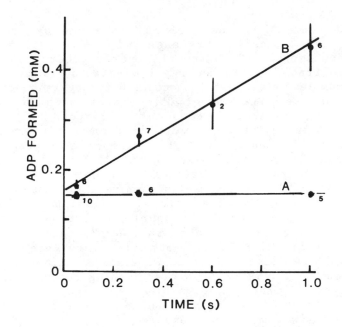

Figure 5. The time course of ATP hydrolysis by glycerinated rabbit psoas muscle fibers after the release of ATP from caged ATP. The line labled A is in the absence of calcium while the line labeled B is in the presence of calcium. Reaction conditions the same as in Fig.4. The size of the data point or the vertical lines imposed on a data point indicate ± one standard error of the mean. The numbers aside each data point indicate the number of measurements.

SUMMARY

    The pattern of energy liberation by tetanically stimulated muscle is reasonably well defined. The energy liberation and ATPase rate are affected by a variety of mechanical factors which, aside from the case of shortening mammalian muscles, are well documented. The amount of ATP consumed by processes associated with the calcium release and sequestration is not trivial, amounting to 30-40% of the energy liberation in an isometric contraction. The energy liberated by isometric and shortening muscles is ultimately accounted for by known chemical reactions. However, there are two instances in which the time course of energy liberation does not correspond to the time course of high energy phosphate utilization. In an isometric tetanus, 30-40 mJ of energy per gram of muscle is produced by reactions probably associated with intracellular circulation of calcium, but not immediately involving ATP hydrolysis. Second, in rapidly shortening muscles, an unknown reaction can produce 6-7 mJ of energy per gram of muscle which is not immediately associated with high energy phosphate splitting. However, immediately after the cessation of shortening, this reaction is reversed by an ATP hydrolysis. Finally, a technique is now available which permits one to perform transient kinetic studies on skinned muscle fibers which are shortening and/or developing force. This development should enable the design of experiments in which the effect of mechanical conditions upon specific steps of the ATPase mechanism can be examined.

Acknowledgement

Support of this work was provided by an NIH grant AM 30988 and a grant from the Muscular Dystrophy Association of America, C79112.

References

Kushmerick, M.J. and R.J. Paul. (1976). Relationship between initial chemical reactions and oxidative recovery metabolism for single isometric contractions of frog sartorius at 0 C. J. Physiol. 254:711.
Curtin, N.A. and R.C. Woledge (1978). Energy changes and muscular contraction. Physiol. Rev. 58:690.
Homsher, E. and C.J.C. Kean (1978). Skeletal muscle energetics and metabolism. Ann. Rev. Physiol. 40:93.
Aubert, X. (1956). "Le couplage energetique de la contraction musculaire", Editions Arscia, Brussels.
Paul, R.J. (1983). Physical and biochemical energy balance during an isometric tetanus and steady state recovery in frog sartorius at 0 C. J. Gen. Physiol. 81:337.
Infante, A.A., D. Klaupiks, and R.E. Davies (1964). Length, tension and metabolism during short isometric contractions of frog sartorius muscles. Biochim. Biophys. Acta. 88:215.
Sandberg, J. and F.D. Carlson (1966). The length dependence of

phosphorylcreatine hydrolysis during an isometric tetanus. Biochem. Z. 345:212.

Homsher, E., W.F.H.M. Mommaerts, N.V. Ricchiuti, and A. Wallner (1972). Activation heat, activation metabolism, and tension related heat in frog semitendinousus muscles. J. Physiol. 220:601.

Smith, I.C.H. (1972). Energetics of activation in frog and toad muscle. J. Physiol. 220:583.

Curtin, N.A. and R.C. Woledge (1981). Effect of muscle length on energy balance in frog skeletal muscle. J. Physiol. 316:453.

Homsher, E. and C.J.C. Kean (1982). Unexplained enthalpy production in contracting skeletal muscle. Fed. Proc. 41:149.

Curtin, N.A. and R.C. Woledge (1979). Chemical change and energy production during contraction of frog muscle: how are their time courses related? J. Physiol. 288:353.

Homsher, E., C.J.C. Kean, A. Wallner, and V. Sarian-Garibian. (1979). J. Gen. Physiol. 73:553.

Gosselin-Rey, C. and C. Gerday (1977). Parvalbumins from frog skeltal muscle (Rana temporaria L.). Biochim. Biophys. Acta. 492:53.

Robertson, S.P., J.D. Johnson, and J.D. Potter (1981). The time course of Ca^{+2} exchange with calmodulin, troponin, parvalbumin, and myosin in response to transient increases in Ca^{+2}. Biophys. J. 34:559.

Gibbs, C.L. and W.R. Gibson (1972). Energy production of rat soleus muscle. Amer. J. Physiol. 223:864.

Wendt, I. and C.L. Gibbs (1973). Energy production of rat extensor digitorum longus muscle. Amer. J. Physiol. 224:1081.

Crow, M.T. and M.J. Kushmerick (1982). Chemical energetics of slow- and fast-twitch muscles of the mouse. J. Gen. Physiol. 79:147.

Ebashi, S., M. Endo, and I. Ohtsuki (1969). Control of muscle contraction. Q. Rev. Biophys. 2:351.

Hill, A.V. (1938). The heat of shortening and the dynamic constants of muscle. Proc. Roy. Soc. B. 126:136.

Hill, A.V. (1964). The effect of load on the heat of shortening of muscle. Proc. Roy. Soc. B. 159:297.

Homsher, E., M. Irving, and A. Wallner (1981). High-energy phosphate metabolism and energy liberation associated with rapid shortening in frog skeletal muscle. J. Physiol. 321:423.

Homsher, E., T. Yamada, A. Wallner, and J. Tsai (1982). Energy balance studies in muscles shortening a 1/2 V_{max}. J. Biophys. 37:123a.

Gordon, A.M., A.F. Huxley, and F.J. Julian (1966). The variation in isometric force with sarcomere length in vertebrate muscle fibers. J. Physiol. 184:170.

Homsher, E., M. Irving, and J. Lebacq (1983). Sarcomere length dependence of shortening heat in frog muscle. J. Physiol. 345:107.

Kushmerick, M.J. and R.E. Davies (1969). The chemical energetics of muscle contraction. Proc. Roy. Soc. B. 174:315.

Curtin, N.A., C. Gilbert, K.M. Kretzschmar, and D.R. Wilkie (1974). The effects of the performance of work on total energy output and metabolism during musclular contraction. J. Physiol. 238:455.

Rall J.A., E. Homsher, A. Wallner, W.F.H.M. Mommaerts (1976). A temporal dissociation of energy liberation and high energy phosphate splitting during shortening in frog skeletal muscles. J. Gen. Physiol. 68:13.

Huxley, A.F. (1973). A note suggesting that the crossbridge attachment during muscular contraction might take place in two stages. Proc. Roy. Soc. B. 183:83.

Taylor, E.W. (1979). Mechanism of actomyosin ATPase and the problem of muscular contraction. Crit. Rev. Biochem. 6:103.

Lymn, R.W. and E.W. Taylor (1971). Mechanism of adenosine triphosphate hydrolysis by actomyosin. Biochem. 10:4617.

Stein, L.A., R.P. Schwartz, P.B. Chock, and E. Eisenberg (1979). Mechanism of actomyosin adenosine triphosphatase. Evidence that adenosine 5'-triphosphate hydrolysis can occur without dissociation of the actomyosin complex. Biochem. 18:3895.

Kaplan, J.H., B. Forbush III, and J.F. Hoffman.(1978). Rapid photolytic release of adenosine 5'-triphosphate from a protected analogue: utilization by the Na:K pump of human red blood cell ghosts. Biochem. 17:1929.

Mc Cray, J., L. Herbette, T. Kihara, and D.R. Trentham (1980). A new approach to time resolved studies of ATP-requiring biological systems: laser flash photolysis of caged ATP. Proc. Natl. Acad. Sci. USA. 77:7237.

Goldman, Y.E., M.G. Hibberd, J.A. McCray, and D.R. Trentham (1982). Relaxation of muscle fibers by photolysis of caged ATP. Nature. 300:701.

Ferenczi, M.A., E. Homsher, and D.R. Trentham (1983). Transient kinetics of MgATP cleavage in single glycerinated muscle fibers. Biophys. J. 41:147a.

ISOZYMES OF CREATINE KINASE IN MAMMALIAN MYOCARDIAL CELL CULTURE

Maria W. Seraydarian and Takenori Yamada

School of Nursing and Department of Physiology
Center for the Health Sciences
University of California at Los Angeles
Los Angeles, CA 90024

INTRODUCTION

The high resting metabolism of the myocardium, a precise coupling of energy production to energy utilization and an efficient access to the available energy in the process of contraction are the functional characteristics of adult myocardium. The mechanisms which subserve these parameters are investigated.

A high steady state ATP concentration at the contractile site in muscle is accomplished by transphosphorylation reaction catalyzed by creatine kinase (CK) located at the contractile site (Jacobs et al., 1964). Phosphocreatine (PCr), thus split at the site of energy utilization leaves creatine as the de facto end product of muscle contraction (Seraydarian and Abbott, 1976). The binding of ATP to myosin is thus favored and a concentration gradient of creatine is established between the myofibrils and mitochondria. Evidence is accumulating that in the myocardium the phosphorylation of creatine to PCr takes place at the mitochondria catalyzed by the bound mitochondrial CK (e.g., Bessman and Fonyo, 1966; Vial et al., 1972,; Jacobus and Lehninger, 1973; Saks et al., 1974, Seraydarian et al., 1974; Jacobus and Ingwall, 1980). Creatine, therefore, might play the role of an effector molecule in coupling the energy utilization at the myofibrils to the energy production in the mitochondria. Furthermore, creatine phosphorylated at the mitochondria functions in the intracellular energy transport. The efficiency of this system is greatly enhanced by the binding of CK to cellular organelles (e.g., myofibrils and mitochondria) which imposes an effective functional compartmentalization of ATP. At the site of energy utilization the

41

reverse CK reaction operates: ADP + PCr $\rightarrow$ ATP + creatine; while
PCr is synthesized mainly at the mitochondria in the forward CK
reaction, ATP + creatine $\rightarrow$ ADP + PCr. It is, therefore, the
creatine- PCr-mitochondrial CK system which subserves a regulatory
function in the coupling of energy production to energy utilization
and in the energy shuttle from the mitochondria to the myofibrils,
providing for the efficient access of energy (from PCr) to the
"bound" nucleotide at the myofibrils catalyzed by myofibrillar CK
(e.g. McClellan et al., 1983).

Using myocardial cells in culture as a model system we have
made numerous observations consistent with the presence of the
energy shuttle and of the specific mitochondrial CK in the cultured
cells (Seraydarian et al., 1974; Seraydarian and Artaza, 1976).
However, since mitochondrial CK was not found in fetal hearts of
several species (Hall and DeLuca, 1975) its presence in the
myocardial cell culture remained to be demonstrated. The
mitochondrial CK isozyme was now demonstrated in the myocardial
cell culture, supporting the previously implied essential role of
mitochondrial CK in the myocardial energy metabolism. The
dependence of the phosphorylation of creatine on aerobic metabolism
in the myocardial cell culture was demonstrated indirectly in
previous studies (Seraydarian and Artaza, 1976). In an attempt to
do so directly, a Lucite attachment which permitted the measurement
of oxygen consumption in cells in culture without manipulating the
cells was constructed. The attachment fitted over commercially
available dishes for cell culture and had an oxygen electrode built
into it. Oxygen uptake of cells was thus measured while the cells
were attached to the substrate of the culture dish and could be
observed in an inverted phase microscope. The rates of oxygen
consumption at different intracellular concentrations of creatine
are currently under investigation.

MATERIALS AND METHODS

Cell Cultures

The primary cultures of cardiac cells were prepared according
to a modification of the method of Harary and Farley (1963).
Myocardial and non-muscle cells derived from the same hearts were
separated as described previously (Van Brussels et al., 1983).
Cells derived from 2 to 6 days old newborn rats (unless specified
otherwise) were cultured in Ham F-10 medium enriched with 10%
newborn calf serum and 1 mM $CaCl_2$ at 37°C, 95% air plus 5% CO_2,
water saturated; medium was changed every 24 h. Two mammalian cell
lines, L6 myoblasts, which retained the ability to fuse and to
synthesize characteristic muscle proteins (Merlie et al., 1977;
Shainberg et al., 1971) and HeLa cells, were also used. Cell lines
were maintained by trypsinization using a solution of 0.25%

bactotrypsin. The cells were suspended in growth medium (Ham F-10 medium containing 10% newborn calf serum and 1 mM $CaCl_2$) and plated in culture dish as for heart cells. Protein of cultured cells was determined by Lowry's method (Lowry et al., 1951), using bovine serum albumin as a standard.

Creatine Kinase

Extraction and measurement of total CK were based on the method of Nielsen and Ludvigsen (1963). Cells from one or more plates were scraped on ice in 2 ml of 10 mM Tris buffer, 0.2 mM dithiothreitol (DTT), pH 7.5 and homogenized 15 s in Tekmar Tissumizer, four times. CK was measured, on aliquots, using the coupled enzyme assay. CK isozymes were separated by electrophoresis on cellulose acetate strips (Gelman Sepraphore III) according to Hall and DeLuca (1975). Samples usually 10 to 20 mU total CK were applied to the cellulose acetate strips, in the presence of 1% NP-40 (Nomidet, non-ionic detergent). The electrophoresis was performed in the cold room for about 90 min, 150 V, 60 mM Tris-barbital buffer, 1 mM DTT, pH 8.8. The strips were treated with 2x concentrated Gelman Sciences, Inc. CK isozyme U.V. Reagent Set with the addition of P^1, P^2 - diadenosine -5' - pentaphosphate, final concentration 10 μM to 20 μM (Miranda et al., 1979). Bands were located using the electrophoretic mobility of MM, BB and mitochondrial CK (prepared from adult rat heart) on accompanying strips. The percent activities of the isozymes were obtained from electrophoretograms by measuring the area for each isozyme and the activities of each isozyme can be obtained by multiplying the percent activity by total CK activity. Turner fluorometer was used to scan the cellulose acetate strips stained for CK activity, and the sensitivity of the method allows for the detection of 0.1 mU CK.

Oxygen Consumption Measurements

Oxygen consumption was measured by using a specially designed attachment. A schematic drawing of the Lucite attachment is shown in Fig. 1. The attachment was constructed to fit over a Falcon #3002 culture dish. A polarographic oxygen electrode, Yellow Spring Instrument Co., YSI 5331, was installed in the attachment. The electric signal from the electrode was amplified by an oxygen monitor, Yellow Spring Instrument Co., YSI53, and recorded by a recorder, Sargent & Co., SRLG. A small circular stirring chamber, affixed at the bottom of the attachment, was equipped with a magnetic stirring bar. A uniform level of oxygen in the medium of the culture dish was maintained by forcing the solution through four 2.5 mm diameter holes cut out tangentially to increase the efficiency of mixing the medium. The attachment had two long 1.0 mm diameter holes in order to remove any air bubbles formed in the medium either in the stirring chamber or in the culture dish. The

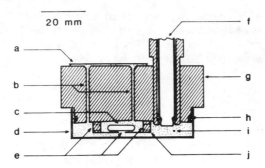

Fig. 1. Attachment for measuring oxygen uptake of cells in
culture (cross sectional view). a) Parafilm, b) holes, 1 mm
diameter, c) magnetic stirring bar, d) culture dish (Falcon
#3002), e) holes, 2.5 mm diameter, f) polarographic oxygen
electrode, g) Lucite attachment, h) 0-ring, i) medium in
culture dish, and j) circular stirring chamber.

whole assembly was immersed in a water bath, temperature was
regulated at 37°C with a water thermostat, Radiometer VTS13.
Solutions of EGTA or KCN were applied with 100 μl or 200 μl
Hamilton microsyringes into the stirring chamber through the hole
located at the center of the Lucite attachment. The added
solutions were mixed with the medium in the culture dish via the
small holes by stirring. The top of the Lucite attachment was
covered during measurements with a sheet of Parafilm to minimize
any leakage of oxygen. The rate of spontaneous contractions of the
myocardial cells was recorded prior to and immediately following
the measurements of the oxygen consumption. The beating rate did
not change detectably following the measurements.

RESULTS AND DISCUSSION

Isozymes of Creatine Kinase

Muscle and non-muscle heart cells in culture contain
comparable levels of PCr, but the nonmyocardial cells have a lower
CK activity. The total CK activity in the four cell types at 96h
in culture was approximately 1,500 mU·mg^{-1} protein in myocardial
cells, 200 mU·mg^{-1} protein in heart non-muscle cells, 2 mU·mg^{-1}
protein in L6 cells and 150 mU·mg^{-1} protein in HeLa cells (Van
Brussel et al., 1983).

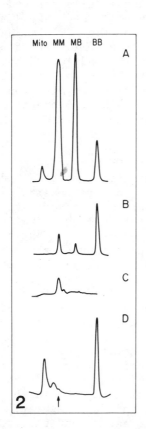

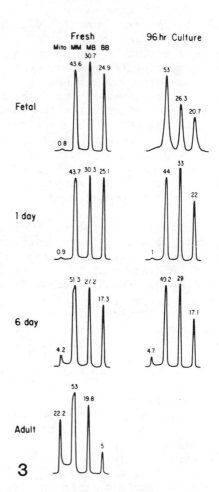

Fig. 2.   Electrophoretogram of CK isozymes on cellulose acetate
strips from 96 h cultures. A, rat myocardial cells, 18 μg
protein; B, rat non-muscle cells derived from the same hearts
as A, 17 μg protein; C, L6 muscle cells, 100 μg protein; D,
HeLa cells, 20 μg protein.

Fig. 3.   Electrophoretogram of CK isozymes on cellulose acetate
strips from fresh tissues and corresponding 96 h cultures.
Fetal rat, 18 days gestation, fresh heart and cultured
myocardial cells; 1-day-old newborn rat, fresh heart and
cultured myocardial cells; 6-day-old rat, fresh heart and
cultured myocardial cells; adult rat 5 months old, fresh
heart. Approximately 10 mU CK per strip.

Four CK isozymes were identified in the cultured myocardial cells: the mitochondrial CK, MM, MB, and BB; the mitochondrial CK moves cathodically, MM remains close to the origin, MB moves between BB and MM and BB moves furthest anodically (Fig. 2A). The mitochondrial isozyme was absent in non-muscle cells derived from the same neonatal rat hearts (Fig. 2B); L6 cells had only 2 mU CK mg^{-1} protein predominantly the MM-CK isozyme (Fig. 2C) and HeLa cells had predominantly the BB-CK isozyme (Fig. 2D). It is evident that in the cells, which do not have the mitochondrial CK the creatine-PCr-mitochondrial CK system cannot subserve the function suggested for the myocardial cells. The absence of mitochondrial CK in non-muscle cells derived from the neonatal rat heart, and in L6 cell line is not surprising, but the mitochondrial CK in HeLa cells was not expected.

Fig. 3 shows the electrophoretogram of CK isozymes of myocardial cell cultures prepared from fetal rat hearts, 18 days gestation, 1 day old rat hearts and 6 days old rat hearts, and the corresponding fresh tissue. Adult rat heart CK isozyme pattern is also shown. The MM isozyme is predominant at all the developmental stages of myocardial cells. Fig. 3 also demonstrates that the CK isozymes of cultured cells tend to correspond to the isozyme patterns typical of the developmental stage of tissue from which the cultures were derived; the percent isozyme distribution approximates the fresh tissue, though total CK of the fresh tissue is much higher than the activity in cultured cells at 96h, i.e., 6.2 $U \cdot mg^{-1}$ protein in fetal heart, 7.3 $U \cdot mg^{-1}$ protein in 1 to 6 days old rat heart and 21.4 $U \cdot mg-1$ protein in 5 months old rats. The percentage of mitochondrial CK increased with the age of the newborn rats from which the culture was derived, suggesting that the majority of cells might be derived from myocytes and not from embryonic cells. The absence of the mitochondrial CK in the fetal hearts (Hall and DeLuca, 1975) indicates that the regulation of energy production at the mitochondria by creatine and energy transport by PCr develop postnatally. The rat myocardial cells in culture could serve as an appropriate model for the study of the trigger mechanism for the synthesis of mitochondrial CK. Similar results were obtained with myosin isozymes separated by electrophoresis on polyacrylamide gels, i.e., the post-natal (6 days) rat myocardial myosin pattern of predominant V_1 isozyme was also characteristic in the cultured cells derived from neonatal hearts; rat fetal myocardial cells are characterized by predominant V_3 isozyme (Lompre et al., 1981 and Van Brussels et al., 1983).

Figure 4 shows the increase of the percentage of mitochondrial CK in myocardial cells with time in culture. Each point is a mean of 10 experiments. The changes in mitochondrial CK are masked by the increase of the non-muscle cell population with time in

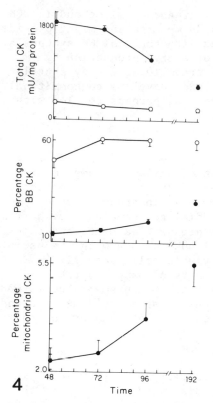

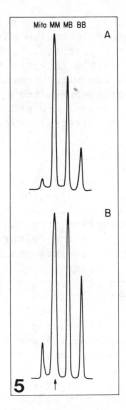

Fig. 4. Total CK and percentage distribution of BB and
mitochondrial CK in cultured myocardial (●) and non-muscle
cells(o) derived from the same rat heart. Each point is a
mean value of 10 experiments ± SEM.

Fig. 5. Electrophoretogram of CK isozymes on cellulose acetate
strips from 96 h myocardial cell culture. A, myocardial cells
in control medium; B, myocardial cells in medium containing
20 mM creatine.

culture, as evidenced by the increase in percentage BB and decrease
of the total CK mU·mg^{-1} protein in the non-muscle cells. The
estimated population of myocardial cells at 96h in culture is only
50%. When cells were cultured in the presence of 20 mM creatine
the mitochondrial CK increased (3.6% to 6.5% in the electrophoretogram at 96h myocardial cell cultures, Fig. 5). In a series of 20
experiments the mean increase of mitochondrial CK (when cells were
grown in 20 mM creatine) was 44% (between 48h and 192h in culture)

with P < 0.005 in paired t-test. The increase of mitochondrial CK in cells grown in medium enriched with 20 mM creatine might provide a clue to the postnatal trigger for the mitochondrial CK synthesis. It is conceivable that the regulation of energy production by creatine at the mitochondria and the intracellular energy shuttle by the creatine–PCr–mitochondrial CK system develops concomitantly with the increased myocardial energy demand, perhaps coupled with the increased arterial oxygen tension.

Oxygen Consumption

Up till now, the basic measurement of oxygen consumption in cultured cells called for manipulations of the cells with potential damage to the cell membrane. Most commonly, in order to study oxygen consumption, the cultured myocardial cells were removed from the substrate of the culture dish by protease treatment, and the oxygen consumption was measured in cell suspensions with the use of a commercial oxygraph. The number of viable cells actually decreased in the course of the measurements of oxygen uptake and the myocardial cells were always quiescent. Measurements performed on myocardial cells still attached to the substrate of the dish and contracting spontaneously could provide important data on the rate of oxygen consumption and the synthesis of PCr over a range of concentrations of creatine.

The trace A in Fig. 6 shows the stability of oxygen level in air-saturated F-10 medium in a culture dish without cells and the time change of oxygen level when nitrogen-saturated F-10 medium has been introduced (trace C of Fig. 6). The uptake of oxygen by cultured myocardial cells in air-saturated F-10 is shown in the trace B of Fig. 6 (till arrow). The decrease of oxygen level with time indicates that oxygen was consumed at a rate of about 1700 nmoles . h^{-1}. The addition of 2 mM KCN (at arrow) to the medium stopped the oxygen uptake of the cells completely.

It was of interest to measure the relative rates of oxygen consumption of quiescent and beating myocardial cells. It is known that in the absence of external calcium myocardial cells stop beating (Langer, 1973). The averaged beating rate of myocardial cells in culture in the present study was 213 ± 4 (S.E.M.) beats.min^{-1} (n=16). When 3 mM EGTA was added (chelating free calcium) to the F-10 medium the myocardial cells immediately stopped beating as observed in the inverted phase microscope and showed an immediate decrease in the rate of oxygen uptake (Fig. 7B). As expected the addition of 3mM EGTA to the medium prior to the measurement showed a decreased rate of oxygen consumption from the start of the measurement (Fig. 7A).

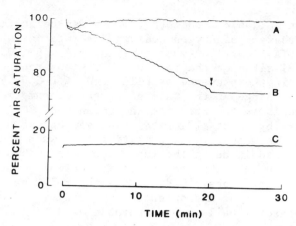

Fig. 6. Typical traces of the changes of oxygen level in the medium at 37°C. A, air-saturated F-10 medium without cells; B, air-saturated F-10 medium with myocardial cells 72 h in culture (646 µg total protein). 2 mM KCN added at arrow. C, nitrogen-saturated F-10 medium without cells.

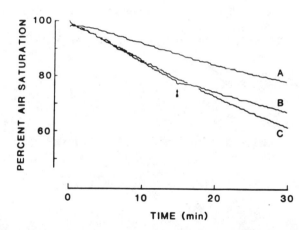

Fig. 7. Typical traces of oxygen uptake of myocardial cells in culture at 37°C in the presence and absence of EGTA. A, B and C are measurements in different culture dishes, each about 72 h in culture, with 689 µg, 710 µg and 798 µg total protein, respectively. A, myocardial cells in F-10 + 3 mM EGTA; B, myocardial cells in F-10, 3 mM EGTA added at arrow; C, myocardial cells in F-10.

As shown in Table 1 the other mammalian cells did not show significant changes of oxygen consumption rate in the presence and absence of EGTA (heart non-muscle cells, $0.4 < P < 0.5$; HeLa cells, $0.2 < P < 0.3$) although the reason for the apparent increase in the L6 cell line in the presence of EGTA ($0.05 < P < 0.1$) is not clear. Therefore the change in the rate of oxygen consumption of myocardial cells in the presence and absence of EGTA is attributed to the higher (by about 47%) rate of oxygen uptake of myocardial cells in culture when cells are beating than when they are quiescent. In adult heart the rate of oxygen uptake is known to increase by about 35% when the heart is beating compared to a non-beating heart (Gibbs, 1978). Thus the relative rates of oxygen consumption of beating and quiescent myocardium and of cultured neonatal myocardial cells are comparable.

The rate of oxygen uptake per mg protein of myocardial cells, non-muscle cells derived from the same hearts, HeLa cells and L-6 cells in culture is summarized in Table 1. Heart non-muscle, HeLa and L6 cells showed almost the same rate of oxygen consumption. Beating myocardial cells had the rate of oxygen consumption of 40.5 nmoles min^{-1} mg^{-1} protein which was approximately four times higher

TABLE 1.   Oxygen Uptake of Various Cells in Culture at 37°C.

Cell Type	Rates of oxygen uptake, nmoles $O_2 \cdot min^{-1} \cdot mg^{-1}$ protein		
	F-10	F-10 + 3 mM EGTA	F-10 + 2 mM KCN
Myocardial	40.5 ± 1.3 (19)	27.6 ± 0.6 (13)	0.1 ± 0.6 (3)
Non-muscle (heart)	11.3 ± 0.7 (6)	12.8 ± 1.9 (5)	0.1 ± 0.9 (3)
HeLa	11.7 ± 1.3 (10)	14.0 ± 1.7 (7)	0.0 ± 0.3 (2)
L-6 muscle	12.0 ± 1.3 (8)	16.2 ± 1.5 (6)	0.0 ± 0.6 (5)

The cells were cultured between 72 and 96 h.

All values are means ± S.E.M. Number in parenthesis indicates the number of experiments.

than the other mammalian cells examined in the present study. The
oxygen uptake was completely inhibited in all the cells examined
when 2 mM KCN was added.

The reported oxygen uptake of non-beating whole heart (Gibbs,
1978) is about 2.5 ml.100 g^{-1} wet wt.min.$^{-1}$ (or 15.5
nmoles.min^{-1}.mg^{-1} protein), which is considerably less than the
quiescent myocardial cells in culture (Table 1). The relatively large population of non-muscle cells (about 75%) in adult
hearts (Marsh, 1983) might account for this difference. The oxygen
uptake rate of cardiac myocytes has been reported to be 69.5
nmoles.min^{-1}.mg^{-1} protein (Burns and Reddy, 1978) in conditions
roughly comparable to the present study. Therefore the present
result, 40.5 nmoles.min^{-1}.mg^{-1}, is significantly smaller than that
of myocytes. The difference in the oxygen uptake of heart cells in
culture derived from newborn rat and that of myocytes derived from
adult myocardium might be explained in the light of the difference
in the content of mitochondrial creatine kinase in the two cell
populations. Adult heart cells have a high level of mitochondrial
creatine kinase (Saks et al., 1974) compared with heart cells of
newborn rat (Van Brussel et al., 1983). These results are
consistent with the view that mitochondrial creatine kinase plays
an important role in the coupling of energy utilization and energy
production in heart cells and its low concentration in the neonatal
cell in culture might be limiting the respiratory activity. It is
expected that the rates of oxygen consumption will change in
parallel with various concentrations of creatine in myocardial
cells but not in either non-muscle heart cells or L6 muscle cell
line.

Oxygen consumption of quiescent myocardial cells was about
twice that of the heart non-muscle cells, HeLa or L-6 cells as
shown in Table 1, consistent with the data that heart has a high
resting level of energy metabolism (Gibbs, 1978). It is reasonable
to assume that specific regulatory mechanisms are needed to prevent
a possible depletion of ATP resulting from a further energy demand
during activity superimposed on the high resting level.

REFERENCES

Bessman, S.P., and Fonyo, A. (1966) The possible role of the
    mitochondrial bound creatine kinase in regulation of
    mitochondrial respiration. Biochem. Biophys. Commun.,
    22:597-602.

Burns, A.H. and Reddy, W.J. (1978) Amino acid stimulation of oxygen and substrate utilization by cardiac myocytes. Am. J. Physiol., 235:E461-E466.

Gibbs, C.L. Cardiac energetics. (1978) Physiol. Rev. 58:174-254.

Hall, N., and DeLuca, M. (1975) Developmental changes in creatine phosphokinase isoenzymes in neonatal mouse hearts. Biochem. Biophys. Res. Commun., 66:988-994.

Harary, I., and Farley, B. (1963) In vitro studies of beating heart cells in culture. I. Growth and organization. Exp. Cell Res., 29:451-465.

Jacobs, M., Heldt, H.W. and Klingenberg, M. (1964) High activity of creatine kinase in mitochondria from muscle and brain and evidence for a separate mitochondrial isoenzyme of creatine kinase. Biochem. Biophys. Res Commun. 16:516-521.

Jacobus, W.E. and Ingwall, J.S., eds. (1980) Heart Creatine Kinase. The Integration of Isozymes for Energy Distribution. Baltimore, Williams & Williams.

Jacobus, W.E. and Lehninger, A.L. (1973) Creatine kinase of rat heart mitochondria. J. Biol. Chem., 248:4803-4810.

Langer, G.A. (1973) Heart: Excitation-contraction coupling. Ann. Rev. Physiol. 35, 55-86.

Lompré, A.M., Mercadier, J.J., Wisnewsky, C., Bouveret, P., Pantaloni, C., D'Albis, A., and Schwartz, K. (1981) Species and age-dependent changes in the relative amounts of cardiac myosin isozymes in mammals. Dev. Biol., 84:286-290.

Lowry, O.H., Rosenbrough, N.J., Farr, A.L., and Randall, R.J. (1951) Protein measurement with the Folin phenol reagent. J. Biol. Chem. 193:265-275.

Marsh, J.D. (1983) The cultured heart cell: A useful model for physiological and biochemical investigation. Int. J. Cardiol. 3:465-468.

McClellan, G., Weisberg, A., and Winegrad, S. (1983) Energy transport from mitochondria to myofibril by a creatine phosphate shuttle in cardiac cells. Am. J. Physiol., 245:C423-C427.

Merlie, J.P., Buckingham, M.E., and Whalen, R.G. (1977) Molecular aspects of myogenesis. Current Topics Dev. Biol., 11:61-114.

Miranda, A.F., Somer, H., and Dimauro, S. (1979) Isoenzyme as markers of differentiation. In: Muscle Regeneration. A. Mauro, R. Bischoff, B. Carlson, S. Shafiq, I. Konigsberg, and B. Lipton, eds. New York, Raven Press, pp. 453-473.

Nielsen, L., and Ludvigsen, B. (1963) Improved method for determination of creatine kinase. J. Lab. Clin. Med., 62:159-169.

Saks, V.A., Chernousova, G.B., Voronkov, U.I., Smirnov, V.N., and Chazov, E.I. (1974) Study of energy transport mechanism in myocardial cells. Circ. Res., 34-35 (Suppl. III): 138-149.

Seraydarian, M.W., and Abbott, B.C. (1976) The role of the creatine-phosphocreatine system in muscle. J. Mol. Cell Cardiol., 8:741-746.

Seraydarian, M.W., and Artaza, L. (1976) Regulation of energy
    metabolism by creatine in cardiac and skeletal muscle cells in
    culture. J. Mol. Cell. Cardiol., 8:669-678.
Seraydarian, M.W., Artaza, L., and Abbott, B.C. (1974) Creatine
    and the control of energy metabolism in cardiac and skeletal
    muscle cells in culture. J. Mol. Cell. Cardiol., 6:405-413.
Shainberg, A., Yagil, G., and Yaffe, D. (1971) Alterations of
    enzymatic activities during muscle differentiation in vitro.
    Dev. Biol., 25:1-29.
Van Brussel, E., Yang, J.J., Seraydarian, M.W. (1983) Isozymes of
    creatine kinase in mammalian cell cultures. J. Cell.
    Physiol. 116:221-226.
Vial, C., Godinot, G., and Gautheron, D. (1972) Creatine Kinase
    (EC 2.7.3.2.) in pig heart mitochondria. Properties and role
    in phosphate potential regulation. Biochimie, 54:843-852.

MICROCOMPARTMENTATION AT THE MITOCHONDRIAL SURFACE:

ITS FUNCTION IN METABOLIC REGULATION

D. Brdiczka, G. Knoll, I. Riesinger, U. Weiler,
G. Klug, R. Benz and J. Krause

Universitat Konstanz
D-7750 Konstanz

About 10 years ago it was observed by Gots and Bessman[1] in liver and later by Inui [2] in brain that the mitochondrial bound hexokinase had a higher activity with ATP supplied by the oxidative phosphorylation as compared to ATP added from the outside. Experiments with labelled phosphate showed that the newly synthesized ATP was directly used by hexokinase and did not equilibrate with the extramitochondrial pool [1]. Therefore, a function of hexokinase and glucose as acceptor for high energy phosphate analogue to creatinekinase and creatine in muscle has been postulated, namely, to increase maximal efficiency of oxidative phosphorylation in resting muscle and in nonmuscular tissues [3].

The structural basis for this functional compartmentation between the surface bound hexokinase and the oxidative phosphorylation was at least partially elaborated recently. The numerous data focusses upon two most important observations. First, the outer mitochondrial membrane is exclusively permeable for polar molecules along a pore protein. This pore protein specifically binds so far known hexokinase and glycerolkinase. Secondly, the outer and inner membrane form close contacts which correlate in frequency to the degree of coupling of the oxidative phosphorylation. There exists some evidence that the pore protein is localized in the contact regions.

I shall describe some experimental results concerning these two points in more detail.

PROPERTIES OF THE MITOCHONDRIAL PORE AND KINASE BINDING PROTEIN

The pore protein of the outer membrane has been characterized in neurospora [4], yeast [5] and liver [6-8] mitochondria. The purified

protein consists of a single polypeptide of Mr 30 000. How many subunits form the active pore in the intact membrane is not yet clear.
The pore could be reconstituted from the isolated protein within planar bilayers and liposomes. It is the only protein amongst all other
investigated outer membrane proteins which made the membranes permeable for ions and ADP [8]. Electronmicroscopic investigations of neurospora outer membranes applying negative staining suggest a pore
diameter of 2 nm and the existance of positive charges at the mouth
or inside the pore [9]. This is consistent with our results obtained
by conductance measurements with the reconstituted pore in planar bilayers. We have calculated a similar diameter and need positive
charges to explain the weak anion selectivity of the pore. Another
interesting property of the pore which has first been described by
Colombini [10] is a voltage dependent change in single channel conductance. This is shown in Table 1 where the decrease in average single
channel conductance is used to calculate the resultant decrease in
diameter. Increasing the voltage from 5 to 100 mV leads to a decrease
of the pore diameter from 20 to 5 Å. This is a magnitude which can
hinder the penetration of polar molecules as ADP, succinate etc.

TABLE I: AVERAGE CONDUCTANCE INCREMENT $\overline{\Lambda}$ ON FOR THE ISOLATED PORE
PROTEIN AS A FUNCTION OF APPLIED MEMBRANE POTENTIAL

Membrane potential mV	$\overline{\Lambda}$on ns	N-on	Calculated diameter (d=2r) Å
5	4.3	431	20
10	3.0	142	16
20	2.4	157	14
50	0.75	221	[8]
100	0.45	35	[5]

The potential was negative on the side at which the protein was added.
The membranes were formed from Asolectin dissolved in n-decane;
T = 25°C. The aqueous phase contained 1M NaCl. N-on are the numbers
of pores from which $\overline{\Lambda}$on was determined. The diameter was calculated
based on the assumption that the pores were filled with an aqueous
solution of the same conductance (σ) as the external bulk phase ac-
cording to the equation $\overline{\Lambda} = \sigma \Pi r^2 /L$. For small diameters σ might be
different from the medium. A pore length (L) of 75 Å was assumed
corresponding to the thickness of the outer membrane.

We suggest that an intrinsic membrane potential may regulate the pore diameter physiologically. An intrinsic membrane potential could be created by an asymmetric distribution of fixed charges between both membranes and surfaces. In this respect it is interesting to mention that the pore protein is asymmetric. This becomes evident when the protein is inserted from one side only into a planar bilayer. The current decreases if the side where the protein was added is negative. Whereas it shows no decay when the polarity of the applied voltage is inverted [8]. One can imagine that an asymmetric cAMP dependent phosphorylation and concommitant dephosphorylation [11] could be a means of influencing the transport across the pore either directly by altering the charges in the entrance of the pore and therefore the ion selectivity or indirectly by changing the trans-membrane potential and/or the polarity and therefore the diameter of the pore.

The hexokinase binding protein characterized by Felgner et al. [13] is identical with the pore protein. This has been proved by two dimensional elcectrophoresis and peptide maps of the two purified proteins [14]. As well as by comparing the biochemical and biophysical properties [15]. Upon purification of the pore protein the binding capacity for hexokinase increased 140-fold in comparison to isolated mitochondria. This agrees with the observation that the mitochondrial pore protein in liver amounts to approximately 0.5% of the mitochondrial protein[15].

Glycerolkinase binds to the mitochondrial porin as well, with an affinity comparable to the hexokinase. Both kinases seem to compete for the same binding protein because glucose-6-phosphate must be added for glycerolkinase binding to be observed when hexokinase is also present [16]. When mitochondria are preincubated with antibodies against the mitochondrial porin the binding of both kinases is inhibited. This is shown for hexokinase in Fig. 1.

DYNAMIC INTERACTIONS OF THE MITOCHONDRIAL BOUNDARY MEMBRANES

Contacts between the two boundary membranes have first been described by Hackenbrock in thin sections [17]. In these preparations large parts of the two boundary membranes have become separated which is an artificial mitochondrial structure. In situ by applying rapid freezing and freeze substitution both membranes appear almost in close contact [18] as in freeze fractured isolated mitochondria after pure physical fixation by the cryogen jet method [19]. The structure of those freeze fractured mitochondria is characterized by an irregular course of the fracture plane jumping back and forth between two different layers (Fig. 2). It has become widely accepted [20-22] that the fracture plane jumps between the interior of the outer and inner membrane as schematically shown in Fig. 2. An interpretation like that implicates that the fracture plane has to cross the outer mitochondrial compartment. For biophysical reason the fracture plane does not cross a space filled with

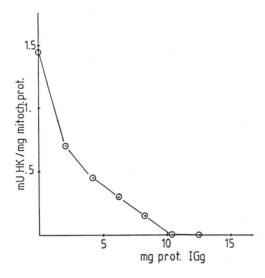

Fig. 1: Displacement of hexokinase from the mitochondrial surface by antibodies against mitochondrial pore protein.
Isolated rat liver mitochondria were preincubated with increasing amounts of purified IgG fraction. After washing and subsequent incubation with 4 mU of hexokinase I from rat brain the mitochondria were again centrifuged and measured for bound hexokinase activity. The antibodies did neither react with free hexokinase nor inactivate bound enzyme.

water but does follow hydrophobic regions. Therefore, it is reasonable to assume that the deflections can occur in zones of intimate contact between the two boundary membranes. Van Venetië and Verkleij 23 freeze fractured mitochondria have proposed a semifusion model for the contact sites in which non-bilayer lipids are involved. Indeed Malhotra has described a 5 layer pattern as a result of close apposition of the two limiting membranes in freeze substituted specimen of the liver, which is in contrast to the commonly observed 7 layer structure in isolated mitochondria [18].

Considering these observations we suggested that the frequency of fracture plane jumps could correlate with the number of contacts. Therefore, determining this parameter would provide a method of estimating the frequency of contacts. As a means of measuring the frequency of fracture plane deflections we determined the length of the fracture plane edge per standard area (Fig. 2b). By comparing isolated mitochondria in state 4 (orthodox) to those in state 3 (condensed) we observed a 4-fold increase of this length parameter in the latter mitochondria. This suggested that in phosphorylating mitochondria the frequency of the fracture plane jumps had increased and, therefore, also the frequency of the membrane contacts [24].

The data is summarized in Table II. This table in addition, contains values for mitochondria which were uncoupled with DNP. According to the very low value of fracture plane deflections determined there, uncoupling leads to a reduction of contacts below that in state 4.

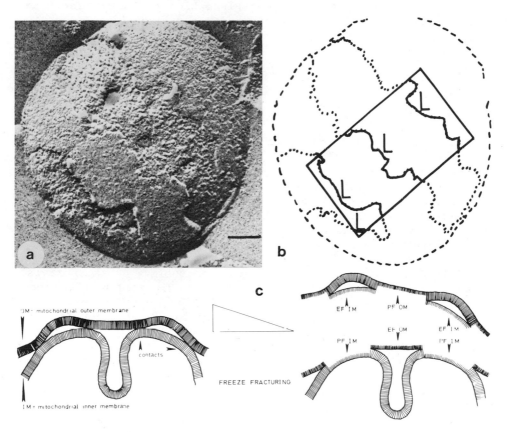

Fig. 2: (a) Freeze-fracture of a mitochodrium (state 1). Bar=0.1μm
(b) Scheme of the evaluation procedure. Isolated mitochondria were
adjusted to the respective energetic state, frozen and freeze-fractured. From each preparation 10-20 detailed micrographs were taken
showing mitochondria with fracture plane deviations and surveys with
approximately 100 fractured mitochondrial membranes. As a means of
quantifying the difference in fracture plane deviations, we measured
the length of the edge where the fracture plane deflects (solid line
on b) as related to the corresponding area (shown in b). The obtained
values were a certain length (L) per area $(\mu m/\mu m^2)$. The length of the
edges was determined in an area where the platinimum carbon was eva-
porated at an angle of approx. 45° to the plane of the specimen. In
order to perform an analysis which takes into consideration the
different amount of smooth membrane fractures in the respective mitochondrial fractions we determined on survey pictures the total area
of smooth membrane fractures (M_s) and patchy membrane fractures (M_p).
The single values, L, were then weighted by the factor $M_p/(M_p+M_s)$ for
the particular preparation [24]. (c) Diagrammatic representation of
how the freeze-cleaved half-membranes arise from the outer and inner
membranes, respectively. The different layers are designated according to the nomenclature in Ref. [25].

59

TABLE II: Length of the Fracture-Plane Edge in Freeze-Fractured
Mitochondria in Different States and After Uncoupling.

	State 1	State 4	State 3	uncoupled
L $\mu m/\mu m^2$	5.1±2.7	5.9±2.4	14.2±7.0	1.8±1.6
probability level	n.s.	n.s.	p<0.01	p<0.01

The isolated mitochondria were incubated in 0.12 M sucrose,
Na-phosphate 10 mM pH 7.5, $MgCl_2$ 5 mM. State 1 = freshly isolated
mitochondria, State 4 = energized by succinate 10 mM, State 3 =
phosphorylating in the presence of succinate and ADP 1 mM, uncoupled
by addition of 50 μM 2,4.-dinitrophenol. Statistical differences of
the measured parameter between the experimental groups and controls
(state 1) are shown as p values. n.s. = no significant difference even
at the level p = 0.1.

From this data we concluded that the coupling of phosphorylation
to the electrochemical potential might be correlated to the frequency
of contacts. This has been investigated in vitro and in vivo. In the
in vitro experiment the mitochondria were partially uncoupled by incubation with palmitate and subsequently recoupled by washing with
albumin. As may be seen from Table III the morphological parameter
representative for the frequency of contacts strictly correlates with
the coupling of oxidative phosphorylation determined by the ADP/O and
acceptor control ratios. The frequency of contacts decrease when the
oxidative phosphorylation becomes partially uncoupled.

TABLE III: Effect of Reversible Uncoupling by Palmitate on the Frequency of Fracture Plane Deflections in Freeze-Fractured Mitochondria.

As a measure for this parameter the length of the fracture plane
edge μm/um² was determined. Isolated liver mitochondria were incubated
for 10 min at room temperature with 50 μM palmitate. Subsequently
half of the pelleted mitochondria were washed with sucrose medium containing 5 % albumin. Washing of untreated mitochondria with albumin
had no effect when the mitochondria were in state 1.

	incubated with 50 μM palmitate	50 μM palmitate and albumin wash
ADP/O	0.57	1.9
AC	1.3	4
State 3 $\mu m/\mu m^2$	2	15

LOCALIZATION OF THE PORE PROTEIN AT THE MITCHONDRIAL SURFACE

In contrast to neurospora and plant mitochondria [26,27] it was not possible to visualize the pore in liver mitochondria by negative staining. By applying immunocytochemical methods to isolated mitochondria we observed that the pore protein as well as the bound hexokinase is localized exclusively within areas of the outer membrane which are in proximity to the inner membrane.

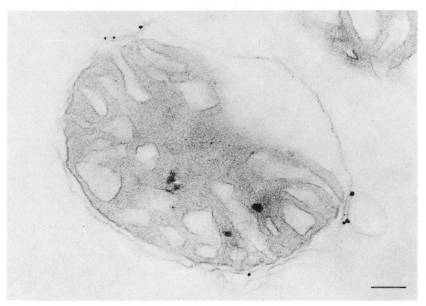

Fig. 3: Gold labelled hexokinase bound to the mitochondrial surface as described in Table IV. Bar = 0.09 μm.

As shown in Fig. 3 hexokinase labelled with colloidal gold binds to the mitochondrial surface. No label is bound where the two boundary membranes have become separated, whereas all label is bound where the two membranes are closely apposed. We have determined the amount of gold label attached to these different areas of the mitochondrial surface. The data is listed in Table IV. Almost no label is bound where the boundary membranes are separated. The same result is obtained whether labelled hexokinase or labelled antibodies against the binding protein are used. This suggests that the distribution of the pore within the outer membrane is regulated by the contacts or vice versa.

Fig. 4 schematically summarizes our interpretation of the results described above. We propose a microcompartment between hexokinase and oxidative phosphorylation in which the pore protein and the contacts between the two limiting membranes are involved. This microcompartment can have two important consequences in metabolic regulation. First, the effective concentrations of metabolites in the

TABLE IV: Localization of Hexokinase and Pore Protein at the
Mitochondrial Surface.

| | boundary membranes | | | |
| | attached | | separated | |
	Length of Sur-face per mito. µm	Grains per µm	Length of Sur-face per mito. µm	Grains per µm
Hexokinase-Gold (23)	1.3	1.8	1.0	0.47
Probability level		p < 0.001		
Antiporin-Prot.A-Gold (19)	1.7	0.9	0.59	0.18
Probability level		p < 0.001		

Isolated mitochondria washed with 10 mM EDTA were incubated with gold labelled hexokinase isoenzyme I in the presence of 10 mM $MgCl_2$. In a second experiment the same mitochondria were decorated with antibodies against the pore protein and were subsequently incubated with gold labelled protein A. All samples were centrifugated and the pellets were fixed by glutaraldehyde 2.5 % and postfixed with osmium 2 %. The fixed samples were embedded in Spurr's expoxy resin.

Mitochondria in thin sections exhibiting attached and separated boundary membranes were selected, numbers in brackets. In these mitochondria the length of the surface with closely apposed or separated membranes was determined and correlated to the number of gold grains bound to the respective part of the surface. The statistical difference of gold grains per different surface section is significant at the given p value.

---

active centres of the respective enzymes can be higher as in the bulk phase to maintain high activity rates and secondly, the flow of metabolites between enzymes which compete for the same substrate can be regulated. I want to give a few examples for that. Adenylatekinase (AdK) and hexokinase (HK) can compete for ATP, glycerolphosphate-oxidase (GPOX) and glycerolphosphate-acyl-transferase (GPAT) can compete for glycerolphosphate. And the latter enzyme (GPAT) and carnitine-acyl-transferase (CAT) can both utilize acyl-CoA.

COMPARTMENTATION OF METABOLITES AT THE MITOCHONDRIAL PERIPHERY

The first example whether adenylatekinase and hexokinase share the same ATP/ADP pool was investigated in the following way. We determined the rate of glucose-phosphorylation by bound hexokinase in

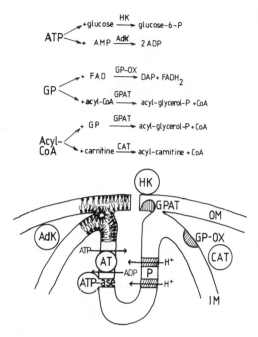

Fig. 4: Hypothetical model of the microcompartment at the mitochondrial periphery.

The contacts between the two boundary membranes are suggested
to form microcompartments which regulate between enzymes competing
for the same substrates: ATP, glycerolphosphate, acyl-CoA. The model
is based on the formation of hexagonal II_{II} cylinders by non-bilayer lipids [28], and refers to the mosaic chemiosmosis [29].

Abbreviations: HK:hexokinase [E.C. 2.7.1.1], AdK = adenylatekinase [E.C. 2.7.4.3], GP-OX = glycerolphosphate-Oxidase E.C.[1.1.99.5],
GPAT = glycerolphosphate-acyl-transferase [E.C. 2.3.1.15], CAT =
carnitine acyltransferase [E.C. 2.3.1.21], AT = ATP/ADPtranslocator,
P = proton-pump, GP = glycerolphosphate, DAP = dihydroxyacetonephos-
phate.

intact well coupled mitochondria. The ATP necessary for this reaction
was provided by 3 different ways: 1. added from outside; 2. produced
by the oxidative phosphorylation in the presence of ADP, phosphate
and succinate; and 3. produced via adenylatekinase from added ADP in
the absence of anorganic phosphate and substrate for the oxidative
phosphorylation. As is shown in Table V the glucose-6-phosphate production from ATP provided by the adenylatekinase is very low and

TABLE V: ATP/ADP Compartmentation at the Mitochondrial Surface.

Mitochondria	ATP provided by			
	1 added from outside	2 oxid. phosphoryl.	3 adenylate kinase	4 adenylate kinase + inhibitor
	nmole glucose-6-P/min x mg			
Control	0.51±0.36	0.75±0.51	0.15±0.15	0.08
low Ca^{2+}	0.92±0.26	0.87±0.19	1.92±0.75	n.d.
low Ca^{2+} + 5 µM Ca^{2+}	0.46±0.12	0.78±0.12	0.0	n.d.

Mitochondria were prepared in 0.25M sucrose, 10 mM Hepes pH 7.4 = Control or in the same medium with addition of 0.1 mM EGTA = low Ca^{2+}. Glucose-6P production was determined in sucrose medium without EGTA in the presence of 4 mM $MgCl_2$ and 1 mM glucose. ATP was supplied by: 1 = 1 mM ATP; 2 = 1 mM ADP + 4 mM phosphate + 5 mM succinate, 3 = 1 mM ADP, 4 = 1 mM ADP + 2 mM P^1, P^5-Di (adenosine 5') pentaphosphate. n.d. = not determined.

sensitive to Di (adenosine 5') pentaphosphate an inhibitor of this enzyme. The rate of glucose phosphorylation from ATP generated by the oxidative phosphorylation is about twice that from ATP supplied from outside. The latter result has already been described by several authors [1,2].

From this data we conclude that formation of the microcompartment between hexokinase and the oxidative phosphorylation can exclude adenylatekinase in the intermembrane space from the ATP/ADP exchange with the inner compartment. It is interesting to note that Ca^{2+} seems to be necessary for the formation of the microcompartment because the microcompartment was not observed in mitochondria isolated with EGTA and could be reestablished by addition of Ca^{2+} to these mitochondria. Ca^{2+} has the capacity to induce a transition of the phoshilipids into non-bilayer structures as a consequence of electrostatic interaction with negatively charged lipids [28]. It might therefore cause the formation of hexagonal H_{II} tubes as proposed in Fig. 4.

THE MICROCOMPARTMENT IN DIFFERENT METABOLIC STATES

If a microcompartment between hexokinase pore protein and adenylate translocator in the inner membrane is assumed it is worthwhile to investigate whether this functional microcompartment is subjected to metabolic regulation. The observation of a correlation between the activity of the bound hexokinase and the number of contacts would give some indication for this.

In collaboration with G. Klug we analyzed liver mitochondria from rats which had been forced into an extreme ketogenic and gluco-neogenic metabolic situation by exhaustive exercise. As can been seen from Table VI exercise when compared to the controls produced a 50% decrease in ADP/O ratios and acceptor control index as well as a 4-fold decrease in hexokinase bound to the mitochondrial surface. We also determined the length of the fracture plane edge ($\mu m/\mu m^2$) in freeze fractured samples of these mitochondria as a means of deter-mining the frequency of boundary membrane contacts. As shown in Table VII no differences exist between mitochondria from exercised and con-trol animals in state 1 and after addition of succinate (state 4). Upon addition of ADP to the energized control mitochondria (state 3) the value increased 3 to 4-fold indicating a significant increase in contacts. Conversely, when mitochondria isolated from the fasted-exhausted group are measured in state 3, the length of the fracture plane edge remained unchanged. Hence, there is no increase in the frequency of membrane contacts upon transition to state 3 in these partially uncoupled mitochondria.

TABLE VI: Effect of Running to Exhaustion upon ADP/O Ratio, Acceptor Control Index and Hexokinase Binding in Liver Mitochondria.

Group	ADP/O	AC	Bound Hexokinase mU/mg protein
Control	(8) 1.6 ± 0.15	(8) 6.4 ± 1.6	(3) 8.4 ± 1.1
Exhausted	(5) 1.1 ± 0.31	(5) 2.8 ± 1.7	(4) 2.0 ± 0.4
Probability level	$p < 0.005$	$p < 0.001$	$p < 0.05$
Fasted Exhausted	(13) 0.92 ± 0.37	(13) 2.5 ± 1.1	(6) 1.83 ± 0.9
Probability level	$p < 0.01$	$p < 0.01$	$p < 0.05$

The mitochondrial respiration was determined at 23°C by polar-graphic techniques. The reaction medium contained 0.25 M sucrose, 10 mM Hepes pH 7.4, 5 mM sodium phosphate, 5 mM $MgCl_2$, 5 mM succinate. ADP/O ratios were determined by addition of 200 nmole ADP several times. Maximal oxidation rates were measured in the presence of 1 mM ADP. The acceptor control index was calculated by dividing the rate of oxygen consumption in the presence of 1 mM ADP and 5 mM succinate (state 3) by the rate of oxygen consumption in the presence of succi-nate (state 4).

Values are given as mean ± standard deviation. The numbers in brackets indicate the number of different mitochondrial fractions measured. Statistical differences of the measured parameters between experimental groups and controls are shown as p values.

TABLE VII: Frequency of Fracture Plane Jumps Between Boundary Membranes as Determined in Freeze-Fractured Mitochondria from Exercised and Control Animals.

		state 1	state 4	state 3
control	$\mu m/\mu m^2$	3.0	3.1	11.7
fasted exhausted	$\mu m/\mu m^2$	2.6	3.6	4.2

For the purposes of quantification, the length of the fracture plane edges of the exoplasmic faces of both boundary membranes were determined(see Fig. 2). Isolated mitochondria from control and exercised, fasted animals were adjusted to the various metabolic states, as described in Table II.

CHANGES OF ISOENZYMES BOUND TO THE MITOCHONDRIAL SURFACE UNDER DIFFERENT METABOLIC REGIMES

Katzen and Schimke [30] pointed out a correlation between the presence of hexokinase type II and the insulin sensitivity of the tissue. It has on the other hand been observed by Borrebaek [31] in fat pads that insulin increases the activity of isoenzyme II bound to the mitochondrial surface.

We have studied the binding of the isolated isoenzymes to liver mitochondria and observed that isoenzyme I,II and III bind to the same saturation whereas isoenzyme IV does not bind. This suggests that the isoenzymes I - III interact with the same limited amount of binding protein. When we studied the effect of carbohydrate rich diet we observed no further increase of the total bound activity. Therefore, we assume that the amount of binding protein is not metabolically regulated. However, the pattern of the bound isoenzymes was dramatically altered in the different metabolic situations. As can be seen from Table VIII the bound activity of isoenzyme II and III decreased about 10-fold by fasting, while isoenzyme I did slightly increase. The importance of this change in metabolic regulation became apparent when we observed a pronounced activation of the free enzymes upon binding to the mitochondrial membrane. Isoenzyme II was activated by a factor of 39, isoenzyme I became activated 5.6-fold and isoenzyme III 1.3-fold. On the basis of these results we calculated the effective activity at the mitochondrial surface. The values shown in Table VIII emphasize the importance of the mitochondrial fraction of low-Km hexokinase because their activity surmounts that of the soluble isoenzyme I - III. Furthermore, the data in Table VIII points to an important function of isoenzyme II in the formation of the microcompartment. It is interesting to ask how the binding of this enzyme is regulated. Because in contrast to isoenzyme I the desorption of type II hexokinase from the mitochondrial surface is apparently unaffected by glucose-6-phosphate [32].

TABLE VIII: Changes of Isoenzymes Bound to the Mitochondrial Surface
Under Different Metabolic Regimes

Hexokinase isoenzymes		Carbohydrate rich diet		Fasted	
		in vitro determined	in vivo effective	in vitro determined	in vivo effective
		mU/mg		mU/mg	
bound	I	1.3	7.3	1.88	10.5
	II	0.51	20.0	0.074	2.9
	III	0.51	0.66	0.04	0.05
free	I-III	12.7		5.2	
	IV	27.3		0.1	

In vitro quantities of hexokinase types bound to the mitochondrial
surface were determined from the distribution in the isoenzyme-electro-
phoresis and the total activity in the mitochondrial fraction. The in
vivo effective activity was calculated by multiplying the in vitro
activity of the hexokinases by the following factors: type I 5.6,
type II 39, type III 1.3. These factors consider the degree of activation which was observed upon binding of the isoenzyme types to the
mitochondrial surface.

THE REGULATION OF THE MICROCOMPARTMENT

An increase in negative surface charge was observed in mitochondria from the aforementioned exercised rats as well as in control
mitochondria when incubated with 80μM palmitate. This change of the
surface charge density was measured by fluorescence titration with 8-
Anilino-1-naphthalene sulfonate [33]. We therefore assume that the
formation of the above described microcompartment may be regulated by
changes in the surface charge of the mitochondrial membranes.

An increase in net negative surface potential by free fatty
acids desorbs hexokinase in vitro from the outer membrane [33]. It
may therefore provide an explanation for the observed decrease in
hexokinase activity bound to the mitochondria from exercised animals.
Since at physiological pH all hexokinase isoenzymes comprise negative
charges increasing from isoenzyme I to IV. Furthermore, the increase
in negative surface charge at the surface of both limiting membranes
may result in repulsion of the membranes from one another and by this,
cause a decrease in contacts between the membranes.

Under the condition of exhaustive exercise where the insulin level is low and glucose phosphorylation in the liver is of little importance to the organism the described microcompartment may be reduced. The level of free fatty acids which is high during exhaustive exercise and fasting could be a mechanism by which hormones such as insulin and glucagon regulate the functional compartmentation at the mitochondrial surface. cAMP dependent phosphorylation of the mitochondrial membranes as observed recently [11] could provide an additional mechanism active in the same metabolic situation. We have recently observed that in vitro phosphorylation of isolated mitochondria reduces the binding capacity for hexokinase but has little effect on the coupling of oxidative phosphorylation. This is because the regulatory mechanism of cAMP dependent phosphorylation is different compared to that of free fatty acids. It is asymmetric and presumably acting exclusively at the surface of the outer membrane.

REFERENCES

1. Gots, R.E. and Bessman, S.P. Arch.Biochem.Biophys., 163:7-14 (1974)
2. Inui, M. and Ishibashi, S. J.Biochem., 85:1151-1157 (1979)
3. Bessman, S.P., Am.J.Medicine, 40:740-748 (1966)
4. Freitag, H., Neupert, W. and Benz, R. Eur.J.Biochem., 234:629-636 (1982)
5. Mihara, K., Blobel, G. and Sato, R. Proc.Natl.Acad.Sci., 779: 7102-7106 (1982)
6. Zalman, L.S., Niakaido, H. and Kagawa, Y. J.Biol.Chem., 255: 1771-1774 (1980)
7. Lindén, M., Gellerfors, P. and Nelson, B.D., Biochem.J., 208: 77-82 (1982)
8. Roos, N., Benz, R. and Brdiczka, D., Biochim.Biophys.Acta, 688:204-214 (1982)
9. Mannella, C.A. and Frank, J. Biophys.J., 37:3-4 (1982)
10. Colombini, M. Nature, 279:643-645 (1975)
11. Famulski, K.S., Nalecz, M.J. and Wojtczak, L. FEBS-Lett., 157: 125-128 (1983)
13. Felgner, P.L., Messer, J.L. and Wilson, J.E., J.Biol.Chem., 254:4946-4949 (1979)
14. Lindén, M., Gellerfors, P. and Nelson, B.D. FEBS-Lett., 141: 189-192 (1982)
15. Fiek, Ch., Benz, R., Roos, N. and Brdiczka, D. Biochim.Biophys. Acta, 688:419:440 (1982
16. Östlund, A.K., Göhring, U., Krause, J. and Brdiczka, D. Biochim. Med., 30:231-245 (1983)
17. Hackenbrock, C.R., Proc.Natl.Acad.Sci.USA, 61:598-605 (1968)
18. Malhotra, S.K. and van Harreveld, A. J.Ultrastruc.Res., 12: 473-487 (1965)
19. Knoll, G. Oebel, G. and Plattner, H. Protoplasma, 111:161-176 (1982)
20. Wrigglesworth, J.M., Packer, L. and Branton, D., Biochim.Biophys. Acta, 205:125-135 (1970)

21. Melnick, R.L. and Packer, L. Biochim.Biophys.Acta, 253: 503-508 (1971)
22. Tewari, J.P., Tu, J.C. and Malhotra, S.K. Cytobios, 5:261-273 (1972)
23. Van Venetië, R. and Verkleij, A.J. Biochim.Biophys.Acta, 692: 379-405 (1982)
24. Knoll, G. and Brdiczka, D., Biochim.Biophys.Acta, 733:102-110 (1983)
25. Branton, D.S., Bullivant, S., Gilula, N.B., Karnovsky. M.J., Moor, H., Muehlthaler, K., Northconte, D.H., Packer, L., Satir, P., Speth, V., Staehlin, L.A. Steere R.L. and Weinstein, R.S. Science, 190:54-56 (1979)
26. Mannella, c.A. J.Cell.Biol., 94:680-687 (1982)
27. Parsons, D.F., Williams, G.R. and Chance, B. Ann.N.Y.Acad.Sci., 137:643-666 (1966)
28. De Kruijff, B., Cullis, P.R. and Verkleij, A.J. Trends in Biochem.Sci., 5:79-81 (1980)
29. Van Dam, K. Woelders, H., Colen, A. and Westerhoff, H.V. Biochem. Soc.Transact. 1983 (in press)
30. Katzen, H.M. and Schimke, R.T., Proc.Natl.Acad.Sci.USA, 54: 1218-1225 (1965)
31. Borrebaek, B. Biochem.Med., 3:485-497 (1970)
32. Weiler, U., Riesinger, I. and Brdiczka, D. unpublished results.

ACKNOWLEDGEMENTS

We wish to thank Dr. K. Allmann for his help in electronmicroscopy and Ms P. Voise for expert technical assistence. The work was supported by the Deutsche Forschungsgemeinschaft (Br 773/1).

THE EFFECT OF INORGANIC PHOSPHATE ON

MITOCHONDRIAL, CREATINE KINASE

Norman Hall and Marlene DeLuca*

Departments of Medicine and Chemistry
University of California, San Diego
La Jolla, California 92093

Since the last meeting at Johns Hopkins in 1979, there has
been a continued interest and a great deal of progress made in our
understanding of the role of mitochondrial creatine kinase in
muscle cells. The existence of the creatine phosphate shuttle
as discussed by Bessman and Geiger (1) is now known to be an important aspect of muscle metabolism. There have been numerous
studies on the effect of creatine kinase on respiration in heart
muscle mitochondria. It is now well-documented that mitochondrial
creatine kinase is responsible for stimulating respiration by
utilizing ATP produced by oxidative phosphorylation and maintaining
a constant high level of ADP available for continued phosphorylation. There has been much discussion about whether the ATP produced by oxidative phosphorylation is preferentially used by the
mitochondrial creatine kinase. This aspect will be addressed by
many of the other speakers here.

In addition to the studies with intact mitochondria, the mitochondrial creatine kinase has now been purified from a variety of
sources and one recent report deserves particular mention. Studies
by Blum et al. (2) have shown that antibodies raised against human
heart mitochondrial creatine kinase did not cross react with mitochondrial creatine kinase from beef, pig, rabbit, rat or chicken,
but cross reacted only with the monkey enzyme. This observation
is particularly surprising since the amino acid composition of the
human enzyme is virtually the same as that reported by Dr. Hall

*This work was supported by National Institutes of Health Grant
HL17682.

and myself for the beef heart mitochondrial enzyme (3). However,
the enzymes appear to be immunologically distinct and, at this
time, it is not clear whether the enzymes from various sources may
be quite different proteins.

What I would like to discuss is the effect of inorganic phosphate on the mitochondrial creatine kinase and what possible physiological implications these effects might have. There have been
many reports dealing with the effects of phosphate, and I will try
to summarize these as well as presenting some recent data from my
laboratory.

For the purposes of discussion, the effects of inorganic phosphate on mitochondrial creatine kinase can be divided into two
major categories: (I) Effects on the purified enzyme, (II) effects
on the enzyme in the mitochondria. This may be an artificial
division since these are undoubtedly overlapping areas.

Let me start by considering the purified or partially purified
enzyme. Almost ten years ago, Saks et al. reported that the enzyme
from rat heart exists in two electrophoretically separable forms
(4). We subsequently found (3) that the beef heart mitochondrial
creatine kinase exists in two electrophoretically distinguishable
forms, both of which migrate toward the cathode at pH 8.8. The
molecular weights of these forms were found to be approximately
80,000 and 190-200,000. We suggested that the larger form might
be an oxidized enzyme in which a disulfide bond had been formed
between two dimers. Since these earlier studies, there have been
reports from many other laboratories in which more than one form

Table I. Molecular Weights of Mitochondrial Creatine Kinases

Source	M.W.	# of Subunits
Beef Heart	42,000	1
	87,000	2
	250,000	6
	340,000	8
	360,000	8
	452,000	10
Dog Heart	80,000	2
	200,000	4 (?)
Human Brain	65,000	2
	184,000	6
Human Heart	80,000	2
	350,000	8

of the enzyme has been observed. The species and molecular weights
are summarized in Table I. As can be seen, the beef heart enzyme
has a subunit molecular weight of 42,000 as determined by SDS gel
electrophoresis. Farrell et al. (6), using a Sephadex G-200 chroma-
tographic determination, estimated the molecular weight for this
enzyme at 250,000 daltons. Jacobs and Graham obtained a molecular
weight of 340,000 by equilibrium sedimentation (7). We have found
molecular weights of 87,000, 360,000 and 452,000 daltons (5). The
enzyme from other species has also been found in multiple forms.
Roberts and Grace (8) report 80,000 and 200,000 for dog heart,
Wevers et al. (9) found two forms for the human brain enzyme, and
Kanemitsu et al. (10) have evidence for two forms of the human
heart enzyme. Regardless of the source, this enzyme has the ability
to self associate producing aggregates of varying molecular weights
from 87,000 to 450,000. At least some of these forms seem to be
interconvertible depending upon the concentration of the enzyme.
Higher protein concentration seems to favor higher molecular weights
and a strong reducing environment produces lower molecular weight
species. It is not at all clear which form of the enzyme is associated with the mitochondrial membrane or whether these various
forms may have physiological significance.

We have found that inorganic phosphate has a marked influence
on the size of the purified enzyme. Figure 1 shows the elution
profile of mitochondrial creatine kinase from a Sephacryl S-300
column as a function of increasing concentration of inorganic phosphate in MOPS buffer pH 7.0, 5 mM β-mercaptoethanol, at constant
ionic strength. At very low or no inorganic phosphate, the enzyme
elutes in the void volume, bound to the marker protein, ferritin.
Recovery of activity is only about 5%. AT 2 mM inorganic phosphate,
it starts moving toward a peak at fraction number 55, molecular
weight 350,000, which would correspond to eight subunits. By 25 mM
inorganic phosphate, it has an apparent molecular weight of 420,000.
In this case, we recovered the total amount of activity applied
to the column. In the absence of inorganic phosphate, addition of
0.5 mM ATP and Mg++ produced an elution profile which was the
same as that obtained in the presence of 25 mM inorganic phosphate.
Figure 2 shows the elution of creatine kinase in 25 mM inorganic
phosphate; it can be seen that the activity corresponds nicely with
the protein and all of the activity applied was recovered. Based
on these experiments, it appears that inorganic phosphate in the
range of 1-25 mM can effect the size of the purified enzyme. This
range of phosphate concentrations is the same as has been used
to solubilize or release the mitochondrial creatine kinase from
the inner mitochondrial membrane or mitoplasts. We have also found
that the enzyme is capable of aggregating when it is kept at concentrations above 0.15 mg/ml. In 25 mM phosphate after a few days at
4° C a white precipitate is formed. This precipitate could be completely dissolved in 0.1 M phosphate with full recovery of active
enzyme.

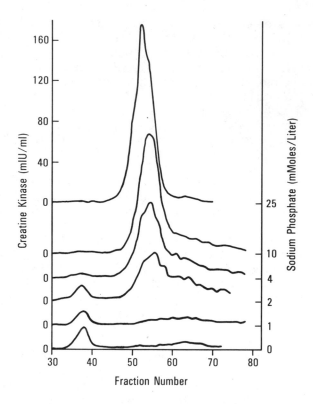

Fig. 1. Elution pattern of mitochondrial creatine kinase from a Sephacryl S-300 column as a function of increasing concentration of inorganic phosphate.

With regard to the effect of inorganic phosphate on the inter- action of the enzyme with the mitochondrial membrane, there have been several studies reported. Jacobus et al. (11) and Vial et al. (12) independently studied the effect of inorganic phosphate on the release of creatine kinase from the mitochondria. Both groups arrived at essentially the same conclusions, that the enzyme release occurs at concentrations of 5 mM phosphate or greater and the solu- bilization is very pH dependent. More enzyme is released at more alkaline pH's. This release appears to be dependent on mitochon- drial swelling since more enzyme is solubilized in hypotonic phos- phate than in isotonic phospate (12). It is not known what the molecular weight of this released enzyme is. Vial et al. also demonstrated that the release of creatine kinase is reversible. If the inorganic phosphate concentration was diluted to 2 mM within approximately 10 minutes, the enzyme would rebind to the mitochon- dria or mitoplasts. It would not rebind to sonicated mitoplasts which are inverted vesicles.

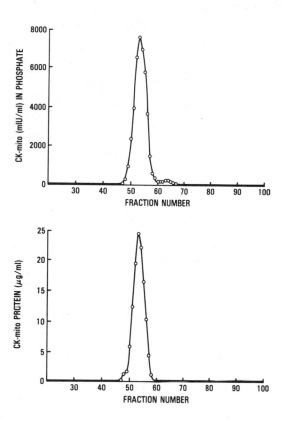

Fig. 2. Elution pattern of mitochondrial creatine kinase in 25 mM inorganic phosphate. Upper figure is enzymatic activity; lower figure is protein concentration.

We extended these studies and demonstrated that after inorganic phosphate extraction there were two electrophoretic forms of the enzyme present (13). The extracted mitochondria in low inorganic phosphate, 2 mM, would rebind either creatine kinase from the crude extract or a purified creatine kinase. There was some degree of specificity for the enzyme since addition of large amounts of MM creatine kinase did not interfere with the binding of mitochondrial creatine kinase. However, there was an apparent lack of specificity with regard to the membrane since heart mitochondrial creatine kinase would bind to liver mitochondria which do not normally con-tain any appreciable amount of mitochondrial creatine kinase. All of these studies only measured the physical release or binding of the enzyme and it is not known if the rebound enzyme is function-ally the same as the original enzyme.

Saks and Jacobus (14) in a subsequent report addressed the question of whether the enzyme behaved differently in the bound vs. soluble state. They measured rates of PCr production from normal heart mitochondria and compared these with liver mitochondria to

75

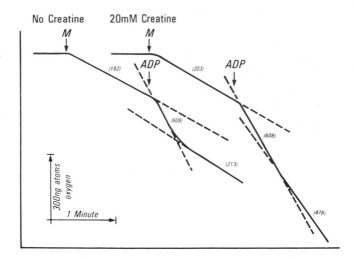

Fig. 3.   Mitochondrial respiration in 5 mM inorganic phosphate
in the presence or absence of creatine.

which had been added heart mitochondrial creatine kinase. They
found that the heart mitochondria with the bound creatine kinase
produce PCr about 3x faster than the liver mitochondria with added
soluble enzyme. They also found that the Km for ATP in the creatine
kinase reaction was 6x lower for the bound enzyme when oxidative
phosphorylation is the source of ATP rather than a soluble ATP
generating system. All of these results suggest the bound enzyme
is more efficiently coupled to oxidative phosphorylation than the
solubilized form.

    We have studied the effect of increasing concentrations of
inorganic phosphate on heart mitochondrial respiration in the presence
and absence of creatine (15). Figure 3 shows the oxygen consumption
by rat heart mitochondria with 5 mM inorganic phosphate in the
absence and presence of 20 mM creatine. In the presence of creatine
the post ADP-state 4 respiration is significantly stimulated.

    Figure 4 shows the effect of increasing inorganic phosphate
on initial respiration rate, state-3 respiration, and post-ADP
state-4 respiration with and without creatine. In the absence
of creatine, increasing inorganic phosphate above 5 mM has no effect
on either the initial state-4 or post ADP state-4 respiration rate.
Above 20 mM inorganic phosphate there is a slight inhibition of
state-3 respiration. In the presence of creatine, there is a stimulation of post ADP-state 4 respiration, which is maximal at about
5 mM inorganic phosphate. This post ADP-state 4 respiration decreases significantly with increasing inorganic phosphate. We
believe this decrease in post ADP-state 4 respiration at high

76

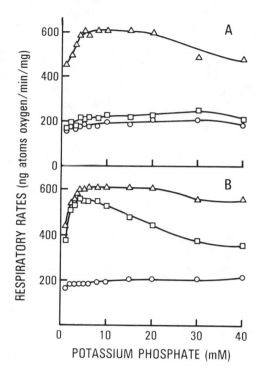

Fig. 4. Effect of increasing concentrations of inorganic phosphate on mitochondrial respiration: A, no creatine; B, 20 mM creatine; O, initial respiration rate; Δ, state 3 respiration; □, post ADP state 4 respiration (15).

inorganic phosphate is due to the release of creatine kinase from the membrane which is reflected by a less efficient utilization of ATP for the synthesis of PCr. This would be indicated by a decreased rate of oxygen consumption since ADP levels are not as high. In order to test this directly, we measured PCr production by respiring mitochondria in 5 mM or 45 mM inorganic phosphate. At the higher inorganic phosphate concentration, the rate of PCR synthesis is only about half that obtained with 5 mM inorganic phosphate, Figure 5. We also measured the apparent Km's for ADP in the coupled reaction (PCr formation) with either 5 mM or 25 mM inorganic phosphate. In 5 mM inorganic phosphate, the Km for ADP is 0.07 mM, which is consistent with the value reported by Jacobus and Saks (16). In 25 mM inorganic phosphate, the Km was about 0.45 mM or a six-fold increase. Under these same conditions there was an increase in Vmax of about 1.8 fold. These results are consistent with the oxygen consumption data and support the hypothesis that the bound enzyme is more efficient in the synthesis of PCr when it is utilizing ATP produced by oxidative phosphorylation. This could result from a close functional relationship with the translocase as has been proposed by others, or to a locally high concentration

77

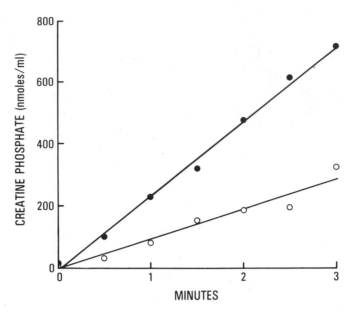

Fig. 5. Creatine phosphate synthesis by mitochondria in the presence of 5 mM phosphate, ●-●; or 45 mM phosphate, O-O.

of ATP in the microenvironment or a combination of these two effects.

Some more recent experiments carried out in collaboration with Vicki Bennett and Dr. Clarence Suelter on chicken heart and breast mitochondria have shown that in these mitochondria there is no apparent effect of inorganic phosphate on either respiration or the rate of PCr formation (17). Figure 6 shows these data. In the case of the chicken breast muscle, there is a large amount of mitochondrial creatine kinase, which we normalized to succinate INT reductase activity. We believe these results demonstrate that, if there is a large excess amount of mitochondrial creatine kinase present so that it is able to use all of the ATP being produced, then it does not matter if the enzyme is bound or soluble. Similarly, if there is very little creatine kinase, as is the case in chicken heart, it does not make any difference where the enzyme is located since the amount of PCr synthesized is only a small percent of the ATP present. Therefore in tissues in which there is either a large excess or a very limited amount of mitochondrial creatine kinase present respiration will not be sensitive to the concentration of inorganic phosphate and/or creatine but will be regulated by the availability

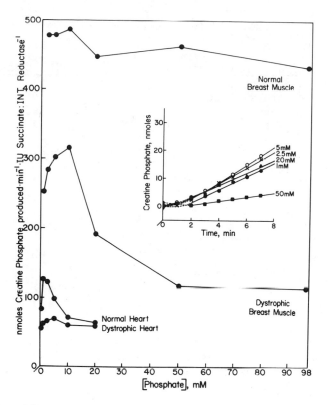

Fig. 6. Creatine phosphate synthesis in normal and dystrophic breast and heart mitochondria with increasing phosphate concentration (17).

of ADP. Table II shows a survey of several tissues for mitochondrial creatine kinase activity normalized to INT reductase, a mitochondrial marker. It can be seen that all of the heart tissues, except the chicken, have a high ratio of CK/INT and would be subject to regulation by inorganic phosphate or creatine. Liver mitochondria generally have very little creatine kinase while skeletal muscle has about as much as heart.

One other study is of interest in this regard, that is the creatine kinase isozyme distribution in certain human tumors (18). We have found that mitochondrial creatine kinase is significantly elevated in some of these tumors, as shown in Table III. Some of these tumors are from tissues which would not ordinarily have any mitochondrial creatine kinase. Unfortunately, when we made these measurements, we did not normalize the amount of mitochondrial creatine kinase to an independent mitochondrial marker, like the INT reductase. We do not understand what the physiological implications of these elevated mitochondrial creatine kinases might be; however, it would be anticipated, based on other experiments, that

Table II. Mitochondrial Creatine Kinase in Various Tissues

	Source Mitochondria	CK/INT Reductase
Rat	Skeletal muscle	45
	Liver	4.8
	Heart	37
Beef	Heart	61
	Liver	3.2
Rabbit	Skeletal muscle	45
	Heart	25
	Brain	69
Chicken	Breast	100
	Heart	4
	Leg	40

these tumors are probably not subject to regulation by inorganic phosphate or creatine and are probably exporting almost entirely PCr from the mitochondria. It would be of particular interest to measure the cellular concentration of inorganic phosphate, creatine and ATP in these tumors.

Finally, one can ask whether it is likely that in a normal muscle cell phosphate concentrations are variable enough to effect the position of the mitochondrial creatine kinase? Lipskaya et al. (19) concluded that, under physiological conditions, only part of the creatine kinase is bound to the mitochondrial membrane. If this is true, then a small change in concentration of inorganic

Table III. Creatine Kinase Isozymes in Human Tumors

Tumor	Total U/gm	BB (%)	Mito (%)
Colon	87	100	---
	12	70	15
	11	20	70
	7	40	50
	6	14	70
Lung	20	30	40
	3	40	35
Melanoma	2	---	60
	1.6	5	50
	1.0	50	35

phosphate might have a large effect on the synthesis of phosphocreatine. Certainly in the case of the ischemic cell, increases in
phosphate concentration are well-documented. It is important in
this regard to determine whether prolonged exposure to high phosphate
alters the binding of the enzyme in an irreversible manner. These
studies are in progress.

REFERENCES

1. S.P. Bessman and P.J. Geiger, Transport of energy in muscle:
    The phosphorylcreatine shuttle, Science 211:448 (1981).
2. H.E. Blum, B. Deus, and W. Gerok, Mitochondrial creatine kinase
    from human heart muscle: Purification and characterization
    of the crystallized isoenzyme, J. Biochem. 94:1247 (1983).
3. N. Hall, P. Addis, and M. DeLuca, Mitochondrial creatine kinase.
    Physical and kinetic properties of the purified enzyme from
    beef heart. Biochemistry 18:1745 (1979).
4. V.A. Saks, G.B. Chernousova, I.I. Voronkor, V.N. Smirnov, and
    E.I. Chazov, Study of energy transport mechanism in myocardial
    cells, Circ. Res. (Suppl. III) 34-35:138 (1974).
5. N. Hall and M. DeLuca, unpublished observations.
6. E.C. Farrell, N. Baba, G.P. Brierly, and H-D. Grumer, On the
    creatine phosphokinase of heart muscle mitochondria, Lab
    Invest. 27:209 (1972).
7. H.K. Jacobs and M. Graham, Physical and chemical characteriza-
    tion of mitochondrial creatine kinase from bovine heart,
    Fed. Proc. 37:1574 (1978).
8. R. Roberts and A.M. Grace, Purification of mitochondrial crea-
    tine kinase. Biochemical and immunological characterization,
    J. Biol. Chem. 255:2870 (1980).
9. R.A. Wevers, C.P.M. Reutelingsperger, B. Dam, and J.B.J. Soons,
    Mitochondrial creatine kinase in the brain, Clin. Chim. Acta
    119:209 (1981).
10. F. Kanemitsu, I. Kawanishi, and J. Mizushima, Characteristics
    of mitochondrial creatine kinases from normal human heart
    and liver tissues, Clin. Chim. Acta 119:307 (1982).
11. W.E. Jacobus, J.A. Bittl, and M.L. Weisfeldt, Loss of mitochon-
    drial creatine kinase in vitro and in vivo: A sensitive index
    of ischemic cellular and functional damage, in: "Heart Creatine
    Kinase, the Integration of Isozymes for Energy Distribution,"
    W.E. Jacobus and J.S. Ingwall, eds., Williams and Wilkins,
    Baltimore (1980).
12. C. Vial, B. Font, D. Goldschmidt, and D.C. Gautheron, Dissocia-
    tion and reassociation of creatine kinase with heart mito-
    chondria; pH and phosphate dependence, Biochem. Biophys.
    Res. Comm. 88:1352 (1979).
13. N. Hall and M. DeLuca, Binding of creatine kinase to heart
    and liver mitochondria in vitro, Arch. Biochem. Biophys.
    201:674 (1980).

14. V.A. Saks, V.V. Kupriyanov, G.V. Elizarova, and W.E. Jacobus, Studies of energy transport in heart cells: The importance of creatine kinase localization for the coupling of mitochondrial phosphorylcreatine production to oxidative phosphorylation, J. Biol. Chem. 255:755 (1980).

15. N. Hall and M. DeLuca, The effect of inorganic phosphate on creatine kinase in respiring rat heart mitochondria, Arch. Biochem. Biophys. (1984) in press.

16. W.E. Jacobus and V.A. Saks, Creatine kinase of heart mitochondria: Changes in its kinetic properties induced by coupling to oxidative phosphorylation, Arch. Biochem. Biophys. 219: 167 (1982).

17. V.D. Bennett, N. Hall, M. DeLuca, and C.H. Suelter, Decreased mitochondrial creatine kinase activity alters the function of the creatine phosphate shuttle in dystrophic chicken breast muscle, submitted to J. Biol. Chem. (1984).

18. M. DeLuca, N. Hall, R. Rice, and N.O. Kaplan, Creatine kinase isozymes in human tumors, Biochem. Biophys. Res. Comm. 99:189 (1981).

19. T.Y. Lipskaya, V.D. Templ, L.V. Belovsova, E.V. Molokova, and I.V. Rybina, Investigation of the interaction of mitochondrial creatine kinase with the membranes of the mitochondria, Biochemistry - New York (translation of Biokhimiya) 45:877 (1980).

HORMONAL REGULATION OF CREATINE KINASE BB

Alvin M. Kaye, Nachum A. Reiss*, Yosef Weisman**, Itzhak
Binderman*** and Dalia Sömjen***

Departments of Hormone Research and *Chemical Immunology
The Weizmann Institute of Science, Rehovot
** Vitamin Research Laboratory and ***The Hard Tissues
Unit, Ichilov Hospital, Tel-Aviv Medical Center
Sackler School of Medicine, University of Tel-Aviv
Tel-Aviv, Israel

The induction of increased synthesis of creatine kinase BB (EC
2.7.3.2) now appears to be a response produced by a variety of hormones. The list includes steroid and polypeptide hormones, prostaglandin E_2, bone derived growth factor, and dibutyryl cAMP. This
survey is the first summary of the breadth of the phenomenon and
will concentrate on examples from work which is still in press or
is yet unpublished.

STEROID HORMONES: Estrogens

Creatine kinase BB was shown by Reiss and Kaye (1981) to be the
overwhelming component of the "estrogen induced protein" (IP) originally described by Notides and Gorski (1966). IP has become a fa-
vorite marker protein for the study of estrogen and antiestrogen
action because of its early response (increased synthesis within 40
min) to the hormone in vivo (Barnea and Gorski, 1970) and in vitro
using physiological concentrations of estradiol-17, i.e. 10^{-9}M to
3×10^{-8}M (Katzenellenbogen and Gorski, 1972; Amroch et al. 1984).
Within 1 h of estrogen injection into immature rats, the concentration of mRNA for uterine CKBB is doubled (Walker and Kaye, 1981).
CKBB synthesis is stimulated by estrogen in all the organs of the
female reproductive tract tested, as well as in the estrogen recep-
tor-rich regions of the hypothalamus (Malnick et al., 1983), and in
normal and neoplastic mammary gland in vitro (Amroch et al., 1984).
Further details of the identification of IP as CKBB as well as
characteristics of the induction of uterine CKBB can be found in

83

recent reviews (Kaye 1983a,b). A study using ^{31}P-NMR to assess the implications of the rapid stimulation of CKBB synthesis on uterine energetics is in press (Degani et al., 1984).

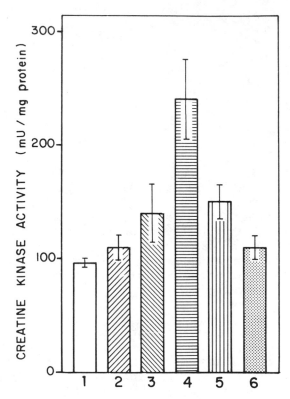

Fig. 1. Stimulation of CK activity in micro-mass chick embryo limb-bud cell cultures. 4×10^5 embryonic chick limb bud mesenchymal cells in a 20 μl drop were placed in a 35 mm diameter tissue culture dish and allowed to attach before adding the medium (Eagle's minimum essential medium [MEM] supplemented with 10% fetal calf serum). After 4 h incubation with the test hormone, cells were extracted and assayed as described previously (Kaye et al., 1981). The assay mixture contained in 1 ml; 50 mM imidazole acetate pH 6.7, 25 mM creatine phosphate, 2 mM ADP, 10 mM Mg acetate, 20 mM D-glucose, 2 mM NAD, 5 mM EDTA, 50 μM diadenosine pentaphosphate (myokinase inhibitor), 20 mM N-acetyl cysteine, 2 mM DTT, 10 μg/ml bovine serum albumin, 2.4 units of glucose-6-phosphate dehydrogenase and 1.6 units of hexokinase. Results are means $\pm$ SEM for n $\geqslant$ 5. 1) Control; 2) 25(OH)D_3, 12 nM; 3) 1α,25(OH)$_2D_3$, 12 nM; 4) 24R,25(OH)$_2D_3$, 12 nM; 5) 24S,25(OH)$_2D_3$, 12 nM; 6) triamcinolone acetonide, 1.0 nM (from Sömjen et al., 1984a).

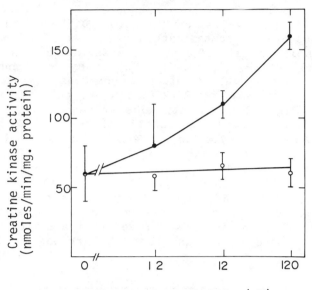

Fig. 2. Concentration dependent stimulation of CK activity by
$24R,25(OH)_2D_3$ in micro-mass chick embryo limb-bud cultures. Cells were treated with $24R,25(OH)_2D_3$ (●) or
$1\alpha,25(OH_2)D_3$ (o) for 4 h. The CK assay is described in
Fig. 1. Results are means ± SEM for n ≥ 3 (drawn from
data in Sömjen et al., 1984a).

Vitamin D metabolites

Both $1\alpha,25(OH)_2$ cholecalciferol [$1\alpha,25(OH)_2D_3$], the active metabolite of vitamin D involved in calcium transport (Norman et al.,
1982), and $24R,25(OH)_2D_3$, implicated in development of embryonic
bone (Corvol et al., 1978; Ornoy et al., 1978) and cartilage (Corvol et al., 1980; Sömjen et al., 1982a,b, 1983; Binderman and Sömjen, 1984), are trophic hormones which stimulate DNA (Majeska and
Rodan, 1982; Sömjen et al., 1983) and protein synthesis, including
the enzyme responsive to a host of stimuli (Russell, 1980; Bachrach, 1984) ornithine decarboxylase (ODC) (Shinki et al., 1981;
Sömjen et al., 1983; Binderman and Sömjen, 1984).

Micro-mass chick embryo limb bud cultures (Binderman et al.,
1979), which develop into nodules of cartilage cells, surrounded by
mesenchymal cells, were tested for their response to vitamin D metabolites (Figs. 1-3). These cultures contain specific receptors
for $24R,25(OH)_2D_3$ (Sömjen et al., 1982a). The presence of 12 nM

24R,25(OH)$_2$D$_3$ caused a 2.5 fold increase in CK activity (Fig. 1) within 4 h.[3] The inactive isomer 24S,25(OH)$_2$D$_3$ had a much smaller effect (attributable to contamination with 24R,25(OH)$_2$D$_3$ in this preparation), while no significant increase was caused by 25 hydroxy calciferol [25(OH)D$_3$], 1α,25(OH)$_2$D$_3$ or by triamcinolone acetonide, which promotes calcification of cartilage. The specific stimulation of CK activity by 24,25(OH)$_2$D$_3$ in this system is both time and dose (Fig. 2) dependent. The increase was shown to be due, at least in part, to an increase in the rate of CK synthesis, by fluorography of polyacrylamide gel electropherograms (not shown) of cytosols from ^{35}S-methionine labeled cells, 1 h after exposure to 24R,25(OH)$_2$D$_3$ or to vehicle.

Isozyme analysis by DEAE cellulose chromatography (Fig. 3) revealed that chick embryo limb bud cultures contained almost exclusively CKBB and that the increase in specific activity stimulated by 24R,25(OH)$_2$D$_3$ was due predominantly to an increase in CKBB.

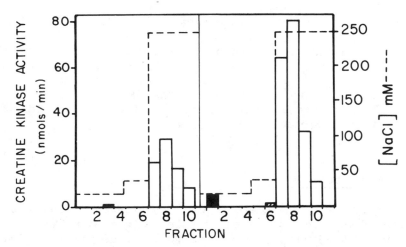

Fig. 3.   CK isozyme distribution in micro-mass chick embryo limb-bud cell cultures. Extracts were prepared from either untreated (control) cells (left panel) or cells treated with 12 nM 24R,25(OH)$_2$D$_3$ for 4 h, (right panel). Supernatant (38,000xg) fractions of extracts were applied to a DEAE-cellulose column (1 ml) in 20 mM NaCl, 100 mM Tris HCl pH 7.9, 5 mM Mg acetate and 0.4 mM EDTA. The MM (muscle type) isozyme of CK (■) was not absorbed to the column, the MB (hybrid) isozyme (▨) was eluted with 40 mM NaCl in 100 mM Tris-HCl pH 6.4 and the BB (brain type) isozyme (▢) with 250 mM NaCl in the same buffer. Fractions were assayed as described in Fig. 1 (from Sömjen et al., 1984a).

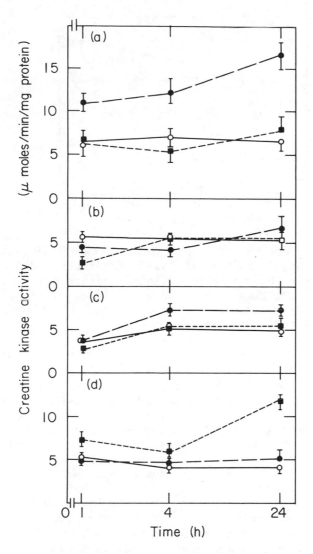

Fig. 4. Time course of CK response in organs of vitamin D depleted rats. Changes in (a) renal, (b) duodenal, (c) diaphysial and (d) epiphysial creatine kinase activity were measured after intraperitoneal injection of 60 ng of $1\alpha,25(OH)_2D_3$ (●); 300 ng of $24R,25(OH)_2D_3$ (■) or vehicle (o). CK assays were performed as described in Fig. 1. Results are means ± SEM for N=5 (from Sömjen et al., 1984b).

In 5-week old rats, maintained on the same vitamin-D deficient diet their mothers had received since the age of 4 weeks, vitamin D metabolites stimulated CKBB activity in bone and in kidney (Fig. 4).

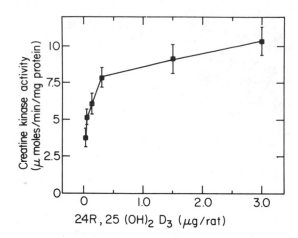

Fig. 5. Dose-dependence of the stimulation of CK activity by
24R,25(OH)$_2$D$_3$ in the epiphyses of vitamin D-depleted rats.
24R,25(OH)$_2$D$_3$ was injected intraperitoneally, and the animals were killed 24 h later. The CK assay is described in
Fig. 1. Results are means $\pm$ SEM for N=4 (from Somjen et
al., 1984b).

The epiphyses (growth region, rich in chondroblasts) of rat ti
biae responded to 24R,25(OH)$_2$D$_3$ but not to 1α,25(OH)$_2$D$_3$ with a 2.6
fold increase in CK specific activity (Fig. 5). Contrariwise,
1α,25(OH)$_2$D$_3$, but not 24R,25(OH)$_2$D$_3$, caused a 1.5 fold increase in
CK specific activity in the diaphyses. This specificity of response parallels the corresponding localization of specific receptors for vitamin D metabolites (Sömjen et al., 1982a).

1α,25(OH)$_2$D$_3$ caused a 2.5 fold increase in CK specific activity
in kidney, which also contains receptors for 1α,25(OH)$_2$D$_3$ (Colston
and Feldman, 1979). Neither metabolite of vitamin D affected the
CK specific activity of intestinal mucosa, an unexpected and as yet
unexplained finding,since intestinal mucosa is a classical responsive tissue to 1α,25(OH)$_2$D$_3$ (Tsai and Norman, 1973; Emtage et al.,
1974).

The activity of epiphysial CK showed a steep dose response (Fig.
5) to 24R,25(OH)$_2$D$_3$ up to 300 ng/rat (in the range in which other
responses to this metabolite have been observed).

In all three tissues which responded to vitamin D metabolites by
increased CK, the BB isozyme, as expected (see reviews by Watts,
1973; and Kenyon and Reed, 1983) was the overwhelming form in both
the unstimulated and stimulated tissues (Fig. 6).

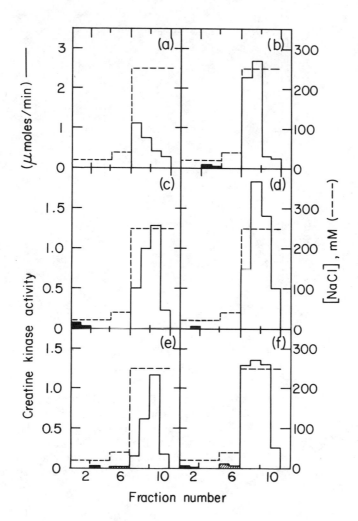

Fig. 6. CK isozyme distribution in organs of vitamin D-depleted rats. $24R,25(OH)_2D_3$ (300 ng), $1\alpha,25(OH)_2D_3$ (60 ng) or vehicle was injected intraperitoneally and the rats were killed 24 h later. Isozymes of CK were separated as described in Fig. 3 and fractions assayed as described in Fig. 1. ■ , MM isozyme; ▨ , MB isozyme; ▭ , BB isozyme. a) kidney, untreated; b) kidney, $1\alpha,25(OH)_2D_3$ treated; c) diaphyses, untreated; d) diaphyses, $1\alpha,25(OH)_2D_3$ treated; e) epiphyses, untreated; f) epiphyses, $24R,25(OH)_2D_3$ treated (from Sömjen et al., 1984b).

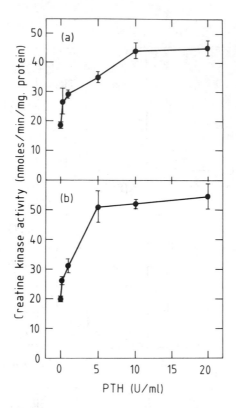

Fig. 7. Dose dependent stimulation of CK activity by parathyroid hormone (PTH). Osteoblast enriched cultures grown in low $[Ca^{2+}]$ (a) or normal cell cultures, grown in standard $[Ca^{2+}]$ (b) were treated with PTH for 24 h. The CK assay is described in Fig. 1. Results are means $\pm$ SEM for N $\geqslant$ 3. (D. Somjen, A.M. Kaye and I. Binderman, in preparation).

PEPTIDE HORMONES AND PROSTAGLANDIN E_2

Parathyroid hormone

Parathyroid hormone (PTH), the primary hormonal regulator of plasma calcium via its action on bone and kidney, has been postulated to act using calcium, in conjunction with cyclic AMP, as an intracellular mediator (Rasmussen et al., 1963) to cause the cellular responses leading to resorption of calcified bone matrices. PTH has also been shown to stimulate ^{3}H thymidine incorporation into DNA (Binderman et al., 1982).

In parallel, PTH also increased ODC activity in bone cells (Söm-jen et al., 1982c). Therefore, PTH was tested (Fig. 7) on bone

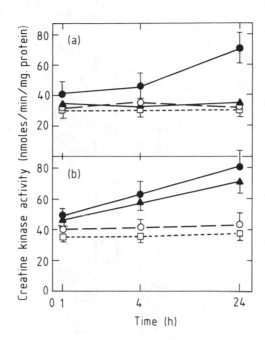

Fig. 8.   Time course of stimulation of CK activity in cultured bone
cells.   Osteoblast enriched cultures grown in low $[Ca^{2+}]$
(a) or normal cell cultures grown in standard $[Ca^{2+}]$ (b)
were untreated (□) or treated with PTH (10 units/ml, ●),
PGE_2 (500 ng/ml, ▲), or CT (100 ng/ml, ○).   The CK assay
is described in Fig. 1.   Results are means $\pm$ SEM for N $\geqslant$ 5
(D. Somjen, A.M. Kaye and I. Binderman, in preparation).

cell cultures prepared from calvaria (top of skull) of 19-20 day
old rat embryos (Binderman et al., 1974) and was found to more than
double CK activity, both in standard cultures and cultures enriched
in osteoblasts as a result of growth in low $[Ca^{2+}]$.   This increase
in CK activity began within 1 h after PTH treatment and continued
up to 24 h, the longest time tested (Fig. 8).

Prostaglandin E_2

Since prostaglandin E_2 (PGE_2) also stimulates ODC activity (Sömjen et al., 1982c) and DNA synthesis (Binderman et al., 1982).
PGE_2 was tested and found to stimulate CK activity to nearly the
same extent as PTH, in standard bone cell cultures, but to have no
effect in osteoblast enriched cultures (Fig. 8), indicating that
PTH and PGE_2 may act on different cell types.

Calcitonin (see review by Austin and Heath, 1981) another peptide hormone, to which bone cells are responsive by an increase in

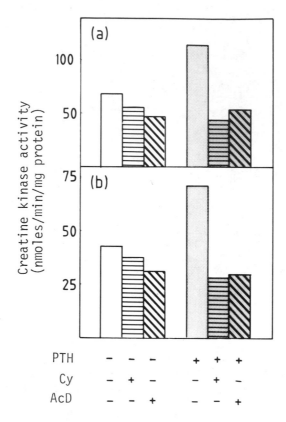

Fig. 9. Inhibition by cycloheximide (Cy) and actinomycin D (AcD) of the stimulation of CK by parathyroid hormone (PTH). Osteoblast enriched cultures grown in low [Ca^{2+}] (a) or normal cell cultures grown in standard [Ca^{2+}] (b) were grown in PTH (10 units/ml) for 24 h. The CK assay is described in Fig. 1. Actinomycin D (5 μg/ml) and cycloheximide (10 μg/ml),were added at the same time as the hormone. The CK assay is described in Fig. 1 (From Sömjen et al., 1984c).

ODC (Sömjen et al., 1982c) but not by increased ^{3}H thymidine incorporation into DNA (Binderman et al., 1982), failed to stimulate CK activity in bone cells in culture (Fig. 8).

To obtain evidence for a mechanism of induction of CK, similar to the stimulation of CKBB mRNA found in the estrogen-treated rat uterus (Walker and Kaye, 1981), bone cultures were treated with PTH in the presence of cycloheximide and actinomycin D. Both inhibitors completely prevented the stimulation of CK by PTH (Fig. 9) consistent with the hypothesis that the stimulation of CKBB depends at least in part on activation of mRNA transcription.

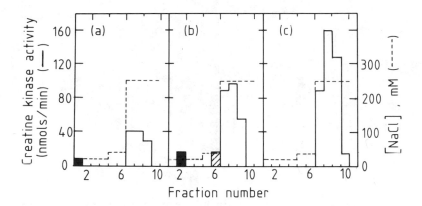

Fig. 10.   CK isozyme distribution in cultured bone cells.   Normal
cell cultures were grown in standard $[Ca^{2+}]$.   Extracts
were prepared from untreated control cultures (a) or cultures treated for 24 h with PTH (10 units/ml) (b) or PGE_2
(500 ng/ml) (c).   Isozymes of CK were separated as described in Fig. 3 and fractions assayed as described in
Fig. 1. ▰ , CKMM; ▨ , CKMB; ▭ , CKBB. (From Sömjen
et al., 1984c).

That the isozyme of CK induced by both PTH and PGE_2 is indeed
the BB type was confirmed by separation of the isozymes on a mini-
column of DEAE cellulose (Fig. 10). As shown above, for chick embryo limb bud cells and rat bone and kidney, the cultured calvaria
cells contained preponderantly the BB isozyme. As in the previous
cases, a small amount of MM isozyme was detected in these cells,
likewise the MB isozyme in some cases. In both PTH and PGE_2 stimulated cultures the increase in CK activity was due preponderantly
or exclusively to an increase in the BB form (Fig. 10).

In contrast, when a rat osteogenic sarcoma line was analyzed by
DEAE cellulose chromatography (Fig. 11), CKMM was found to be a
substantial albeit minor component of CK activity. Upon stimulation of these sarcoma cells with PTH, which caused a 60% increase
in CK activity, the proportion of CKBB to CKMM increased (Fig. 11).
The appearance of a substantial proportion of CK activity as the MM
isozyme may occur in many tumor types (Shatton et al., 1979) originating from cells showing a very small proportion, if any, of this
isozyme. Some human mammary tumors (Meyer et al., 1980; De Luca et
al., 1981; Amroch et al., 1984) show this phenomenon very strikingly.

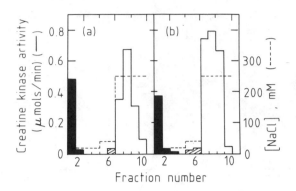

Fig. 11.   CK isozyme distribution in rat osteogenic sarcoma sub-
clone 17/2.   Extracts were prepared from untreated cells
(a) or cells treated with PTH (10 units/ml), for 24 h
(b).   Isozymes of CK were separated as described in Fig.
3 and fractions assayed as described in Fig. 1. ■■ ,
CKMM; ▨▨ , CKMB; ▭▭ , CKBB (From Sömjen et al., 1984c).

Growth factors and fluoride

In addition to PTH and prostaglandins, other agents which increase ^{3}H thymidine incorporation into DNA – bone derived growth
factor 1 (BDGF1) (J. Termine, personal communication), NaF (Farley
et al., 1983) and fetal calf serum (FCS) were also tested for stimulation of CK activity in bone cell cultures.   The newly discovered
growth factor BGDF1, extracted from rat long bones, as well as fetal calf serum (the usual source of hormones and growth factors for
growing cells in culture) stimulated CK activity when measured after 24 h exposure (Table 1).   Sodium fluoride at a concentration of
10^{-5}M caused a 70% increase in CK activity in normal BGJ$_b$ medium,
and an 86% increase in osteoblast enriched cultures.

Growth hormone

In the light of the previous results and effects on ODC (Hurley
et al., 1980) it might be expected that growth hormone would also
be able to stimulate CK activity in organs bearing growth hormone
receptors (Li, 1982; Isaksson et al., 1982; Eden et al., 1983).

Table 1. Stimulation of CK activity in rat calvaria cells in culture by NaF, bone derived growth factor (BDGF) and fetal calf serum (FCS).

Treatment	Normal cultures (standard $[Ca^{2+}]$)	Osteoblast enriched cultures (low $[Ca^{2+}]$)
	(Specific activity, E/Specific activity, C)	
BDGF 1 (1 μg/ml)	1.88	–
FCS (5%)	1.64	–
NaF (10^{-6}M)	1.06	1.28
NaF (10^{-5}M)	1.70	1.86

Cells were incubated in BGJ$_b$ medium (C) or in medium plus test agent (E) for 24 h, and CK was assayed in cell extracts as described in Fig. 1. NaF was tested in medium containing 10% FCS. Bone derived growth factor was the generous gift of Dr. John Termine, Bethesda, MD. CK was assayed as described in Fig. 1 (D. Sömjen, A.M. Kaye and I. Binderman, unpublished results).

Indeed human growth hormone (1 μg/g body weight) when injected into rats, causes, 24 h later, a 78% increase in CK activity in epiphyses, and a 40% increase in liver, but no increase when the whole brain is analyzed (compare results on hypothalamus versus whole brain concerning estrogen-stimulated CK; Malnick et al., 1983).

An increase in circulating growth hormone may be one of several factors which cause the increased CK activity observed in regenerating rat liver (Shatton et al., 1979). After removal of 2/3 of this organ (D. Russell, S. Malnick and A.M. Kaye, unpublished observations) there is an increase in the rate of synthesis of CK (detected by PAGE fluography of ^{35}S labeled cytosols) accompanied by increased CK specific activity, 4 h after partial hepatectomy, which reaches more than twice the control value after 16 h and more than 3 times the control value at 24 h. The corticosteroids released by the stress of the operation might also contribute to stimulating hepatic CK.

Prolactin

Parallel to the attempt to reveal the broad range of organs responsive to vitamin D metabolites, human placenta and associated

Table 2. Stimulation of CK activity in human placenta and associated tissues by bone seeking hormones and prolactin.

Treatment	Placenta	Decidua	Amnion
	(Specific activity, E/Specific activity, C)		
$1\alpha,25(OH)_2D_3$ (15 ng/ml)	1.37	0.91	2.67
$24,25(OH)_2D_3$ (75 ng/ml)	0.50	1.86	4.70
Prolactin (1 µg/ml)	1.16	0.72	2.20
HPL (1µg/ml)	0.28	0.28	1.18
PTH (1µg/ml)	1.24	0.61	3.48
CT (100 ng/ml)	0.53	0.84	0.71
HGH (1 µg/ml)	0.18	0.17	0.68

Explants (approximately 2x2 mm) of human tissues were cultured for 24 h in RPMI1640 medium (control, C) or in medium plus hormones (experimental, E) and CK assayed in cell extracts as described in Fig. 1. (D. Somjen, A. Golander, I. Binderman, A.M. Kaye and Y. Weisman, unpublished results).

tissues were challenged with a series of hormones including the structurally related hormones, ovine prolactin (Flückinger et al., 1982), human placental lactogen (HPL; Varner and Hauser, 1981), and human growth hormone (HGH; Gluckman et al., 1981). In addition to a greater than 4-fold stimulation of CK activity in amnion caused by $24,25(OH)_2D_3$ (Table 2) and a slightly lesser response to $1\alpha,25(OH)_2D_3$ (note that exceptionally this tissue responds to both vitamin D metabolites), prolactin but not HPL or HGH caused a 2.2-fold increase in CK activity. The amnion also shows a 3.5-fold response to PTH. The decidua responds to $24,25(OH)_2D_3$ while the placenta responds slightly to $1\alpha,25(OH)_2D_3$ with increased CK activity. Both CT and HGH, on the contrary, caused a decreased CK specific activity in all three tissues. Thus each tissue shows a characteristic pattern of specific interaction between hormone(s) and the receptors it contains, leading to the response of modulation of CK specific activity.

Luteinizing hormone releasing hormone (LHRH)

It has been suspected that LHRH has trophic properties. The use of the longer acting synthetic LHRH agonist, Buserelin, and a synthetic antagonist (Clayton and Catt, 1981) permitted a test for LHRH regulation of CK activity in incubated rat hemipituitaries.

Table 3. Stimulation of CK activity in rat organs by
luteinizing hormone releasing hormone (LHRH).

Treatment	E/C
LHRH agonist[a] (10 ng/ml)	1.38
LHRH antagonist[b] (50 ng/ml)	0.53
LHRH agonist (10 ng/ml) + LHRH antagonist (50 ng/ml)	0.55

E/C, ratio of experimental to control value of CK specific activity assayed as described in Fig. 1.
[a] $[DSer(Bu^t)^6]des\ Gly^{10}$ LHRH ethylamide (Buserelin).
[b] $DpGlu^1,DPhe^2,DTrp^{3,6}$ LHRH.
(D. Sömjen, N. Ben Aroya, A.M. Kaye and Y. Koch, unpublished results).

While Buserelin produced a 38% increase in CK activity after 8 h,
the LHRH antagonist halved CK activity within this time period (Table 3), even in the presence of the stimulating concentration of
Buserelin.

CYCLIC AMP

    The involvement of cAMP in the mechanism of action of many pep-
tide hormones led to the testing of a system directly responsive to
dibutyryl cAMP for its stimulation of CKBB. Neurite extension and
biochemical differentiation in neuroblastoma cell lines (Kimhi,
1981) and changes associated with glial cell differentiation (Nicklas and Browning, 1983), e.g. extension of processes, are stimulated by dibutyryl cAMP as well as a variety of other agents (Kimhi,
1981).

    In both mouse neuroblastoma (N18TG-2) and rat glioma (C6BU-1)
cell lines, and hybrids of mouse neuroblastoma with rat glioma or
rat liver cells, grown in 1mM dibutyryl cAMP for 4 days, there was
a 2 to 7-fold increase in CK activity (A. Zutra, A.M. Kaye and U.
Littauer, unpublished results). The glioma line which showed the
highest stimulated activity (2.7 μmoles/mm/mg protein, 7 times control) also exhibited the highest basal activity. The BB isozyme of
CK was the only form found in the dibutyryl cAMP stimulated cultures of these neuroblastoma, glioma and hybrid cells. DMSO and
mixed brain gangliosides (Sigma) were also capable of stimulating
CK activity in NI8TG-2 neuroblastoma, suggesting that a stimulus to
differentiation (not necessarily via dibutyryl cAMP) may be responsible for the increase in CK activity.

CONCLUSION

The impetus for this survey was the interest in discovering the breadth of the phenomenon of rapid stimulation of synthesis of CKBB from the point of view of the hormone or growth factor involved. The data obtained provide a new convenient marker for the specific interaction between a variety of stimulating molecules and their responsive cells, parallel to the widespread use of cAMP and ODC. In addition, the rapidity of the response and the involvement of gene activation (as established for estrogen stimulation in the rat uterus) provide an advantageous test system for exploring regulation of gene expression, in this case of a key enzyme of energy regeneration. The growing use of immunocytochemistry to study the cellular localization and microcompartmentation of CKBB and the further applications of ^{31}P NMR techniques to cellular energetics hold the promise of growing integration of our knowledge of CKBB at the molecular, enzymic and cellular levels.

ACKNOWLEDGEMENTS

We thank Mrs. E. Berger for excellent technical help and Mrs. M. Kopelowitz and R. Levin for skilled preparation of the MS. This work was supported in part by grants from the Rockefeller Foundation and the Ford Foundation to the late Prof. H.R. Lindner. A.M. Kaye is the incumbent of the Joseph Moss Professorial Chair in Molecular Endocrinology.

REFERENCES

Amroch, D., Cox, S., Shaer, A., Malnick, S., Chatsubi, S., Hallowes, R., and Kaye, A.M., 1984, Estrogen responsive creatine kinase in normal and neoplastic human breast, in: "Hormones and Cancer", Vol. 2, F. Bresciani, R.J.B. King, M. Lippman and J.P. Raynaud, eds., Raven Press, N.Y. in press.

Austin, L.A., and Heath, H.III, 1981, Calcitonin: physiology and pathophysiology, N. Eng. J. Med. 304:269.

Bachrach, U., 1984, Physiological aspects of ornithine decarboxylase, Cell Biochem. and Function, 2:6.

Barnea, A., and Gorski, J., 1970, Estrogen-induced protein. Time course of synthesis, Biochemistry, 9:1899.

Binderman, I., and Sömjen, D., 1984, 24R,25 dihydroxycholecalciferol induces the growth of chick cartilage cells in vitro. Endocrinology, (in press).

Binderman, I., Duksin, D., Harell, A., Katchalsky, E., and Sachs, L., 1974, Formation of bone tissue in culture from isolated bone cells. J. Cell. Biol. 61:427.

Binderman, I., Greene, R.M., and Pennypacker, J.P., 1979, Calcification of differentiating skeletal mesenchyme in vitro. Science, 206:222.

Binderman, I., Sömjen, D., Shimshoni, Z., and Harell, A., 1982, The role of prostaglandins (PGE$_2$) in mechanically induced bone remodelling, in: "Osteoporosis", J. Menczel, G.R. Robin and M. Maikin, eds., Wiley and Sons, London, pp. 195.

Clayton, R.H., and Catt, K.J., 1981, Gonadotropin-releasing hormone receptors: characterization, physiological regulation and relationship to reproductive function. Endocrine Revs. 2:186.

Colston, K.W., and Feldman, D., 1979, Demonstration of a 1,25-dihydroxycholecalciferol cytoplasmic receptor-like binder. J. Clin. Endocrinol. Metab, 49:798.

Corvol, M.T., Dumontier, M.F., Garabedian, M., and Rappaport, R., 1978, Vitamin D and cartilage. II. Biological activity of 25-hydroxycholecalciferol and 24,25,- and 1,25-dihydroxycholecalciferols on cultured growth plate chondrocytes, Endocrinology, 102:1269.

Corvol, M., Ulmann, A., and Garabedian, M., 1980, Specific nuclear uptake of 24,25-dihydroxycholecalciferol, a vitamin D$_3$ metabolite biologically active in cartilage, FEBS Lett. 116:273.

Degani, H., Shaer, A., Victor, T.A., and Kaye, A.M., 1984, Estrogen-induced changes in high-energy phosphate metabolism in rat uterus:^{31}P NMR studies. Biochemistry, In press.

DeLuca, M., Hall, N., Rice, R. and Kaplan, N.O., 1981, Creatine kinase isozymes in human tumors, Biochem. Biophys. Res. Commun. 99:189.

Eden, S., Isaksson, O.G.P., Madsen, K., and Friberg, U., 1983, Specific binding of growth hormone to isolated chondrocytes from rabbit ear and epiphyseal plate. Endocrinology 112:1983.

Emtage, J.S., Lawson, D.E.M., and Kodicek, E., 1974, The response of the small intestine to vitamin D. Correlation between calcium-binding-protein production and increased calcium absorption, Biochem. J., 144:339.

Farley, J.R., Wergedal, J.E., and Baylink, D.J., 1983, Fluoride directly stimulates proliferation and alkaline phosphatase activity of bone-forming cells, Science, 222:330.

Flückiger, E., del Pozo, E., and von Werder, K., 1982, Prolactin: physiology, pharmacology and clinical findings, Monogr. Endocrinol., 23:1.

Gluckman, P.D., Grunbach, M.M., and Kaplan, S.M., 1981, The neuroendocrine regulation and function of growth hormone and prolactin in the mammalian fetus, Endocr. Revs., 2:363.

Hurley, T.W., Thadani, P., Kuhn, C.M., Schanberg, S.M., and Handwerger, S., 1980, Differential effects of placental lactogen, growth hormone and prolactin on rat liver ornithine decarboxylase activity in the perinatal period. Life Sci. 27:2269.

Isaksson, O.G.P., Jansson, J.-O. and Gause, I.A.M., 1982, Growth hormone stimulates longitudinal bone growth directly. Science 216:1237.

Katzenellenbogen, B.S., and Gorski, J., 1972, Estrogen action in vitro. J. Biol. Chem., 247:1299.

Kaye, A.M., Reiss, N., Shaer, A., Sluyser, M., Iacobelli, S., Amroch, D., and Soffer, Y., 1981, Estrogen responsive creatine kinase in normal and neoplastic cells, J. Steroid Biochem., 15:69.

Kaye, A.M., 1983a, Sequential regulation of gene expression by estrogen in the developing rat uterus, in: "Regulation of Gene Expression by Hormones", K.W. McKerns, ed., Plenum Pub. Co., N.Y., p. 103.

Kaye, A.M., 1983b, Enzyme induction by estrogen, J. Steroid. Biochem. 19:33.

Kenyon, G.L., and Reed, G.H., 1983, Creatine kinase: structure-activity relationships, Adv. Enz., 54:367.

Kimhi, Y., 1981, Nerve cells in clonal systems, in: "Excitable Cells in Tissue Culture", P.G. Nelson and M. Lieberman, Plenum Press, N.Y., p. 173-245.

Li, C.H., 1982, Human growth hormone: 1974-1981, Mol. Cell. Biochem. 46:31.

Majeska, R.J., and Rodan, G., 1982, The effect of $1,25(OH)_2D_3$ on alkaline phosphatase in osteoblastic osteosarcoma cells, J. Biol. Chem., 257:3362.

Malnick, S.D.H., Shaer, A., Soreq, H. and Kaye, A.M., 1983, Estrogen-induced creatine kinase in the reproductive system of the immature female rat, Endocrinology, 113:1909.

Meyer, I.J., Thompson, J.A., Kiser, E.J., and Haven, G.T., 1980, Observation of a variant creatine kinase isoenzyme in sera and breast tumor cytosols. Am. J. Clin. Path., 74:332.

Nicklas, W., and Browning, E.T., 1983, Glutamate uptake and metabolism in C-6 glioma cells: alterations by potassium ion and dibutyryl cAMP. J. Neurochem. 41:179.

Norman, A.W., Roth, J., and Orci, L., 1982, The vitamin D endocrine system: Steroid metabolism, hormone receptors, and biological response (calcium binding proteins), Endocr. Revs., 3:331.

Notides, A., and Gorski, J., 1966, Estrogen-induced synthesis of a specific uterine protein, Proc. Natn. Acad. Sci. U.S.A., 56:230.

Ornoy, A., Goodwin, D., Noff, D., and Edelstein, S., 1978, 24,25-Dihydroxy vitamin D is a metabolite of vitamin D essential for bone formation, Nature, 276:517.

Rasmussen, H., De Luca, H.F., Arnaud, C., Hawker, C., and von Steding, K.M., 1963, The relationship between vitamin D and parathyroid hormone, J. Clin. Invest., 42:1940.

Reiss, N.A., and Kaye, A.M., 1981, Identification of the major component of the estrogen induced protein of rat uterus as the BB isozyme of creatine kinase, J. Biol. Chem., 256:5741.

Russell, D.H., 1980, Ornithine decarboxylase as a biological and pharmacological tool, Pharmacology, 20:117.

Shatton, J.B., Morris, H.D., and Weinhouse, S., 1979, Creatine kinase activity and isozyme composition in normal tissues and neoplasms of rats and mice, Cancer Research, 39:492.

Shinki, T., Takahashi, N., Miyaura, C., Samejima, K., Nishii, Y., and Suda, T., 1981, Ornithine decarboxylase activity in chick duodenum induced by 1α,25-dihydroxycholecalciferol, Biochem. J., 195:685.

Sömjen, D., Binderman, I., Harell, A., and Weismann, Y., 1982a, Biologic action of 24,25(OH)$_2$D$_3$: Induction of growth in developing skeletal tissue, in: "Current Advances in Skeletogenesis: Development, Biomineralization, Mediators and Metabolic Bone Disease", Excerpta Medica, Amsterdam, p. 185.

Sömjen, D., Sömjen, G.J., Harell, A., Mechanic, G.L., and Binderman, I., 1982b, Partial characterization of a specific high affinity binding macromolecule for 24R,25 dihydroxyvitamin D$_3$ in differentiating skeletal mesenchyme, Biochem. Biophys. Res. Commun. 106:644.

Sömjen, D., Korenstein, R., Fischler, H., and Binderman, I., 1982c, Effects of intensity of electric field on the response of cultured bone cells to parathyroid hormone and prostaglandin E$_2$, in: "Current Advances in Skeletogenesis: Development, Biomineralization, Mediators and Metabolic Bone Disease", Excerpta Medica, Amsterdam, p. 412.

Sömjen, D., Binderman, I., and Weisman, Y., 1983, The effects of 24R,25 dihydroxycholecalciferol and of 1α,25 dihydroxycholecalciferol on ornithine decarboxylase activity and on DNA synthesis in the epiphysis and diaphysis of rat bone and in the duodenum, Biochem. J., 214:293.

Sömjen, D., Kaye, A.M., and Binderman, I., 1984a, 24R,25-dihydroxy vitamin D stimulates creatine kinase BB activity in chick cartilage cells in culture, FEBS Lett. 167:281.

Sömjen, D., Weisman, Y., Binderman, I., and Kaye, A.M., 1984b, Stimulation of creatine kinase BB activity by 1α,25-dihydroxycholecalciferol and 24R,25-dihydroxycholecalciferol in rat tissues, Biochem. J., (in press).

Sömjen, D., Kaye, A.M., and Binderman, I., 1984c, Hormonal regulation of creatine kinase in normal and transformed bone cells, in: "Proc. 6th Int. Workshop Calcified Tissues", Kiryat Anavim, A. Ornoy, ed., Elsevier, Amsterdam, In press.

Tsai, H.C., and Norman, A.W., 1973, Studies on calciferol metabolism. VIII. Evidence for a cytoplasmic receptor for 1,25-dihydroxy-vitamin D$_3$ in the intestinal mucosa, J. Biol. Chem. 248:5967.

Varner, M.W., and Hauser, K.S., 1981, Current status of human placental lactogen, Semin. Perinatol. 5:123.

Walker, M.D., and Kaye, A.M., 1981, mRNA for the rat uterine estrogen induced protein: translation in vitro and regulation by estrogen, J. Biol. Chem., 256:23.

Watts, D.S., 1973, Creatine kinase (adenosine 5' triphosphate-creatine phosphotransferase), in: "The Enzymes", P.D. Boyer, ed., vol. 8, part 2, p. 383, Academic Press, N.Y.

COMPARTMENTATION OF ADENINE NUCLEOTIDES AND PHOSPHO-CREATINE SHUTTLE IN CARDIAC CELLS: SOME NEW EVIDENCE

Valdur A. Saks, A.V. Kuznetsov,
Z.A. Huchua and V.V. Kupriyanov

Bioenergetics, USSR Research Center for Cardiology
3 Cherepkovskaya street 15, Moscow 121552

1. INTRODUCTION

The concept of the phosphocreatine shuttle for intracellular energy channelling in muscle cells (1-6) assumes compartmentation of adenine nucleotides in mitochondrial and myofibrillar compartments and around membranes. The link between these compartments is considered to be performed by phosphocreatine molecules due to heterogeneous distribution of creatine kinase isoenzymes functioning in mitochondria in direction of creatine phosphorylation and in myofibrils in direction of phosphocreatine dephosphorylation. While different isoenzymes of creatine kinase are well characterized, adenine nucleotide compartmentation still remains to be an unsolved question. In our recent studies described below a competitive enzyme method was used to show the existence of rather closed functional cycles of adenine nucleotides in mitochondria and in myofibrils due to activation of creatine kinase in those structures. Also, ^{31}P-NMR saturation transfer method was used to show the role of those coupled creatine kinases inside mitochondrial and myofibrillar compartments in the integrated intracellular energy fluxes in isolated perfused rat hearts at different workloads.

2. Mitochondrial compartment

Mitochondrial isoenzyme of creatine kinase first described by Jacobs et al. (7) was shown by Jacobus and Lehninger (4) and by Saks et al. (8,9) to produce phos-

103

phocreatine from mitochondrial ATP with high rates and efficiency. Detailed kinetic analyses have revealed the specific effect of mitochondrial oxidative phosphorylation on the kinetics of the membrane-bound creatine kinase reaction: the process of oxidative phosphorylation decreases by an order of magnitude the value of dissociation constant for MgATP from the productive ternary enzyme-substrate complex E·creatine·MgATP and in the lesser extent the value of the dissociation constant for MgATP from the binary complex E·MgATP at practically unchanged kinetic constants for creatine and phosphocreatine (10,11). These changes in the creatine kinase kinetics result in high rates of aerobic phosphocreatine production in cardiac mitochondria and were taken to confirm the concept of functional coupling between mitochondrial adenine nucleotide translocase and creatine kinase (2,9-11). Further evidence for such an interaction was reported by Moreadith and Jacobus who showed that ADP produced by the membrane-bound creatine kinase effectively removes atractyloside from its binding sites on the translocase (5). Radioisotope studies carried out by the Bessman group also did show the privileged access of mitochondrial ATP to creatine kinase (12,13). However, this group interpreted their data as a result of compartmentation of mitochondria-produced ATP in the intermembrane space, since in their experiments the effect of oxidative phosphorylation was lost when the outer mitochondrial membrane was removed (14). Therefore, the nature of the mitochondrial compartment of adenine nucleotides acessible and interacting with creatine kinase became more questinable. To solve the question we repeated the experiments with mitoplasts which were almost completely deprived of the outer membrane (Fig.1) by using a competitive enzyme method. This method was earlier successfully used by several authors to show adenine nucleotide compartmentation in intact mitochondria (11) and their membrane-bound pool in erythrocytes (17). In our experiments with mitoplasts we used the phosphoenolpyruvate-pyruvate kinase (PEP-PK) system of high activity which competes with the translocase for ADP. If mitochondrial creatine kinase and translocase interact via the intermembrane pool of adenine nucleotides, the creatine kinase produced ADP should become entirely accessible to the exogenous PEP-PK system after removal of the outer mitochondrial membrane. However, that does not happen as it is clearly shown in Fig.2.

In control experiments when ADP was produced by added hexokinase-glucose to support fully activated

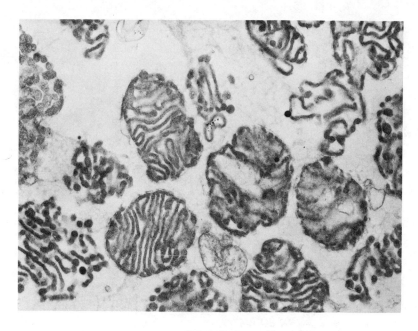

Fig.1.

Electron micrograph of mitoplasts preparation obtained
from rat heart mitochondria by a digitonin procedure.
Respiratory activities were 370 ng-atoms O_2 per min
per mg in State 3 and 130 in State 4, creatine kinase
activity was 1.9 µmoles per min per mg at $30^{\circ}C$, pH 7.4.

oxidative phosphorylation and ADP was therefore produced in the homogeneous medium, addition of pyruvate
kinase completely suppressed oxygen uptake by mitoplasts
due to rapid and complete removal of ADP (trace A,
Fig.2). However, when ADP was produced in the membrane-
bound creatine kinase reaction activated by creatine,
35 mM, addition of pyruvate kinase did not affect oxidative phosphorylation significantly (Fig. 2B). This
experiment shows clearly that ADP in the latter case
is not accessible to pyruvate kinase added into the
medium. Consequently, the phenomenon of coupling between the creatine kinase reaction and oxidative phosphorylation is restricted to the mitochondrial matrix
and inner membrane system, and ADP is undoubtly direc-
ted from creatine kinase to translocase without release
even into the intermembrane space.
    The independence of the coupling between mitochon-
drial oxidative phosphorylation and phosphocreatine production from the events in the medium including intermembrane space are shown also by the results of ther-

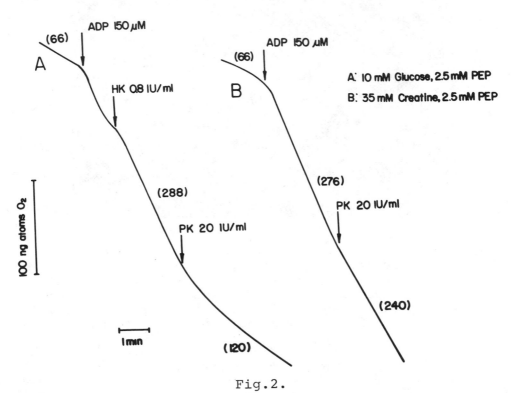

Fig.2.

Recordings of oxygen uptake by rat heart mitoplasts
stimulated by the exogenous hexokinase (HK) reaction
(A) or by endogenous creatine kinase reaction (B).
Oxygraph medium was as described in (11). In both cases
2.5 mM phosphoenolpyruvate was present . At the time
points indicated pyruvate kinase (PK) was added in ex-
cessively high activity to remove ADP from the medium.
Numbers in parentheses indicate the role of respiration
in ng-atoms of O_2 per min per mg. Mitoplast protein
concentration was 0.4 mg/ml.

modynamic approach to the problem. In these experiments, the values of the creatine kinase mass action ratio,

$$\Gamma = \frac{[MgADP]\ [PCr]}{[Cr]\ [MgATP]}$$ and the apparent equilibrium constant,

$K_{eq}^{app} = 0.7 \times 10^{-2}$ at $30^{\circ}C$ and pH 7.4 (11) were compared. When the creatine kinase reaction was not coupled to the oxidative phosphorylation, the creatine kinase reaction always run in the direction of decreasing the difference between Γ and K_{eq}^{app} (in direction of a decrease of free energy of the creatine kinase system), as it is shown in Fig. 3A.

Opposite situation was observed when the creatine kinase reaction in the mitoplasts was coupled to the oxidative phosphorylation (Fig. 3B). In this case the reaction definitely run in the direction of phosphocreatine synthesis and continuous increase in the difference between Γ and K_{eq}^{app} was observed to occure.

These results show again that the mitochondrial aerobic phosphocreatine production is not governed by the thermodynamics characteristics of the surrounding medium but is restricted to the inner membrane system. Such a restriction ensures efficient conversion of the energy released during oxidative phosphorylation into the free energy of the creatine kinase system in the external medium under condition when MgADP concentration is kept low.

These effects as well those described earlier (5, 8,9,11,16) can be explained only by some specific interaction between adenosine nucleotide translocase which connects mitochondrial matrix with the outer space, and creatine kinase localized on the outer surface of the inner membrane. Operation of this coupled system obviously results in the functional compartmentation of adenine nucleotides in the mitochondria concomitant with aerobic production of phosphocreatine.

3. Myofibrillar compartment

Isolated and purified myofibrillar preparations (18) from rat hearts containing equal activities of MgATPase (Ca-sensitive) and creatine·kinase were used in the experiments described below. MgATPase was fully activated by addition of saturating amount of a substrate MgATP to 1 mM.

The route of ADP movement was followed by assessment of the efficiency of competition between added exogenous PEP-PK system and endogenous myofibrillar creatine kinase in utilization of ADP when creatine

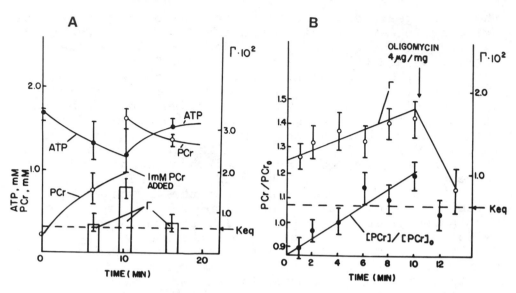

Fig.3.

Changes in the concentrations of creatine kinase substrates and in mass action ratio (Γ) without (A) and
with (B) oxidative phosphorylation catalyzed by rat
heart mitoplasts preparation.
In (A), 10 μM carboxyatractyloside and 4 μg/ml oligomycin were used to inhibit oxidative phosphorylation.
Initially 30 mM creatine and 1.6 mM MgATP were added.
At 10 min 1 mM phosphocreatine was added to shift the
system from the equilibrium. In (B) oxidative phosphorylation was run in oxygenated medium containing initially 4 mM phosphocreatine, 0.12 mM MgATP, 40 mM creatine and 0.05 mM MgADP. Mitoplasts were added to concentration 3 mg/ml. At time points indicated samples
were withdrawn, reaction was stopped by $HClO_4$ and mixture analyzed for ATP, ADP, creatine and phosphocreatine.

kinase was activated by addition of a substrate, phosphocreatine, 10 mM. As a homogeneous control system,
glucose + hexokinase were used as MgATPase, soluble
skeletal muscle creatine kinase was added and the activities of enzymes were fitted to those in the myofibrillar system. To both systems pyruvate kinase in increasing amount was added (Fig.4).

In the control soluble hexokinase - creatine kinase system the addition of PK to 5 IU/ml resulted in
complete inhibition of the creatine kinase reaction
(creatine release from phosphocreatine coupled to the
ATPase activity of system) and the rate of pyruvate release was symmetrically activated (Fig. 4A). However,
in the myofibrillar system the same activity of PK, 50
IU/ml, was not able to inhibit the creatine kinase
reaction coupled to MgATPase, and pyruvate release was
not higher than 50% of the MgATPase activity. Both those
degrees of the creatine kinase reaction inhibition and
activation of PK reaction were approached asymptotically (Fig. 4B). In conclusion, the inability of PK to inhibit the creatine kinase reaction coupled to myofibrillar MgATPase reaction demonstrates unequivocally
that significant part of ADP produced in the myofibrillar MgATPase reaction is not accessible to PK and is
directly channelled to the particulate creatine kinase
and rapidly rephosphorylated in the presence of phosphocreatine into MgATP in the local myofibrillar pool
of adenine nucleotides. These biochemical data showing
myofibrillar compartmentation of adenine nucleotides
are entirely consistent with the results of physiological data described recently almost simultaneously in
three laboratories (20-22) which have demonstrated much
more efficient relaxation of the skeletal muscle or cardiac muscle skinned fibers from their rigor state in
the presence of phosphocreatine than in the presence of
ATP. Among these authors, McCellan et al. (21) were
able to demonstrate directly the existence of specific
myofibrillar pool of ATP not accessible to mitochondria
in cardiac muscle cells.

4. Demonstration (inderect) of coupled creatine kinases
   in mitochondrial and myofibrillar compartments in
   heart cells in vivo by ^{31}P-NMR saturation transfer
   technique

Recently, the ^{31}P-NMR spectroscopy has successfully been used to study the phosphorus metabolism in perfused hearts (23-28). This powerful method is able to
provide information of the metabolic fluxes in the li-

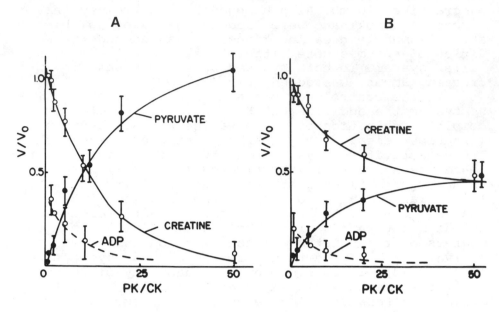

Fig.4A.

The effect of increasing pyruvate kinase/creatine kinase activity ratio (PK/CK) on the rate of creatine and pyruvate release in the homogeneous system.
The reaction mixture (25 mM Tris-HCl, pH 7.4, 20 mM glucose, 5 mM $MgCl_2$) contained 0.1-0.15 IU/ml both of hexokinase and skeletal muscle creatine kinase, 1 mM MgATP and 10 mM phosphocreatine, 1 mM phosphoenolpyruvate and different amounts of pyruvate kinase. Mean values for 5 experiments and standard deviations are shown. The reaction rates were determined by analysis of the creatine and pyruvate concentration in the reaction mixture after termination of the reaction by $HClO_4$. ADP concentrations were determined in the same samples. V_0 - the rate of creatine release without pyruvate kinase; v - the rate determined at given PK/CK ratio.

Fig.4B.

The effect of increasing pyruvate kinase/creatine kinase activity ratio (PK/CK) on the rate of creatine release in the myofibrillar creatine kinase reaction. The reaction mixture contained 1.0-1.5 mg of myofibrillar protein per ml, 1 mM MgATP, 10 mM phosphocreatine, 1 mM phosphoenolpyruvate and different amounts of pyruvate kinase. Determinations were performed as described in the legend to Fig.4A.

ving undisrupted cells and therefore may be considered
as a method for final judgement of correctness of biochemical concepts developed by conventional procedures.
An attempt has been made by two groups of investigators
to study the relationship between metabolic fluxes
through creatine kinase and the work performed by perfused rat heart, and the results are conflicting (26-
28). According to reports by Mathews et al. an increased
workload only slightly accelerates the metabolic fluxes
through creatine kinase (26,27) while Kobayashi et al.
(28) observed substantial increase (about 1.7 times) in
the rate of creatine kinase reaction at enhanced workload. In our studies we used the CXP-200 NMR spectrometer (Bruker, FRG) for ^{31}P-saturation transfer measurements of energy fluxes through creatine kinase in isolated Wistar rat hearts perfused with a Krebs-Hanseleit
bicarbonate buffer, pH 7.4 containing 11 mM glucose with
10 IU/L insulin, without phosphate and aerated by 95%
O_2, 5% CO_2 mixture, 37°C. At zero workload perfused
hearts were arrested with 20 mM_3KCl in the perfusate.
Maximal workload (up to 40 x 10^3 mm Hg/min) was obtained
at high perfusate flow rates (18-28 ml/min). Oxygen
consumption was measured by Clarck oxygen electrode in
the separate experiments under conditions similar to
those in NMR studies. The ^{31}P-NMR spectra were recorded
at 80.98 MHz. Selective saturation was evoked by "Dante"
method using long pulses (0.3, 0.6 and 4.2 s) at resonance frequencies of γ-phosphate of ATP. The saturating
pulse was followed by a 90° observing pulse (76 us),
acquisition time and relaxation delay - 3 s, number of
scans - 150-180, memory size 16 K. The NMR spectra
measured at off-resonance saturation at maximal duration
(4.2 s) were observed as controls. To obtain M_z° for
phosphocreatine and γ-P(ATP) quantitative spectra
with 6 s relaxation delay were accumulated. From exponential dependences of phosphocreatine magnetization
versus saturation time the exchange rate constants K_1
was calculated and the value of the energy flux was
found as $F=k_1(PCr)$, where (PCr) is a phosphocreatine
tissue content determined by a biochemical method (29).

Creatine kinase reaction as it is well-known proceeds via formation of binary and ternary enzyme substrate complexes. Chemical shifts of ^{31}P signals of PCr
and γ-P(ATP) in binary and ternary complexes are practically the same as those of their free forms (3).
Therefore, selective saturation (or exitation) of PCr
of γ-P(ATP) signals lead also to saturation (or exitation) of those from bound forms. It means that steps
of formation and breakdown of binary and ternary comp-

lexes are masked due to this phenomenon. In general,
this will cause some overestimation of fluxes. Fortunately, the rate-limiting step of creatine kinase reaction at physiological temperatures is phosphoryl group
transfer (31,32). Therefore, possible overestimation
of real fluxes cannot be significant and measured fluxes
should be close to real ones. The results of determinations of energy fluxes in perfused heart are given in
Table 1. These data indicate significant (35%) enhancement of the flux through the creatine kinase reaction
during rest-high work transition. At the rest the flux
PCr $\longrightarrow$ ATP occurs obviously due to the equilibrium
creatine kinase (33). During activation of mitochondrial ATP production in oxidative phosphorylation (that
is equal to the ATP utilization for contraction in the
steady state) the flux through the creatine kinase reaction is increased concomitantly, and the most important
observation is that Δ Flux (PCr $\longrightarrow$ ATP)$/\Delta F_{(ATP)} > 1$.
The same ratio could be calculated from data by Kobaya-
shi et al. (28), given in the Table 1 for comparison,
who observed almost doubled flux PCr $\longrightarrow$ ATP at high
workload in the working heart preparation. Could the
data given in Table 1 be explained by the equilibrium
creatine kinase reaction in the cytoplasm due to changes
in the substrate concentration (27)? To answer this
question, we have repeated the ^{31}P-NMR saturation transfer experiments in vitro using the equilibrium reaction
mixture composed of soluble skeletal muscle creatine
kinase (800 IU/ml), 24 mM HEPES, pH 7.4, 8 mM ATP, 10 mM
magnesium acetate, 0.5 mM dithiothreitol, 110 mM potassium acetate, 30 mM KCl and 20% D_2O, different amounts
of creatine and phosphocreatine at constant total creatine (PCr + Cr) concentration equal to 30 mM. The PCr /
 Cr value varied from 0.15 to 9.0 to cover exceedingly
the range of the value of this ratio observed in vivo,
where it is altered from 2.0 to 1.0 (34, Table 1). Table
2 shows the determined fluxes through the equilibrium
creatine kinase at different equilibrium concentrations
of substrates presented by different PCr / Cr ratios.
The fluxes in the equilibrium system as evidenced by data in Table 2 are suprisingly stable and do not practically vary with changes in PCr / Cr ratio. Obviously,
changes in PCr / Cr ratio are compensated for by opposite changes in MgADP / MgATP ratio in equilibrium
system.
       The comparison of data from Tables 1 and 2 leads
to the following conclusion: while the creatine kinase
fluxes in the resting state could be ascribed to the
enzyme action in the equilibrium state, the workload

Table 1.

The dependence of energy fluxes in perfused rat heart on workload and intensity of oxidative metabolism.

Our data

Conditions	PCr content, μmol/g dr.wt.	Oxygen consumption, μmol/min g dr.wt.	Calculated $\frac{F\,ATP \to Pi=6}{}$ VO$_2$ μmol/min·g dr.wt.	Flux PCr→ATP, μmol/min·g dr.wt.	Flux PCr→ATP, μmol/min·g dr. wt.
1. High work, WL*=31.7+4.6 mm Hg min 10³, (6)	35.5+5.0	46.4+10.4	229	1614+240	426
2. 25 mM KCl-arrest	38.8+6.2	8.3+3.1		1188+174	

Data of Kobayshi et al. (personal commun., Biophys.J., 1982, 37, 123a)

Conditions	PCr content, μmol/g dr.wt.	Flux ATP→Pi, μmol/min·g dr.wt.	Calculated VO$_2$, μmol/min· g dr.wt.	Flux PCr→ATP, μmol/min· g dr.wt.	Flux PCr → ATP
A.Langendorff prep. WL=26.1+0.3 mm Hg/min	30.3+0.6	330+42	55+7	1980+78	630
B.Working heart prep. WL=40.5+0.8	26.8+0.9	546+18	91+3	2580+138	1230
KCl - arrest	35.9+1.4	–	–	1350+108	

Table 2.

Dependence of values of fluxes through creatine kinase on PCr / Cr in vitro.

Phosphocreatine, mM	4	10	13	17	21	27
Creatine, mM	26	20	17	13	9	3
$\dfrac{\text{Phosphocreatine}}{\text{Creatine}}$	0.15	0.5	0.8	1.3	2.3	9.0
Normalyzed flux, $\text{flux}/V_m^f \cdot E_o$	0.17	0.35	0.40	0.35	0.35	0.22

The flux F, determined at 37°, pH 7.4, was expressed in umol/s·ml related to the maximal rate of forward creatine kinase reaction, expressed in umol/s·ml ($V_m^f \cdot E_o$).

induced increase in the energy fluxes, Flux(PCr → ATP), cannot be explained by the same concept. On the contrary, this increase, Flux(PCr → ATP), is consistent with the concept of unidirectional functioning of mitochondrial creatine kinase and myofibrillar creatine kinase in steady-state in the opposite directions at high workload, and thus, with the concept of the phosphocreatine shuttle. The necessary prerequisite for this pathway, Δ Flux(PCr → ATP) $/\Delta F_{(ATP)} \geqslant 1$ is experimentally observed to be met.

ACKNOWLEDGEMENTS

The results reported here were obtained in collaboration with Drs.W.E.Jacobus and M.Miceli, the Johns Hopkins University, Baltimore, USA, and with Dr.Renee Ventura-Clapier, University Paris-Sud, Orsey, France and are fully described in our joint communications (35,36).

REFERENCES

1. S.Gudbjarnason, P.Mathes, K.G.Ravens, J.Mol.Cell. Cardiol. 1:325-339 (1970).
2. V.A.Saks, L.V.Rosenshtraukh, V.N.Smirnov, E.I.Chazov, Can.J.Physiol.Pharmacol.56:691-706 (1978).
3. S.P.Bessman, P.J.Geiger, Science 211:448-452, 1981.
4. W.E.Jacobus, A.L.Lehninger, J.Biol.Chem. 248:4803-4810 (1973).
5. R.W.Moreadith, W.E.Jacobus, J.Biol.Chem. 257:889-905 (1982).

6. M.W.Seraydarian, B.S.Abbott, J.Mol.Cell.Cardiol. 8:741-746 (1976).
7. H.Jacobs, H.W.Heldt, H.Klingenberg, Biochem.Biophys. Res.Comm. 16:516-521 (1964).
8. V.A.Saks, G.B.Chernousova, Y.I.Voronkov, V.N.Smirnov, E.I.Chazov, Circulation Res. 34, suppl.3,138-149 (1974).
9. V.A.Saks, G.B.Chernousova, D.E.Gukovsky, V.N.Smirnov, E.I.Chazov, J.Biochem. 57:273-290 (1975).
10. V.A.Saks, V.V.Kupriyanov, G.B.Elizarova, W.E.Jacobus, J.Biol.Chem. 255:755-763 (1980).
11. W.E.Jacobus, V.A.Saks, Arch.Biochem.Biophys. 219: 167-178 (1982).
12. W.C.T.Yang, P.J.Geiger, S.P.Bessman, B.Borrebaeck, Biochem.Biophys.Res.Comm. 76:882-887 (1977).
13. S.Erickson-Viitanen,P.Viitanen, P.J.Geiger, W.C.T. Yang, S.P.Bessman, J.Biol.Chem. 257:14395-14404 (1982).
14. S.Erickson-Viitanen, P.J.Geiger, P.Viitanen, S.P. Bessman, J.Biol.Chem. 257:14405-14411 (1982).
15. C.Schnaitman, J.W.Greenwalt, J.Cell Biol. 38:158-175 (1968).
16. F.Gellerich, V.A.Saks, Biochem.Biophys.Res.Comm. 105:473-81 (1982).
17. R.W.Mercer, P.B.Dunham, J.Gen.Physiol. 78:547-568 (1981).
18. V.A.Saks, G.B.Chernousova, R.Fetter, V.N.Smirnov, E.I.Chazov, FEBS Lett. 62:293-296 (1976).
19. F.Savabi, P.J.Geiger, S.P.Bessman, Biochem.Biophys. Res.Comm. 144:785-790 (1983).
20. G.McCellan, A.Weisberg, S.Winegrad, Am.J.Physiol. 245:C433-C427 (1983).
21. V.Veksler, V.I.Kapelko, Biochem.Biophys.Acta , in press (1984).
22. W.E.Jacobus, G.Taylor, D.P.Hollis, R.L.Nunnaly, Nature 265:756-758 (1977).
23. P.B.Garlick, G.K.Radda, P.J.Seeley, B.Chance, Biochem.Biophys.Res.Comm.74:1256-1262 (1977).
24. E.T.Fossel, H.E.Morgan, J.S.Ingwall, Proc.Natl.Acad. Sci.USA 77:3654-3658 (1980).
25. P.M.Matthews, T.L.Bland, D.G.Gadian, G.K.Radda, Biochim.Biophys.Acta 721:312-320 (1982).
26. P.M.Matthews, J.L.Bland, D.G.Gadian, G.K.Radda, Biochem.Biophys.Res.Comm. 103:1052-1059 (1981).
27. K.Kobayashi, E.Fossel, J.S.Ingwall, Biophys.J.37: 123a (1982).
28. W.Lamprecht, P.Stein, in: "Methods of Enzymatic Analysis", H.U.Bergmeyer, ed., p.1777-1785, Academic Press, New York (1964).

29. B.D.N.Rao, M.Cohn, J.Biol.Chem. 256:1716-1721 (1981).
30. W.W.Cleland, in: "The Enzymes", Boyer P.D., ed., vol.2, pp.1-66, Acad.Press, New York (1970).
31. J.F.Morrison, E.James, Biochem.J. 97:37-52 (1965).
32. V.V.Kuprianov, E.R.Seppet, I.V.Emelin, V.A.Saks, Biochem.Biophys.Acta 592:197-210 (1980).
33. J.R.Williamson, C.Ford, K.Kobayashi, J.Illingworth, Circulation Res. 38, suppl.1, 39-48 (1976).
34. V.A.Saks, R.Ventura-Clapier, Z.A.Kuchua, A.N.Preobrazhensky, I.V.Emelin, Biochim.Biophys.Acta, in press (1984).
35. V.A.Saks, A.V.Kuznetsov, V.V.Kupriaynov, M.V.Miceli, W.E.Jacobus, in preparation.

COMPARTMENTATION OF HORMONE ACTION

IN ADULT MAMMALIAN CARDIOMYOCYTES

Iain L.O. Buxton and Laurence L. Brunton

Divisions of Pharmacology and Cardiology, M-013H
University of California, San Diego
La Jolla, California 92093

"He is short-sighted who looks only on the path he treads and the wall on which he leans."

Kahlil Gibran

INTRODUCTION

Our interests in hormone action on mammalian heart have led us to explore the hormonal responsiveness of purified adult ventricular cardiomyocytes. In this report, we shall describe cardiomyocytes from both rat and rabbit that retain excellent biochemical homology with the intact heart and possess an abundance of receptors for adrenergic and cholinergic hormones that regulate the metabolism and contraction of cardiac muscle. Our data demonstrate the utility of the purified cardiomyocyte preparation in questions about the distribution of hormonal responsiveness between myocyte and non-myocyte elements of cardiac tissue. In addition, our data demonstrate the subcellular basis of hormone-specific compartmentation of cyclic AMP (cAMP) and cAMP-protein kinase (cAMP-PK) in cardiomyocytes, implying that the expression of cAMP-PK activity is regulated intracellularly by factors in addition to cAMP.

EXPERIMENTAL PROCEDURES

We prepare freshly isolated adult mammalian cardiomyocytes of rabbit and rat by collagenase perfusion in the absence of added calcium, by the method of Frangakis (1980), as we have recently described in detail (Buxton and Brunton, 1983). Suspensions of purified myocytes ($1-2 \times 10^6$/ml) are maintained in complete medium equilibrated with oxygen/carbon dioxide (95%/5%), pH 7.2-7.4,

containing millimolar calcium and 0.01% bovine serum albumin at 32°.
Following hormonal stimulation, myocytes are rapidly centrifuged and
the cell pellets frozen in liquid nitrogen, powdered and stored at
-70°. Biochemical assays are performed using frozen tissue powder.
Binding studies employ myocytes incubated with ligands as required
for 120-240 minutes, followed by filtration (see Weiland and
Molinoff, 1981, and Weiland et al., 1981 for details). Binding data
are analyzed using the non-linear fitting program, LIGAND, (Munson
and Rodbard, 1980). Cyclic AMP was measured from acid extracts by
the method of Gilman (1970). Cyclic AMP-protein kinase was measured
by the method of Corbin (1977) using histone HF2B as substrate.
Glycogen phosphorylase was assayed in soluble extracts by the coupled
fluorescent method of Hardman (1965). Soluble and particulate fractions were prepared by centrifugation (3000 x g x 5 min, 4°).

RESULTS

Characteristics of Cardiomyocytes

The myocyte preparation we employ is a relatively pure population of cardiac muscle cells (>90% homogenous visually) that remain
viable (as judged by exclusion of trypan blue) for at least 20 hours
following their preparation. These cardiomyocytes display a number
of properties that mimic whole ventricle. Their rod-shaped, branched
appearance is identical to that of the myocyte in situ, with average
dimensions of 17 x 138 µm (rabbit; rat, $\sim$10% smaller). The cells
maintain normal ATP contents (14-16 nmol/mg protein) and can synthesize cAMP in response to beta-adrenergic agonists and prostaglandin E_1 (Buxton and Brunton, 1983). Incorporation of $[^{35}S]$methionine
into myocyte proteins proceeds rapidly for at least six hours and is
doubled in the presence of 100 nM insulin. Myocytes readily incorporate $[^{32}P]$inorganic phosphate into ATP. Cells thus labelled will
incorporate $[^{32}P]$ into discrete domains of phosphoproteins in
response to hormones (beta and muscarinic), to phorbol ester (activation of calcium-phospholipid-dependent protein kinase) and to oxygen
deprivation.

Hormone Receptors on Ventricular Myocytes

With a view toward learning the potential of the ventricular
myocyte for hormonal responsiveness, we have exmployed radioligand
binding methods to study both adrenergic and cholinergic receptors
on intact cardiomyocytes from both rat and rabbit (Table 1). Myocytes from both species possess approximately 2 x 10^5 beta-adrenergic
receptors per cell as determined by specific $[^{125}I]$iodocyanopindolol
binding ($[^{125}I]$ICYP). Similar data have been gathered employing
$[^3H]$prazosin to identify alpha receptors and $[^3H]$quinuclidinyl benzi-
late ($[^3H]$QNB) to quantify cholinergic muscarinic receptors.

Our studies of beta-adrenergic receptors on the intact myocyte reveal an interesting feature of compartmentation at the cellular level in heart. In rat heart we have measured the presence of both beta-1 and beta-2 receptors (Table 1). Does this mean that responses of the ventricle following isoproterenol treatment of rat heart result from the stimulation of both receptor types? Do both beta-1 and beta-2 receptors co-exist on ventricular myocytes? Comparison of receptor distribution in whole heart, non-myocyte and myocyte elements offers definitive answers to these sorts of questions.

Table 1. Characteristics of Adrenergic and Cholinergic Receptors on Adult Mammalian Cardiomyocytes.

	Receptor Type				
	Beta $[125_I]$ICYP		Alpha $[^3H]$prazosin	Muscarinic $[^3H]$QNB	
	Rat	Rabbit	Rat	Rat	Rabbit
Affinity for radioligand (K_D in pM)	70±12	26±1	82±3	95±13	102
Affinity for agonist (K_D)	--	80nM (1-INE)	3µM (1-NE)	117µM (Carbachol)	--
Receptor number (site/cell x 10^4)	21±2	26±3	8+.5	16±2	9
Receptor density (site/µm^2)	33±3	33±5	13±1	25±3	11
Subtype	beta-1	beta-1	alpha-1	--	--

Isolated myocytes were incubated with radioligand and agonist or antagonist drugs under equilibrium conditions in medium plus BSA and Ca^{++} as described in Experimental Procedures. Scatchard analysis of saturation isotherms was employed to obtain number and affinity of receptors. For $[125_I]$ICYP binding to both whole ventircle and non-myocyte membranes normally discarded during myocyte preparation, competition with subtype specific antagonists practolol and zinterol revealed the presence of 30 and 50% beta-2 receptors, respectively. Data are mean+SEM, n=3-6. Values for density of receptors were obtained by expressing receptor number as a function of surface area of a cylinder with dimensions of 17 x 138 µm (average dimensions for rabbit myocytes).

Competition of $[^{125}I]$ICYP binding to purified myocytes or to membranes made from non-myocytes by the beta subtype specific antagonists practolol (beta-1) and zinterol (beta-2), reveals that beta-2 receptors are enriched in the portion of ventricle normally discarded during myocyte purification and that only beta-1 receptors can be detected on the myocyte (within the limits of discrimination of such an assay, ∿10% of either receptor type). We conclude that the responses measured in myocytes following isoproterenol stimulation occur via a single receptor type, beta-1. We presume that cardiac beta-2 receptors occur on non-moycyte elements, such as fibroblasts and vascular smooth muscle cells. Thus, the effects of beta agonists are compartmented between or among different cardiac cell types as a result of the multicellular distribution of beta-adrenergic receptors.

We should note that the beta-1 receptors on myocytes may not be homogeneous, even though equilibrium binding studies indicate only a single populaton of sites. $[^{125}I]$ICYP dissociates from myocytes in a biphasic manner (k_{-1} = 0.026/min, k'_{-1} = 0.0009/min), a heterogeneity that we believe is not related to use of the racemate of radiolabeled CYP (Hoyer et al., 1982) but to actual beta-1 receptor heterogeneity that may represent receptors at different surface locations (sarcolemma vs. t-tubules).

Alpha and muscarinic receptors on cardiac myocytes also have interesting properties. On rat myocytes, alpha receptors are of the alpha-1 subtype, ∿8 x 10^4/cell. Remarkably, the affinity of these receptors for norepinephine (the physiologic agonist) is decreased by GTP (Fig. 1). Although the GTP shift is slight (two-fold), it is readily demonstrated and statistically significant. One implication of a GTP shift is coupling of a receptor to a GTP-binding membrane transducer protein, as originally described by Maguire et al. (1976) for beta-responsive adenylate cyclase. An alpha effect on cAMP metabolism may occur, since we find evidence for alpha inhibition of cAMP-PK activity (Fig. 2). The occurrence of both alpha and beta receptors linked to cAMP and cAMP-PK on a single cell suggests the possible coordination, in time, of beta then alpha influences to aid in terminating a pulse of beta stimulation, or considering the poorer affinity of the alpha receptors for norephinephrine, a mechanism at high agonist concentrations to protect agonist excessive beta stimulation.

Muscarinic cholinergic receptors, 1.5 x 10^5/cell, are quite clearly linked to adenylate cyclase in an inhibitory manner (Fig. 3),

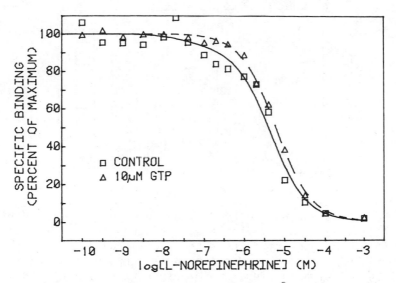

Figure 1. L-Norepinephrine Competition of $[^3H]$Prazosin Binding in Rat Myocyte Membranes. Membranes were prepared from frozen myocyte powder as described in Experimental Procedures. Competition of $[^3H]$-prazosin binding by agonist was performed in the absence ($\square$-$\square$; K_I=1.3μM) and presence ($\triangle$-$\triangle$; K_I=2.4μM) of 10μM GTP. Data from several experiments yield a highly significant difference between l-norepinephrine competition with and without added GTP.

consistent with the negative inotropic effects expected of acetylcholine. Whether depressed adenylate cyclase is the single primary response of ventricular myocytes to cholinergic stimultion is not clear: in conjunction with Dr. Joan Heller Brown at the University of California, San Diego we have found cholinergic enhancement of phosphatidylinositol turnover in these cells (unpublished observation).

We believe that these preliminary but provocative data demonstrate the potential of purified myocytes for biochemical studies of the hormonal regulation of ventricular metabolism. We now turn to a specific example of the utility of the isolated cardiomyocyte for studying compartmentation and hormone action at a subcellular level.

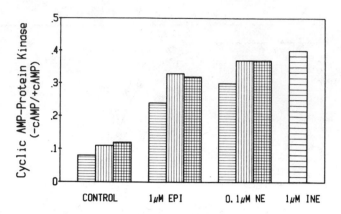

Figure 2. Alpha Adrenergic Effects on Myocyte cAMP-dependent Protein Kinase Activity. Protein kinase was measured in homogenates of myocytes in the presence of diluent (horizontal bars), 10^{-5} M phentolamine (verticle bars) or 10^{-8} M prazosin (hatched bars). Protein kinase was stimulated with nothing, 10^{-6} M epinephrine, 10^{-7} M norepinephrine or 10^{-6} M isoproterenol as shown.

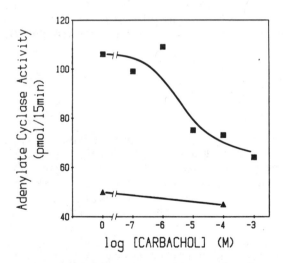

Figure 3. Carbachol Inhibition of Myocyte Adenylate Cyclase. Adenylate cyclase activity was measured at 37° in homogenates of myocytes using $[\alpha^{-32}P]ATP$ as substrate. Activity was measured in the presence (■-■) and absence (▲-▲) of 3×10^{-5} M isoproterenol.

Functional Compartmentation of Cyclic AMP and Protein Kinase

Keely (1979) and Hayes et al. (1979) have demonstrated that PGE_1 can elevate cAMP and cAMP-PK in isolated perfused mammalian hearts without causing any of the usual sequelae of cAMP elevation (phosphorylation of phosphorylase kinase, glycogen synthase and troponin I; see Brunton et al., 1981) Whether this anomalous effect of PGE_1 occurs because PGE_1 responsive cells are distinct from cells with substrates for cAMP-PK (i.e., the beta responsive cells) could not be determined in isolated heart. Clearly, this is the sort of experimental dilemma in which a homogeneous population of cardiomyocytes is very useful.

Incubation of rabbit cardiomyocytes with PGE_1 or INE produces exactly the same pattern noted in the isolated perfused heart. Both agents cause cAMP accumulation and consequent activation of soluble cAMP-PK. Only INE causes the activation of glycogen phosphorylase (Table 2).

This distinction between the effects of PGE_1 and INE seems unrelated to differential activation of the two isozymes of cAMP-PK (Hayes et al., 1980), but apparently results from actual subcellular compartmentation of cAMP and cAMP-PK. Using the simple centrifuged fractionation suggested by Corbin et al. (1977) to separate soluble and membrane-bound cAMP-PK activities of rabbit heart, 3000 x g x 5 min, we have made soluble and particulate fractions from homogenates of frozen, powdered cardiomyocytes. Remarkably, the specificity of INE and PGE_1 to activate cAMP-PK fractionates cleanly by the same simple scheme (Table 2). INE causes a large increase in particulate cAMP, a concomitant decrease in cAMP-PK activity remaining in the particulate fraction (translocation of active subunit to soluble fraction) and a marked activation of glycogen phosphorylase. PGE_1 treatment, however, does not alter either the cAMP content or the cAMP-PK activity. Rather, PGE_1 elicits cAMP accumulation and cAMP-PK activation only in the soluble fraction, activation of a fraction of cAMP-PK that does not lead to phosphorylase b $\rightarrow$ a conversion. The combination of maximal PGE_1 and INE give the same result as INE alone, ruling out inhibitory effects of PGE_1 on expression of soluble cAMP-PK and on activation of particulate cAMP-PK. A lower concentration of INE (1 nM) that produces the same effects in the soluble fraction as 10 µM PGE_1 also causes particulate responses and phosphorylase activation, indicating that the failure of PGE_1 to cause expected effects is not due simply to the modest size of cAMP accumulation in response to PGE_1. INE, on the other hand, causes the rapid appearance of cAMP and activation and translocation of C subunit of cAMP-PK from the particulate to the soluble fraction (Fig. 4).

Table 2. Effects Of Isoproterenol And Prostaglandin E_1 On Soluble And Particulate Fractions Of Rabbit Cardiomyocytes

	Control	PGE$_1$ (10μM)	INE (1μM)
Soluble cAMP-PK (-cAMP/+cAMP)	0.21±.02	0.39±0.04*	0.66±0.05*
Particulate cAMP-PK (% of total)	47.00±.70	45.00±1.20	30.00±0.70*
Particulate cAMP (pmol/mg protein)	3.00±.40	3.20±0.40	9.20±1.00*
Soluble cAMP (pmol/mg protein)	2.30±.43	5.80±0.40**	7.70±0.50*
Phosphorylase (- AMP/+ AMP)	0.15±.02	0.14±0.02	0.47±0.04*

Myocytes were incubated at $32°$ with INE or PGE$_1$ for 15 min. Incubations were terminated by rapid (20-30 sec) centrifugation. The myocyte pellet was frozen immediately in liquid nitrogen. Soluble and particulate fractions were prepared from frozen tissue powders by centrifugation (3000 x g x 5 min) of homogenates prepared in phosphage buffer (pH 6.8) described in detail by Buxton and Brunton (1983). Particulate protein kinase activity is expressed as a percentage of total protein kinase activity (soluble + particulate). Values are the mean + SEM of eight experiments. Asterisks indicate values differeing significantly from control: * p<.003, ** p <.03, by analysis of variance.

Thus, INE treatment causes effects in two compartments of the myocyte and results in phosphorylation of glycogen phosphorylase. The cellular response to PGE$_1$ seems confined to a distinct fraction of the myocyte homogenate, the soluble compartment, and does not include activation of glycogenolysis, a response one might have thought to be obligatory when intracellular cAMP was elevated. By comparison of the effects of PGE$_1$ and INE, we conclude that the activation of particulate cAMP-PK is responsible for activation of phosphorylase and by analogy to results from isolated perfused heart, for cAMP-mediated phosphorylation of glycogen synthase and troponin I (Brunton et al., 1981).

124

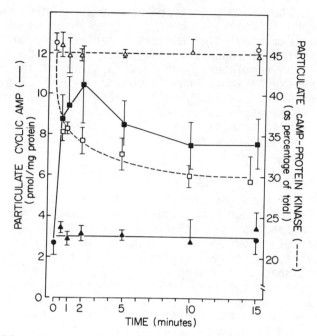

Figure 4. Time Course of Translocation of Particulate Protein Kinase
Following Stimulation of Myocytes by Isoproterenol. INE (1μM □,■),
PGE₁ (10μM, △,▲) or diluent (o,●) was added at zero time. Aliquots
were withdrawn, frozen, separated into soluble and particulate fractions and assayed for cAMP (——) and cAMP-PK (---) as described.
cAMP-PK activity disappearing from particulate fraction appeared in
soluble fraction. Values are the mean ± range of two separate experiments.

CONCLUSIONS

These data demonstrate the usefulness of purified ventricular
myocytes for biochemical studies of adrenergic and cholinergic hormone action on cardiac tissue. For instance, the cells can be used
to localize receptors and responses to the cardiomyocyte, distinct
from other cell types present in heart. Myocytes have high densities
of adrenergic and cholinergic receptors, suggesting that these cells
will be an excellent starting material for studies of receptor regulation as well as more distal consequences of receptor occupation.

The architectural complexity of the myocytes affords additional experimental opportunities, such as the likelihood of observing structural compartmentation of hormone receptors and subsequent responses in isolatable and functionally relevant subcellular fractions (such as the regulatory membranous systems of the myocyte - sarcolemma, transverse tubule and sarcoplasmic reticulum). As an example of hormone action in which this level of compartmentation may be important, we have presented data on hormonally specific effects of PGE_1 and the beta agonist, INE. These data demonstrate that within a cell, not all cAMP interacts with all pools of cAMP-PK and that not all cAMP-PK can interact with the kinase's classical substrates.

We do not yet know the structural basis of this compartmentation of cAMP and cAMP-PK. Our data suggest the testable hypothesis that hormonal responsiveness via cAMP depends on cAMP accumulation at discrete subcellular loci, with subsequent phosphorylation not of all possible proteins, but of a limited number of substrates. We believe that a distinct spatial and temporal organization of the reactive components (receptor, cyclase, cAMP-PK, substrates) accounts for this observed compartmentation and that compartmentation very likely begins at the level of receptor-adenylate cyclase complexes within the sarcolemma and transverse tubules. Purified ventricular myocytes will be essential in probing this speculative hypothesis.

ACKNOWLEDGEMENTS

Supported by the National Science Foundation (PCM 81-10116) and National Institutes of Health (RCDA HL 00935 to Dr. Brunton).

REFERENCES

Brunton, L.L., Hayes, J.S., and Mayer, S.E., 1981, Functional compartmentation of cyclic AMP and protein kinase in heart, Adv. Cyclic Nuc. Res. 14:391-397.
Buxton, I.L.O., and Brunton, L.L., 1983, Compartmentation of cyclic AMP and protein kinase in cardiac myocytes, J. Biol. Chem. 258:10233-10239.
Corbin, J.D., Snyden, P.H., Lincoln, T.M., and Keely, S.C., 1977, Compartmentalization of adenosine 3':5'-monophosphate and adenosine 3':5'-monophosphate-dependent protein kinase in heart tissue, J. Biol. Chem. 252:3854-3861.
Frangakis, C.J., Bahl, J.J., McDaniel, H., and Bressler, R., 1980, Tolerance to physiological Ca^{++} by isolated myocytes from the adult heart rat: an improved cellular preparation, Life Sci. 27:815-825.

Gilman, A.G., 1970, A protein binding assay for adenosine 3':5'-
     cyclic monophosphate, Proc. Nat'l Acad. Sci. U.S.A. 67:305-
     312.
Hardman, J.G., Mayer, S.E., and Clark B.J., 1965, Cocaine potentia-
     tion of the cardiac inotropic and phosphorylase responses to
     catecholamines as related to the uptake of ^{3}H-catecholamines,
     J. Pharm. Exp. Therap. 150:341-348.
Hayes, J.S., Brunton, L.L, Brown, J.H., Reese, J.B., and Mayer, S.E.,
     1979, Hormonally specific expression of cardiac protein
     kinase activity, Proc. Natl Acad. Sci. U.S.A. 76:1570-1574.
Hoyer, D., Engel, G., and Berthold, R., 1982, Binding characteristics
     of (+)-, (+)- and (-)-[^{125}Iodo] cyanopindolol to guinea pig
     left ventricle membranes, Naunyn-Schmiedeberg's Arch. Phar-
     macol. 318:319-329.
Keeley, S.L., 1979, Prostaglandin E_1 activation of heart cAMP-
     dependent protein kinases: Apparent dissociation of protein
     kinase activation from increases in phosphorylase activity
     and contractile force, Mol. Pharmacol. 15:235-245.
Maguire, M.E., Van Arsdale, P.M., and Gilman, A.G., 1976, An agonist
     specific effect of guanine nucleotides on binding to the beta
     adrenergic receptor, Molec. Pharmacol. 12:335-339.
Munson, P.J., and Rodbard, D., 1980, LIGAND: A versatile computerized
     approach for characterization of ligand binding systems,
     Anal. Biochem. 107:220-239.
Wieland, G.A., and Molinoff, P.B., 1981, Quantitative analysis of
     drug-receptor interactions: I. Determination of kinetic and
     equilibrium properties, Life Sci. 29:313-330.
Wieland, G.A., Wolfe, B.B., and Molinoff, P.B., 1981, Quantitative
     analysis of drug-receptor interactions: II. Determination of
     the properties of receptor subtypes, Life Sci. 29:427-443.

FUNCTION OF CREATINE KINASE LOCALIZATION IN MUSCLE CONTRACTION

S. Koons and R. Cooke

Dept. of Biochemistry & Biophysics and
Cardiovascular Research Institute
University of California, San Francisco
San Francisco, California 94143

Introduction

The creatine phosphate shuttle hypothesis, a central theme of
the Congress, suggests that mitochondrial creatine kinase (CK)
produces phosphocreatine (PCr) from ATP, that CK on or near the
sarcomere produces ATP from PCr, and that energy is shuttled from
mitochondria to the myofibrils via PCr. According to the
hypothesis the CK reaction is crucial to the control of
respiration and to the control of the microenvironment of the
contractile apparatus. The nucleotide concentrations in the
region of the myosin ATPase are thought to depend on the
localization of CK on the sarcomere (Bessman and Geiger, 1981).
Many studies have addressed the issue of CK localization on the
mitochondrial membrane, and of the effects of nucleotide and PCr
on oxidative respiration (Jacobus and Lehninger, 1973; Saks et
al., 1980). At the opposite end of the shuttle, the sarcomere,
there is evidence for CK localization on the M-line structure
(Turner et al., 1973). This result motivated several
investigations of CK interactions with myosin and with other
M-line proteins. Although some studies came to the intriguing
conclusion that CK binds to the head region of myosin, others
failed to confirm this observation (Houk and Putnam, 1973; Botts
et al., 1975; Mani et al., 1980; Woodhead and Lowey, 1983). The
possibility of a direct interaction of CK with the myosin head
suggests that the contractile mechanism may depend upon CK
binding, and thus upon the CK concentration. However, the
functional significance of the binding of CK to either myosin or

the M-line has not been previously explored by physiological measurements of fiber contraction.

Our work addresses the question of whether the tightly bound M-line CK provides ATP more effectively than does additional CK, which may be either soluble or weakly bound to the sarcomere. We measured the retained CK activity of glycerinated rabbit psoas fibers. These fibers retained approximately 3% of total CK following two weeks storage in 50% glycerol-rigor solution and subsequent washing in a rigor solution. This CK must be tightly bound within the protein matrix of the fibers and it is most probably the CK that has been shown to be localized at the M-line. The ability of this bound CK to provide ATP for contraction was compared to that of CK added to the medium bathing the fibers, as described below. Our data address two questions. Does the tightly bound CK provide a better ATP regeneration system than added CK, and does added CK bind to myosin and alter the contractile interaction?

At low ATP and high PCr, contractile velocity is limited by the availability of ATP (Cooke and Bialek, 1979). By measuring contractile velocity as a function of added CK, the dose-response curve can distinguish the effectiveness of intrinsic CK versus that of added CK at providing ATP for contraction. If CK binds to the myosin heads, we would expect ATP to be supplied more directly by that bound CK, than by soluble CK. If the bound CK is enmeshed in the M-line, then it may provide ATP less effectively than does soluble CK.

Methods

Bundles of rabbit psoas muscle were disected into 1-2mm bundles, tied to supports at rest length and incubated in 50% glycerol-rigor solution (0.12M KCl, 5mM $MgCl_2$, 5mM EGTA, 20mM TES, pH 7.0). Fibers were stored in the above solution at -20°C for up to 1 month. Individual fibers of diameters 50-90 μm and length 1cm were dissected for velocity measurements, which were conducted with a computer-controlled tensiometer described by Crowder and Cooke (1984). Fibers were immersed directly into an activating solution containing: 0.12M KCl, 5mM $MgCl_2$, 2mM EGTA, 1.6mM $CaCl_2$, 100μM ATP, 20mM PCr, and 20mM TES, pH 7.0. In this solution, contractile velocities were very low and slack-velocity measurements of maximum velocity were unreliable. Extrapolation of force velocity relations to zero tension to estimate the maximum contraction velocity were made, however the large curvature of some force-velocity relations introduced considerable error to the estimate of the maximum velocity. The most reliable comparison of fiber performance was obtained by using measurements

130

of the velocity at 10% of initial tension (V_{10}), using the tension clamp program of the tensiometer.

Experimental conditions for velocity measurements were chosen to best demonstrate the dependence of contraction on the CK ATP regeneration system. At 100μM ATP, no contractile velocity could be measured in the absence of PCr. 20mM PCr was employed for most measurements, to saturate the system. As in the experiments of Cooke and Bialek (1979) a small but measurable velocity was present with PCr, but no added CK.

Fiber CK activities were measured on single glycerinated fibers from the same batches used for velocity measurements. The fibers were washed for 5 min. in rigor solution, immersed in .5M KCl, 20mM TES, pH 7.6, and sonicated. The protein concentration of the muscle suspension was measured by the method of Bradford (1976), and the CK activity was measured by determination of the rate of ATP production using a luciferase-luciferin coupled assay at pH 7.6, and 25°C. By determining the volume of the fibers introduced into the assay, we could calculate the CK activity per unit volume inside the fibers.

Results

The glycerinated fiber system is a sensitive assay of the ability of CK to replenish ATP for contraction. Cooke and Bialek (1979) showed that fiber velocity is a linear function of ATP concentration at low ATP levels. As a control experiment, to demonstrate that CK was not limiting in their conditions, they measured fiber velocity as a function of CK in the fiber bath. The fibers retained sufficient CK to support contraction in the absence of added CK. Our present experiments take advantage of improved CK activity assays, to perform similar measurements, calibrated to internal CK activity rather than CK concentration in the surrounding solution.

To measure the intrinsic fiber CK, fibers were dissected to bundles of no more than five fibers, and washed for five minutes to ensure that CK was not carried into the assay from the glycerol-rigor solution. The activity of CK in a fiber suspension was assayed, as described in the methods section, giving an activity per mg of protein. With the measured fiber protein concentration of 210 mg/ml, the intrinsic fiber CK was determined. Measurements were stable over a period of one week, while the measured activity decayed significantly over several months due to slow loss or inactivation of CK. The fibers used in this study had been incubated in glycerol-rigor for two weeks. The activity of the intrinsic bound CK of these fibers used was 120 units/ml (1 unit = 1 μ mole ATP produced/min).

To determine to what extent added CK diffused into the fibers, assays of fiber CK activity were performed as a function of the time incubated in a solution containing CK. Fiber bundles of no more than 5 fibers were incubated in 500 units/ml CK, removed after 1, 3, 5 and 10 minutes, blotted on filter paper, suspended and assayed . At 3 minutes, the fiber CK activity per ml was about 50% of external. Within five minutes the activity/ml of the fibers had saturated at 70% of the solution CK. It is therefore clear that CK did diffuse into the fibers, and the 70% inclusion of CK was used in subsequent calculations of internal CK activity. These data argue that added CK does not bind strongly to the proteins of the sarcomere. Approximately 30% of the volume of the fibers is occupied by the proteins of the myofibril along with their hydration layers. Thus, the measured CK activity is close to that expected if little CK is bound to the myofibril and the concentration of CK in the aqueous region within the fiber is the same as that in the external solution. The rate of CK diffusion into fibers, may be compared to the time course of the increase in fiber velocities following addition of CK to the surrounding solution. Following addition of CK, both tension and contraction velocity increased over a period of 30-60 seconds. It is not clear why the increase in fiber performance occurs more quickly than the time for complete equilibration of the fiber interior with CK.

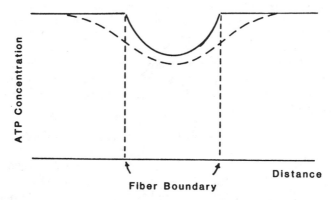

Figure 1: Fiber ATP profiles in stirred and unstirred solutions. The ATP concentration is shown as a function of distance from the center of the fiber. The fiber occupies the region between the two vertical dashed lines in the center of the figure. The solid line shows the ATP concentration calculated with the assumption that there is no significant unstirred layer at the fiber surface. The dashed curve shows how an extensive unstirred layer is expected to lower the ATP concentration within the fiber.

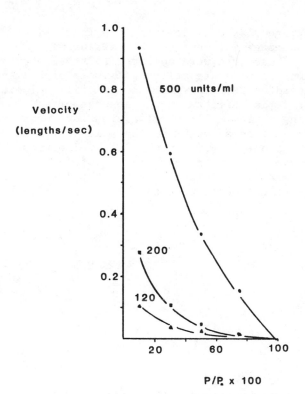

Figure 2: Force velocity relationships at different internal CK
activities. The velocity of contraction measured during isotonic
load clamps is shown as a function of the tension exerted by the
fiber. The lowest curve gives the velocities measured in the
absence of added CK. In this batch of fibers the activity of
retained CK was 120 units/ml (1 unit=1μmole/min). Addition of CK
to the medium to produce total internal concentrations given in
the figure increases the velocity of contraction. Each point
represents the mean of measurements from at least five fibers.
Omission of PCr resulted in no measurable velocity.

   Although the fiber bath was stirred, microscopically there
always exists an unstirred layer, which, if large, would alter the
interpretation of the results. In the presence of a large
unstirred layer, CK in the unstirred layer would affect the ATP
concentration at the fiber boundary and throughout the fiber,
replenishing ATP consumed by contraction. Figure 1 illustrates
ATP profiles in the presence and absence of the unstirred layer.
To test the significance of this effect under our experimental
conditions, we increased the unstirred layer by omitting stirring,

and decreased the unstirred layer by removing the incubation
solution from the tensiometer well and quickly measuring
contractile velocity. These data were compared to those obtained
in our normal conditions of moderate stirring. These experiments
were performed with no added CK because the contractile velocity
is most sensitive to stirring effects in the absence of an
external CK regenerating system. Fiber velocities were measured
in 100μM ATP, 20mM PCr, but no added CK. Fibers in unstirred
solutions averaged a decrease in V_{10} of only 10%, while those
removed from solution averaged an increase in V_{10} of only 6%. The
very small differences measured confirm that the unstirred layer
effect is small, and does not contribute to the effects of added
CK that we measured.

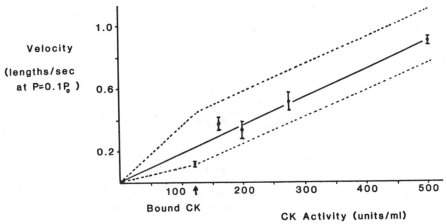

Figure 3: V_{10}, the velocity of contraction at 10% of maximum
tension is shown as a function of fiber CK activity. Error bars
represent the standard error of the mean for 5-10 measurements.
Omission of PCr, which eliminates all CK activity, results in very
low velocities, providing a point at the origin. All other
measurements were performed in 100μM ATP, 20mM PCr. The upper
dashed line represents the case where tightly bound CK is twice as
effective as soluble CK at ATP regeneration. The lower dashed
line represents the case in which soluble or weakly bound CK is
half as effective as tightly bound CK at supplying ATP. The
straight line represents the data expected if bound and soluble CK
are equally effective at supplying ATP to the contractile
proteins. The observed data shown in figure 3 is best fit by this
model.

    Figure 2 illustrates force-velocity relationships at
different CK activities. The velocity increases and the curvature
of the force-velocity relationship decreases as fiber CK is
increased. The contractile velocity at 10% of initial tension
(V_{10}) is plotted as a function of CK in Figure 3. Although there

is scatter in the data, the points are roughly linear, with the values for little or no added CK lying on the same line as those for greater concentrations. Data plotted are from a group of fibers incubated for two weeks in glycerol-rigor. A second batch of fibers incubated for the same time yielded comparable results.

Discussion

There is strong evidence for CK localization in the sarcomere, and this localization was expected to be reflected in the physiological measurements. The hypothetical dose-response profiles shown by the dashed lines of Figure 3 demonstrate two possibilities. If bound CK is more effective by a factor of two at promoting contraction, the top profile would result. Bound CK that is only half as effective as soluble CK would generate the lower curve, and a linear plot given by the solid line would reflect bound CK indistinguishable from soluble. Although there is some scatter in the data, there are no systematic deviations from a linear dependence of V_{10} on the CK content of the fiber. The data lie entirely within the dashed profiles representing the results expected for CK one half as effective or twice as affective as added CK. Therefore localization of CK affects its ability to regenerate ATP for the contractile interaction by less than a factor of two.

A great deal of energy has been invested in the technically difficult problem of measuring the binding of CK to muscle proteins. Our measurements of CK diffusion into fibers does not support the hypothesis that added CK binds to the protein array of the fiber. However if such binding does occur, any interaction of CK with the contractile apparatus results in little or no direct effect on the velocity of contraction. Although we cannot exclude the possibility on the basis of our results, it would be surprising if CK would bind directly to the myosin head, but not influence the mechanism of contraction.

Our results are especially relevant to those of Savabi et al. (1983). These investigators measured the rate of tension development and relaxation in large bundles of glycerinated rabbit psoas fibers, and showed that PCr contributed to both the contraction and relaxation of the fibers in the presence of 250μM ADP. They concluded that CK in the permeable fibers was localized near the myosin ATPase and was particularly effective in supplying ATP for the actomyosin interaction. Wallimann et al. (1984) have very recently shown that chicken myofibrils retain sufficient M-line CK to regenerate ATP consumed by the actin-activated Mg^{2+} ATPase. These workers also concluded that the localization of CK on the M-line was of physiological significance. In nonmuscle cells, the discovery of CK localization in the mitotic spindle

(Koons et al., 1982) led to the demonstration that CK could function to supply ATP for mitosis (Koons et al., 1982; Cande, 1983). These results again suggested that localization of CK on cytoskeletal proteins might be linked to function. The hypothesis that localization of CK makes it more effective at ATP regeneration, however, is not supported by the data presented here.

The M-line localization of CK is well established and, almost certainly, it was this CK that was retained by the glycerinated fibers. It remains uncertain whether its presence at the M-line is one of structural economy, but the CK retained by the fiber does not provide a special source of ATP for contraction. Our data suggest that models of energy transport should incorporate the shuttling of PCr and creatine between CK in two compartments: one localized in the mitochondria and a second which is either soluble or bound in the remaining cytoplasm. Localization of CK on elements within this cytoplasmic compartment does not play a significant role.

Acknowledgement

This work was supported by grants from the USPHS: HL-06707 to SK and HL32145, AM30868 and AM00479 to RC.

References

Bessman, S.P., and Geiger, P.J., 1981, Transport of energy in muscle: the phosphorylcreatine shuttle, Science, 211:448.
Botts, J., Stone, D.B., Wang, A.T.L., and Mendelson, R.A., 1975, Electron paramagnetic resonance and nanosecond fluorescence depolarization studies on creatine-phosphokinase interaction with myosin and its fragments, J. Supramol. Str., 3:141.
Bradford, M., 1976, Rapid and sensitive method for quantitation of microgram quantities of protein utilizing the principle of protein-dye binding, Anal. Biochem., 72:248.
Cande, W.Z., 1983, Creatine kinase role in anaphase chromosome movement, Nature 304:557.
Cooke, R., and Bialek, W., 1979, The contraction of glycerinated muscle fibers as a function of the ATP concentration, Biophys J., 28:241
Crowder, M.C., and Cooke, R., 1984, Effects of sulfhydryl modification on the mechanics of fiber contraction, J. Mus. Res. and Cell Mot., 5:131.
Houk, T.W., Jr., and Putnam, S.V., 1973, Location of creatine phosphokinase binding site of myosin, Biochem. Biophys. Res. Commun., 55:1271.
Jacobus, W.E., and Lehininger, A.L., 1973, Creatine kinase of rat heart mitochondria. Coupling of creatine phosphorylation to electron transport, J. Biol. Chem., 248:4803.
Koons, S.J., Eckert, B.S., and Zobel, C.R., 1982,

Immunofluorescence and inhibitor studies on creatine kinase and mitosis, Exp. Cell. Res., 140:401.

Mani, R.S., Herasymowych, O.S., and Kay, C.M., 1980, Physical, chemical and ultrastructural studies on muscle M-line proteins, Int. J. Biochem., 12:333.

Saks, V.A., Kupriyanov, V.V., Elizarova, G.V., and Jacobus, W.E., 1980, Studies of energy transport in heart cells. The importance of creatine kinase localization for the coupling of mitochondrial phosphorylcreatine production to oxidative phosphorylation, J. Biol. Chem., 255:755.

Savali, F., Geiger, P.J., and Bessman, S.P., 1983, Kinetic properties and functional role of creatine phosphokinase in glycerinated muscle fibers - further evidence for compartmentation, Biochem. Biophys. Res. Commun., 114:785.

Turner, D.C., Wallimann, T., and Eppenberger, H.M., 1973, A protein that binds specifically to the M-line of skeletal muscle is identified as the muscle form of creatine kinase, Proc. Natl. Acad. Sci. USA, 70:702.

Wallimann, T., Schlosser, T., and Eppenberger, H.M., 1984, Function of M-line bound creatine kinase as intramyofibrillar ATP regenerator at the receiving end of the phosphorylcreatine shuttle in muscle, J. Biol. Chem., 259:5238.

Woodhead, J.C., and Lowey, S., 1983, An in vitro study of the interactions of skeletal muscle M-protein and creatine kinase with myosin and its subfragments, J. Mol. Biol., 168:831.

ISOTOPE LABELING RATIOS:

A TOOL FOR THE EXPLORATION OF METABOLIC COMPARTMENTS

Joanne K. Kelleher and Robert T. Mallet

Department of Physiology
The George Washington University
Washington, D.C.

INTRODUCTION

Reports of metabolic compartmentation often stem from data viewed as unfortunate by the reporters. Namely, an investigation of a metabolic pathway by isotopic tracer techniques yields results incompatible with the starting assumption that a single pool of each metabolite is present in the system. Thus compartmentation is added so that the data are consistent. A reader offered a specific compartmentalized arrangement in the closing paragraphs of a paper may wonder what other possible compartmental arrangements might have been uncovered if, from the onset of the project, multiple compartments of each metabolite had been assumed. Our goal is to describe techniques for determining the information available from steady state isotopic tracer studies if we assume that multiple pools of each metabolite exist which mix when the system is analyzed. Essentially we assume that the specific radioactivity (SA) of metabolite pools cannot be determined by experiment. We are particularly interested in the application of these techniques to investigations of oxidative energy metabolism and pathways involving metabolic cycles. Our previous studies have focused on the TCA cycle (Kelleher, 1984; Mallet et al., 1984). In this area of metabolism, the presence of enzyme aggregates and a variety of compartments including mitochondrial and cytoplasmic spaces render the estimation rates from isotopic tracer studies especially perilous.

METHODS

Before proceeding to general questions of metabolic compartmentation we will review the methodology used in our laboratory

for calculating the SA of a metabolic pool and attacking problems
of isotope distribution in pathways where compartmentation of
metabolite pools may exist. This presentation is confined to systems in isotopic and metabolic steady state. Once steady state is
reached, the SA of any metabolic intermediates remains constant;
fluxes are constant, and the rate of accumulation of label in end
products is linear with time. Under these conditions the SA of
any pool, P, equals the labeled flux into P divided by the total
flux into P, or:

$$SA\ P\ =\ \frac{\sum\limits_{i=1}^{m} (Fpi\ SAi)}{\sum\limits_{i=1}^{m} Fpi} \qquad\qquad Eq.\ 1$$

where m is the number of pools inputing to pool, p, and Fpi equals
the flux from pool i to pool p. This equation has been used by
other investigators of intermediary metabolism including Heath
(1968). If the compound, P, is a precursor of compound, S, and is
the only labeled precursor of S the following relationship is also
available:

$$If\ P \rightarrow S \qquad\qquad SA\ P\ =\ \frac{SA\ S\ \sum\limits_{i=1}^{m} Fsi}{Fsp} \qquad\qquad Eq.\ 2$$

We find both forms of this relationship useful in assessing the
possibility of compartmentation within a steady state metabolic
system. Throughout this paper we use F1, F2, etc. to represent
fluxes and other uppercase letters to indicate various metabolites; symbols following letters indicate specific pools of the
metabolite.

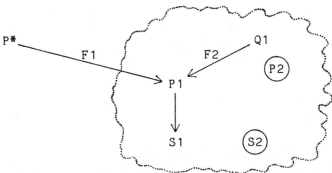

Fig. 1. * indicates a labeled metabolite added to the system enc-
losed in a membrane which contains the metabolic pathway
$Q \rightarrow P \rightarrow S$. F1 and F2 are fluxes.

Figure 1 illustrates a common experimental situation. A labeled
metabolite, P*, is added external to a membrane bound metabolic

system.   Since the system is   capable of synthesizing P,   isotope
dilution occurs and the SA S is   less than the SA P*,   the isotope
pool outside the membrane.   Often the investigator wishes to estimate the rate of synthesis of the end product, S,   using the relationship:

   rate of synthesis of S = rate of labeling of S / SA P1

which requires that the investigator determine the SA of P1,   the
pool of P which is the precursor of S1.   Because of the possible
existence of pool P2,   and the difficulty in separating pools P*
and P1,   inaccurate estimates may   occur.   Perhaps the best known
example of the situation displayed in Fig. 1 is gluconeogenesis.
Since endogenously produced oxaloacetate mixes with the oxaloacetate produced by pyruvate carboxylation,   rates of gluconeogenesis
based   of the SA of 3 carbon precurors of glucose necessarily
underestimates the   true rate.   Methods of correcting for this
effect have been proposed by Hetenyi (1982) and Radziuk (1982).

   Another   important   feature   of steady   state metabolism is
illustrated by Fig. 1. and Eq. 1.   When a labeled metabolite must
cross a memebrane to participate in a pathway, the dilution of the
SA of the labeled metabolite by endogenously synthesized metabolite is determined by the flux through the endogenous pool relative
to the movement of label across the membrane, not by the size of
the endogenous metabolite pool. From Eq. 1 we calculate, SA P1 =
SA P* F1/(F1+F2).   Thus,   the contribution of the endogenous pool
may be ignored only if F1 is known to be much greater than F2 or
the SA of S1 is measured and found to be approximately equal to SA
P*.   As an example, consider gluconeogenesis where the endogenous
oxaloacetate pool may be quite small and yet produce significant
isotope dilution because of the relatively large TCA cycle flux.

   The methodology described in this manuscript enables investigators to   identify "kinetically distinct" compartments which we
define as follows:

$$P \longleftarrow S1 \longleftrightarrow S2 \longrightarrow R$$

Two pools of a metabolite S,   S1 and S2,   occupy kinetically distinct compartments if the probability of efflux to any product of
S (P or   R) is not identical   for molecules in either pool of S.
Alternatively, if these two   pools exchange material with each
other so rapidly that the probability of flux to any product is
the same for molecules in both pools, the pools are not kinetically distinct.   Using this definition,   it is possible that two
pools in physically distinct compartments such as cytoplasm and
mitochondria will comprise only one "kinetically distinct" compartment.   And,   it is also possible that kinetically distinct

pools will be found for which no structural basis of compartmentation exists.

An interesting feature of metabolic pathways is that metabolites often travel around in circles whether they be metabolically important ones such as the TCA cycle or the urea cycle, futile cycles such as pyruvate → oxaloacetate → PEP → pyruvate, or simply reversible reactions. Although these events complicate the interpretation of tracer metabolite studies, they also provide an opportunity to obtain information about these cycles. Our method for accommodating such cycles is described as follows:

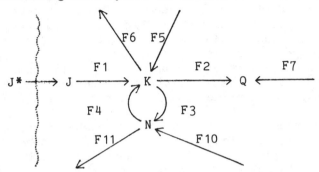

Fig. 2. Hypothetical flux path containing loop.

Consider as a model the flux path shown in Figure 2 where labeled J is added to the system in metabolic and isotopic steady state. To write an expression for the SA of Q in terms of the SA of J we write a series of equations proceeding backwards from Q to J, using Eq. 1 to determine the SA of each pool.

SA Q = SA K x F2/(F2+F7)

SA K = [SA J x F1/(F1+F4+F5)] + [SA K x F3/(F3+F10) x F4/(F1+F4+F5)]

   let L = F3/(F3+F10) x F4/(F1+F4+F5)

$$\text{SA K} = \frac{\text{SA J x F1}}{(1-L)(F1+F4+F5)}$$ therefore,

$$\text{SA Q} = \frac{\text{SA J x F1 x F2}}{(1-L)(F1+F4+F5)(F2+F7)}$$ Eq 3.

Note that the term, 1-L, appears in the final two equations to account for flux through the loop K → N → K. The term, L, actually equals the probability at any moment that a molecule in pool K will travel around this route rather than any of the other exit paths from pool K such as F6 or F2 or F3, F11. Of course, if a molecule travels this route and returns to pool K, it once again will have the chance to flow through any of the paths leading from pool K. Thus, the cumulative effect of loop L on the SA of pool K is described by a convergent geometric series which approaches the value 1/(1–L). Using this procedure to write equations for the SA of each pool enables us to avoid the tormenting task of repeatedly calculating flux around the cycle (Exton and Park, 1967).

COMPARTMENTATION – A GENERALIZED CASE

To apply these methods to the analysis of compartmentalized metabolic pathways, consider the models described by Figures 3a and 3b. Two pathways, A $\longrightarrow$ B and D $\longrightarrow$ E, share a common chemical intermediate, C. If the ratio of the amount of each product (B:E) formed from the first precursor (A) is not identical to the ratio of the amount of each product formed from the second precursor (D), kinetically distinct pools of the intermediate are indicated as shown in Figure 3b.

3a)   3b)

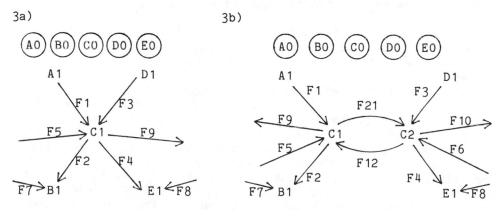

Fig. 3. Models used to test the hypothesis that metabolite C is compartmentalized into two pools, C1 and C2, which are precursors of the products, B and E. Encircled metabolite pools represent pools of each metabolite which do not participate in the pathways indicated by the arrows.

Figure 3 contains the essential features of metabolic systems where little a priori information about metabolic compartments is assumed. Pools of each metabolite are included which, even in steady state, never label. Isotope dilution may occur in each limb of the pathway. Material may enter or leave intermediate pools (C1 and C2) by fluxes (F5, F6, F9, F10) which cannot be measured; therefore, expressions equating the steady state influx and efflux are not available. We do assume that the ammount of label in metabolites B, C and E can be measured in steady state in the presence of labeled A or D. Although an actual pathway may contain more pools between precursor and product or additional fluxes into and out of each pool, it may still conform to either Model 3a or 3b and be affected by the limitations which apply to these two models. Determining if a system conforms to Model 3a or 3b requires two separate experiments using a medium of identical chemical composition but containing different tracers. Using Fig. 3 as a model, we expose the system to labeled A or labeled D and measure the steady state dpm in both products, B and E. If the ratio, dpm B : dpm E, does not vary with the choice of label, no evidence of compartmentation of the metabolite C appears and the model shown as Figure 3a is appropriate. It is equally appropriate to compare the ratios:

dpm Ba : dpm Bd and dpm Ea : dpm Ed

where a and d are used to designate results with labeled A and D respectively. This latter method has been used by others to indicate metabolic compartmentation (Blum, 1978; Katz and Rognstad, 1978). Using either method of ratio comparison, if the two ratios are not equal, kinetically distinct pools of the common intermediate are indicated as shown in Figure 3b.

We now consider the question: What information about the system can be obtained if these ratios are not equal? First, consider what cannot be determined from this type of steady state analysis. Direct fluxes between metabolic intermediates, C1 and C2 cannot be determined. This limitation is serious since the answer to a basic question such as: Is there net synthesis of E from A? requires that the difference between F12 and F21 is known. In this example, the answer is yes if F21 > F12. However, with steady state analysis we can obtain a value for a term which indicates the extent to which the two pathways are interconnected. Specifically, we can determine the value of relative flux between the pools C1 and C2; which equals F21/(F3+F6+F21) x F12/(F1+F5+F12). Let L equal the product of these two fractions which is the probability of flux between the two pools of C. To derive an expression for the experimental determination of L, we first write equations for the SA of each product pool. If A is the tracer in the system, let (SA B1a) and (SA E1d) equal the SA of the product pools; thus:

$$(SA\ B1a) = \frac{(SA\ A1a)\ F1\quad F2}{(F1+F5+F12)(F2+F7)(1-L)} \qquad Eq.\ 4$$

$$(SA\ E1a) = \frac{(SA\ A1a)\ F1\quad F21\quad F4}{(F1+F5+F12)(F3+F6+F21)(F4+F8)(1-L)} \qquad Eq.\ 5$$

The comparable equations when D is the source of label are:

$$(SA\ B1d)\ =\ \frac{(SA\ D1d)\ F3\quad F12\quad F2}{(F3+F6+F21)(F1+F5+F12)(F2+F7)(1-L)} \qquad Eq.\ 6$$

$$(SA\ E1d)\ =\ \frac{(SA\ D1d)\ F3\quad F4}{(F3+F6+F21)(F4+F8)(1-L)} \qquad Eq.\ 7$$

Combining Eqs. 4, 5, 6, and 7 yields:

$$\frac{SA\ E1a}{SA\ B1a}\ x\ \frac{SA\ B1d}{SA\ E1d}\ =\ \frac{F21}{(F3+F6+F21)}\ \frac{F12}{(F1+F5+F12)}\ =\ L \qquad Eq.\ 8$$

However, the four SA terms on the left in Eq. 8 cannot be obtained experimentally due to the possibility of unlabeled pools of each product. If SA Be = experimentally measured SA of metabolite B, note that:

$$SA\ Be\ =\ dpm\ B1/(moles\ B1\ +\ moles\ B0)$$

while $\quad SA\ B1\ =\ dpm\ B1/moles\ B1$

But, by substituting the relationship above for all SA terms in Eq. 8 we obtain:

$$\frac{dpm\ Ea}{dpm\ Ba}\ x\ \frac{dpm\ Bd}{dpm\ Ed}\ =\ \frac{F21}{(F3+F6+F21)}\ x\ \frac{F12}{(F1+F5+F12)}\ =\ L \qquad Eq.\ 9$$

Now all four terms on the left can be determined experimentally and the value of L calculated. If the value of L approaches 1, the flux between pools is large and the system collapses to the model described in Figure 3a. At the opposite extreme, if the value of dpm Ea = 0, F21 = 0 and if dpm Bd = 0, F12 = 0 (within the detection limits of the labeling procedure). But what can be learned about the system when L is greater than 0 but less than 1? Obviously, the minimum possible value for either term, F12/(F1+F5+F12) or F21/(F3+F6+F21), is L while the maximum value of either fraction is 1. Figure 4 demonstrates the relationship between these two fractions. Thus, if L is large, the value of L is limited to a small range of values. However, if L is small, the range of possible values for each fraction is limited only slightly by this calculation.

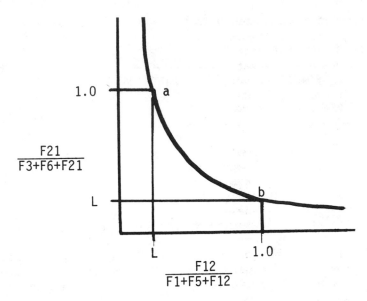

Fig. 4. Graph of possible values of each fraction comprising probability of flux between pools C1 and C2. Value of L limits the value of each fraction to the curve between points a and b.

What is the value of determining L if one cannot determine either net flux between the two pools or the value of the two fractions plotted in Figure 4 ? Suppose an investigator wishes to determine whether transamination of alanine to pyruvate occurs in the cytoplasmic or mitochondrial space. Although most glutamate pyruvate transaminase activity is cytoplasmic, mitochondrial transamination has been suggested based on the effects of a drug which blocks transport of pyruvate across the mitochondrial membrane (Mendes-Mourao, et al., 1975). The investigator interested in this problem might set up an experimental model based on Figure 3b. Let glucose represent compound A which is metabolized to the cytoplasmic pools of pyruvate (C1) and lactate (B1). (B). Let alanine represent compound D which we hypothesize is metabolized to the mitochondrial pyruvate (pool C2) and the acetate derived carbons of citrate (pool E1). Exposing the system to labeled glucose or alanine will result in labeled citrate and lactate. Of course, we are not surprised to find some labeled citrate when the system is provided with labeled glucose and some labeled lactate when the system is provided with labeled alanine (even if all alanine transamination is mitochondrial) because pyruvate will cross the mitochondrial membrane. However, determining the value of L, as indicated in Eq. 9, may provide information about the site of alanine transamination. A value for L of less than 1.0 indicates that all alanine transamination does not occur in the same compartment as glycolysis; presumably then, some transamination is mitochondrial. A value for L of 1.0 indicates either that alanine transamination does take place in the same compartment as glycolysis or that flux between the two pyruvate pools is so rapid that model 3a (and not 3b) is appropriate for this experimental system. Thus, Eq. 9 may be useful in specific experimental situations. However, it is important to note that the procedure described above is valid only for an experimental system which conforms to model 3b.

Another useful piece of information obtained from analysis of the generalized pathway shown as Figure 3b is a series of mathematical expressions for determining the dpm in each of two pools of the same metabolite (C1 and C2) in a system conforming to the model presented as Figure 3b. To utilize these expressions in an experimental system, an investigator need measure only the steady state dpm present in each of three compounds, B, C, and E, in two samples which are identical except that A is the source of label in one sample, D in the other. Physical separation of the two pools, C1 and C2, is not required. The derivation of these expressions is as follows: Recall that metabolite C may be located in any of the 3 pools, C1, C2 or C0, which mix together on isolation. Label, however, is present only in pools C1 and C2. Let mC1 and mC2 equal the amount, in moles, of each pool, C1 and C2, present in the experimental sample. When A is the label source, the sample's total dpm in compound C (dpm Ca) is:

dpm Ca = dpm C1a + dpm C2a

dpm Ca = (SA C1a) mC1 + (SA C2a) mC2   or

dpm Ca = (SA C2a)mC1(F3+F6+F21)/F21 + (SA C2a)mC2   Eq. 10

(SA C2a) mC2 = dpm Ca - (SA C2a) mC1 (F3+F6+F21)/F21   Eq. 11

When two sources of label are used, the relationship between the specific activities of the pool of compound C which is the precursor for compound E, C2, is:

(SA C2d)/(SA C2a) = (SA Ed)/(SA Ea)   or,

(SAC2d) = (SA C2a) (dpm Ed)/(dpm Ea)   Eq. 12

Likewise,   (SAC1d) = (SA C1a) (dpm Bd)/(dpm Ba)   Eq. 13

When D is the source of label, total dpm in pool C (dpmCd) is:

(dpm Cd) = (SA C1d) mC1 + (SAC2d) mC2   Eq. 14

substituting Eq. 12 and Eq. 13 into Eq. 14 yields:

$$\text{dpm Cd} = \frac{(SA\ C1a)\ mC1\ (dpm\ Bd)}{(dpm\ Ba)} + \frac{(SA\ C2a)\ mC2\ (dpm\ Ed)}{(dpm\ Ea)} \qquad \text{Eq. 15}$$

From Eq. 1, the relationship, (SA C2a) = (SA C1a) F21/(F3+F6+F21) is obtained and substituted into Eq. 15 yielding Eq. 16 (below)

$$\text{dpm Cd} = \frac{(SA\ C2a)\ mC1\ (F3+F6+F21)(dpm\ Bd)}{F21\ (dpm\ Ba)} + \frac{(SA\ C2a)\ mC2\ (dpm\ Ed)}{(dpm\ Ea)}$$

substituting Eq. 11 into Eq. 16 produces Eq. 17 (below)

$$\frac{(SA\ C2a)mC1(F3+F6+F21)}{F21} = \frac{dpm\ Ba[(dpm\ Cd)(dpm\ Ea)-(dpm\ Ca)(dpm\ Ed)]}{(dpm\ Bd)(dpm\ Ea) - (dpm\ Ba)(dpm\ Ed)}$$

Notice that the left side of Eq. 17 equals the contribution of pool C1a (dpm C1a) to the total dpm Ca as described in Eq. 10. Equally important, the right side of Eq. 17 contains only terms which can be found experimentally without separating pools C1 and C2. Thus, dpm C1a is found from Eq. 17. If the total dpm in compound C (dpm Ca) is measured experimentally, the value of dpm C2a can be determined from Eq. 11. Knowing the value of dpm C1a and dpm C2a, the value of dpm C1d and dpm C2d may be found using Eq. 12 and Eq. 13.

What is the value of knowing dpm C1a, dpm C2a, dpm C1d and dpm C2d since we cannot differentiate between a large pool of low SA and a small pool of high SA? Using these expressions to calculate the dpm in each pool of C may be useful in the evaluating the effectiveness of experimental techniques which aim to separate two endogenous pools of the same compound, C1 and C2. Current methods for the physical separation of cytoplasmic and mitochondrial metabolite pools include freeze-stop homogenization in non aqueous media (Soboll, et al., 1979) and the digitonin and cell cavitation procedure (Zuurendonk, et al., 1979). Proponents of both methods recommend the use of marker enzymes or added labeled compounds which remain in the "cytoplasmic" compartment to assess the effectiveness of the procedures in separating metabolite pools from these two compartments. We suggest that investigators might also evaluate these techniques by including tracers and comparing the values for dpm C1 and dpm C2 found with these experimental techniques to the values predicted from the equations above. The principle advantage in using the equations is that this theoretical method does not assume that metabolites follow the same distribution pattern as enzymes. A potential disadvantage is that not all pathways conform to the model (Figure 3b).

CONCLUSIONS

   We have described the information available, and some that is
not available, when two simple, interconnected pathways are analyzed, assuming the SA of each metabolite cannot be measured (Fig.
3b). Our major conclusions are that one can determine (1) the
product of the relative fluxes between the two pools, L, and (2)
the amount of label in each of the two pools which interconnect
the pathways. We cannot determine net flux between the two pathways. Mathematical expressions derived from the model (Figure 3b)
may be useful in evaluating experimental techniques for separating
metabolic pools and in resolving questions concerning the location
of specific enzyme reactions. In developing these techniques we
do not wish to imply criticism of isotopic techniques based on
different assumptions or direct measurements of pool sizes and
fluxes. In dealing with real systems we need to collect many
pieces of information so that the conclusions we draw are derived
from as large a data base as possible. As a final note, we offer

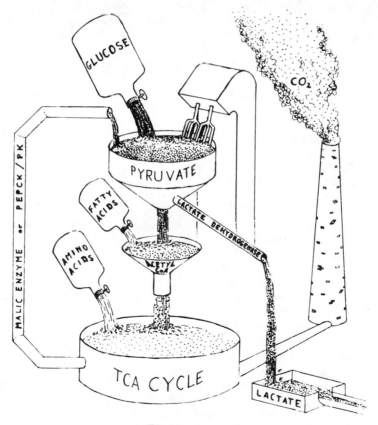

Figure 5.

149

Figure 5 as a reminder of the complexity of well known pathways and the challenges isotopic labeling patterns still present.

Acknowledgment: This research was supported by NIH S01-RR-5359-22. to J.K.K. and a GWU Medical School Graduate Scholarship to R.T.M.

REFERENCES

Blum, J.J. 1978. Influence of metabolic compartmentation on the quantitative analysis of intermediary metabolism, in: dMicroenvironments and Metabolic Compartmentation,d R. Estabrook and P. Srere, ed., Academic, New York.

Exton, J.H, and C.R. Park. 1967. Control of gluconeogenesis in liver: I. General features of gluconeogenesis in the perfused livers of rats. J. Biol. Chem., 242: 2622.

Heath, D.F. 1968. Redistribution of carbon label by reactions involved in glycolysis, gluconeogensis, and the tricarboxylic acid cycle in rat liver. Biochem. J., 110: 313.

Hetenyi, G., Jr. 1982. Correction for the metabolic exchange of 14C for 12C atoms in the pathway of gluconeogenesis in vivo, Fed. Proc. 41: 104.

Katz, J. and R. Rognstad. 1978. Compartmentation of glucose metabolism in liver, in: dMicroenvironments and Metabolic Compartmentation,d R. Estabrook and P. Srere, ed., Academic, New York.

Kelleher, J.K. 1984. Analysis of the tricarboxylic acid cycle using citrate 14C specific activity ratios, Am. J. Physiol., (in press).

Mallet, R.T., J.K. Kelleher, and M.J. Jackson. 1984. Substrate metabolism by rat jejunal epithelium: The role of glutamine. Fed. Proc., 43: 446.

Mendes-Mourao, J., A.P. Halestrap, D.M. Crisp, and C.I. Pogson. 1975. The involvement of mitochondrial pyruvate transport in the pathways of gluconeogenesis from serine and alanine in isolated rat and mouse liver cells. FEBS Letters 53: 29.

Radziuk, J. 1982. Sources of carbon in hepatic glycogen synthesis during absorption of an oral glucose load in humans, Fed. Proc. 41: 110.

Soboll, S.,R. Elbers, and H.W. Heldt. 1979. Metabolite measurements in mitochondria and in the extramitochondrial compartment by fractionation of freeze-stopped liver tissue in nonaqueous media. Methods in Enzymol. 56: 201.

Zuurendonk, P.F., M.E. Tischler, T.P.M. Akerboom, R. Van Der Meer, J.R. Williamson, and J.M. Tager. 1979. Rapid separation of particulate and soluble fractions from isolated cell preparations (Digitonin and cell cavitation procedures). Methods in Enzymol. 56: 207.

THE MITOCHONDRIAL CREATINE PHOSPHOKINASE IS

ASSOCIATED WITH INNER MEMBRANE CARDIOLIPIN

Michele Müller, Dominique Cheneval
and Ernesto Carafoli

Laboratory of Biochemistry
Swiss Federal Institute
of Technology (ETH)
8092 Zurich, Switzerland

INTRODUCTION

Inorganic phosphate (P_i) and negatively charged SH-group reagents solubilize the membrane bound mitochondrial creatine phosphokinase (m-CPK) into the medium (1,2). The rebinding of the solubilized m-CPK to the inner mitochondrial membrane is inhibited by adriamycin, a drug widely used in cancer chemotherapy, (3). Adriamycin binds specifically to mitochondrial cardiolipin (4,5) and has been found to inhibit the activity of cardiolipin-dependent proteins, such as cytochrome c oxidase and the phosphate transport protein (6-8). It has been proposed that m-CPK and the ADP/ATP translocator form a tightly coupled functional complex (9,10). The proposal, however, is not universally accepted (11). In this report we present evidence that m-CPK binds to membrane-associated cardiolipin in a reaction that is inhibited by adriamycin in mitochondria as well as in liposomes.

EXPERIMENTAL PROCEDURES

Membranes and protein preparation

Rat heart mitochondria were isolated as described by Crompton et al. (12) using a medium containing 210 mM mannitol, 70 mM sucrose, 0.1 mM EDTA and enough KOH to adjust the pH to 7.4 (buffer A). Mitochondria were isolated freshly for each experiment. Phospholipid vesicles were prepared from mixtures of dried phospholipids dissolved in 22 mM manitol, 7 mM sucrose, 10 mM Hepes and enough KOH to raise the pH to 7.4 (Buffer B). The lipids were sonicated continuously with a Branson sonifier B-13 for 2 min at 4°C under a N₂ stream at 70 W output. The solution was centrifuged for 60 min at 150,000 xg and the pellet was resuspended in buffer B. m-CPK was isolated from rat heart mitochondria according to the method of Font et al. (1) slightly modified as follows: 80 µl rotenone (0.5 mg/ml), 80 µl oligomycin (1 mg/ml) and 160 µl carboxyatractylate 1 mg/ml) were added to 20 mg of mitochondria suspended in 2.7 ml of Na pi pH 7.2. After 15 min incubation at 10°C the suspension was centrifuged for 7 min at 12,000 xg. The supernatant was again centrifuged for 60 min at 150,000 xg, and the resulting supernatant was then used for activity measurements and binding experiments after a 10-fold dilution with doubly distilled water. m-CPK was released from mitochondria according to the procedure described by Font et al. (1).

Binding of m-CPK to mitochondria and to phospholipid vesicles

The mitochondrial pellet resulting from the first centrifugation after the incubation with mersalyl was used for rebinding experiments. Adriamycin was added to this pellet resuspended in buffer B in the presence of the corresponding supernatant, diluted 10-fold with doubly distilled water containing the m-CPK. The mixture was incubated for 15 min at 10°C and centrifuged 7 min at 18,000 xg. The supernatant was analyzed for m-CPK activity and for protein content and composition.

To test the binding of additional m-CPK to inner mitochondrial membranes, increasing amounts of m-CPK preparation were added to 1 mg of untreated mitochondria resuspended in buffer B in a final volume of 0.5 ml. After incubation for 15 min at 10°C, the solution was centrifuged for 10 min at 12,000 xg and the m-CPK activity was measured in the supernatant.

To test the binding of m-CPK to liposomes, about 300 µl of m-CPK preparation (∿ 250 µg protein/ml) were added to 2 mg of phospholipid vesicles suspended in 160 µl of buffer B and the final volume was adjusted to 0.5 ml with buffer B. The suspension was incubated for 30 min at 10°C and centrifuged for 60 min at 150,000 xg. The supernatant was analyzed for m-CPK activity.

Activity measurements and analytical methods

m-CPK activity was assayed spectrophotometrically by the coupled enzyme system using 550-366 nm as the wavelength couple in an Aminco DW-2a Spectrophotometer. The solution contained 250 mM sucrose, 10 mM Hepes and enough KOH to adjust the pH to 7.4, 1 mM Mg Cl₂, 0.2 mM NADH, 0.5 mM phosphoenolpyruvate, 1 U lactatedehydrogenase/ml, 1 U pyruvate kinase/ml and 0.5 mM ATP. The reaction was started by the addition of creatine (4.8 mM final concentration) in the presence of the m-CPK.

The protein concentration was determined by a biuret procedure or by the method of Bradford (14). In both cases bovine serum albumin was used as standard.

Sodium dodecyl sulfate polyacrylamide gel electrophoresis was performed according to a slight modification of the method of Laemmli (15) described by Müller et al. (16). The gels were stained with Coomassie blue.

MATERIALS

Phosphatidylcholine and phosphatidylethanolamine, grade I, were purchased from Lipid Products, Surrey, England; cardiolipin from Sigma, St. Louis, MO, USA; mannitol and sucrose from BDH Chemicals Ltd., Poole, England. Adriamycin was a generous gift of Farmitalia-Carlo Erba, Milano, Italy.

RESULTS AND DISCUSSION

The treatment of mitochondria with Pi released to the medium a number of proteins, among which m-CPK was by far the most abundant. This can be judged by sodium dodecylsulfate polyacrylamide gel electrophoresis (SDS-PAGE). Pi-released preparations had a specific activity of about 15 µmoles creatine-phosphate synthesized/mg/min. When added back to intact or Pi-(or mersalyl-) treated mitochondria m-CPK rebound to the inner mitochondrial membrane. In the presence of 250 nmoles adriamycin/mg mitochondrial protein, the rebinding was inhibited completely. The inhibition was specific for m-CPK, as judged by SDS-PAGE. Other proteins present in the m-CPK preparation were always found in the supernatant at the end of the rebinding experiment regardless of the presence of adriamycin. Adriamycin per se failed to release m-CPK activity from mitochondria.

Intact mitochondria incubated with m-CPK were able to bind approximately twice the amount of m-CPK originally present in them. This indicates that the inner mitochondrial membrane contains additional binding receptors for m-CPK which are normally not occupied by it.

Binding experiments carried out with unilamellar vesicles composed of phosphatidylcholine bound some m-CPK, but vesicles composed of phosphatidylcholine/cardiolipin bound much more of it (Table 1). Addition of adriamycin to the phosphatidylcholine/cardiolipin vesicles prior to the incubation with m-CPK, inhibited its binding to the membranes up to 80%. This indicates that m-CPK is associated with membrane-bound cardiolipin of the inner mitochondrial membrane.

153

Table 1. Binding of the mitochondrial creatine phosphokinase
to phospholipid vesicles

Phospholipids	activity recovered in the supernatant %
control without phospholipids	100
phosphatidylcholine[a]	57
phosphatidylcholine/cardiolipin[a] (3:1)[b]	0.2
phosphatidylcholine/phosphatidylethanolamine/ cardiolipin[a] (4:3.5:2.5)[b]	0
phosphatidylcholine[a] + adriamycin[c]	74
phosphatidylcholine[a]/cardiolipin[a] (3:1) + adriamycin[c]	81
phosphatidylcholine/phosphatidylethanolamine/ cardiolipin[a] (4:3.5:2.5)[b] + adriamycin	72

[a] Total phospholipid concentration: 10 mg/ml
[b] Weight ratios
[c] Adriamycin concentration: 100 nmoles /mg lipid

The ADP/ATP translocator has been considered as a possible
binding receptor for m-CPK. However, the following findings mili-
tate against their possibility. Carboxyatractylate, a very specific
inhibitor of the ADP/ATP translocator which binds to it through
ionic interactions from the cytoplasmic side of the protein, does
not release m-CPK to the medium under hypotonic conditions (necessary to make the outer membrane permeable to m-CPK). The translocator and m-CPK are both basic proteins, making their (ionic) interaction unlikely. The specific activity of m-CPK in intact mitochondria is about 10-15 times higher than that of the ADP/ATP translocator. Considering that almost all of the ATP produced by mitochondria is used to phosphorylate creatine, and that m-CPK will
diffuse on the membrane much rapidly than the ADP/ATP translocator
in the membrane, a fixed complex between the two proteins seems
improbable.

REFERENCES

1. B. Font, C. Vial, D. Goldschmidt, D. Eichenberger, and
    D.C. Gautheron, Heart mitochondrial creatine kinase
    solubilization, Arch. Biochem. Biophys. 212, 195:203
    (1981).
2. B. Font, C. Vial, D. Goldschmidt, D. Eichenberger, and
    D.C. Gautheron, Effect of SH-Group reagents on creatine
    kinase interaction with mitochdonrial membrane, Arch.
    Biochem. Biophys. 220, 541:548 (1983).
3. R.A. Newman, M.P. Hacker, and M.A. Fagan, Adriamycin media-
    ted inhibition of creatinephosphokinase binding to heart
    mitochondria, Biochem. Pharm. 31, 109:111 (1980).
4. E. Goormaghtigh, P. Chatelain, J. Caspers, and J.M.
    Ruysschaert, Evidence of a specific complex between
    adriamycin and negatively charged phospholipids, Bio-
    chim. Biophys. Acta 597, 1:14 (1980).
5. M. Müller, D. Cheneval, R. Toni, S. Ruetz, and E. Carafoli,
    Adriamycin as a probe for the transversal distribution
    of cardiolipin in the inner mitochondrial membrane,
    submitted.
6. E. Goormaghtigh, R. Brasseur, and J.M. Ruysschaert, Adria-
    mycin inactivates cytochrome c oxidase by exclusion of
    the enzyme from its cardiolipin essential environment,
    Biochem. Biophys. Res. Comm. 104, 314:320 (1982).
7. D. Cheneval, M. Müller, and E. Carafoli, The mitochondrial
    phosphate carrier reconstituted in liposomes is inhibi-
    ted by doxorubicin, FEBS Lett. 159, 123:126 (1983).
8. M. Müller, D. Cheneval, and E. Carafoli, Doxorubicin inhi-
    bits the phosphate transport protein reconstituted in
    liposomes: a study on the mechanism of the inhibition,
    Eur. J. Biochem., in press.
9. V.A. Saks, V.V. Kupriyanov, G.V. Elizarova, and W.E.
    Jacobus, Studies of energy transport in heart cells,
    J. Biol. Chem. 255, 755:763 (1980).
10. R.W. Moreadith, and W.E. Jacobus, Creatine kinase of heart
    mitochondria, J. Biol. Chem. 257, 899:905 (1982).
11. K.K. Vandergaer, and W.E. Jacobus, Evidence against direct
    transfer of the adenine nucleotides by the heart mito-
    chondrial creatine-kinase-adenine nucleotide translo-
    case complex, Biochem. Biophys. Res. Comm. 109, 442:448
    (1982).
12. M. Crompton, M. Capano, and E. Carafoli, The sodium induced
    efflux of calcium from heart mitochondria, Eur. J. Bio-
    chem. 69, 453:462 (1976).

13. A.G. Gornall, G.J. Bardawill, and M.M. David, Determination of serum protein by means of the Biuret Reaction, J. Biol. Chem. <u>177</u>, 751:766 (1949).

14. M. Bradford, A rapid and sensitive method for the quantities of protein utilizing the principles of protein-dye binding, Anal. Biochem. <u>72</u>, 248:254 (1976).

15. U.K. Laemmli, Cleavage of structural proteins during the assembly of the head of Bacterioplage T4, Nature (London) <u>227</u>, 680:685 (1970).

16. M. Müller, J. Krebs, R.J. Cherry, and S. Kawato, Selective labeling and rotational diffusion of the ADP/ATP translocator in the inner mitochondrial membrane, J. Biol. Chem. <u>257</u>, 1117:1120 (1982).

A ROLE FOR MITOCHONDRIA IN MYOCARDIAL ADENOSINE PRODUCTION

Richard D. Bukoski, Harvey V. Sparks and
Leena M. Mela-Riker*

Department of Physiology, Michigan State
University, East Lansing, MI 48824 and
*Department of Surgery, Oregon Health
Sciences University, Portland, OR 97201

INTRODUCTION

It is now generally accepted that the purine nucleoside, adenosine, is a potent modulator of cardiac function. For instance, adenosine probably participates in the regulation of coronary blood flow (Berne and Rubio, 1979) and Bellardinelli et al (1982) have demonstrated that adenosine decreases the rate of sinoatrial node depolarization and the rate of conduction through the atrioventricular node. Schrader et al (1977) have shown that adenosine decreases cyclic AMP mediated increases in inotropy caused by isoproterenol treatment. Finally, it has been shown that adenosine limits norepinephrine release from sympathetic nerve endings (Verhaege, 1978). It is possible that during periods of increased oxygen demand or mild ischemia, adenosine may cause an increase in coronary blood flow to meet the increased oxygen demand. Under more severe periods of anoxia or ischemia, adenosine may have negative inotropic and chronotropic effects, reducing myocardial oxygen needs and thus having a protective effect. A similar mechanism of action for the cardioprotective effect of calcium channel blockers has recently been proposed (Cheung et al, 1984).

Unfortunately, our knowledge of the subcellular source of adenosine and the exact trigger of its production and release is incomplete. Berne (1980) has proposed that as the rate of ATP hydrolysis increases, there is an increase in ADP and concomitantly in AMP, through the adenylate kinase equilibrium. AMP is then thought to be dephosphorylated (forming adenosine) and simultaneously transported out of the cell by an ecto-5'-nucleotidase in the cell membrane (Frick and Lowenstein, 1978).

157

The vectorial transport was proposed because of the high adenosine deaminase activity and the low K_m of adenosine kinase for adenosine in the cytosol of cardiac muscle (Rubio and Berne, 1975).

Subsequently Olsson et al (1982) have demonstrated that adenosine is present within the myocardium, perhaps bound to the adenosine binding protein, S-adenosylhomocysteine hydrolase (SAH hydrolase). Similarly, Schutz et al (1981), provided evidence that during hypoxia in isolated perfused guinea pig hearts, adenosine is formed intracellularly and is subsequently transported out of the cell across the cell membrane. In addition, Schrader et al (1981), have been able to decrease adenosine release from isolated perfused guinea pig hearts during hypoxia by infusing homocysteine thiolactone. Homocysteine thiolactone is thought to drive newly formed adenosine into SAH within the cell.

Finally, there is circumstantial evidence that adenosine may be formed from the pool of AMP resulting from the action of phosphodiesterase on cellular cAMP (Schrader et al, 1976). For example, the increase in adenosine release caused by catecholamines is greater than that caused by increased heart rate or afterload (Manfredi and Sparks, 1982) and adenosine release in response to catecholamine infusion is phasic (DeWitt et al, 1983), as is the elevation in cAMP (Clark et al, 1982).

Taken together, the above studies support the view that there is at least one store of adenosine within the cell and that there may be at least three intracellular pathways for the production of adenosine: (1) ATP $\rightarrow$ ADP $\rightarrow$ AMP $\rightarrow$ ADO, (2) SAH $\rightarrow$ ADO and (3) ATP $\rightarrow$ cAMP $\rightarrow$ ADO. They also indicate that the flux through each of these pathways can be increased, in response to a specific class of stimuli.

In an effort to identify a subcellular site of adenosine production, related to oxygen supply and demand, we examined isolated rat heart mitochondria to determine if they produce adenosine (Bukoski et al, 1983). This work was stimulated by (1) the fact that mitochondria are the site of oxygen consumption within the cell and as such may serve as cellular "oxygen sensors" (see also Wilson et al, 1978); (2) the finding that greater than 90% of the AMP within the cell is associated with the mitochondrial fraction (Bunger et al, 1983) and (3) the work of Nuutinen et al (1982,1983) which indicates that mitochondria may play a role in the regulation of coronary blood flow.

We found that there is a time dependent production (or release) of adenosine by isolated mitochondria and this production (or release) is inhibited by conversion from state 4 to state 3 respiration upon the addition of ADP, by oligomycin (an inhibitor of the mitochondrial ATPase), by 1799, an uncoupler of mitochondrial oxidative phosphorylation and by atractyloside (an inhibitor of the mitochondrial adenine nucleotide translocase). These data are consistent with the hypothesis that adenosine is formed within the matrix or is present within the mitochondrial matrix from the beginning of the isolation procedure and is subsequently transported out, possibly by the adenine nucleotide translocase. A second hypothesis, which was also discussed, states that adenosine is formed outside of the mitochondrial matrix by an extramitochondrial 5'-nucleotidase, with the substrate (AMP) being derived from the matrix nucleotides.

The work presented here examines these alternative hypotheses and indicates that adenosine appearance is the result of an active production by the mitochondrial suspension. The data also indicate that the adenosine production may be the result of the activity of an intramitochondrial 5'-nucleotidase enzyme. The implications of adenosine production by mitochondria in light of the current knowledge of control of myocardial oxidative metabolism are discussed.

METHODS

Subcellular Fractionation

Mitochondrial fractions of rat heart were prepared as previously described (Bukoski et al, 1983). Briefly, male rats (250-300g) were beheaded and the hearts rapidly removed and placed in 10ml of 120mM KCl/1mM EGTA, rinsed with this solution three times, and then added to 10ml of 120mM KCl/1mM EGTA with 5 mg Nagase. The mince was homogenized with two strokes of a Potter-Elvehjem homogenizer, diluted with 20ml of 120mM KCl/1mM EGTA, then homogenized with two more strokes of the homogenizer. The homogenate was then centrifuged at 1,800 rpm for 5 minutes and the supernatant was filtered through two layers of cheesecloth, then centrifuged at 8,000 g for 10 minutes. The pellet (unwashed mitochondria) was then washed three times by resuspending in 120mM KCl and centrifuging at 8,000 g for 10 minutes. Microsomes were isolated by centrifuging the original 8,000 g supernatant at 100,000 g for 60 minutes. The final mitochondrial and microsomal pellets were resuspended in 120mM KCl. Protein was determined by the Biuret method. Mitochondrial oxygen consumption was measured polarographically using a Clark oxygen electrode in a temperature controlled cuvette at 30°C with a volume of 1 ml.

Mitochondrial Adenosine Production

Mitochondria (1.5-3 mg protein/ml) were incubated at 30°C in 120mM KCl/10mM TrisP$_i$/10mM TrisCl, pH 7.4 in a temperature controlled cuvette. At specified times, 150 μl aliquots were removed, and then added to the top layer of a microcentrifuge tube containing from top to bottom, 500 μl of a solution of 0.1M sucrose/1mM EGTA/10 mM HEPES, pH 7.4; 300 μl bromododecane and 100μl 2N perchloric acid (PCA). The tubes were centrifuged at 10,000 g for 1.5 minutes in an Eppendorf centrifuge and 500 μl of the top layer were removed, added to 50 μl 5N PCA, then neutralized with

K_2CO_3. In some experiments, the bromododecane layer was removed, 1ml cold H_2O was added to the PCA layer and allowed to incubate for 15 minutes. This layer was removed and neutralized with K_2CO_3. Adenosine content of the supernatant and the pellet extract were determined using high performance liquid chromatography as previously described (DeWitt et al, 1983).

Enzyme Assays

5'-nucleotidase activity was determined by measuring the amount of inorganic phosphate liberated from 5'-AMP in a mixture of 100mM Tris HCl, pH 7.4; 10mM $MgCl_2$; protein and 0.3mM AMP at $30°C$. Inorganic phosphate was measured colorimetrically by the method of Rockstein and Herron (1951). Nonspecific phosphatase activity in the preparation was accounted for by measuring the release of inorganic phosphate from p-nitrophenyl phosphate (pNPP) under the conditions described above and subtracting pNPPase activity from 5'-AMPase activity.

Adenyl cyclase was determined by incubating protein for 10 minutes at $30°$ in a mixture of 10mM TrisCl, pH 7.4; 10mM $MgCl_2$; 6mM KCl; 5mM aminophylline; 5mM Na_2ATP and an ATP regenerating system consisting of 20mM phosphoenolpyruvate and 9.8 units of pyruvate kinase (ATP:pyruvate 2-0-phosphotransferase). Cyclic AMP in the deproteinized sample was determined radioimmunochemically after removal of nucleotides by eluting the samples over a column of Dowex 50W as described by Steiner (1974).

RESULTS

Figure 1 shows the results of an experiment designed to determine whether the adenosine which appears in a suspension of isolated mitochondria at $30°C$ is the result of an efflux of a store of adenosine present within the mitochondrial matrix at the time of isolation, or is the result of a production of adenosine by mitochondria. After separating the mitochondria from the suspending medium by centrifugation through an organic layer (see Methods), the adenosine content of the medium and of the mitochondrial pellet (matrix content) was measured. Figure 1a shows the effect of time on the concentration of adenosine in the suspending medium and in the mitochondrial pellet (calculated using 1.6 µl matrix H_2O/ mg mitochondrial protein). There is a time dependent increase in the concentration of adenosine in the supernatant and a decrease of adenosine concentration in the matrix. However, it can be seen from the relative masses of adenosine in the two fractions (Fig. 1b), that the appearance of adenosine in the supernatant cannot be accounted for by a simple mass transfer from the matrix. For example, five times as much adenosine is present in the suspension (1.5 nmoles adenosine/mg protein) after 5 minutes as was present within the mitochondrial matrix (.28 nmoles adenosine/mg protein) at

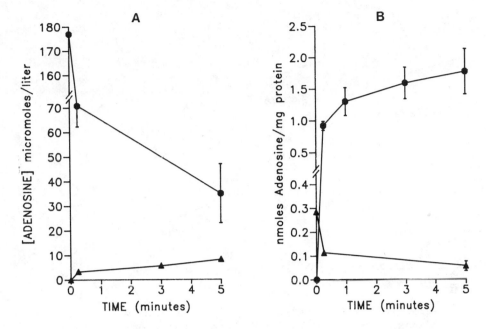

Fig. 1. This figure illustrates the rate of change of adenosine
concentration (1a) in the mitochondrial matrix (●) and in
the suspending medium (▲) and the rate of change of the mass
of adenosine (1b) in the matrix (▲) and suspending medium
(●). Adenosine concentration of the matrix was calculated
assuming a value of 1.6 μl matrix H_2O/ mg mitochondrial
protein. Adenosine in the pellet and in the medium were
measured as described in the Methods. Values are mean ± SEM,
n = at least 5. Please note the break in the scale of the
ordinate in both graphs.

the beginning of the incubation. These data indicate that adenosine
was present within the mitochondria when the incubation period was
begun, however, they also demonstrate that isolated mitochondria
produce adenosine.

We next wished to determine if adenosine was being formed by a
5'-nucleotidase enzyme located outside of the mitochondrial matrix.
The effect of   α,β methylene adenosine diphosphate (AOPCP), a
potent inhibitor of 5'-nucleotidase activity, on adenosine
production was examined. We found that 0.1mM AOPCP inhibited
adenosine appearance by 74%, n=5. To determine whether AOPCP acts
only on the 5'-nucleotidase enzyme, or has other effects on
mitochondrial function, the effect of AOPCP on ADP stimulated
respiration of mitocondria was examined. Figure 2 shows that AOPCP
stimulates state 4 respiration with pyruvate and malate as

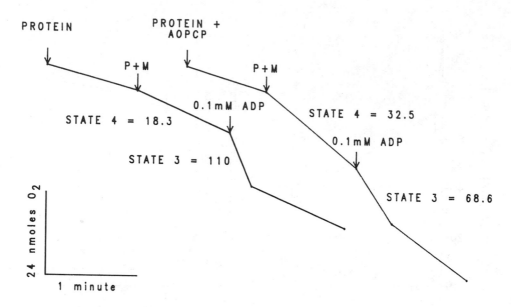

Fig. 2. This figure illustrates the effect of 1mM α,β methylene
adenosine diphosphate (AOPCP) on respiratory activity of
isolated rat heart mitochondria. Mitochondria (0.59 mg
protein) were added to a 1 ml cuvette containing 120mM KCl,
10mM TrisP$_i$, and TrisHCl, pH 7.4 + 1mM AOPCP. State 4
respiration was induced by the addition of 6mM pyruvate and
2mM malate, and conversion to state 3 respiration was
induced by the addition of 0.5mM ADP. Values nmoles O_2
consumed/mg protein min. and similar results were obtained
from 5 preparations.

substrates and subsequently inhibits the rate of state 3
respiration. These results indicated to us that in addition to an
effect of AOPCP on 5'-nucleotidase activity, it may also inhibit
adenosine production by a secondary effect on the mitochondrion,
perhaps within the intermembrane space (see Discussion).

The results obtained in the experiments using AOPCP indicated
that there is a 5'-nucleotidase enzyme present in the mitochondrial
fraction. We therefore compared 5'-nucleotidase activity in
themitochondrial fraction with 5'-nucleotidase activity in a
microsomal fraction. There is an 8-9 fold greater specific activity
of 5'-nucleotidase in the microsomal fraction than in the
mitochondrial fraction (Table 1). If one assumes that mitochondria
have no 5'-nucleotidase activity of their own, then a calculation
can be made to estimate the amount of microsomal material which must
be present in the mitochondrial fraction to account for the
activity. Given this assumption, we calculate that as much as 12% of

Table 1. 5'-Nucleotidase and Adenyl Cyclase Activities of
Mitochondrial and Microsomal Fractions of Rat Heart

	Mitochondrial Fraction	Microsomal Fraction	Contamination*
5'-nucleotidase (μmol P_i/mg min)	0.69 $\pm$ 0.07	5.86 $\pm$ 0.33	12%
Adenyl Cyclase (pmol cAMP/mg min)	0.93 $\pm$ 0.18	2.90 $\pm$ 0.08	34%

* % Contamination is the percentage of microsomal material
(based on specific enzyme activity) which must be present in the
mitochondrial fraction to account for the observed
5'-nucleotidase or adenyl cyclase activity. Values are mean $\pm$
SEM, n = 5.

the protein in the mitochondrial fraction could be microsomal in
origin. The possibility of significant microsomal contamination of
our preparation lead us to examine the distribution of another
sarcolemmal marker enzyme (adenyl cyclase), between the two
fractions. Making the same calculation as described above for
5'-nucleotidase activity, we found that up to 34% of the protein in
the mitochondrial fraction could be microsomal (Table 1). These data
support the hypothesis that adenosine production by the
mitochondrial fraction may involve both mitochondrial and microsomal
activity. For instance, mitochondria may provide substrate (AMP)
which can be converted to adenosine by microsomal a 5'-nucleotidase
enzyme.

DISCUSSION

It is clear that adenosine is an important modulator of cardiac
function Berne and Rubio (1979). However, the subcellular site of
adenosine production and the trigger for its release are poorly
understood. Previous work from our laboratory demonstrated that
adenosine appears in a suspension of isolated rat heart mitochondria
and that its rate of appearance is altered by agents which are known
modulators of mitochondrial function (Bukoski et al, 1983). The
experiments reported here were designed to test the hypothesis that
the adenosine appearance is the result of an efflux of previously
formed adenosine out of the mitochondrial matrix. We also tested the
hypothesis that adenosine formation by mitochondria requires the
presence of a sarcolemmal 5'-nucleotidase.

The experiments illustrated in Figure 1 clearly demonstrate that most of the adenosine appearing in the suspension is newly formed during the incubation. There is an apparent concentration gradient for adenosine from the matrix to the extramitochondrial volume (Fig. 1a), but the mass of adenosine in the pellet at zero time is too small to account for the mass of adenosine which appears in the suspension (Fig. 1b). If the adenosine associated with the pellet is distributed in the mitochondrial matrix, its concentration is much higher than in the supernatant. This suggests that the newly formed adenosine moves from the matrix space to the extramitochondrial compartment. This is consistent with the presence of an intramitochondrial 5'-nucleotidase enzyme. Earlier work, demonstrating that adenosine appearance is inhibited by atractyloside, is also consistent with intramitochondrial adenosine formation and indicates that its export may require a functional adenine nucleotide carrier (Bukoski et al, 1983).

We wanted to determine if the adenosine production could be inhibited by AOPCP, an inhibitor of 5'-nucleotidase. We reasoned that if AOPCP could not cross the inner mitochondrial membrane, it would not be able to inhibit an intramitochondrial 5'-nucleotidase enzyme. The results showed that there was only a 74% inhibition of adenosine production by 0.1mM AOPCP, a supramaximal concentration of this drug (IC_{50} = 6nM, Lowenstein et al, 1983). Assuming that AOPCP did not cross the inner membrane, and its only effect is on 5'-nucleotidase, these findings are consistent with a production of adenosine by both an intra- and an extramitochondrial 5'-nucleotidase enzyme (since the inhibition was not 100%). Further experiments, however, demonstrated that AOPCP stimulates state 4 and inhibits state 3 respiratory activity (Fig.2). It is possible that AOPCP may enter the intermembrane space and there have an unspecific uncoupling effect (resulting in the observed respiratory effects) and also inhibited the adenine nucleotide translocase at the outer transport site. If AOPCP inhibits the translocase, then it could attenuate adenosine production either by decreasing substrate availability or adenosine efflux from the matrix compartment. The effect of AOPCP on mitochondrial respiratory activity is a new observation and could lead to the use of AOPCP or similar compounds as tools to study mitochondrial nucleotide transport. Although the data obtained using AOPCP are not unequivocal, they indicate that there is 5'-nucleotidase activity present intramitochondrially as well as extramitochondrially.

We next tested the hypothesis that a portion of the adenosine formation we have observed results from cooperation between the mitochondria and a sarcolemmal 5'-nucleotidase, i.e. mitochondria provide the substrate (AMP) and a sarcolemmal 5'-nucleotidase dephosphorylates it, producing adenosine. To test this, we compared the distribution of 5'-nucleotidase activity and adenyl cyclase activity in the mitochondrial and microsomal fractions. The results indicate that there is microsomal material present within the mitochondrial fraction which can account for the 5'-nucleotidase activity that we observe. Although the microsomal fraction itself exhibits 5'-nucleotidase activity, it cannot produce adenosine in the absence of added AMP. These results therefore support the hypothesis that mitochondria are the source of substrate (AMP) for any adenosine production by sarcolemmal 5'-nucleotidase in the mitochondrial fraction. However, our finding that there is microsomal 5'-nucleotidase activity in the mitochondrial fraction does not address the question of the presence of 5'-nucleotidase activity in the mitochondrial matrix. There are, however, three lines of evidence which suggest that there is an intramitochondrial 5'-nucleotidase, (1) the observation that there is adenosine in a pellet of freshly isolated mitochondria (Fig. 1), (2) the finding that 26% of the 5'-nucleotidase activity in the mitochondrial fraction is insensitive to AOPCP inhibition (Fig. 2) and (3) our previous demonstration that atractyloside inhibits adenosine production in the mitochondrial fraction (Bukoski et al, 1983).

The above experiments have lead us to develop a working hypothesis linking mitochondrial production of adenosine to delivery of oxygen to the myocardium. It is currently thought that the rate of mitochondrial respiration is regulated by either the cytosolic phosphorylation potential, [ATP]/[ADP][P$_i$], (Erecinska and Wilson, 1982) or by the extra- or intramitochondrial ATP/ADP ratio where the activity of the adenine nucleotide translocase is rate limiting (Tager et al, 1983). In either hypothesis, the phosphorylation potential or extramitochondrial ratio of ATP/ADP decreases as a result of increased ATP hydrolysis. Wilson et al, 1983 have recently demonstrated that the intramitochondrial ratio of free ATP/ADP is slightly greater than or equal to the extramitochondrial ratio of ATP/ADP indicating that there is an equilibrium of the adenylate system across the mitocondrial inner membrane mediated by the nucleotide translocase. Therefore an increase in cytosolic ADP could result in an increase in intramitochondrial ADP and hence AMP. The AMP could then serve as substrate for a mitochondrial 5'-nucleotidase enzyme which would then produce adenosine either inside or outside of the matrix. The adenosine formed within the matrix could then be transported out, possibly in conjunction with the adenine nucleotide translocase (Fig. 1) and the adenosine could then be exported out of the cell by a nucleoside carrier in the cell membrane causing an increase in interstitial adenosine. The resulting vasodilation would then increase oxygen delivery to mitochondria. This hypothesis is particularly attractive when one thinks of the mitochondria as the "cellular oxygen sensors". It remains to be determined, of course, if this series of events occurs in vivo.

Summary

The results from the previous work (Bukoski et al, 1983) and those presented here indicate that mitochondria from rat heart are capable of producing adenosine in concert with a sarcolemmal

5'-nucleotidase. In addition, and perhaps more importantly, these data also indicate that mitochondria can produce adenosine in the presence of inhibition of sarcolemmal 5'-nucleotidase. Given the current understanding of the regulation of mitochondrial respiration and thus oxygen consumption, mitochondria may be uniquely situated to sense increases in myocardial oxygen demand and respond to this with a feedback signal (adenosine) which can return the system to a state of balance.

REFERENCES

Bellardinelli, L., Fenton, R., West, A. Linden, J. and Berne, R.M., 1982, Extracellular action of adenosine and antagonism by aminophylline on the atrioventricular conduction in isolated perfused guinea pig and rat heart, Circ. Res., 51:569.

Berne, R.. and Rubio, R., 1979, Coronary circulation, in: "Handbook of Physiology, the Cardiovascular System, R.M. Berne and N. Sperelakis, eds., American Physiological Society, Washington, p. 873.

Berne, R.M., 1980, The role of adenosine in the regulation of coronary blood flow, Circ. Res., 47:807.

Bunger, R., Soboll, S. and Permanetter, B., 1983, Effects of norepinephrine on coronary flow, myocardial substrate utilization, and subcellular adenylates, in: "Ca^{2+} Entry Blockers, Adenosine and Neurohumors", G.F. Merrill and H.R. Weiss, eds., Urban and Schwarzenberg, Baltimore, p. 267.

Bukoski, R.D., Sparks, H.V. and Mela, L.M., 1983, Rat heart mitochondria release adenosine. Biochem. Biophys. Res. Comm., 113:990.

Cheung, J.Y., Leaf, A. and Bonventre, J.V., 1984, Mechanism of protection of verapamil and nifedipine from anoxia injury in isolated cardiac myocytes, Am. J. Physiol., 240:C323.

Clark, M.G., Patten, G.S. and Filsell, O.H., 1982, Evidence for an $\alpha-$ adrenergic receptor-mediated control of energy production in heart. J. Molec. Cell. Cardiol., 14:313.

DeWitt, D.F., Wangler, R.D., Thompson, C.I. and Sparks, H.V., 1983, Phasic release of adenosine during steady state metabolic stimulation in the isolated guinea pig heart, Circ. Res., 53:636.

Erecinska, M. and Wilson, D.F., 1982, Regulation of cellular energy metabolism, J. Membrane Biol., 70:1.

Frick, G.P., Lowenstein, J.M., 1978, Vectorial production of adenosine by 5'-nucleotidase in the perfused rat heart, J. Biol. Chem., 253:1240.

Lowenstein, J.M., Yu, M.-K. and Naito, Y., 1983, Regulation of adenosine metabolism by 5'-nucleotidases, in: "Regulatory Function of Adenosine", R.M. Berne, T.W. Rall and R. Rubio, eds., Martinus Nijhoff, Boston, p. 117.

Manfredi, J.P. and Sparks, H.V., 1982, Adenosine's role in coronary vasodilation induced by atrial pacing and norepinephrine. Am. J. Physiol., 243:H536.

Nuutinen, E.M., Nishiki, K., Erecinska, M. and Wilson, D.F., 1982, Role of mitochondrial oxidative phosphorylation in regulation of coronary blood flow, Am. J. Physiol., 243:H159.

Nuutinen, E.M., Nelson, D., Wilson, D.F. and Erecinska, M. Regulation of coronary blood flow: effects of 2,4-dinitrophenol and theophylline. Am. J. Physiol., 244:H369.

Olsson, R.A., Saito, D. and Steinhardt, C.R., 1982, Compartmentalization of the adenosine pool of dog and rat hearts, Circ. Res., 50:617.

Rockstein, M., Herron, P.W., 1951, Colorimetric determination of inorganic phosphate in microgram quantities, Anal. Chem., 23:1500.

Rubio, R. and Berne, R.M., 1975, Regulation of coronary blood flow, Prog. Cardiovasc. Dis., 18:105.

Schrader, J. and Gerlach, E., 1976, Compartmentation of cardiac adenine nucleotides and formation of adenosine, Pflugers Arch., 367:129.

Schrader, J., Baumann, G. and Gerlach, E., 1977, Adenosine as an inhibitor of mitocardial effects of catecholamines, Pfleugers Arch. 372:29.

Schrader, J., Schutz, W. and Bardenheuer, H., 1981, Role of S-adenosyl homocysteine hydrolase in adenosine metabolism in mammalian heart, Biochem. J., 196:65.

Schutz, W., Schrader, J. and Gerlach, E., 1981, Different sites of adenosine formation in the heart, Am. J. Physiol., 240:H963.

Steiner, A.L., 1974, Assay of cyclic nucleotides by radioimmunoassay methods, Methods Enzymol., 38:96.

Tager, J.M., Wanders, R.J.A., Groen, A.K., Kunz, W., Bohnensack, R., Kuster, U., Letko, G., Bohne, G., Duszynski, J. and Wojczak, L., 1983, Control of mitochondrial respiration, FEBS Lett., 151:1.

Verhaege, R.H., Lorenz, R.R., McGrath, M.A., Shepherd, J.T. and Vanhoutte, P.M., 1978, Metabolic modulation of neurotransmitter release-adenosine, adenine nucleotides, potassium, hyperosmolarity and hydrogen ion, Fed. Proc., 37:208.

Wilson, D.F., Erecinska, M., Drown, C. and Silver, I.A., 1978, The oxygen dependence of cellular energy metabolism, Arch. Biochem. Biophys., 195:485.

Wilson, D.F., Erecinska, M. and Schramm, V.L., 1983, Evaluation of the relationship between intra- and extramitochondrial [ATP]/[ADP] ratios using phosphoenolpyruvate carboxykinase, J. Biol. Chem. 258:10464.

ASPECTS OF HEART RESPIRATORY CONTROL

BY THE MITOCHONDRIAL ISOZYME OF CREATINE KINASE

William E. Jacobus[*], Koenraad M. Vandegaer, and
Randall W. Moreadith

Departments of Medicine and Physiological Chemistry
The Johns Hopkins University School of Medicine
Baltimore, Maryland 21205

INTRODUCTION

The isolation of intact mitochondria by Claude (1,2), the refinements by Hogeboom et. al (3), and the recognition by Kennedy and Lehninger (4) that these organelles were the site of oxidative phosphorylation heralded the modern era of cellular bioenergetics. Shortly thereafter, Siekevitz and Potter (5) and others (6-10) began to explore the regulation of mitochondrial respiratory rates

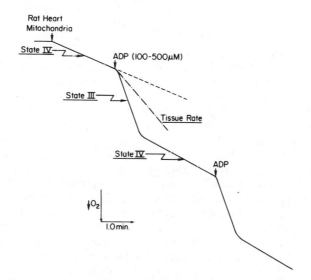

Fig. 1. **Mitochondrial respiratory control.**

and oxidative phosphorylation. The reason for this rather extended quest is straightforward. As seen in Fig. 1, when intact mitochondria are incubated in respiratory medium, oxygen is consumed at an endogenous rate termed State IV. With substrate and Pi present, the addition of ADP (phosphate acceptor), even at micromolar concentrations, results in a marked stimulation of respiration to near-maximum velocity called State III. From the view of cellular physiology, neither State IV or State III are relevant, since the normal rate of oxygen consumption by a tissue, e.g. the heart, lies between these two in vitro rates. Only under conditions of extreme stress does heart oxygen consumption ever come close to maximum respiratory rates. Therefore, the biologically important issue is to determine how a cell modulates oxygen consumption and, thus, high-energy phosphate production, at intermediate rates. The achievement of this involves the notion of respiratory control.

In 1955 Chance and Williams (11) suggested that the kinetics of mitochodrial oxidative phosphorylation could be described by the availability of ADP. This was an idea which predated our knowledge of the adenine nucleotide translocase (12). Klingenberg (13) subsequently postulated that the extramitochondrial phosphorylation potential, [ATP]/[ADP]x[Pi], was the parameter which determined the immediate rates of oxygen consumption. Since that time, this hypothesis has received much experimental and theoretical support (14-24). In 1973, Slater et al. (25) proposed that mitochondrial respiratory control was simply a function of the [ATP]/[ADP] ratio, independent of the tissue content of Pi. This theory has likewise achieved considerable support (26-35). Control by the phosphorylation potential is based on near equilibrium thermodynamic considerations, while the ATP/ADP ratio theory is founded on the kinetics of the adenine nucleotide translocase.

The need for these additional theories arose from from the observations that the tissue content of ADP appeared to be considerably higher than the apparent K_m of the adenine nucleotide translocase for ADP. For example, the acid-extracted content of ADP in the heart is almost 1.0 mM, while the translocase K_m is about 20 to 30 uM. Under these conditions, the translocase would clearly be saturated with ADP, so other control theories were required. Recent 31-P NMR data on the in vivo rat brain (36), our own studies on the perfused heart, computer calculations of heart nucleotides (37), and a recent re-estimation of tissue phosphorylation potentials (38) all cast considerable doubt on both of these theories for adenine nucleotide control. These data (36-38) suggest that the concentrations of free ADP in tissues are much lower than that estimated from freeze extraction, and potentially within the ADP kinetic control range. Therefore, it appeared that this problem merited reinvestigation.

170

A recent publication from our laboratory (39) supported the concept that ADP availability was the primary adenine nucleotide parameter (11) controlling the rates of oxydative phosphorylation. These studies were conducted with rat liver mitochondria, using hexokinase as the enzymatic source for ADP generation. In this communication, the work is extended and two important and separate concepts are now discussed. These are the adenine nucleotide control of mitochondrial respiration, and the kinetics of the heart mitochondrial adenine nucleotide translocase. The data in the first section clearly demonstrate that under conditions of mitochondrial creatine kinase control, the phosphorylation potential and ATP/ADP ratio control theories can not adequately describe respiratory control. An analysis of the kinetics of the adenine nucleotide translocase suggest that the translocase has the highest affinity for ADP generated by the endogenous mitochondrial creatine kinase reaction operating in the forward direction. This is consistent with the view that the ADP generated by mitochondrial creatine kinase has "privileged access" to the translocase (40,41).

MATERIALS AND METHODS

Materials

The adenine and pyridine nucleotides, Tris and HEPES buffers, EGTA, phosphoenolpyruvate, and coupling enzymes used in the analytical procedures were purchased from Sigma. The adenine nucleotides were the substantially vanadium-free grades. The specific designations for the coupling enzymes have been previously reported (39). Sucrose and glucose were obtained from J. T. Baker, and all other reagents were of the highest commercial purity. Solutions were prepared in deionized water of low conductivity. HEPES and EGTA are abbreviations for 4-(2-hydroxyethyl)-1-piperazineethanesulfonic acid, and ethylene glycol bis (beta-amino ether)-N,N,N′,N′-tetraacetic acid, respectively. Agarose-bound yeast hexokinase was purchased from Sigma.

Experimental Methods

Mitochondrial Isolations. The mitochondrial fraction was isolated from the livers of female retired breeder Sprague-Dawley rats according to a modification of the proceedure of Vercesi et al. (42), as previously described in detail (39). Heart mitochondria were isolated from rats using Nagarse protease to minimally pre-digest the tissue (42). In both cases, standard methods of differential centrifugation were employed (43).

Oxygraph Proceedures. Respiratory traces were obtained using a Clark-type oxygen electrode (Yellow Springs Inst. Co.) in a 3.0 ml water-jacketed closed oxygraph chamber maintained at 37° C by a

Haake E12 circulator-heater. Voltage changes were recorded with a
Heath-Schlumberger recorder, with a polarizing electrode voltage
of 0.8 V. The oxygraph medium contained 0.25 M sucrose, 3.0 mM
HEPES, 2.0 mM KHPi, 5.0 mM K-succinate, 0.5 mM EGTA, 11 mM $MgCl_2$,
and 5 uM rotenone, at pH 7.2. In the liver mitochondrial
experiments presented in the initial section, respiratory control,
ATP was always added 1.0 min prior to the additions of creatine
kinase to phosphorylate any ADP present in the ATP solution. The
orders of additions and sequence of events are essentially the
same as reported for our hexokinase studies (39). In all cases,
creatine was present at 20 mM. In the kinetic experiments,
section 2, creatine or glucose were present at 20 mM
concentrations. Steady-state rates of respiration were initiated
by ATP addidions. After 1 min of steady-state respiration,
samples were removed for acid extraction, and the analysis of ADP.
All samples were corrected for the endogenous ADP content in the
matrix. Apparent K_m values were obtained from double reciprocal
plots of respiration rate versus 1/[ADP].

Sample Extractions. Samples (2.5 ml) were removed from the
oxygraph chamber 1.0 min after steady-state rates of respiration
were achieved. The sample was quickly mixed with 0.75 ml of 18%
$HClO_4$. The mixture was quickly filtered through 0.45 u Millipore
filters, neutralized to a methyl orange end point with K_2CO_3, and
centrifuged to remove $KClO_4$ crystals. The resultant solution was
decanted and frozen for nucleotide and Pi analysis.

Quantitation of Metabolites. The exact conditions for the
quantitation of ATP, ADP, and Pi have been previously reported in
detail (39). The methods used in these experiments were exactly
duplicated.

Protein concentrations were determined by the method of
Bradford (44), using nitrogen-calibrated, crystallized bovine
serum albumin as the primary protein standard.

RESULTS

Adenine Nucleotide Control of Mitochondrial Respiration

Studies to define the nature of the adenine nucleotide
control of respiration have traditionally employed three
approaches. In the first, samples are removed from the oxygraph
chamber at different points during the State III to State IV
transition, the period of "dynamic control" (14,16). Another
approach has been to use translocase inhibitors to selectively
inhibit the translocase, and note the results on rates of
respiration (19,30,32). The third method has been to preincubate
mitochondria in media containing fixed concentrations of ATP and
Pi, and initiating steady-state rates of respiration by the graded

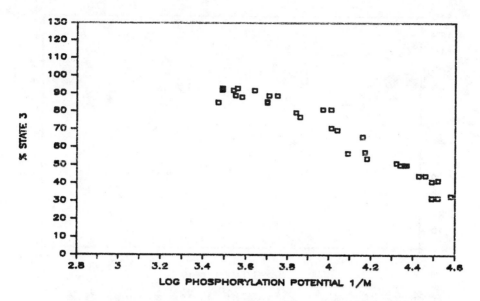

Fig. 2A. **Correlation of liver mitochondrial respiratory rates to log phosphorylation potential at fixed ATP (1.0 mM) and variable skeletal muscle creatine kinase.** Respiratory rates were calculated from steady-state rates. Samples were removed 1.5 min after enzyme addition, extracted and assayed as described in **MATERIALS AND METHODS.** The chamber contained 3.0 mg protein.

additions of either an ATPase enzyme, or an ADP generating system like hexokinase (26-28). A non-experimental approach has used computer modeling (17,18,23,29,35). From these combined approaches, arguments have been generated as to the degree to which mitochondrial respiratory rates are controlled by the extramitochondrial phosphorylation potential, by [Pi], by the kinetics of the translocase, by the [ATP]/[ADP] ratio, by oxygen, by substrate availability, or by the rates of electron transport, exclusively or in some combination (45). The focus of this report is not on the multiplicity of control, but only on the nature of the adenine nucleotide regulation.

In our recent work, data were presented for the control of liver mitochondrial respiration, using hexokinase as the ADP generating system (39). In that report, we used two protocols, constant ATP with variable enzyme, and constant enzyme with variable concentrations of ATP. Using the same experimental approaches, we now wish to report the data for heart and liver respiratory control, when creatine kinase is utilized as the exogenous ADP generating reaction, Figs. 2, 3, and 4. In Fig. 2A, data are shown for the relationships between respiratory rates and

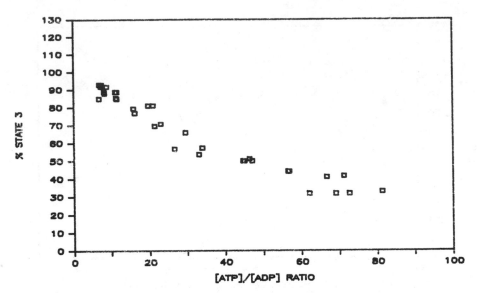

Fig. 2B. **Correlation of liver mitochondrial respiratory rates to [ATP]/[ADP] ratios at fixed ATP and variable skeletal muscle creatine kinase.** Conditions are the same as in Fig. 2A.

the log of the phosphorylation potential. Comparable to previous reports by us (39) and others, we note that as the log phosphorylation potential decreased, there is an increase in the rate of respiration. A similar correlation is seen with the [ATP]/[ADP] ratio data, Fig. 2B. In this figure, we also note that respiratory rates increase as the [ATP]/[ADP] ratio declines. In other words, the standard approach provided the expected results.

One of the basic assumptions of phopshorylation potential, or [ATP]/[ADP] ratio control is that under all conditions the rates of respiration could be correlated to the calculated value for either parameter, and are independent of how the conditions were established. This is the rationale for freeze-extracting tissue, measuring nucleotide levels, calculating ratios, and projecting information on its metabolic status. However, such does not appear to be the case. When the liver mitochondrial respiratory studies are conducted under more "physiological" conditions a markedly different picture is seen, Fig. 3.

In Fig. 3A we see the data for the rates of respiration as a function of the log phosphorylation potential, obtained when the concentration of creatine kinase was constant, and graded rates of respiration were obtained by ATP titrations. These conditions are considered more "physiological", since the cell usually operates

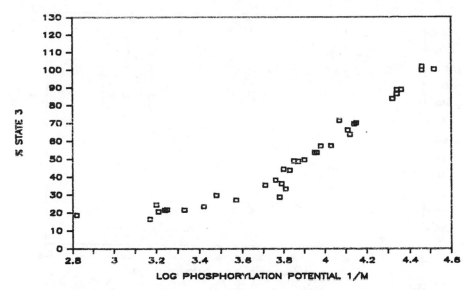

Fig. 3A. **Correlation of liver mitochondrial respiratory rates to log phosphorylation potential at fixed concentrations of skeletal muscle creatine kinase (0.3 IU) and variable [ATP].** Conditions are the same as in Fig. 2A except that the concentrations of ATP are varied from 0.005 to 10.0 mM.

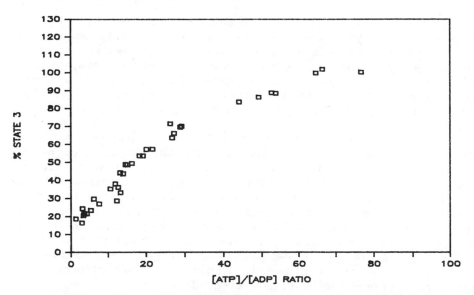

Fig. 3B. **Correlation of liver mitochondrial respiratory rates to [ATP]/[ADP] ratios at fixed skeletal muscle creatine kinase and variable [ATP].** Conditions are as in Fig. 3A.

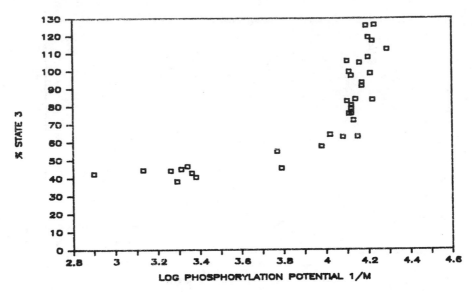

Fig 4A. **Correlation of heart mitochondrial respiratory rates to log phosphorylation potential using endogenous mitochondrial creatine kinase and variable [ATP].** The oxygraph chamber contained 0.5 mg rat heart mitochondrial protein. All other conditions were as in Fig. 3A.

with fixed concentrations of enzyme and variable concentrations of substrate. When the experiment is conducted in this manner, we note an almost mirror image correlation between respiratory rates and phosphorylation potentials. Now the rate of respiration increases as the phopsporylation potential increases: compare Figs. 2A versus 3A. A similar paradoxical correlation is also seen for the [ATP]/[ADP] ratios: compare Figs. 2B and 3B.

When the control of respiration is studied in heart mitochondria, using the endogenous mitochondrial isozyme of creatine kinase, a similar paradoxical picture is seen, Fig. 4. Since the amount of creatine kinase is fixed by its mitochondrial activity, we were left with little option but to grade the rates of respiration by alterations in [ATP]. We see in Fig. 4A a similar correlation between respiratory rate and log phosphorylation potential as noted in liver under similar conditions, Fig. 3A. Likewise, the data in Fig. 4B are similar in profile to the trend noted in Fig. 3B. Thus, there is a consistency between the heart and liver data.

When taken together, these data leave little doubt that neither the extramitochondrial phosphorylation potential, or the [ATP]/[ADP] ratios are primary signals **per se** for the regulation

176

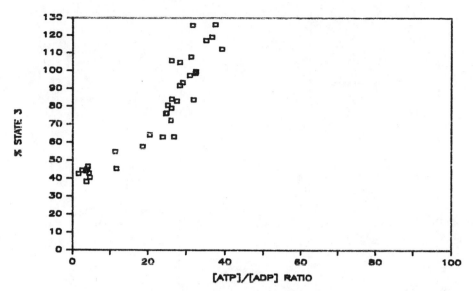

Fig. 4B. **Correlation of heart mitochondrial respiratory rates to [ATP]/[ADP] ratios using endogenous mitochondrial creatine kinase and variable [ATP].** Conditions are as in Fig. 4A.

of mitochondrial respiration. Some other aspect of the adenine nucleotides must be the controlling feature. In data not shown, in all cases there was a direct and hyperbolic correlation between the rates of respiration and the concentration of ADP. In other words, the data strongly suggest that ADP availability at the translocase is the key regulating parameter. The results are totally consistent with our previous data (39), and the concept initially postulated by Chance and Williams (11).

Kinetics of Heart Mitochondrial ADP Transport

The experimental results outlined above lead to a second interesting question. Is it possible that the kinetics of ADP transport by the translocase are influenced by the site of ADP formation? If so, this could represent a rather unique form of microcompartmentation. To explore this possibility, the kinetics of ADP transport were studied using 3 enzymatic systems for ADP formation, Fig 5. In the first, representative of cytoplasmic ADP formation, hexokinase immobilized to agarose beads was used, Fig. 5A. In the second condition, we employed normal soluble yeast hexokinase for ADP generation, Fig. 5B. The third system was the endogenous mitochondrial isozyme of creatine kinase, generating ADP in the mitochondrial intermembrane space, rather close to the translocase, Fig. 5C. In these experiments, heart mitochondria

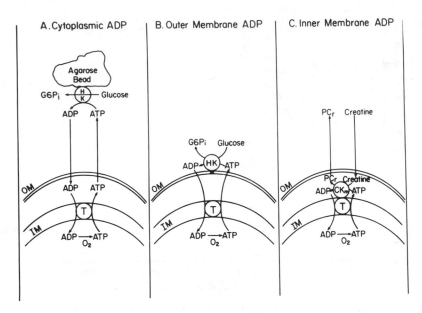

Fig. 5. **Cartoon drawing representing three ADP generating systems.** <u>A.</u> The use of agarose bound yeast hexokinase to generate "cytoplasmic" ADP. <u>B.</u> The use of soluble hexokinase (HK) to generate ADP at the outer mitochondrial membrane (OM). <u>C.</u> The use of endogenous creatine kinase (CKm) to generate ADP at the inner membrane (IM), in close proximity to the adenine nucleotide translocase (T). In all cases, ATP regeneration is via oxidative phosphorylation (O_2).

were incubated in sucrose oxygraph medium, with succinate as the substrate. Either glucose or creatine, the secondary phosphate acceptors, were present at 20 mM concentrations. The amount of hexokinase added was carefully titrated so that the maximal rates of respiration were not greater than 95 per cent of ADP-stimulated State III. This is crucial, since we did not want the ADP generating system to potentially produce ADP faster than it could be transported by the translocase. The maximum rates of creatine stimulated respiration were also about 95 per cent of State III. The reactions were initiated by the addition of ATP. After a short period, about 1.5 min, a sample was removed, acid extracted, and assayed for the content of ADP. The rates of respiration were then plotted in double-reciprocal format versus 1/[ADP], Fig. 6. The data for the fourth line of Fig. 6 were obtained by the direct additions of ADP to the respiratory medium, in the absence of a secondary acceptor. The apparent K_m for ADP stimulated respiration was then derived from the extrapolated data, Table I.

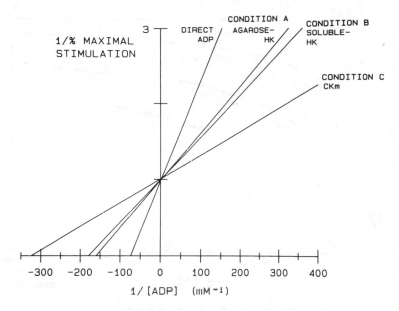

Fig. 6. **Double reciprocal plot of ADP kinetic data.**

TABLE I

**Apparent K$_m$ values for ADP stimulated respiration
as a function of the site of ADP formation.**

	Apparent K$_m$ (uM)
Direct ADP additions.	13.2
Agarose insoluble hexokinase (A).	7.0
Soluble yeast hexokinase (B).	5.9
Mitochondrial creatine kinase	2.8

The data of Fig. 6 and Table I show an almost 5-fold difference in the apparent K$_m$ for ADP stimulated respiration, an effect which is dependent upon the site of ADP formation. The clearest conclusion from these results is that the adenine nucleotide translocase appears to have the highest affinity for ADP generated by mitochondrial creatine kinase. This is quite consistent with the documentation of the functional coupling of ADP transport from mitochondrial creatine kinase to the adenine nucleotide translocase (40,41).

In a companion series of experiments, data not shown, the effects of ATP on the inhibition of ADP stimulated respiration were determined. The experiments yielded values for K$_i$, the

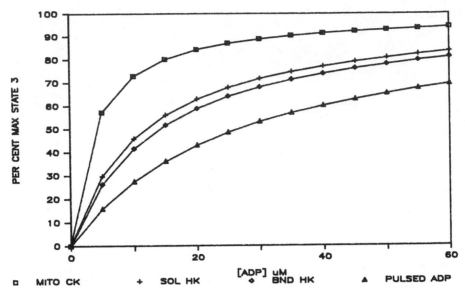

Fig. 7. **Theoretical curves for heart mitochondrial respiration as a function the site of ADP formation.** The rates are calculated from the apparent K_m data, Table I, and ATP K_i values, assuming a cytoplasmic concentration of 10 mM ATP.

inhibitory strength of ATP. Knowing the ADP K_m values, and the ATP K_i values, these numbers can be subsituted into the rate equation for competitive inhibition, known to be the case for the translocase (46). It is then possible to mathematically generate curves for the rates of heart mitochondrial respiration as a function [ADP] and dependent upon the site of ADP generation, Fig. 7. The curves presented in Fig. 7 clearly show that heart mitochondrial respiration is most responsive when ADP is generated by the endogenous creatine kinase reaction. This pathway is capable of stimulating respiration to the highest levels. At low concentrations of ADP, the rates of respiration induced by mitochondrial creatine kinase are markedly above those produced by any other generating system. Thus, the data are also quite consistent with the idea that in heart, the forward activity of the mitochondrial creatine kinase reaction (phosphocreatine and ADP formation) may be the dominant reaction controlling the rate of oxidative phosphorylation, and thus the rate of tissue oxygen consumption. The data underscore the crucial importance of this phosphotransferase reaction in myocardial high-energy phosphate metabolism.

DISCUSSION

The data presented in this paper shed new light on two

180

related areas of cell physiology. First, they are consistent with our previous observations on the adenine nucleotide control of respiration (39). The results suggest that under conditions which approximate those in a cell, the mitochondrial adenine nucleotide translocase is under kinetic control and dependent upon the availability of ADP, be it cytoplasmic or generated in the mitochondrial intermembrane space. A major revelation of the past few years, which initiated the reconsideration of respiratory control, is the observation that the concentration of free ADP in the cell represents only about 2 per cent of the measured ADP. At this concentration range, 20-40 uM, and at a free ATP concentration of 10 mM, the calculations of Fig. 7 show that these are appropriate conditions for kinetic regulation of the translocase. The data presented in this report also suggest that it is unnecessary to invoke more sophisiticated hypotheses for adenine nucleotide control. Our results appear to be inconsistent with the theory that primary control is exerted by either the extramitochondrial phosphorylation potential, or by the cytoplasmic [ATP]/[ADP] ratio.

From the perspective of the integration of cell high-energy phosphate metabolism, direct control of ATP production by ADP availability makes sense. In order to tightly couple the critical balance between energy supply (metabolism) and energy demand (work), respiration should be controlled by a signal indicative of the magnitude of cell labor. In other words, ATP production rates should be responsive to changes in the rate of ATP turnover. Clearly, the product of increased cellular "work", whether physical (as in the heart with contraction), or biosynthetic (as in liver), is usually the generation of ADP and Pi, or in some cases AMP and PPi. Therefore, changes in the availability of ADP do, in fact, directly reflect the steady-state magnitude of energy demand. Our experiments suggest that such changes act as the primary adenine nucleotide signal to stimulate mitochondrial ATP production.

The second point relates to the topic of this conference, microcompartmentation (Fig. 7), intertwined with the concept of mitochondrial creatine kinase-adenine nucleotide translocase "functional coupling." The idea that inner membrane localization is critical for the integration of phosphocreatine production to oxidative phosphorylation was first expressed by Jacobus and Lehninger (47). Thereafter, kinetic studies documenting alterations in the apparent K_m for ATP (48-51), chemical labeling studies (52), and thermodynamic experiments (53) all support the view that there is a unique interaction between mitochondrial creatine kinase and ATP supplied by the adenine nucleotide translocase. These observations have been challenged (54,55) to some degree. In addition, recent work using translocase inhibitors (40), or pyruvate kinase competition for ADP (41), have

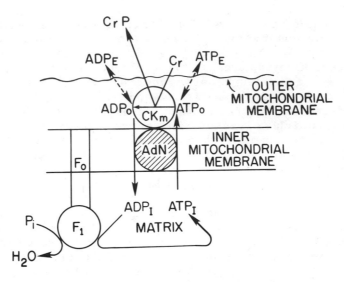

Fig. 8. **Model for the integration of heart mitochondrial creatine kinase (CK_m) to the adenine nucleotide translocase (AdN).** The abbreviations used are: F_oF_1, the proton translocating ATPase; ADP_e and ATP_e, exogenous adenine nucleotides; ADP_o and ATP_o, nucleotides in close proximity to CK_m; ADP_I and ATP_I, the matrix adenine nucleotide pool; Cr and CrP, creatine and phosphocreatine, respectively. [From Jacobus et al. (40). With permission from **Journal of Biological Chemistry.**]

also shown a unique interaction between the translocase and the ADP generated by mitochondrial creatine kinase. A model for these interactions is presented in Fig. 8. The concept of "functional coupling" does not in any way include the requirement for **exclusive access** by either ATP or ADP. This is clearly shown in Fig. 8, where both endogenous and exogenous nucleotides are shown to interact with either the translocase or creatine kinase.

What is the nature of this effect? Mosbach (56) has stated that the kinetic enhancement of a multi-step enzyme system could be explained by four properties of an enzymatic microenviornment. They are: 1) enzyme-enzyme proximity, 2) the establishment of Nernst unstirred layers, 3) other diffusional restrictions, and 4) exclusive effects imposed by structured water. For reasons previously detailed (40), we feel that unstirred layers and structured water play only a minor role. Data from our laboratory have also shown that there is no concerted or "direct" transfer of the nucleotides (57). More likely, functional coupling is the result of proximity, the consequence of the fact that the enzyme is bound to the exterior surface of the inner mitochondrial membrane, the membrane also containing the translocase. As a result of this localization, the translocase is positioned to efficiently supply ATP to the active site of creatine kinase, and the enzyme effectively supplies ADP to the carrier. Since the translocase operates by obligatory exchange (antiport), these processes would occur almost simultaneously. Therefore, the translocase activity could effectively induce local concentration gradients, increasing [ATP] and decreasing [ADP] in the enviornment of the enzyme. As a result, the forward direction of the reaction will be favored. The magnitude of such gradients has yet to be determined. It is also quite possible that the outer membrane acts as a moderate barrier for diffusion, thus contributing to "functional coupling" (58). Independent of its mechanism, "functional coupling" is a very interesting process. The reason is that the coupling of the translocase and creatine kinase potentially represent a very unique form of a multi-enzyme complex. It appears to be the singular example of a transport process coupled to enzymatic catalysis, where the transport system functions to both supply substrate (ATP) and remove product (ADP). With respect to respiratory control and the maintenance of the reaction exclusively in the forward direction, ADP removal is probably the more important aspect of the coupling. ADP removal minimizes the reversibility of the reaction to a degree which, under physiological conditions, has yet to be defined.

As readers of this volume will note, mitochondrial respiration and high-energy phosphate production are not controlled by an exclusive step. We have purposely focused on exogenous adenine nucleotide control. However, a unique contribution by Tager's group (59) has been the application of control theory (60-63) to mitochondrial respiratory control. The important outcome of this work is the documentation that respiratory control is actually a shared process, and that the degree of control by a single step depends upon the respiratory state (59). Under State III conditions, control is primarily exerted by the dicarboxylate carrier and the translocase. However, at lower rates or respiration, eg. 50 per cent State III, the rate of the ADP generating reaction (hexokinase) becomes the dominant control parameter (ref. 59, Fig. 3). Control by ADP generation is quite consistent with the data presented in this report, and supports the notion that the activity of mitochondrial creatine kinase may play a major physiological role in the control of heart oxygen consumption. The degree to which other steps, Pi transport, oxygen, transmembrane pH gradients, substrate transport, nucleotide pool sizes, and relative intramitochondrial versus extramitochondrial energy demands, all interact to regulate respiration (64-74) clearly remains an issue of open controversy. It is anticipated that future uses of innovative experimental approaches will yield new data about these matters. Such a technique appears to be 31-P NMR. Using saturation transfer methods, Matthews et al. (75) have estimated the flux rates for ATP systhesis and calculated an in vivo ADP/O ratio. This methodology opens the door to much more sophisiticated analyses of tissue bioenergetics. In a similar manner, 13-C NMR holds promise for investigations about the substrate control of respiration.

ACKNOWLEDGEMENTS

The authors wish to acknowledge the use of WordStar and Lotus 1-2-3 in the preparation of this manuscript. This work was supported by United States Public Health Service Grant HL-20658. W.E.J. was an Established Investigator of the American Heart Association during the time these experiments were conducted. R.W.M. current address: Duke University School of Medicine, Durham, North Carolina 27710.

*Author to whom inquiries should be addressed, at:

Division of Cardiology
538 Carnegie Building
The Johns Hopkins Hospital
600 North Wolfe Street
Baltimore, Maryland 21205

REFERENCES

1. A. Claude, Fractionation of mammalian liver cells by differential centrifugation I. Problems, methods and preparation of extract. J. Exp. Med. **84**:51-59 (1946).

2. A. Claude, Fractionation of mammalian liver cells by differential centrifugation II. Experimental procedures and results. J. Exp. Med. **84**:61-89 (1946).

3. G. H. Hogeboom, W. C. Schneider and G. E. Palade, Cytochemical studies of mammalian tissues I. Isolation of intact mitochondria from rat liver; some biochemical properties of mitochondria and submicroscopic particulate material. J. Biol. Chem. **172**:619-636 (1948).

4. E. P. Kennedy and A. L. Lehninger, Oxidation of fatty acids and tricarboxylic acid cycle intermediates by isolated rat liver mitochondria. J. Biol. Chem. **179**:957-972 (1949).

5. P. Siekevitz and V. R. Potter, Intramitochondrial regulation of oxidative rate, J. Biol. Chem. **210**:1-13 (1953).

6. H. Niemeyer, R. K. Crane, E. P. Kennedy and F. Lippmann,

Observations on respiration and phosphorylation with liver mitochondria of normal, hypo-, and hyperthyroid rats. Fed. Proc. **10**:229 (1951).

7. H. A. Lardy and H. J. Wellman, Oxidative phosphorylations: role of inorganic phosphate and acceptor systems in control of metabolic rates. J. Biol. Chem. **195**:215-224 (1952).

8. M. Rabinovitz, M. P. Stulberg and P. D. Boyer, The control of pyruvate oxidation in a cell-free rat heart preparation by phosphate acceptors. Science **114**:641-642 (1951).

9. V. R. Potter, R. O. Recknagel and R. B. Hurlbert, Intracellular enzyme distribution: interpretation and significance. Fed. Proc. **10**:646-653 (1951).

10. W. W. Kielley and R. K. Kielley, Myokinase and adenosinetriphosphatase in oxidative phosphorylation. J. Biol. Chem. **191**:485-500 (1951).

11. B.Chance and G. R. Williams, Respiratory enzymes in oxidative phosphorylation. I. Kinetics of oxygen utilization. J. Biol. Chem. **217**:385-393 (1955).

12. M. Klingenberg and E. Pfaff, Structural and functional compartmentation in mitochondria, in: "Regulation of Metabolic Processes in Mitochondria," J. M. Tager, S. Papa, E. Quagliariello and E. C. Slater, eds., American Elsevier Publishing Co., New York, pp. 180-201 (1966).

13. M. Klingenberg, Zur reversibilitat der oxydativen phosphorylierung. IV. Die beziehung zwischen dem redoxzustand des cytochrome c und dem phyosphorylierungs-potential des adenosintriphosphates. Biochem. Zeit. **335**:263-272 (1961).

14. C. S. Owen and D. F. Wilson, Control of respiration by the mitochondrial phosphorylation state. Arch. Biochem. Biophys. **161**:581-591 (1974).

15. D. F. Wilson, M. Stubbs, R. L. Veech, M. Erecinska and H. A. Krebs, Equilibrium relations between the oxidation-reduction reactions and the adenosine triphosphate synthesis in suspensions if isolated liver cells. Biochem J. **140**:57-64 (1974).

16. A. Holian, C. S. Owen and D. F. Wilson, Control of respiration in isolated mitochondria: quantitative evaluation of the dependence of respiratory rates on [ATP], [ADP], and [Pi]. Arch. Biochem. Biophys. **181**:164-171 (1977).

17. K. Nishiki, M. Erecinska and D. F. Wilson, Energy relationships between cytosolic metabolism and mitochondrial respiration in rat heart. Am. J. Physiol. 234:C73-C81 (1978).

18. M. Erecinska, D. F. Wilson and K. Nishiki, Homeostatic regulation of cellular energy metabolism: experimental characterization in vivo and fit to a model. Am. J. Physiol. 234:C82-C89 (1978).

19. M. Stubbs, P. V. Vignais and H. A. Krebs, Is the adenine nucleotide translocator rate-limiting for oxidative phosphorylation? Biochem J. 172:333-342 (1978).

20. M. Erecinska, T. Kula and D. F. Wilson, Regulation of energy metabolism: evidence against a primary role of adenine nucleotide translocase. FEBS Lett. 87:139-144 (1978).

21. R. van der Meer, T. P. M. Akerboom, A. K. Groen and J. M. Tager, Relationship between oxygen uptake of perfused rat-liver cells and the cytosolic phosphorylation state calculated from indicator metabolites and a redetermined equilibrium constant. Eur. J. Biochem. 84:421-428 (1978).

22. D. F. Wilson, M. Erecinska, C. Drown and I. A. Silver, The oxygen dependence of cellular energy metabolism. Arch. Biochem. Biophys. 195:485-493 (1979).

23. D. F. Wilson, C. S. Owen and M. Erecinska, Quantitative dependence of mitochondrial oxidative phosphorylation on oxygen concentration: a mathematical model. Arch. Biochem. Biophys. 195:494-504 (1979).

24. A. Holian and D. F. Wilson, Relationship of transmembrane pH and electrical gradients with respiration and adenosine 5°-triphosphate synthesis in mitochondria. Biochem. 19:4213-4221 (1980).

25. E. C. Slater, J. Rosing and A. Mol, The phosphorylation potential generated by respiring mitochondria. Biochim. Biophys. Acta 292:543-553 (1973).

26. E. J. Davis and L. Lumeng, Relationships between the phosphorylation potentials generated by liver mitochondria and respiratory state under conditions of adenosine diphosphate control. J. Biol. Chem. 250:2275-2282 (1975).

27. U. Kuster, R. Bohnensack and W. Kunz, Control of oxidative phosphorylation by the extra-mitochondrial ATP/ADP ratio. Biochim. Biophys. Acta 440:391-402 (1976).

28. E. J. Davis and W. I. A. Davis-van Thienen, Control of mitochondrial metabolism by the ATP/ADP ratio. Biochem. Biophys. Res. Commun. **83**:1260-1266 (1978).

29. R. Bohnensack and W. Kunz, Mathematical model of regulation of oxidative phosphorylation in intact mitochondria. Acta. Biol. Med. Ger. **37**:97-112 (1978).

30. E. N. Christiansen and E. J. Davis, The effects of coenzyme A and carnitine on steady-state ATP/ADP ratios and the rate of long-chain free fatty acid oxidation in liver mitochondria. Biochim. Biophys. Acta **502**:17-28 (1978).

31. M. Reichert, H. Schaller, W. Kunz and G. Gerber, The dependence on the extramitochondrial ATP/ADP ratio of the oxidative phosphorylation in mitochondria isolated by a new procedure from rat skeletal muscle. Acta. Biol. Med. Ger. **37**:1167-1176 (1978).

32. J. J. Lemasters and A. E. Sowers, Phosphate dependence and atractyloside inhibition of mitochondrial oxidative phosphorylation. The ADP-ATP carrier is rate-limiting. J. Biol. Chem. **254**:1248-1251 (1979).

33. G. Letko and U. Kuster, Competition between extramitochondrial and intramitochondrial ATP-consuming processes. Acta Biol. Med. Germ. **38**:1379-1385 (1979).

34. C. D. Stoner and H. D. Sirac, Steady-state kinetics of the overall oxidative phosphorylation reaction in heart mitochondria. J. Bioenerg. Biomemb. **11**:113-146 (1979).

35. R. Bohnensack, Control of energy transformation in mitochondria: Analysis by a quantitative model. Biochim. Biophys. Acta **634**:203-218 (1981).

36. J. J. H. Ackerman, T. H. Grove, G. G. Wong, D. G. Gadian and G. K. Radda, Mapping of metabolites in whole animals by ^{31}P NMR using surface coils. Nature **283**:167-170 (1980).

37. M. C. Kohn, M. J. Achs and D. Garfinkel, Distribution of adenine nucleotides in the perfused rat heart. Am. J. Physiol. **232**:R158-R163 (1977).

38. R. L. Veech, J. W. R. Lawson, N. W. Cornell and H. A. Krebs, Cytosolic phosphorylation potential. J. Biol. Chem. **254**: 6538-5647 (1979).

39. W. E. Jacobus, R. W. Moreadith and K. M. Vandegaer, Mitochondrial respiratory control. Evidence against the regulation of respiration by extramitochondrial phosphorylation potentials or by [ATP]/[ADP] ratios. J. Biol. Chem. 257:2397-2402 (1982).

40. R. W. Moreadith and W. E. Jacobus, Creatine kinase of heart mitochondria. Functional coupling of ADP transfer to the adenine nucleotide translocase. J. Biol. Chem. 257:899-905 (1982).

41. F. Gellerich and V. A. Saks, Control of heart mitochondrial oxygen consumption by creatine kinase: the importance of enzyme localization. Biochem. Biophys. Res. Commun. 105:1473-1481 (1982).

42. A. Vercesi, B. Reynafarge and A. L. Lehninger, Stoichiometry of H^+ ejection and Ca^{2+} uptake coupled to electron transport in rat heart mitochondria. J. Biol. Chem. 253:6379-6385 (1978).

43. W. C. Schneider, Methods for the isolation of particulate components of the cell, in: "Manometric Techniques," W. W. Umbreit, R. Burris and F. J. Stauffer, eds. Burgess Publishing Co., Minneapolis, Chapter 11 (1972).

44. M. Bradford, A rapid and sensitive method for the quantitation of microgram quantities of protein utilizing the principle of protein-dye binding. Anal. Biochem. 12:248-254 (1976).

45. J. M. Tager, R. J. A. Wanders, A. K. Groen, W. Kunz, R. Bohnensack, U. Kuster, G. Letko, G. Bohme, J. Duszynski and L. Wojtczak, Control of mitochondrial respiration. FEBS Letters 151:1-9 (1983).

46. E. Pfaff and M. Klingenberg, Adenine nucleotide translocation of mitochondria. 1. Specificity and control. European J. Biochem. 6:66-79 (1968).

47. W. E. Jacobus and A. L. Lehninger, Creatine kinase of rat heart mitochondria. Coupling of creatine phosphorylation to electron transport. J. Biol. Chem. 248:4803-4810 (1973).

48. V. A. Saks, N. V. Lipina, V. N. Smirnov and E. I. Chazov, Studies of energy transport in heart cells. The functional coupling between mitochondrial creatine phosphokinase and ATP-ADP translocase: Kinetic evidence. Arch. Biochem. Biophys. 173:34-41 (1976).

49. V. A. Saks, E. K. Seppet and V. N. Smirnov, Does oxidative phosphorylation increase the rate of creatine phosphate synthesis in heart mitochondria or not? J. Mol. Cell. Card. 11:1265–1273 (1979).

50. V. A. Saks, V. V. Kupriyanov, G. V. Elizarova and W. E. Jacobus, Studies of energy transport in heart cells. The importance of creatine kinase localization for the coupling of mitochondrial phosphorylcreatine production to oxidative phosphorylation. J. Biol. Chem. 255:755–763 (1980).

51. W. E. Jacobus and V. S. Saks, Creatine kinase of heart mitochondria: Changes in its kinetic properties induced by coupling to oxidative phosphorylation. Arch. Biochem. Biophys. 219:167–178 (1982).

52. W. C. T. Yang, P. J. Geiger, S. P. Bessman and B. Borrebaek, Formation of creatine phosphate from creatine and ^{32}P-labeled ATP by isolated rabbit heart mitochondria. Biochem. Biophys. Res. Commun. 76:882–887 (1977).

53. R. A. DeFuria, J. S. Ingwall, E. T. Fossel and M. K. Dygert, Microcompartmentation of the mitochondrial creatine kinase reaction, in: "Heart creatine kinase: The integration of isozymes for energy distribution," W. E. Jacobus and J. S. Ingwall, eds., Williams and Wilkins, Baltimore, pp. 135–141 (1980).

54. R. A. Altschuld and G. P. Brierley, Interaction between the creatine kinase of heart mitochondria and oxidative phosphorylation. J. Mol. Cell. Card. 9:875–896 (1977).

55. B. Borrebaek, The lack of direct coupling between ATP-ADP translocase and creatine phosphokinase in isolated rabbit heart mitochondria. Arch. Biochem. Biophys. 203:827–829 (1980).

56. K. Mosbach, The microenviornment of immobilized multistep enzyme systems, in: "Microenviornments and metabolic compartmentation," P. A. Srere and R. W. Estabrook, eds, Academic Press, New York, pp. 381–400 (1978).

57. K. M. Vandegaer and W. E. Jacobus, Evidence against direct transfer of the adenine nucleotides by the heart mitochondrial creatine kinase-adenine nucleotide translocase complex. Biochem. Biophys. Res. Commun. 109:442–448 (1982).

58. S. Erickson-Viitanen, P. J. Geiger, P. Viitanen and S. P. Bessman, Compartmentation of mitochondrial creatine phosphokinase. II. The importance of the outer

mitochondrial membrane for mitochondrial compartmentation. J. Biol. Chem. **257**:14405–14411 (1982).

59. A. K. Groen, R. J. A. Wanders, H. V. Westerhoff, R. v. d. Meer and J. M. Tager, Quantification of the contribution of various steps to the control of mitochondrial respiration. J. Biol. Chem. **257**:2754–2757 (1982).

60. R. Heinrich and T. A. Rapoport, A linear steady-state treatment of enzymatic chains. General properties, control and effector strength. Eur. J. Biochem. **42**:89–95 (1974).

61. R. Heinrich and T. A. Rapoport, A linear steady-state treatment of enzymatic chains. Critique of the crossover theorem and a general procedure to identify interaction sites with an effector. Eur. J. Biochem. **42**:97–105 (1974).

62. T. A. Rapoport, R. Heinrich, G. Jacobasch and S. Rapoport, A linear steady-state treatment of enzymatic chains. A mathematical model of glycolysis of human erythrocytes. Eur. J. Biochem. **42**:107–120 (1974).

63. H. Kacser and J. J. Burns, Molecular democracy: Who shares the controls? Biochem. Soc. Trans. **7**:1149–1160 (1979).

64. M. Erecinska, M. Stubbs, Y. Miyata, C. M. Ditre and D. F. Wilson, Regulation of cellular metabolism by intracellular phosphate. Biochim. Biophys. Acta **462**:20–35 (1977).

65. D. F. Wilson, C. S. Owen and A. Holian, Control of mitochondrial respiration: A quantitative evaluation of the roles of cytochrome c and oxygen. Arch. Biochem. Biophys. **182**:749–762 (1977).

66. P. Schonfeld and U. Kuster, Functional investigations of isolated mitochondria under steady-state conditions by means of a perifusion technique. Acta Biol. Med. Germ. **38**:1307–1314 (1979).

67. G. Letko, U. Kuster, J. Duszynski and W. Kunz, Investigation of the dependence of the intramitochondrial [ATP]/[ADP] ratio on the respiration rate. Biochim. Biophys. Acta **593**:196–203 (1980).

68. F. Brawand, G. Folly and P. Walter, Relation between extra- and intramitochondrial ATP/ADP ratios in rat liver mitochondria. Biochim. Biophys. Acta **590**:285–289 (1980).

69. G. K. Asimakis and J. R. Aprille, In vitro alteration of the size of the liver mitochondrial adenine nucleotide pool:

Correlation with respiratory functions. <u>Arch. Biochem.</u> <u>Biophys.</u> **203**:307–316 (1980).

70. W. Kunz, R. Bohnensack, G. Bohme, U. Kuster, G. Letko and P. Schonfeld, Relations between extramitochondrial and intra-mitochondrial adenine nucleotide systems. <u>Arch. Biochem.</u> <u>Biophys.</u> **209**:219–229 (1981).

71. U. Kuster, G. Letko, W. Kunz, J. Duszynsky, K. Bogucka and L. Wojtczak, Influence of different energy drains on the interrelationship between the rate of respiration, proton-motive force and adenine nucleotide patterns in isolated mitochondria. <u>Biochim. Biophys. Acta</u> **636**:32–38 (1981).

72. D. F. Wilson and N. G. Forman, Mitochondrial transmembrane pH and electrical gradients: Evaluation of their energy relationships with respiratory rate and adenosine 5-triphosphate synthesis. <u>Biochemistry</u> **21**:1438–1444 (1982).

73. N. G. Forman and D. F. Wilson, Energetics and stoichiometry of oxidative phosphorylation from NADH to cytochrome c in isolated rat liver mitochondria. <u>J. Biol. Chem.</u> **257**:12908–12915 (1982).

74. N. G. Forman and D. F. Wilson, Dependence of mitochondrial oxidative phosphorylation on activity of the adenine nucleotide translocase. <u>J. Biol. Chem.</u> **258**:8649–8655 (1983).

75. P. M. Matthews, J. L. Bland, D. G. Gadian and G. K. Radda, The steady-state rate of ATP synthesis in the perfused rat heart measured by ^{31}P NMR saturation transfer. <u>Biochem.</u> <u>Biophys. Res. Commun.</u> **103**:1052–1059 (1981).

CONTROL OF RESPIRATION IN INTACT MUSCLE

Michael Mahler
Department of Kinesiology and Jerry Lewis Neuromuscular
Research Center, UCLA
Los Angeles, CA 90024

We believe that the hydrolysis of ATP provides the free energy
for all cell function, and we know that the ultimate source of
almost all ATP produced in muscle is oxidative metabolism (Fig. 1).
We'd like to know, in as much detail as possible, the mechanism
coupling these two fundamental processes, whereby a change in the
rate of ATP utilization leads to a change in the rate of oxidative
phosphorylation. That brings me to my second reason for choosing
the first figure. In what can be thought of as perhaps the first
attempt to model the control of respiration in muscle, Chance and
Connelly[1] used a scheme little more complicated than this. Having
determined the responses of isolated mitochondria to limiting concentrations of ADP or inorganic phosphate (Pi), they assumed that
the rest of the cell could be represented simply as an ATPase. I

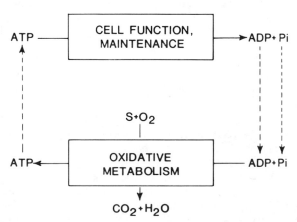

Fig. 1. Schematic diagram of the coupling of oxidative phosphorylation to ATP hydrolysis.

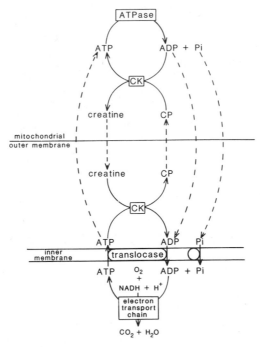

Fig. 2. Simplified schematic diagram of the reactions currently
believed to couple oxidative phosphorylation to extramitochondrial ATP hydrolysis.

mention this not to impugn or embarass two distinguished scientists,
but to illustrate the point that, in general, workers in this field
have shown a surprising lack of awareness of, or concern for, events
occurring outside the mitochondrial inner membrane. To the extent
that this audience shares that attitude, I hope to correct it.
Fig. 2 shows a current, schematic description of the reactions believed to couple oxidative phosphorylation to ATP hydrolysis, which
I hope will meet with everyone's approval. A certain fraction of
the ADP produced by ATP hydrolysis is rephosphorylated via creatine
kinase (CK); the rest of the ADP can presumably diffuse to the mitochondria. ADP is transported into the matrix, and ATP out, by
their translocase, and a carrier also exists for Pi. Within the
matrix, the rate of oxidative phosphorylation is some function of
the concentrations of ADP, Pi, ATP, substrate, and O_2. Since CK is
also present in the intermembrane space of the mitochondrion, a
certain fraction of the ATP leaving the matrix will be used within
the mitochondrion to produce creatine phosphate (CP); the rest will
presumably diffuse to the ATPases.
    Of course, the reason this scheme is acceptable is that it's
merely qualitative; the challenge lies in making it quantitative.
Considerable progress has been made in providing plausible quantitative descriptions of some of the individual steps, and the prevailing opinion seems to be that if we simply learn enough about

the pieces, we'll be able to deduce how the intact system must work.
Certainly, characterization of the individual steps is indispensable,
but it seems to me that the almost exclusive attention given to work
of this sort has brought the field of control of respiration to a
standstill, with no consensus on any major points, and competing
hypotheses appearing equally plausible in the light of selected in
vitro experiments.[2-7] I believe that before the field can progress,
proposed quantitative descriptions of the individual reactions comprising this coupling process must be placed squarely within the
context of the behavior of the process in intact muscle. Fortunately
for us, this behavior provides several provocative clues.

DYNAMIC BEHAVIOR OF THE COUPLING REACTIONS IN INTACT MUSCLE

The dynamic behavior of this coupling in intact muscle can be
demonstrated by analyzing the process as a system whose imput is
the rate of ATP hydrolysis, and whose output is the rate of oxygen
consumption (Q_{O_2}), both considered as functions of time. The
measurements I'll describe here were made on the excised frog
sartorius muscle. The essential features of any system are revealed
by its response to a family of impulse inputs,* and a brief isometric
tetanus produces an impulse-like change in the rate of ATP hydrolysis
in this muscle.[8,9] The method of measuring the subsequent time-
course of Q_{O_2} is based on the previous demonstration[9,10] that the
P_{O_2} profile within the muscle is well described by the diffusion
equation for O_2 in a homogeneous medium:

$$D\alpha\left(\frac{\partial^2 P}{\partial x^2} + \frac{\partial^2 P}{\partial y^2}\right) - \alpha\frac{\partial P}{\partial t} = Q, \tag{1}$$

where x and y are spatial coordinates, t is time, Q(t) is the Q_{O2},
P(x,y,t) is the P_{O_2}, D is the diffusion coefficient for O_2, and α
is the solubility of O_2 in the tissue. The principle of the method
is that from the measured time course of P_{O_2} at the closed, lower
surface of the muscle, obtained while the P_{O_2} at the upper surface
is held constant, we can numerically solve the diffusion equation
to find the corresponding time-course of the Q_{O_2}.[11] Two recent
modifications have been made in the method. Previously, I had assumed the frog sartorius muscle could be treated as a plane sheet.
However, a much better description of its configuration is given
by a hemi-elliptical cylinder (Fig 3), and the two-dimensional
diffusion equation, with elliptical boundary, is now used for the

---

* If the responses are essentially identical after normalization
  by impulse area, the system is linear, and its transfer function
  is the inverse Laplace transform of the response to an impulse
  of unit area.

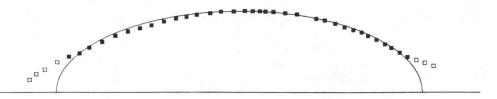

Fig. 3.   Points digitized from perimeter of a transverse section of
          frog sartorius muscle.   Smooth curve: best-fitting hemi-
          ellipse.

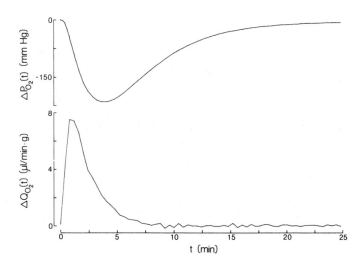

Fig. 4.   Top trace: time-course of P_{O_2} at closed, lower surface of
          sartorius of R. temporaria during and after an isometric
          tetanus of 0.5 s at 20°C.   The P_{O_2} at the upper surface
          was held constant at 446 mm Hg.   Bottom trace: time-course
          of ΔQ_{O_2} obtained by numerical solution of the diffusion
          equation for O_2.

determination of the Q_{O_2}.   We have also made direct measurements of
the solubility of O_2 in the frog sartorius.[9]   Fig. 4 shows results
of a typical experiment.   We're now quite confident of the accuracy
of this method.   Fig. 5 shows a check on this: the filled symbols
give the mean time-course of the rate of heat production in the
sartorius of R. temporaria after a 0.5 s tetanus at 20°C, measured
by Earl Homsher; we knew that the Q_{O_2} should closely match this,[12,13]
and, as shown by the open symbols, the time-course obtained by the
diffusion method did pass this test.

     As shown in Fig. 6, it was evident that the time-course of the
Q_{O_2} after a tetanus--i.e., the impulse response of the reaction
scheme coupling the Q_{O_2} to the rate of ATP hydrolysis, was very
similar to that of a simple first order system.   After a rapid rise
to a peak, the Q_{O_2} declined with a course that could be well fit by

196

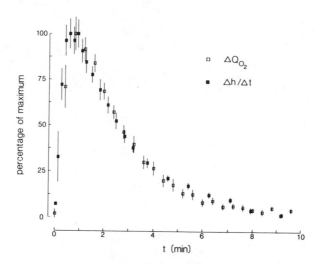

Fig. 5. Filled symbols: nondimensionalized mean time-course of the rate of suprabasal heat production, $\Delta h/\Delta t$, in the sartorius of R. temporaria after a 0.5 s tetanus at 20°C. Open symbols: nondimensionalized mean time-course of ΔQ_{O_2} as measured by the diffusion method, for the same conditions. Error bars designate $\pm$ SEM.

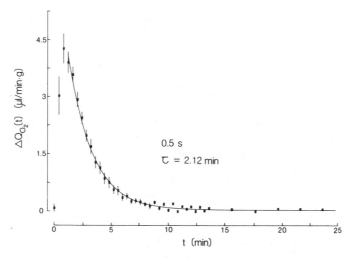

Fig. 6. Mean time-course of ΔQ_{O_2} in the sartorius of R. temporaria after a 0.5 s tetanus at 20°C. Smooth curve: best-fitting monoexponential. Error bars designate $\pm$ SEM.

a monoexponential. An equally important point is that when we increased the duration of the tetanus over a 100-fold range, for which the amount of ATP split during the contraction varied 20-fold, the value of this time constant of the Q_{O_2} didn't change.[11] Fig. 7A shows the mean time-course of ΔQ_{O_2} for a 0.2 s tetanus in the sar-

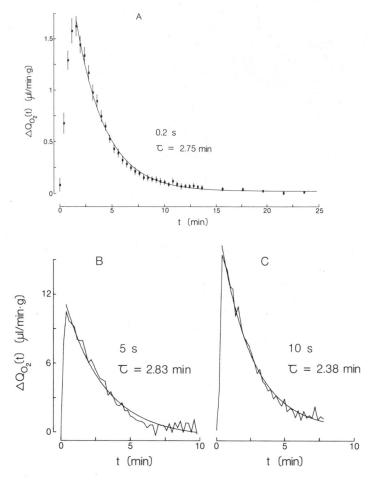

Fig. 7. A: Mean time-course of ΔQ_{O_2} in the sartorius of R. pipiens
after a 0.2 s tetanus at $20^{\circ}C$, with best-fitting monoexponential through descending limb. Error bars designate $\pm$
SEM. B,C: Single measurements of time-course of ΔQ_{O_2}
after tetani of 5 and 10 s at $20^{\circ}C$ in the sartorius of R.
pipiens, with best-fitting monoexponentials.

torius of Rana pipiens at $20^{\circ}C$, with $\tau = 2.75$ min. In a few cases,
we were able to get a relatively complete time course of Q_{O_2} in
this muscle after tetani as long as 5 or 10 s, and although the
data are rather sparse, the form of this time-course appears to be
essentially invariant (Fig. 7B,C). So, except for the brief delay
in reaching the peak response, the coupling process really does
behave like a first order system. Moreover, these kinetics are not
peculiar to frog muscle. On the contrary, they seem to be evident
in all skeletal and cardiac muscle (cf. ref. 11 for review).

198

That the coupling process we're examining should show such linear behavior, let alone first order kinetics, ought to come as a surprise. This branching, looping scheme of reactions (Fig. 2) behaves as if it were an unbranched chain, rate-limited by a single step with apparent first order kinetics, with rate constant $(1/\tau)$.

PROPORTIONALITY BETWEEN $\Delta\{CP\}$ AND ΔQ_{O_2}

The first order kinetics of muscle Q_{O_2} have an implication that's not immediately obvious. It depends also on the well known fact that the ATP content of muscle stays essentially constant, not only during a contraction (demonstrated for amphibian,[14-18] avian,[19] and mammalian[20-22] muscle), but also during recovery.[18-20,23,24] Using the constancy of $\{ATP\}^*$ during recovery, we can deduce that while $Q_{O_2}(t)$ is monoexponential, it must be changing in parallel with the levels of creatine and CP, as stated in Equation 2:

$$\Delta Q_{O_2}(t) \;=\; \frac{-1}{\tau p}\,\Delta\{CP\}(t) \;=\; \frac{1}{\tau p}\,\Delta\{creatine\}(t). \qquad (2)$$

Here $\Delta Q_{O_2}(t)$, $\Delta\{CP\}(t)$, and $\Delta\{creatine\}(t)$ denote the changes in Q_{O_2}, $\{CP\}$, and $\{creatine\}$, respectively, from their basal values, at time t, and p denotes the P:O_2 ratio for oxidative metabolism in vivo. Note that τ, the time constant of ΔQ_{O_2}, now appears in the proportionality constant linking $\Delta\{CP\}$ and ΔQ_{O_2}. The derivation of Equation 2 is straightforward, and is given in the Appendix.

This predicted proportionality between $\Delta\{CP\}(t)$ and $\Delta Q_{O_2}(t)$ was tested by measuring both variables under identical or equivalent conditions, according to two protocols. In the first, measurements were made after a 0.5 s tetanus in the sartorius of R. temporaria (Fig. 8). Using τ = 2.12 min (Fig. 8A) and p = 6.2,[8,22] the predicted proportionality constant was -0.0761 μmol O_2/min·μmol CP. After normalization by total creatine (C_T) content,[25] the observed line of best fit relating $\Delta Q_{O_2}(t)$ to $\Delta\{CP\}(t)$ had intercept not different from zero $[(-1.19\pm2.42)\times10^{-4}]$, correlation coefficient -0.993, and slope -0.0777 ± 0.0055. If the line was constrained to pass through the origin, its slope was -0.0755. No significant changes were observed in $\{ATP\}$ or $\{ADP\}$.

Despite this good overall agreement between prediction and observation, this test of Equation 2 was handicapped by the relatively large variability in the values of $\Delta\{CP\}$. In order to test

---

* The terminology and notation introduced by Hohorst et al.[26] are used, in which the tissue level of substance A, denoted $\{A\}$, designates the total content of A per unit weight. The symbol [A] is reserved for the actual concentration of A in free solution within the tissue or relevant compartment.

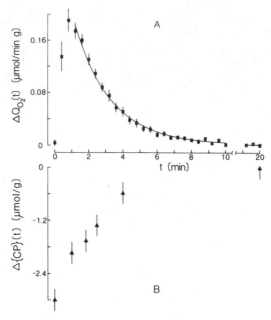

Fig. 8. Simultaneous time-courses of ΔQ_{O_2} (A) and $\Delta\{CP\}$ (B) in the sartorius of R. temporaria after a 0.5 s tetanus at $20^\circ C$. Error bars designate $\pm$ SEM.

the prediction over a wider range of values of $\Delta\{CP\}$ and ΔQ_{O_2}, a second protocol was devised. Sartorii of R. pipiens were tetanized isometrically for up to 10 s. As with shorter tetani, ΔQ_{O_2} could be determined by measuring the time course of P_{O_2} at the closed, lower surface of the muscle while the P_{O_2} at its upper surface was held constant, then numerically solving the diffusion equation for $\Delta Q_{O_2}(t)$. For tetani of longer than 5 s, the P_{O_2} at the lower surface of the muscle usually fell to zero within 2-3 min even when the P_{O_2} at the upper surface exceeded 700 mm Hg (Fig. 9A), but with the proper mathematical precautions, it was possible to calculate $\Delta Q_{O_2}(t)$ for the period during which the muscle was oxygenated, which was always long enough to allow Q_{O_2} to reach its peak (Fig. 9B). A 10 s tetanus presented a severe challenge to the contractile and metabolic capability of the muscle. Tension fell to $42 \pm 2\%$ (n=18) of its initial maximum. $\Delta Q_{O_2}(t)$, measured at 6 s intervals, had a peak value, reached 24 s after the beginning of stimulation, of 0.831 ± 0.047 (n=9) μmol O_2/min·g, nearly 30 times the resting Q_{O_2} [$0.029\overline{4} \pm 0.0015$ (n=12) μmol O_2/min·g]. Using $\tau = 2.6$ min and p = 6.2, Equation 2 predicted that $\{CP\}(t)$ would simultaneously have dropped to about half its resting value. Accordingly, rather than tracking $\Delta\{CP\}$ and ΔQ_{O_2} during a single metabolic episode, measurements were made of $\Delta Q_{O_2}(t)$, including the time at which its peak value was reached (t_{peak}), for five more tetanus durations between 0.2 and 5 s, and in companion experiments $\Delta\{CP\}(t_{peak})$ was measured

200

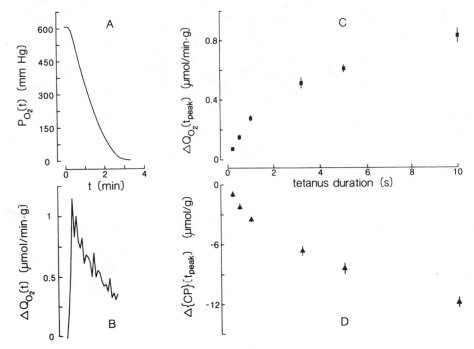

Fig. 9.   A: Time-course of P_{O_2} at closed, lower surface of sartorius
of R. pipiens after a 10 s tetanus at 20°C.   B: Time-course
of ΔQ_{O_2} calculated from the record in A.   C,D: Values of
$\Delta Q_{O_2}(t_{peak})$ and $\Delta\{CP\}(t_{peak})$ in the sartorius of R. pipiens
after tetani of 0.2–10 s at 20°C.   For a given tetanus
duration, t_{peak} denotes the time at which the mean time-
course of ΔQ_{O_2} reached its peak.   Error bars designate $\pm$
SEM.

for each tetanus duration.   Now it was unmistakable that ΔQ_{O_2} and
$\Delta\{CP\}$ closely mirror each other (Fig. 9C,D), and it was again impossible to distinguish statistically between the measured values and
those predicted by Equation 2.   The predicted proportionality constant was -0.0617 μmol O_2/min·μmol CP; after normalization by $\{C_T\}$,
the best-fitting line relating $\Delta Q_{O_2}(t_{peak})$ to $\Delta\{CP\}(t_{peak})$ had
intercept $(-4.88 \pm 11.0)\times10^{-4}$, r = -0.988, and slope -0.0666 $\pm$
0.0055.   If the line was constrained to pass through the origin, its
slope was -0.0646.   No significant changes were observed in $\{ATP\}$ or
$\{ADP\}$.

Again, the proportionality between $\Delta\{CP\}$ and ΔQ_{O_2} is not restricted to frog muscle, but appears to be a general one.   In Fig.
10, using a method suggested by Equation 2, I've plotted my results
together with data from the two other sets of experiments I'm aware
of in which ΔQ_{O_2}, τ, and $\Delta\{CP\}$ were all measured.[27,28]   Equation 2
can be rearranged to give

$$\tau \cdot \Delta Q_{O_2} \;=\; \frac{-1}{P}\,\Delta\{CP\}\,. \tag{2.1}$$

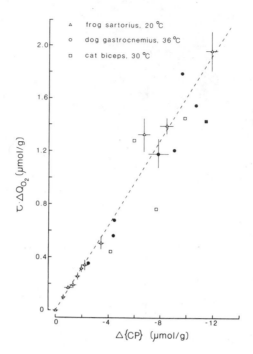

Fig. 10. Relationship between $\Delta\{CP\}$ and $\tau\cdot\Delta Q_{O2}$ in frog sartorius at $20^{\circ}C$,* dog gastrocnemius at $36^{\circ}C$,[27] and cat biceps at $30^{\circ}C$.[28] The dashed line is that predicted by Equation 2.1, using $p = 6.2$. Filled symbols denote steady-state values, and open symbols, non-steady-state values. Error bars designate $\pm$ SEM.

The value of τ can be expected to vary widely, depending on the species, muscle type, temperature, and other factors. In fact, it was 2–3 min in the frog sartorius at $20^{\circ}C$, only 24 s in the dog gastrocnemius at $36^{\circ}C$,[27] and 6.2 min in the cat biceps at $30^{\circ}C$[28]—— a 15-fold range. Similarly, for a given $\Delta\{CP\}$, ΔQ_{O2} can be expected to vary widely for different muscles; however, the $P:O_2$ ratio (p) should be very similar in all cases. Thus it's predicted that for a given $\Delta\{CP\}$, the product $\tau\cdot\Delta Q_{O2}$ should be essentially constant in all cases, and more precisely that it should equal $(-1/p)\Delta\{CP\}$. When plotted in this way, the data cluster encouragingly around the predicted proportionality. Moreover, in this context, a recent observation by Jacobus and co-workers has special significance: they

---

* The values of ΔQ_{O2} used here are 10–15% higher than the measured values shown in Figs. 8,9. Muscles used for measurement of ΔQ_{O2} typically had slightly higher values of $\{C_T\}$ than muscles used for measurement of $\Delta\{CP\}$, probably due to a slight drying of the former muscles in their gaseous environment. To correct for this, values of ΔQ_{O2} were first normalized by $\{C_T\}$, then multiplied by the mean values of $\{C_T\}$ of the muscles used to measure $\Delta\{CP\}$.

showed that when increases in [creatine] in the medium bathing isolated rat heart mitochondria were accompanied by equal decreases in
[CP], steady-state Q_{O_2} changed in parallel with [creatine] over the
entire physiological range,[29,30] just as occurs in intact muscle.

PSEUDO-FIRST ORDER KINETICS OF MITOCHONDRIAL CK

The observed proportionality between $\Delta\{CP\}$ and ΔQ_{O_2} during
recovery, together with the constancy of $\{ATP\}$, have an interesting
implication, stated in Equation 3. The forward CK reaction, which
presumably occurs within the mitochondria (Fig. 2), must be pseudo-
first order in $\Delta\{creatine\}$, with rate constant $1/\tau$:

$$\Delta v_{CK} \approx \frac{1}{\tau}\Delta\{creatine\} = \frac{-1}{\tau}\Delta\{CP\} . \qquad (3)$$

To see this, consider first the arguments summarized in Equation 4:

$$\Delta v_{CK} = \frac{d}{dt}\Delta\{CP\} \approx \begin{array}{c}\text{suprabasal}\\ \text{rate of ATP}\\ \text{utilization}\end{array} \approx \begin{array}{c}\text{suprabasal}\\ \text{rate of ATP}\\ \text{production}\end{array} \approx p\,\Delta Q_{O_2} . \qquad (4)$$

Because $\{ATP\}$ stays fixed, the suprabasal rates of ATP production
and utilization must be closely matched at all times. Of the pathways for suprabasal ATP production, all but oxidative metabolism
can be ignored. The rate of ATP production by the reverse CK reaction (Fig. 2) is normally virtually identical to the rate of ATP
hydrolysis,[14-22] but since suprabasal ATP hydrolysis during recovery
appears to be negligible by the time ΔQ_{O_2} becomes monoexponential,[9]
suprabasal ATP production via extramitochondrial CK is presumably
also negligible. Likewise, the fraction of suprabasal ATP production coupled to lactate formation appears to be no more than 5%.[24]
As for the pathways for ATP utilization, as just noted, suprabasal
hydrolysis of ATP appears to be negligible, and the only other
quantitatively important sink for ATP is the forward CK reaction.
It follows that during the period of interest, suprabasal ATP production results in a virtually stoichiometric increase in $\{CP\}$.
Substituting the observed proportionality between $\Delta\{CP\}$ and ΔQ_{O_2}
(Equation 2) into the rightmost term of Equation 4 yields Equation 3.

TWO HYPOTHESES CONCERNING MITOCHONDRIAL CK

The observation that the forward CK reaction, which we'll
assume to be occurring in the mitochondria, obeys a pseudo-first
order rate law during recovery leads to two hypotheses, one conventional and unenlightening, the other unconventional but quite provocative. Note first that the close match between the mitochondrial

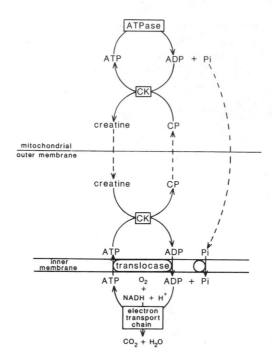

Fig. 11.   Modified schematic diagram of the reactions coupling oxi-
           dative phosphorylation to ATP hydrolysis, necessitated by
           the hypothesis that respiration is rate-limited by the
           mitochondrial CK reaction.   The direct fluxes of ADP and
           ATP between ATPases and mitochondria must be negligible.

CK rate and the rate of ATP production by oxidative metabolism
(Equation 4) is consistent with the conventional assumption that the
mitochondrial CK reaction is rate-limited by oxidative metabolism.
It would then follow immediately from the first order kinetics of
ΔQ_{O2} that Δv_{CK} must also exhibit apparent first order kinetics
(Equation 3), and that $\Delta \{CP\}$ must change in proportion to ΔQ_{O2}
(Equation 2).   With this hypothesis, however, one is still faced
with the task of accounting for the first order kinetics of ΔQ_{O2},
which, as discussed below, appears to be a formidable one.
     The close match between Δv_{CK} and $p \cdot \Delta Q_{O2}$ suggests an alternative
hypothesis: that oxidative metabolism, rather than being rate-limit-
ing for the mitochondrial CK reaction, is rate-limited by it.   This
hypothesis has at least two immediate corollaries that fly in the
face of conventional wisdom.   First, since a metabolic pathway cannot
be rate-limited by a near-equilibrium reaction,[31] it is implied that,
contrary to a widely made assumption, the mitochondrial CK reaction
cannot be continuously near equilibrium.   Second, if the intramitochondrial production of ADP via CK is an obligatory step in the
coupling between ATP hydrolysis and oxidative phosphorylation, it
follows that the direct flux of ADP from extramitochondrial ATPases
to the translocase must be negligible (Fig. 11); in other words,

this hypothesis for the control of respiration has as a direct corol-
lary the controversial "creatine shuttle" hypothesis.

The hypothesis that respiration in muscle is rate-limited by
the mitochondrial CK reaction neatly explains the first order kinetics of muscle Q_{O2}, since the mitochondrial CK reaction is observed
to be pseudo-first order in $\Delta\{creatine\}$ (Equation 3). Of course,
one is then left with the problem of accounting for these pseudo-
first order kinetics of mitochondrial CK from first principles. We
are currently investigating this.

TESTING MODELS FOR THE CONTROL OF RESPIRATION

Let me now pass to the topic of modelling the control of respiration in muscle. The hypotheses just discussed constitute models
only in a rudimentary sense: while they do describe the behavior of
the overall coupling process in terms of properties of its component
reactions, the latter properties themselves are rather hypothetical,
complicated, or mysterious; ideally, these properties should be fundamental ones like rate equations, equilibrium constants, or diffusion coefficients and distances. It's one thing, for example, to
postulate that respiration is rate-limited by mitochondrial CK, and
quite another to demonstrate that this follows from the fundamental
propeties of the underlying reactions.

One thing is certain: no model deserves to be taken seriously
if it fails to account for first order kinetics of ΔQ_{O2}, or a proportionality between $\Delta\{CP\}$ and ΔQ_{O2}. With such a test in mind, I
derived the relationship between $\Delta\{creatine\}$ and ΔQ_{O2} predicted by
the model originally postulated by Chance and co-workers in 1962,[32]
which assumes: 1. a well-stirred cytoplasm; 2. continuous near-equilibrium of CK; 3. determination of Q_{O2} by cytoplasmic [ADP], according to a first order Michaelis-Menten relationship; and 4. constant
([ATP] + [ADP]). Since this model was proposed, many additional
aspects of the control of respiration in muscle have become apparent,
including the chemiosmotic description of oxidative phosphorylation;
[33,34] the existence of the ATP:ADP translocase, and competitive
inhibition by ATP of inward ADP transport;[35-37] and the existence of
the mitochondrial isozyme of CK.[38] Nevertheless, the model assumptions remain plausible. The location of CK near all sinks and sources for ATP functions as a mixing device for the CK reactants, and
is thus consistent with assumptions 1 and 2. The rate of inward
translocation exhibits a first order dependence on [ADP], and is
competitively inhibited by ATP,[35-37] but since cytoplasmic [ATP]
stays essentially constant in muscle under almost any conditions,
[14-24] for a well-stirred cytoplasm the rate of translocation would
be only implicitly dependent on [ATP], via a constant K_M for ADP.
Assumption 3 is thus consistent with the hypothesis that the translocase is rate-limiting for oxidative phosphorylation.[3,5-7] If that
hypothesis is valid, this model would appear to be consistent with
the recent quantitative formulations of Williamson and co-workers.[4,39]

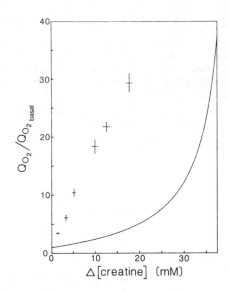

Fig. 12.   Relationships between Δ[creatine] and Q_{O_2}/(basal Q_{O_2}).
Data are those of Fig. 9, with the assumption that [X] =
1.5{X}. Smooth curve: relationship predicted by the model
of Chance et al.,[32] for parameter values given in text.

To place this analysis in the context of the general hypotheses
discussed in the previous section, note that this model is one in
which mitochondrial CK is rate-limited by oxidative metabolism,
rather than vice versa.   It's a matter of simple algebra to show
that the relationship between Δ[creatine] and ΔQ_{O_2} predicted by this
model, valid for both steady and non-steady-states, can be written
in the form

$$\Delta Q_{O_2} \;=\; \frac{C_1\,\Delta[\text{creatine}]}{C_2 - \Delta[\text{creatine}]} \;, \tag{5}$$

where C_1 and C_2 are positive constants (cf. Appendix).   If Δ[creatine]
is much smaller than C_2, this relationship will be approximately
linear.   However, it appears that for any plausible set of parameter
values, this won't be the case. C_2 is only slightly larger than the
resting [CP], which is the upper limit for Δ[creatine]; thus if
Δ[creatine] changes through any appreciable fraction of its physiological range, Equation 5 becomes markedly nonlinear.   As shown in
Fig. 12, for parameter values chosem to simulate the frog sartorius
at 20°C,* the predicted relationship between Δ[creatine] and ΔQ_{O_2}

---

*   The basal values of [ATP], [CP], and [creatine] were calculated
    using {ATP} = 5 mmol/g, {CP} = 25 mmol/g, {creatine} = 8 mmol/g,
    and the assumption that free intracellular water accounts for

differs drastically from that actually observed. Moreover, the predicted curve is remarkably insensitive to uncertainty in the parameter values. I can't see any way to move it up or straighten it out.

It seems fair to conclude that modelling of the control of respiration in muscle is still in a rudimentary stage. To my knowledge, no model exists which can account for these "red flags" the muscle is waving at us—the facts that the respiratory rate changes with first order kinetics, in parallel with the levels of creatine and CP. My challenge to all of you is to begin to produce such models; we won't understand the control of respiration in this tissue until we do. To do so, the assumption of near-equilibrium of CK in a well-stirred cytoplasm, so frequently and so blithely made to calculate increases in [ADP] at the translocase, will almost certainly have to be refined. My intuition is that the crux of the matter is the proper quantitative description of the flux of ADP from extramitochondrial ATPases to the translocase,[41] and of compartmentalization of ADP and ATP in the intermembrane space.[42-46]

APPENDIX

DERIVATION OF EQUATION 2

A formal derivation of Equation 2 for the case of the impulse response shown in Figs. 6,7 is the following. Let T denote the time at which $\Delta Q_{O_2}(t)$ becomes monoexponential. Then for any $t \geq T$,

$$\Delta Q_{O_2}(t) = \Delta Q_{O_2}(T) \cdot e^{-(t-T)/\tau}. \tag{6}$$

As discussed in the text and stated in Equation 4,

$$p \cdot \Delta Q_{O_2}(t) \approx \frac{d}{dt} \Delta\{CP\}(t), \tag{4}$$

or rearranging,

$$\Delta Q_{O_2}(t) \approx \frac{1}{p} \frac{d}{dt} \Delta\{CP\}(t). \tag{4.1}$$

66.7% Of muscle weight, so that $[X](mM) = 1.5\{X\}(\mu mol/g)$. Thus basal [ATP], [CP], and [creatine] were 7.5, 37.5, and 12 mM, respectively. K_{CK} was assumed to be 1/166,[40] and model assumption 2 forced basal [ADP] to be 14.5 μM. From model assumption 3 it follows that $K_M/[ADP]_o = [(max\ Q_{O_2})/(basal\ Q_{O_2})] - 1$, where the K_M is that of the translocase for ADP, and $[ADP]_o$ denotes the basal [ADP]. Measurements showed that $(max\ Q_{O_2})/(basal\ Q_{O_2})$ was at least 30, and it was assumed to be 40. This set K_M at 0.564 mM.

Equating the right hand sides of Equations 6 and 4.1 and integrating from t to ∞ yields Equation 2; the former integral is $\tau \cdot \Delta Q_{O2}(t)$, and the latter is $(1/p)\Delta\{CP\}(t)$.

DERIVATION OF EQUATION 5

Model assumptions 2 and 4 allow $\Delta[ADP]$ to be expressed as a function of $\Delta[creatine]$. Let the concentrations of MgADP, MgATP, CP, and creatine be denoted by D, T, P, and C, respectively, and let the subscript o denote the basal value. Then

$$K_{CK} = (D_o + \Delta D)(P_o + \Delta P)/(T_o + \Delta T)(C_o + \Delta C) \tag{7.1}$$

$$= (D_o + \Delta D)(P_o - \Delta C)/(T_o - \Delta D)(C_o + \Delta C) \tag{7.2}$$

and

$$\Delta D = \frac{(D_o + K_{CK}T_o)\Delta C}{(P_o + K_{CK}C_o) + (K_{CK} - 1)\Delta C} \cdot \tag{8}$$

Let Q denote the Q_{O2}. From assumption 3,

$$\Delta Q = \Delta Q_{max} \cdot \Delta D/[\Delta D + (K_M + D_o)] , \tag{9}$$

where K_M denotes the apparent K_M of the translocase for MgADP. Substituting Equation 8 into Equation 9 yields Equation 5, with

$$C_1 = \frac{\Delta Q_{max}(D_o + K_{CK}T_o)}{K_M(1 - K_{CK}) - K_{CK}(D_o + T_o)} , \tag{10.1}$$

$$C_2 = \frac{(K_M + D_o)(P_o + K_{CK}C_o)}{K_M(1 - K_{CK}) - K_{CK}(D_o + T_o)} \cdot \tag{10.2}$$

Assumption 3 is strictly valid only for steady states. However, the transient-state kinetics of the translocase[47] are evidently rapid enough that only small errors are introduced by making assumption 3 even during non-steady states. For example, the integrated form of Equation 9[48] provides an adequate approximation to the time-course of Q_{O2} or cytochrome a absorbance after addition of varying amounts of ADP to isolated mitochondria[49] (M. Mahler, unpublished).

From Equation 10.2, using the relationships $D_o<<K_M$, $K_{CK}C_o<<P_o$, $K_{CK}<<1$, and $D_o = K_M(\Delta Q_{max}/Q_o)$, it follows that

$$C_2 \simeq \frac{P_o(\Delta Q_{max}/Q_o)}{(\Delta Q_{max}/Q_o) - (P_o/C_o) - 1} \cdot \qquad (11)$$

E.g., for $(Q_{max}/Q_o) = 40$, $P_o = 37.5$, and $C_o = 12$, $C_2 \simeq 1.12\ P_o$.

Equation 11 shows that C_2, which determines the range of linearity of Equation 5, is essentially determined only by the readily measured parameters P_o, C_o, Q_o, and Q_{max}, not by K_M, K_{CK}, D_o, or T_o, which have much higher uncertainty. Similarly, the slope of the linear portion of Equation 5 is

$$C_1/C_2 \simeq (P_o + C_o)Q_o/C_oP_o \cdot \qquad (12)$$

ACKNOWLEDGEMENTS

Supported by NIH grant AM 32199. Portions of the work reported here were also supported by NIH grant HL 11351 and a Senior Investigatorship of the American Heart Association, Greater Los Angeles Affiliate.

REFERENCES

1. B. Chance and C. M. Connelly, A method for the estimation of the increase in concentration of adenosine diphosphate in muscle sarcosomes following a contraction, Nature (London) 179:1235 (1957).
2. E. J. Davis and L. Lumeng, Relationships between the phosphorylation potentials generated by liver mitochondria and respiratory state under conditions of adenosine diphosphate control, J. Biol. Chem. 250:2275 (1975).
3. K. Nishiki, M. Erecinska, and D. F. Wilson, Energy relationships between cytosolic metabolism and mitochondrial respiration in rat heart, Am. J. Physiol. 234:C73 (1978).
4. J. H. Williamson, Mitochondrial function in the heart, Ann. Rev. Physiol. 41:485 (1979).
5. R. G. Hansford, Control of mitochondrial respiration, Curr. Top. Bioenerg. 10:217 (1980).
6. W. E. Jacobus, R. W. Moreadith, and K. M. Vandegaer, Mitochondrial respiratory control. Evidence against the regulation of respiration by extramitochondrial phosphorylation potentials or by [ATP]/[ADP] ratios, J. Biol. Chem. 257:2397 (1982).
7. A. K. Groen, R. Van der Meer, H. V. Westerhoff, R. J. A. Wanders, T. P. M. Akerboom, and J. M. Tager, Control of metabolic fluxes, in: "Metabolic Compartmentation", H. Sies, ed., Academic Press, New York (1982).

8. M. Mahler, The relationship between initial creatine phosphate breakdown and recovery oxygen consumption for a single isometric tetanus of the frog sartorius muscle at 20°C, J. Gen. Physiol. 73:159 (1979).

9. M. Mahler, C. Louy, and E. Homsher, A reappraisal of diffusion, solubility, and consumption of oxygen in frog skeletal muscle, J. Gen. Physiol. (submitted).

10. M. Mahler, Diffusion and consumption of oxygen in the resting frog sartorius muscle, J. Gen. Physiol. 71:533 (1978).

11. M. Mahler, Kinetics of oxygen consumption after a single isometric tetanus of the frog sartorius muscle at 20°C, J. Gen. Physiol. 71:559 (1978).

12. D. K. Hill, The time course of the oxygen consumption of stimulated frog's muscle, J. Physiol. (London) 98:207 (1940).

13. D. K. Hill, The time course of evolution of oxidative recovery heat of frog's muscle, J. Physiol. (London) 98:454 (1940).

14. F. D. Carlson, The mechanochemistry of muscular contraction, a critical review of in vivo studies, Prog. Biophys. 13:262 (1962).

15. W. F. H. Mommaerts, Energetics of muscular contraction, Physiol. Rev. 49:427 (1969).

16. C. Gilbert, K. M. Kretzschmar, D. R. Wilkie, and R. C. Woledge, Chemical change and energy output during muscular contraction, J. Physiol. (London) 218:163 (1971).

17. E. Homsher, J. A. Rall, A. Wallner, and N. V. Ricciutti, Energy liberation and chemical change in frog skeletal muscle during single isometric contraction, J. Gen. Physiol. 65:1 (1975).

18. M. J. Dawson, D. G. Gadian, and D. R. Wilkie, Contraction and recovery of living muscles studied by ^{31}P nuclear magnetic resonance, J. Physiol. (London) 267:703 (1977).

19. P. Arese, R. Kirsten, and E. Kirsten, Metabolitgehalte und -gleichgewichte nach tetanischer Kontraktion des Taubebrustmuskels und des Rattenskeletmuskels, Biochem. Z. 341:523 1965).

20. R. H. T. Edwards, R. C. Harris, E. Hultman, and L. Nordesjo, Phosphagen utilization and resynthesis in successive isometric contractions, sustained to fatigue, of the quadriceps muscle in man, J. Physiol. (London) 224:40P (1972).

21. D. C. Gower and K. M. Kretzschmar, Heat production and chemical change during isometric contraction of rat soleus muscle, J. Physiol. (London) 258:659 (1976).

22. M. T. Crow and M. J. Kushmerick. Chemical energetics of slow and fast-twitch muscles of the mouse, J. Gen. Physiol. 79:147 (1982).

23. J. Piiper and P. Spiller, Repayment of O_2 debt and resynthesis of high-energy phosphates in gastrocnemius muscle of the dog, J. Appl. Physiol. 28:657 (1970).

24. M. J. Kushmerick and R. J. Paul, Aerobic recovery metabolism following a single isometric tetanus in frog sartorius muscle at 0°C, J. Physiol. (London) 254:693 (1976).

25. F. D. Carlson, D. Hardy, and D. R. Wilkie, The relation between heat produced and phosphorylcreatine split during isometric contraction of frog's muscle, J. Physiol. (London) 189:209 (1967).

26. H. J. Hohorst, M. Reim, and H. Bartels, Studies on the creatine kinase equilibrium in muscle and the significance of ATP and ADP levels, Biochem. Biophys. Res. Commun. 7:142 (1962).

27. J. Piiper, P. E. DiPrampero, and P. Cerretelli, Oxygen debt and high energy phosphates in gastrocnemius muscle of the dog, Am. J. Physiol. 215:523 (1968).

28. M. J. Kushmerick, unpublished results.

29. W. E. Jacobus and D. M. Diffley, Regulation of heart mitochondrial respiration by [creatine] and [phosphocreatine], Biophys. J. 41:249a (1983).

30. W. E. Jacobus, Regulation of mitochondrial respiration, (these proceedings).

31. D. F. Wilson. M. Erecinska, and P. L. Dutton, Thermodynamic relationships in mitochondrial oxidative phosphorylation, Annu. Rev. Biophys. Bioeng. 3:203 (1974).

32. B. Chance, G. Mauriello, and X. Aubert, ADP arrival at muscle mitochondria following a twitch, in: "Muscle as a Tissue", K. Rodahl and S. M. Horvath, eds., McGraw-Hill, New York (1962).

33. P. Mitchell, Chemiosmotic coupling in oxidative and photosynthetic phosphorylation, Biol. Rev. Cambridge Phil. Soc. 41:445 (1966).

34. P. Mitchell, Vectorial chemistry and the molecular mechanics of chemiosmotic coupling: power transmission by proticity, Biochem. Soc. Trans. 4:399 (1976).

35. P. V. Vignais, Molecular and physiological aspects of adenine nucleotide transport in mitochondria, Biochim. Biophys. Acta 456:1 (1976).

36. M. Klingenberg, The ADP-ATP translocation in mitochondria, a membrane potential controlled transport, J. Membr. Biol. 56:97 (1980).

37. J. M. H. Souverijn, L. A. Huisman, J. Rosing, and A. Kemp, Jr., Comparison of ADP and ATP as substates for the adenine nucleotide translocator, Biochim. Biophys. Acta 305:185 (1973).

38. H. Jacobs, H. W. Heldt, and M. Klingenberg, High activity of creatine kinase in mitochondria from heart and brain and evidence for a separate mitochondrial isoenzyme of creatine kinase, Biochem. Biophys. Res. Commun. 16:516 (1964).

39. J. A. Illingworth, W. C. L. Ford, K. Kobayashi, and J. R. Williamson, Regulation of myocardial energy metabolism, Recent Adv. Stud. Card. Struct. Metab. 8:271 (1975).

40. J. W. R. Lawson and R. L. Veech, Effects of pH and free Mg^{2+} on the K_{eq} of the creatine kinase reaction and other phosphate hydrolyses and phosphate transfer reactions, J. Biol. Chem. 254:6528 (1979).

41. R. A. Meyer, Am. J. Physiol. (in press).

42. V. A. Saks, N. V. Lipina, V. N. Smirnov, and E. I. Chazov, Studies of energy transport in heart cells. The functional coupling between mitochondrial creatine phosphokinase and ATP-ADP translocase: kinetic evidence, Arch. Biochem. Biophys. 173:34 (1976).

43. V. A. Saks, V. V. Kupriyanov, G. V. Elizarova, and W. E. Jacobus, Studies of energy transport in heart cells. The importance of creatine kinase localization for the coupling of mitochondrial phosphorylcreatine production to oxidative phosphorylation, J. Biol. Chem. 255:755 (1980).

44. R. W. Moreadith and W. E. Jacobus, Creatine kinase of heart mitochondria. Functional coupling of ADP transfer to the adenine nucleotide translocase, J. Biol. Chem. 257:899 (1982).

45. S. Erickson-Viitanen, P. Viitanen, P. J. Geiger, W. C. T. Yang, and S. P. Bessman, Compartmentation of mitochondrial creatine phosphokinase. I. Direct demonstration of compartmentation with the use of labeled precurcors, J. Biol. Chem. 257:14395 (1982).

46. S. Erickson-Viitanen, P. J. Geiger, P. Viitanen, and S. P. Bessman, Compartmentation of mitochondrial creatine phosphokinase. II. The importance of the outer mitochondrial membrane for mitochondrial compartmentation, J. Biol. Chem. 257:14405 1982).

47. E. Pfaff, H. W. Heldt, and M. Klingenberg, Adenine translocation of mitochondria. Kinetics of the adenine nucleotide exchange, Eur. J. Biochem. 10:484 (1969).

48. I. H. Segel, "Biochemical Calculations", Wiley, New York (1967), p. 245.

49. B. Chance and G. R. Williams, Respiratory enzymes in oxidative phosphorylation. VI. The effects of adenosine diphosphate on azide-treated mitochondria, J. Biol. Chem. 221:477 (1956).

ENERGY COMPARTMENTATION AND ACTIVE TRANSPORT

IN PROXIMAL KIDNEY TUBULES

Lazaro J. Mandel, Stephen P. Soltoff and
Peter C. Brazy

Department of Physiology and
Division of Nephrology
Duke University and Durham VA Medical Centers
Durham, North Carolina 27710

INTRODUCTION

The primary work of the kidney is active transport.[1] It is a long-standing observation that a linear relationship exists between the rate of sodium reabsorption by the whole kidney and its rate of oxygen consumption.[2,3] Since the oxygen is consumed at the mitochondria and the energy for active transport is used by the Na,K-ATPase located at the plasma membrane on the basolateral side, a basic question in cellular physiology concerns the mechanism whereby the two processes are linked. The answer to this question leads directly to energy compartmentation.

As shown in Fig 1 for a schematic model of a proximal renal tubule, ATP is hydrolyzed by the Na,K-ATPase into ADP and orthophosphate (P_i), which diffuse to the mitochondria for rephosphorylation into ATP. There is little creatine phosphate present in this tissue,[4] so alterations in the rate of Na,K-ATPase activity would be expected to result directly in concentration changes of ATP and/or its hydrolysis products. Furthermore, these products (ADP and Pi) have been shown to alter the respiratory rate in isolated mitochondria.[5,6] In this communication, we employ various experimental conditions which should be associated with changes in the cellular levels of ATP, ADP and phosphate. As we shall see, the changes we observed will be qualitatively in the expected direction; however, quantitatively, these

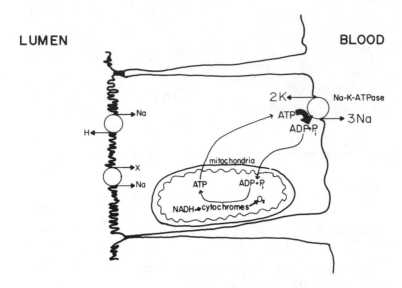

Fig 1. Schematic diagram of a renal proximal cell showing the relationship between mitochondrial ATP production and utilization of ATP by the Na,K-ATPase.

data are difficult to explain unless there is compartmentation, particularly between the cytosol and the mitochondria.

ADP COMPARTMENTATION

About 5 years ago, Balaban et al.,[7] in our laboratory, measured the total ATP and ADP levels in a preparation of proximal tubules in suspension under control conditions and after exposure to 25 µM ouabain. While the total ATP levels did not change much by ouabain addition, the ADP levels decreased by about 20% and the oxygen consumption was inhibited by about 50%. Qualitatively, this is the expected response since the lowered rate of ATP utilization elicited by ouabain would be expected to decrease the ADP levels, and thereby reduce ATP production and oxygen consumption. Whether ADP by itself constitutes the signal for respiratory control or whether it is the ATP/ADP ratio or the $\{ATP\}/\{ADP\}\{P_i\}$ ratio is a matter of intense controversy. Other communications in this volume deal with this fascinating topic in more detail.

In isolated mitochondria, the dependence of respiration on the extramitochondrial concentration of ADP has been measured in the presence of excess P_i. A saturable function of ADP has been described with a K_m in the 15 to 50 μM range.[8,9] If we take the ADP values of Balaban et al.[7] and convert them into concentrations using a value of 2.4 μl/mg protein for cellular water,[10] we obtain 520 μM for the control and 330 μM for ouabain. Both of these would be clearly saturating for the mitochondrial ATP-ADP translocase[8] and would stimulate the mitochondria to their maximal respiratory rate (state 3) in both conditions. This quantitative discrepancy may be due to the difference between an average cellular concentration calculated from a total cellular extract and the actual free cytoplasmic concentration of ADP.

Various types of studies in other tissues suggest that most of the cellular ADP is compartmentalized within the mitochondria and, therefore, only a small percentage of the total ADP is free in the cytosol.[9,11,12] ADP has been reported to be concentrated by factors of 10-1,000 in the mitochondria.[13] Veech et al.[9] found that only 5% of the total ADP in brain, liver, and muscle was metabolically active in the cytosol. If we assume the same proportion for kidney tubules, the control and ouabain-treated free ADP concentrations would be 32 μM and 21 μM, respectively, values close to the K_m for ADP in isolated mitochondria. This calculation is in agreement with ^{31}P NMR spectral analysis of rabbit and rat kidney tissue[14,15] as well as rabbit cortical tubules, showing that the free cytosolic ADP concentration is much smaller than the ATP value. Although these calculations may not quantitatively represent the events occurring in the intact renal cell accurately, they do indicate that the changes in ATP and ADP observed in this study during perturbations of active transport may explain the accompanying changes in QO_2.

OTHER POSSIBLE FORMS OF ENERGY COMPARTMENTATION IN KIDNEY TUBULES

Two types of experiments that we have recently performed suggest various other forms of energy compartmentation in the kidney. In the first experiment, we measured the dependence of Na,K-ATPase activity on the cellular ATP content in intact tubules and found this dependence to be surprisingly different from that found in the isolated enzyme.[16] The second type of experiment relates to the metabolic and transport consequences of phosphate deprivation in the kidney. The first type of experiment stresses the possible compartmentation of ATP within the renal cell, whereas the second one highlights the importance of phosphate compartmentation.

When broken membrane preparations from proximal kidney tubules were bathed in a solution containing 140 mM NaCl and 10 mM KCl, the Na,K-ATPase activity displayed a hyperbolic relationship as a function of Mg ATP concentration, reaching 90% Vmax at about 1.5 mM.[16] The Na,K-ATPase hydrolytic activity was half-maximally activated by about 0.4 mM ATP.[16] These results are similar to those reported for the Na,K-ATPase from other tissues as well as other renal tissue.[17,18]

To investigate the dependence of the Na,K-ATPase activity in intact cells on intracellular ATP, Soltoff and Mandel[16] used a suspension of proximal tubules exposed to graded amounts of rotenone, which inhibits the mitochondrial production of ATP by blocking the NADH dehydrogenase to lower the intracellular ATP content in a graded fashion. The tubules were initially suspended in a K^+-free medium to which rotenone was added, and the extracellular K concentration and the oxygen content were monitored on-line with electrodes. The extracellular potassium concentration that was measured at the beginning of the experiment was 0.2-0.3 mM, which is well below the $K_{1/2}$ of the Na,K-ATPase for potassium.[19] The Na,K-ATPase activity was stimulated two to three minutes after rotenone by the addition of a KCl bolus sufficient to raise the extracellular potassium concentration to about 5 mM. The KCl addition elicited a large increase in the respiratory rate, which was accompanied by the net uptake of potassium, measured by the disappearance of K from the medium. This K uptake represented active ion transport, since it was inhibited by ouabain and displayed kinetic properties that identified it as occurring through the Na,K-ATPase. Samples for ATP determinations were obtained during the period of maximal respiratory stimulation. These results enabled the rate of K uptake to be examined as a function of ATP in the intact tubules.[16]

Interestingly, the potassium uptake rate was a linear function of the ATP content. The intracellular Na+ concentration was about 150 mM during the K+-free incubation and presumably saturated the intracellular Na+ site of the ATPase, so these results singularly reflected the dependence of the Na,K-ATPase on ATP during conditions of maximal stimulation.

The ATP dependence of the Na,K-ATPase (sodium pump) activity of the intact proximal tubule could be quantitatively compared to that of the Na,K-ATPase of the membrane preparation by assuming a K/ATP stoichiometry of 2.[19] The Na,K-ATPase activities of both preparations as a function of ATP concentration are shown in Fig 2.

In these experiments, the maximal Na,K-ATPase activity in the intact tubules was obtained without rotenone present, and that gave ATP concentrations in the 3-4 mM range (Fig 2, highest point on dotted line).

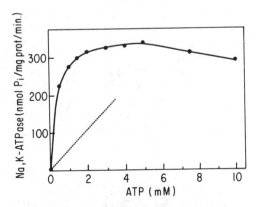

Fig 2.   The dependence of the Na,K-ATPase activity of proximal tubule membranes (solid line) and the sodium pump activity of intact proximal tubules (broken line) on the ATP concentration. Reproduced with permission from ref 16.

Lower ATP values were obtained with the graded rotenone additions. Qualitatively, these results provide important information regarding a novel concept, namely, that the cells do not normally possess a saturating concentration of ATP. This suggests that cellular metabolism may play a controlling role in the regulation of sodium transport.

This finding is consistent with the results of Gullans et al.[20] from our laboratory, who reported that a concentration of rotenone that reduced the ATP content of proximal tubules by only 30% also caused a proportional reduction of fluid reabsorption (J_v) in the isolated perfused proximal convoluted tubule. Other metabolic or pathological conditions which alter metabolism so as to change the production of ATP will similarly affect renal sodium transport.

In these studies, it is quantitatively not possible to evaluate the ATP dependence in terms of alterations in a $K_{1/2}$ value, since the sodium pump is not saturated with ATP in the intact tubule. Nevertheless, the affinity of the sodium pump for ATP appears to be much less than that of the Na,K-ATPase measured in the lysed membrane preparation. Moreover, the maximum Na,K-ATPase activity ($\simeq$ 340 nmol P_i/mg protein·min) for the proximal membranes was approximately twice the calculated maximum observed for the Na,K-ATPase activity ($\simeq$ 185 nmol P_i/mg protein·min) of the tubules in suspension (Fig 2). Thus, there are real quantitative differences between the results obtained in this study using the lysed membranes under specific well-defined assay conditions, and those obtained using a preparation that may be regulated in a more physiological manner. In the intact tubule, it is possible that the microenvironment in the vicinity of the Na,K-ATPase may be different from the one surrounding the lysed membrane fragments. The local concentrations of ATP, ADP, phosphate, magnesium, or vanadate in the vicinity of the pump are unknown. These compounds, singly or in combination, could affect the kinetic properties of the Na pump.[16]

Fig 3 shows the morphological organization of this microenvironment in a transmission electron micrograph of a proximal tubule, demonstrating a multitude of compartments. There is clear mitochondrial vs. cytosolic compartmentation. However, there may be multiple subcompartments; for example, most mitochondria are localized near the basolateral membranes. These mitochon-

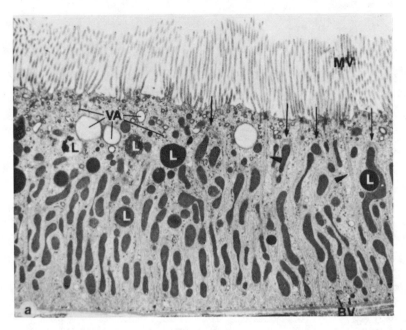

Fig 3. Electron micrograph of a proximal tubular (S1)
        segment from a rabbit kidney. Interdigitating
        cell processes in parallel arrangement contain
        long slender mitochondria that extend into the
        apical region (arrows). MV = microvilli, L =
        lysosomes, VA = vacuolar apparatus, BV = basal
        villi. Magnification is about 6800. Repro-
        duced with permission from ref 29.

dria are larger and more elongated than the ones
located near the apical side; therefore, there may be
more than one mitochondrial compartment. In addition,
at least two sub-compartments may be identified within
the cytoplasm. Notice the numerous invaginations
present on the basolateral surface, essentially paral-
leling the mitochondria as shown schematically in Fig
4. The Na,K-ATPase has been localized to the entire
length of this basolateral surface.[21] The cytosolic
space between the mitochondria and the basolateral membranes probably contains a very different concentration
of metabolic intermediates than the apical cytosolic
space. The feedback regulation of respiration by
active transport probably only involves the small cytosolic compartment between the mitochondria and the
Na,K-ATPase. To really be able to understand the

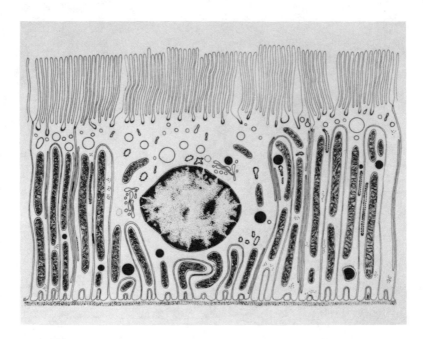

Fig 4. Schematic diagram of a proximal tubular (S1) segment highlighting the close association between the basolateral membrane invagination and the mitochondria. Reproduced with permission from ref 29.

kinetic relationship between these two processes, we would ideally need to know the ATP, ADP and P_i concentrations within that small space. We certainly have not succeeded in making those measurements nor do we know anybody who has. However, it is an important measurement to be made, and we bring it up as a challenge to stimulate creative investigators to obtain this information.

PHOSPHATE COMPARTMENTATION

Finally, we would like to discuss the important role of phosphate (P_i) compartmentation in cellular metabolism, a subject which became evident in experiments with phosphate-deprived tubules. These studies were performed in complementary experiments using individual perfused proximal convoluted tubules, in which net transepithelial fluid (J_v) and solute transport were measured under different experimental conditions, and a suspension of proximal tubules[22] for the metabolic studies. These tubules were prepared in the same manner as those used in the ATPase studies.

As shown by Brazy et al.,[23] perfusion of the tubular lumen with a fluid containing no phosphate completely inhibited fluid transport. In the tubule suspensions, the removal of extracellular phosphate produced appreciable inhibitions in both the control oxygen consumption as well as the QO_2 stimulated by respiratory uncouplers. The effect of phosphate depletion could only be elicited from the lumen, since removal of phosphate from the bath did not inhibit J_v. Thus, phosphate entry across the luminal membrane may be an important source of inorganic phosphate for cellular metabolism.

In this regard, the effect of sugars on the inhibitory actions of the P_i-free medium was very interesting, particularly the observation that the inhibition of J_v required the presence of glucose in the per-

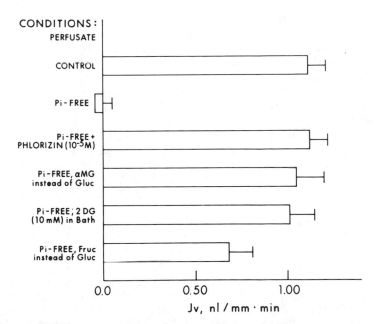

Fig 5. Effect of sugars on the inhibitory action of phosphate depletion on fluid transport (J_v). Adapted from ref 23.

fusate.[23] A series of experiments, shown in Fig 5, examined whether it was the entry of glucose into the cells or the metabolism of glucose that was responsible for this inhibition of fluid transport. Phlorizin, which inhibits the entry of glucose through the luminal membrane,[24] maintained J_v in a phosphate-free medium. Thus, the prevention of glucose entry protected the cells from the inhibiting action of glucose in phosphate-free medium. Similarly, substitution of α-methylglucoside (a sugar that is transported but not metabolized[25]) for glucose also protected the tubule and maintained a normal J_v. Finally, the addition to the bath of 2-deoxyglucose, which blocks glucose metabolism,[26] had a similar protective action.

These results suggest that the entry of glucose through the apical side followed by its metabolism interacts with intracellular phosphate to inhibit oxidative metabolism and transport. The pattern is similar to the Crabtree effect in which phosphate is sequestered by metabolic intermediates of glycolysis in the cytosol and therefore becomes limiting for oxidative metabolism under these conditions of phosphate limitation.[23]

Under these phosphate-deprived conditions, phosphate could become limiting to oxidative metabolism in at least two ways: (1) Directly, since P_i is a substrate of oxidative phosphorylation, reacting with ADP to form ATP; or (2) Indirectly, since intramitochondrial P_i exchanges for dicarboxylic acids that are Krebs cycle intermediates.[13] Therefore, the phosphate concentration in the mitochondrial matrix could be expected to influence the mitochondrial level of these intermediates. We examined the direct dependence of oxidative phosphorylation on cytoplasmic P_i by measuring the State 3 (ADP stimulation) response[6] of the tubule mitochondria as a function of P_i. This experiment was performed with tubules in suspension bathed in a KCl medium. Digitonin was added to permeabilize the plasma membranes to ADP and P_i, and a maximal ADP concentration was added in the presence of varying concentrations of P_i. The results (Fig 6) showed a linear dependence on P_i below 1 mM, and a tendency towards saturation at higher P_i values.[27] How do these values compare with the normal free cytosolic concentration of phosphate? In the presence of normal extracellular phosphate the total phosphate content approximates 5 mM, but most of this is bound.[11] Using NMR measurements, Freeman et al.[28] have estimated the free P_i to

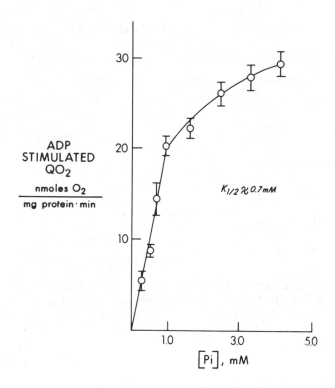

Fig 6.   Dependence of ADP-stimulated oxygen consumption
(State 3 respiration) on cytosolic phosphate of
proximal rabbit tubules. The experiments were
performed in 4 to 7 suspensions of digitonin-
treated tubules. Reproduced with permission
from ref 27.

be about 0.6 mM. Such a low value would suggest that
P_i is normally limiting for oxidative phosphorylation
and that this effect would clearly be magnified further
by P_i depletion.

We explored the indirect dependence of oxidative
phosphorylation on phosphate by determining the effect
of addition of various metabolic substrates to tubules
perfused with a P_i-free medium. As shown in Fig 7,
short chain fatty acids did not improve the situation,
which is not wholly unexpected since their entry into
mitochondria is independent of phosphate transport.[13]

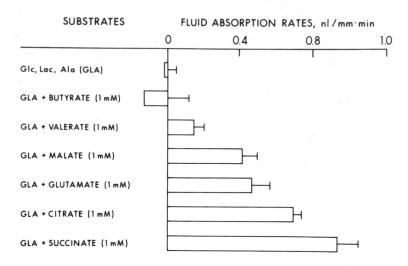

Fig 7. Ability of metabolic substrates to ameliorate the inhibitory action of phosphate depletion on fluid absorption. Adapted from ref 27.

On the other hand, Krebs cycle intermediates, which exchange for phosphate directly or indirectly, provided various degrees of restoration in fluid transport.[27]

We performed metabolic studies in tubule suspensions under these conditions to determine the extent of metabolic restoration afforded by the various substrates under P_i-free conditions.[27] The results with butyrate, which provided no restoration of J_v, and succinate, which provided full restoration, are shown in Table I. With no added substrate (no additional substrate supplementing glucose, lactate, and alanine), the omission of phosphate caused a 40% decline in ATP and oxygen consumption. Addition of a mitochondrial uncoupler increased oxygen consumption substantially, demonstrating that respiration was not necessarily limited by the availability of metabolic substrates even in the absence of phosphate. Rather, the limitation in oxygen consumption and the rate of ATP production was more likely a direct result of P_i limiting oxidative phosphorylation.

Table I. Effects of butyrate and succinate on J_V, ATP content and oxygen consumption rates in the presence and absence of phosphate. Adapted from ref 27.

Substrate Added	J_V (nl/mm·min)		ATP Content (nmoles/mg)		Oxygen Consumption Rates (nmoles/mg·min)			
					Control		Uncoupled	
	$+P_i$	$-P_i$	$+P_i$	$-P_i$	$+P_i$	$-P_i$	$+P_i$	$-P_i$
None	1.01 ±0.18	-0.02* ±0.05	7.51 ±0.7	4.57* ±0.3	20.1 ±0.7	12.6* ±1.0	31.1 ±2.2	24.2* ±1.2
Butyrate (1 mM)	1.04 ±0.15	-0.13* ±0.13	8.74 ±0.7	6.59* ±1.3	26.9 ±0.6	19.4* ±1.2	74.6 ±5.2	63.2* ±5.9
Succinate (1 mM)	1.10 ±0.09	0.93 ±0.16	8.96 ±0.37	7.81* ±0.42	23.9 ±0.6	21.0* ±1.0	50.1 ±2.2	48.4 ±3.6

*Values significantly different ($P < 0.05$) between $+P_i$ and $-P_i$.

The other results in this table indicate that both substrates are able to largely restore the ATP levels and the QO_2 rates toward normal, even if complete restoration is not achieved. Succinate preserves function a little better than butyrate, but it seems that measurement of these overall metabolic variables does not explain the difference between the effects of succinate and butyrate on J_V.

It is still unclear how succinate maintains J_V under conditions of phosphate limitation. Since free cytosolic phosphate may normally be limiting for oxidative phosphorylation, we speculate that succinate induces a redistribution of phosphate within the cell to make it available for metabolism. Phosphate redistribution could in turn induce a redistribution of other key metabolic variables such as Ca^{2+}, ATP and ADP, all of which may in some fashion be linked to each other. This is purely hypothetical, but it underscores the need to have detailed knowledge of compartmentation to begin to understand cellular metabolic processes.

CONCLUSIONS

To recapitulate, ADP, ATP, and P_i appear to be compartmentalized within the renal cell. Various aspects of the compartmentation of each of these were discussed, but more information regarding their compartmentation is needed to fully understand the energetics of this cell. To obtain this information will involve using innovative techniques and experimental approaches. In the next few years, it will be necessary to focus in on more specialized compartments to develop this knowledge.

REFERENCES

1. L. J. Mandel and R. S. Balaban, Stoichiometry and coupling of active transport to oxidative metabolism in epithelial tissues, Am. J. Physiol. 240:F357-F371 (1981).

2. K. Thurau, Renal Na reabsorption and O_2 uptake in dogs during hypoxia and hydrocholorothiazide infusion, Proc. Soc. Exp. Biol. Med. 106:714-717 (1961).

3. G. Torelli, E. Mella, A. Faelli, and S. Costantini, Energy requirements for sodium reabsorption in the in vivo rabbit kidney, Am. J. Physiol. 211:576-580 (1966).

4. P. Needleman, J. V. Passonnau, and O. H. Lowry, Distribution of glucose and related metabolites in rat kidney, Am. J. Physiol. 215:655-659 (1968).

5. H. A. Lardy and H. Wellman, Oxidative phosphorylations: role of inorganic phosphate and acceptor systems in control of metabolic rates, J. Biol. Chem. 195:215-224 (1952).

6. B. Chance and C. M. Williams, The respiratory chain and oxidative phosphorylation. Adv. Enzymol. Relat. Areas Mol. Biol. 17:65-134 (1956).

7. R. S. Balaban, L. J. Mandel. S. Soltoff, and J. M. Storey, Coupling of Na-K-ATPase activity to aerobic respiratory rate in isolated cortical tubules from the rabbit kidney. Proc. Natl. Acad. Sci. USA 77:447-451 (1980).

8. W. E. Jacobus, R. W. Moreadith, and K. M. Vandegaer, Mitochondrial respiratory control. Evidence against the regulation of respiration by extramitochondrial phosphorylation potentials or by {ATP}/{ADP} ratios, J. Biol. Chem. 257:2397-2402 (1982).

9. R. L. Veech, J. W. Randolph, N. W. Cornell, and H. A. Krebs, Cytosolic phosphorylation potential, J. Biol. Chem. 254:6538-6547 (1979).

10. S. P. Soltoff and L. J. Mandel, Active ion

transport in the renal proximal tubule. I. Transport and metabolic studies, J. Gen. Physiol., in press (1984).

11. T. P. M. Akerboom, H. Bookelman, P. R. Zuurendonk, R. van der Meer, and J. M. Tager, Intramitochondrial and extramitochondrial concentrations of adenine nucleotides and inorganic phosphate in isolated hepatocytes from fasted rats, Eur. J. Biochem. 84:413-420 (1978).

12. W. D. Schwenke, S. Soboll, H. J. Seitz, and H. Sies, Mitochondrial and cytosolic ATP/ADP ratios in rat liver in vivo, Biochem. J. 200:405-408 (1981).

13. K. F. LaNoue and A. C. Schoolwerth, Metabolic transport in mitochondria, Ann. Rev. Biochem. 48:871-922 (1979).

14. R. S. Balaban, Nuclear magnetic resonance studies of epithelial metabolism and function, Fed. Proc. 41:42-47 (1982).

15. R. S. Balaban, D. G. Gadian, and G. K. Radda, Phosphorus nuclear magnetic resonance study of the rat kidney in vivo, Kidney Int. 20:575-579 (1981).

16. S. P. Soltoff and L. J. Mandel, Active ion transport in the renal proximal tubule. III. The ATP dependence of the sodium pump, J. Gen. Physiol., in press (1984).

17. P. L. Jorgensen, Regulation of the (Na$^+$ + K$^+$)-activated ATP hydrolyzing enzyme system in rat kidney. I. The effect of adrenalectomy and the supply of sodium on the enzyme system, Biochim. Biophys. Acta 151:212-224 (1968).

18. J. M. Braughler and C. N. Corder, Purification of the (Na$^+$ + K$^+$)-adenosine triphosphatase from human renal tissue, Biochim. Biophys. Acta 481:313-327 (1977).

19. S. I. Harris, L. Patton, L. Barrett, and L. J. Mandel, (Na$^+$, K$^+$)-ATPase kinetics within the intact renal cell, J. Biol. Chem. 257:6996-7002 (1982).

20. S. R. Gullans, P. C. Brazy, S. P. Soltoff, V. W. Dennis, and L. J. Mandel, Metabolic inhibitors: Effects on metabolism and transport in rabbit proximal tubule, Am. J. Physiol. 243:F133-F140 (1982).

21. J. Kyte, Immunoferritin determination of the distribution of (Na$^+$ + K$^+$) ATPase over the plasma membranes of renal convoluted tubules. II. Proximal segment, J. Cell. Biol. 68:304-318 (1976).

22. R. S. Balaban, S. Soltoff, J. M. Storey, and L. J.

Mandel, Improved renal cortical tubule suspension: spectrophotometric study of O_2 delivery, Am. J. Physiol. 238:F50-F59 (1980).

23. P. C. Brazy, S. R. Gullans, L. J. Mandel, and V. W. Dennis, Metabolic requirement for inorganic phosphate by the rabbit proximal tubule. Evidence for a Crabtree effect, J. Clin. Invest. 70:53-62 (1982).

24. P. C. Brazy and V. W. Dennis, Characteristics of glucose-phlorizin interactions in isolated proximal tubules, Am. J. Physiol. 234:F279-F286 (1978).

25. A. Kleinzeller, J. Kolinska, and I. Benes, Transport of monosaccharides in kidney-cortex cells, Biochem. J. 104:852-860 (1967).

26. A. N. Wick, D. R. Drury, H. J. Nakada, and J. B. Wolfe, Localization of the primary metabolic block produced by 2-deoxyglucose, J. Biol. Chem. 224:963-969 (1957).

27. P. C. Brazy, L. J. Mandel, S. R. Gullans, and S. P. Soltoff, Interactions between phosphate and oxidative metabolism in proximal renal tubules, Am. J. Physiol., in press (1984).

28. D. Freeman, S. Bartlett, G. Radda, and B. Ross, Energetics of sodium transport in the kidney. Saturation transfer of ^{P}-NMR. Biochim. Biophys. Acta 762:325-336 (1983).

29. B. Kaissling and W. Kriz, Structural analysis of the rabbit kidney, Advances in Anatomy Embryology and Cell Biology 56:1-123 (1979).

THE OXYGEN DEPENDENCE OF CELLULAR ENERGY METABOLISM

David F. Wilson and Maria Erecińska

Department of Biochemistry and Biophysics
University of Pennsylvania
Philadelphia, PA.   19104

INTRODUCTION

It is well known that supply of oxygen to the heart is equal to the rate of oxygen utilization over a wide range of physical work loads (see Eckenhoff et al., 1947; Alella et al., 1955; Neely et al., 1967; Nuutinen et al., 1982). This precise regulation of oxygen delivery is expressed in the fact that the arterial venous difference in oxygen tension remains essentially constant when the heart work rates increase from minimal to near maximal levels. However, such precise regulation requires a tissue "oxygen sensor" i.e. an oxygen dependent metabolic system which detects changes in tissue oxygen tension in the physiological range and transduces this information into a form which regulates vascular resistance. In the present communication we will summarize data which indicate that the oxygen sensor for regulation of coronary flow is mitochondrial oxidative phosphorylation. We will then demonstrate that this metabolic pathway is oxygen sensitive in the physiological range of oxygen tensions both in vivo and in vitro and thus fulfills the requirements for the tissue "oxygen sensor".

Is coronary flow determined by cardiac oxygen tension per se or by the tissue energy state?

These two possibilities can be distinguished by comparing the effect of inhibitors of mitochondrial oxidative phosphorylation with that of changing mechanical workload on the behavior of isolated perfused rat heart (Nuutinen et al., 1982).

A. Increasing workload: In Langendorff perfusions of electronically paced isolated rat hearts oxygen consumption, which reflects

229

the metabolic energy requirement, increases with increasing perfusion pressure. The observed relationship of coronary flow to oxygen consumption is shown in Figure 1. The hearts were first perfused at a pressure of 70 cm H_2O (6.87 kPa) for 10 minutes and then the pressure was changed to either 100 cm H_2O (9.81 kPa) or 130 cm H_2O (12.8 kPa). Coronary flow increased step wise as did oxygen consumption. The data are best fit by a straight line which extrapolates to near zero flow at zero oxygen consumption. Causing arrest of hearts perfused at 70 cm H_2O by lowering the Ca^{2+} concentration to 0.5 mM supressed both flow and oxygen consumption. In this case the measured changes deviate slightly from proportionality which suggests an additional small direct vasodilatory effect on the vascular smooth muscle. In general, however, oxygen delivery (coronary flow) increases by the same amount as does oxygen consumption, resulting in a constant A/V oxygen difference.

When hearts are freeze clamped at each perfusion pressure and the tissue metabolite concentration measured, the creatine phosphate is found to decrease with increasing pressure while creatine and inorganic phosphate (Pi) rise. This means that the tissue energy

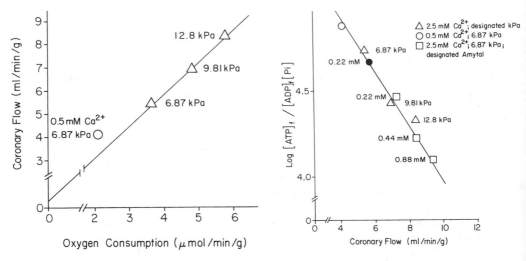

Figure 1. Correlation between oxygen consumption and coronary flow in isolated perfused rat heart. Oxygen consumption rate was varied by changing perfusion pressure ($\triangle$) or by lowering influent Ca^{2+} concentration (o). Linear regression analysis gives a correlation coefficient of 0.999 (taken from Nuutinen et al., 1982).

Figure 2. Relationships between coronary flow and [ATP]/[ADP][Pi] in isolated rat hearts perfused under the conditions indicated in the figure. The solid symbol ($\bullet$) indicates perfusion with 0.5 mM Ca^{2+} and 0.22 mM amytal. Linear regression analysis gives a regression coefficient of 0.982 (taken from Nuutinen et al., 1982).

level ($[ATP]_{free}/[ADP]_{free}[Pi]$), calculated assuming equilibration
of the creatine phosphokinase reaction, also decreases with increasing
perfusion pressure. As shown in Figure 2, coronary flow (and therefore the rate of oxygen consumption) is linearly correlated with the
logarithm of $[ATP]_{free}/[ADP]_{free}[Pi]$. It is worth pointing out
that the respiratory rate of suspensions of isolated mitochondria is
also nearly linearly related to the logarithm of the extramitochondrial $[ATP]_{free}/[ADP]_{free}[Pi]$ (Holian et al.,1977). Moreover, the
relationship of respiratory rate to the energy state for perfused
heart fits the same kinetic equations as does that for suspensions of
isolated mitochondria (Wilson et al., 1977b; 1979b; Erecińska et
al.,1978).

B. Inhibitors of the mitochondrial respiratory chain

Infusion of an inhibitor of the mitochondrial respiratory chain,
such as amobarbitol (amytal), into isolated perfused heart leads to a
rapid increase in coronary flow and decrease in oxygen consumption
(Nuutinen et al., 1982). Measurements of the metabolite levels in
hearts which have been freeze clamped at varying degrees of inhibition
show that increasing inhibitor concentration decreases
$[ATP]_{free}/[ADP]_{free}[Pi]$. The relationship between coronary flow
and the tissue energy level (Figure 2) is the same as that observed
for varied perfusion pressure.

These data show that:
1. Coronary flow is not regulated through tissue oxygen tension
per se since vasodilation occurs both when oxygen consumption
increases due to increasing work load (O_2 tension decreases) and
when oxygen consumption decreases due to amytal infusion (O_2 tension
increases).
2. Tissue energy level correlates with coronary flow for both
conditions suggesting that the latter is regulated in response to
changes in the metabolic products of oxygen reduction by oxidative
phosphorylation.

If mitochondrial oxidative phosphorylation is an important
"sensor" of tissue oxygen tension for regulation of coronary flow then
it must respond to changes in tissue oxygen tension in the same range
as does coronary flow. Since the mean oxygen tension in normoxic rat
heart muscle is reported to be near 35 torr (see for example Reves et
al., 1978), mitochondrial oxidative phosphorylation must be oxygen
dependent to this value and higher in order to effectively "sense" the
need for increased or decreased oxygen delivery.

Oxygen dependence of mitochondrial oxidative phosphorylation in vivo

Evaluation of the oxygen dependence of oxidative phosphorylation
in intact tissues must necessarily be concerned with oxygen diffusion

and spatial heterogeneity of the microcirculation. We have chosen, therefore, to use isolated cells for which in suspension there is a homogeneous milieu with uniform oxygen tension. When suspensions of cells were placed in a sealed reaction vessel, the oxygen tension of the media progressively decreased due to cellular respiration. Continuous measurements of the level of reduction of cytochrome c showed that it became steadily more reduced as the oxygen tension fell below approximately 80 μM (Wilson et al., 1977a; 1979a,b). In addition, the respiratory rate began to decrease below approximately 20 μM as did the cellular [ATP]/[ADP] measured in rapidly quenched aliquots of the cell suspension. These observations have been extended to include several mammalian cell types such as neuroblastoma (Wilson et al., 1979a,b), BHK cells (Wilson et al., 1977a), hepatocytes (Jones and Mason, 1978; Kashiwagura et al., 1984), oligodendroglia (Erecińska et al., unpublished) and Tetrahymena pyriformis (Erecińska et al., 1978). Thus it is a general observation that in intact cells oxidative phosphorylation by mitochondria is oxygen dependent throughout the range of O_2 tensions found in most tissues.

Mitochondrial oxidative phosphorylation in vitro. A. Normoxia

When mitochondria are removed from their cellular environment they are exposed to very different physical and metabolic conditions. Although our goal was to evaluate the oxygen dependence under physiological conditions, suspensions of isolated mitochondria allowed us to manipulate the metabolic state in order to study more effectively the phenomena of interest. In the steady state the rate of oxygen reduction by cytochrome c oxidase is, by definition, always equal to the rate of mitochondrial respiration. Thus we can simplify both measurements and interpretation by restricting electron transport to this portion of the respiratory chain. The non-enzymatic electron donors phenazine methosulfate and N,N,N',N'-tetramethyl-p-phenylene diamine (TMPD) directly donate their reducing equivalents to cytochrome c, bypassing the first two phosphorylation sites. When TMPD is used as electron donor the reactions which are kinetically significant are:

$$\text{TPMD} + c^{3+} \longrightarrow c^{2+} + \text{WB} \qquad (1)$$

In the presence of ascorbate to rereduce rapidly Wursters Blue (WB) to TMPD the donor remains essentially fully as TMPD. The net result is an irreversible second order reaction of TMPD with oxidized cytochrome c (c^{3+}). The rate of respiration is determined by the rate of reoxidation of reduced cytochrome c by molecular oxygen

$$2c^{2+} + 1/2 \ O_2 + 2H^+ + \text{ADP} + \text{Pi} \longrightarrow 2c^{3+} + H_2O + \text{ATP} \qquad (2)$$

This is the minimal reaction with which the regulation of mitochondrial respiration can be studied. The rate of this reaction is dependent on the pH of the medium, level of reduction of cytochrome c,

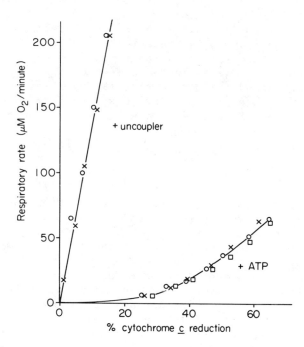

Figure 3. Dependence of mitochondrial respiratory rate on the level of reduction of cytochrome c. Rat liver mitochondria were suspended at a final concentration of cytochrome c of 0.59 μM in a 0.2 M mannitol, 0.05 M sucrose, 0.2 mM EGTA medium buffered with 30 mM Tris-Cl, final pH 8.0. The mitochondria were treated with 8 mM Na ascorbate and the respiratory rate and cytochrome c reduction (550 nm - 540 nm) measured after sequential additions of TMPD (25 uM to 500 uM). For the experimental data labeled + uncoupler 0.2 μM S-13 (5-Cl-3-t-butyl-2'-Cl-4'-nitrosalicylanilide) was added after ascorbate while for the experimental data labeled +ATP 0.05 μM S-13 was added to fully oxidize cytochrome c, the mitochondria were recoupled with 2 mg bovine serum albumin/ml and then 2 mM ATP was added. The reaction chamber was thermostatted at 23 $\pm$ 0.2°C.

[ATP]/[ADP][Pi] and [O_2]. When pH and [ATP]/[ADP][Pi] are held constant, increasing the concentration of TMPD causes reduction of cytochrome c and an increased respiratory rate (see Figure 3). For suspensions of rat liver mitochondria which were fully uncoupled the respiratory rate increased linearly with increasing reduction of cytochrome c with the maximal respiratory rate at 23° corresponding to a cytochrome c turnover of 158 sec^{-1} or a cytochrome a turnover of approximately 300 sec^{-1}. By contrast, when the mitochondria were fully coupled and treated with 4 mM ATP the respiratory rate was much lower at each level of cytochrome c reduction and the relationship was not linear. At 25% reduction of cytochrome c the respiratory rate was 5 μM O_2/min in the presence of ATP and 340 μM O_2/min after uncoupling, giving a respiratory control ratio of 68.

The effect of $[H^+]$ is different in uncoupled and coupled mitochondria. For the former, the relationship of cytochrome c reduction and the respiratory rate is independent of pH between 6.6 and 8.3
whereas for the latter (i.e. in the presence of ATP) a strong pH
dependence is observed (Wilson et al., 1977b). Moreover, the behavior
of mitochondria with excess ATP deviates more from that of uncoupled
mitochondria as the pH is made more alkaline (Wilson et al., 1977b).

Mitochondrial oxidative phosphorylation in vitro: B. Oxygen
concentration dependence

Since reaction 2 is dependent on pH, [ATP]/[ADP][Pi] and the
reduction of cytochrome c these parameters must be considered when
evaluating its oxygen dependence. Indeed the kinetic model previously
described (Wilson et al., 1977b; 1979b; Erecińska et al., 1978)
predicts that when the state of reduction of cytochrome c and
[ATP]/[ADP][Pi] are held constant oxygen dependence increases with
increasing pH and when the state of reduction of cytochrome c and pH
are held constant the oxygen dependence increases with increasing
[ATP]/[ADP][Pi]. These predictions have been tested and found to be
generally correct. In the following we will demonstrate the oxygen
dependence of oxidative phosphorylation at high [ATP]/[ADP][Pi], first
at alkaline pH (8.3) where it is more easily observed and then at pH
7.4.

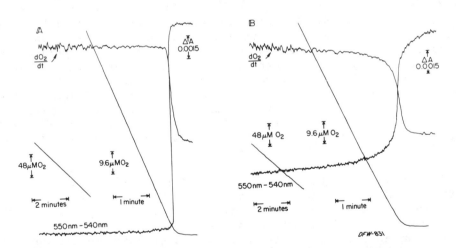

Figure 4A,B. The oxygen dependence of the respiratory rate and
cytochrome c reduction in suspensions of isolated rat liver
mitochondria at pH 7.4. Rat liver mitochondria were suspended at a
cytochrome c concentration of 0.67 μM in a medium containing 0.2 M
sucrose, 0.2 mM EGTA and 30 mM Tris-Cl. A. The mitochondria were
uncoupled with 0.2 μM S-13, 8 mM ascorbate added and then respiration
initiated by adding 30 μM TMPD. B. The same conditions as for A
except that 3 mM ATP was added instead of S-13. The incubation
temperature was $23\pm0.2^{\circ}$C.

234

Suspensions of rat liver mitochondria were treated with uncoupler, respiration was activated by addition of TMPD and ascorbate and· then the respiratory rate and cytochrome c reduction were measured. There was little change in either the respiratory rate or cytochrome c reduction until the oxygen concentration approached zero (Figure 4A). When coupled mitochondria at pH 8.3 in the presence of ATP were used, cytochrome c reduction began when the oxygen concentration fell below approximately 150 μM while the respiratory rate began to decrease below approximately 50 μM (Figure 4B). For either uncoupled or coupled mitochondria addition of oxygen at any point returned both respiratory rate and cytochrome c reduction to their values at the higher oxygen concentration. The marked difference in oxygen dependence between uncoupled and coupled mitochondria for otherwise identical experimental conditions clearly establishes that the difference is of metabolic origin.

In agreement with Figure 3, cytochrome c was much more reduced in coupled mitochondria with ATP than in uncoupled mitochondria when the experimental conditions were selected to give equal respiratory rates (the large difference in respiratory rates precludes experiments at equal reduction of cytochrome c). Since any absorption changes other than cytochrome c reduction and all instrument limitations including response time are contained in experiments such as that in Figure 4A, the latter serve as good controls for studies with coupled mitochondria.

The oxygen dependence at pH 7.4 (Figure 5A,B) was less than that at pH 8.3 but still readily measurable. Cytochrome c reduction began at approximately 50 μM O_2 while the decrease in respiratory rate began by approximately 25 μM O_2.

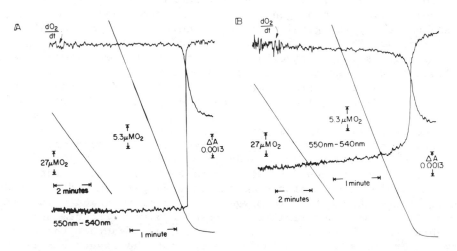

Figure 5A,B. The oxygen dependence of the respiratory rate and cytochrome c reduction in suspensions of isolated rat liver mitochondria at pH 7.4. The reaction conditions were the same as in Figure 4 except that the final pH was 7.4.

DISCUSSION

It has generally been observed that in suspensions of intact
cells (Warburg and Kubowitz, 1929; Longmuir, 1957; Wilson et al.,
1977; 1979a,b; Jones and Mason, 1978) and of isolated mitochondria
(Peterson et al., 1974; Oshino et al., 1974; Sugano et al., 1974) the
rate of respiration is independent of oxygen concentration down to low
values (apparent Km less than 1 uM). On the other hand, measurements
of other metabolic functions related to oxidative phosphorylation
including cytochrome $\underline{c}$ reduction, cellular [ATP]/[ADP][Pi], and
lactate/pyruvate ratio (Wilson et al., 1977; 1979a,b; Jones and Mason,
1978; Jones and Kennedy, 1982) showed that these all begin to change
at much higher oxygen tensions than does the respiratory rate. This
apparent paradox arises from the regulatory mechanisms which control
the rate of mitochondrial respiration combined with the fact that the
ATP utilizing reactions are, for the most part, independent of oxygen
concentration. Decreasing oxygen tension causes a decrease in the
rate of ATP synthesis but does not affect the rate of ATP utilization.
Thus with a decline in [O_2] the rate of ATP synthesis falls below
the rate of ATP utilization and this lowers [ATP]/[ADP][Pi].
Decreasing [ATP]/[ADP][Pi], however, stimulates the rate of ATP
synthesis and the latter quickly rises until it again equals the rate
of ATP utilization. The net effect is that the rate of respiration
(ATP synthesis) remains essentially constant to very low oxygen
tensions but the cellular metabolic parameters such as cytochrome $\underline{c}$
reduction and [ATP]/[ADP][Pi] begin to change at much higher oxygen
tensions.

Two different explanations have been offered for the fact that in
intact cells mitochondrial oxidative phosphorylation is dependent on
oxygen tension above 1-2 torr. One explanation attributes this
behavior directly to the oxygen dependence of mitochondrial cytochrome
$\underline{c}$ oxidase under physiological metabolic conditions (Wilson et al,
1977a; 1979a,b). The other is that mitochondrial oxidative
phosphorylation is insensitive to oxygen tension to very low values
but diffusion of oxygen is restricted by 70-100 fold at the
cytosol/mitochondria interface (Aw and Jones, 1982; Jones and Mason,
1978; Jones and Kennedy, 1982). The observed oxygen dependence would
then be due to the oxygen tension in the mitochondria being less than
that in the cytosol. The first explanation predicts that under
experimental conditions similar to those which the mitochondria
experience $\underline{in}$ $\underline{vivo}$ the oxygen dependence of suspensions of
isolated mitochondria should be similar to that observed in intact
cells. The second explanation predicts that suspensions of isolated
mitochondria are insensitive to oxygen tension to very low values (< 1
μM) even under conditions similar to those $\underline{in}$ $\underline{vivo}$. Experimental
data such as that shown in Figures 4 and 5 clearly support the first
explanation and provide strong evidence against the oxygen barrier
hypothesis.

It is important to emphasize that for a multi-substrate reaction
such as cytochrome c oxidase (reaction 2), the Km (substrate
concentration for 50% maximal respiratory rate) for any one of the
reactants is often strongly dependent on the concentration(s) of the
other reactants. A good example of such an interdependence is
observed in the kinetic equations for a proposed mechanism of oxygen
reduction by cytochrome c oxidase (Wilson et al, 1979b). The
kinetic relationships for this model predict very small Km values ($<$ 1
μM) for uncoupled mitochondria and much larger Km values (to $>$ 50 μM)
when [ATP]/[ADP][Pi] is high. Thus the model is fully consistent with
the oxygen dependence observed in the respiratory rate and energy
relationships of both intact cells (Wilson et al., 1977a; 1979a,b;
Jones and Mason, 1978) and suspensions of isolated mitochondria
(Wilson et al., 1979b; Degn et al., 1974; Peterson et al., 1974; this
paper). This means that there is not a single Km for oxygen but the
Km is strongly dependent on the other reactants of cytochrome c
oxidase. Studies of the oxygen dependence of mitochondrial oxidative
phosphorylation in vivo and in vitro must be equally as
concerned with these variables as with oxygen tension.

SUMMARY

   1. In isolated perfused rat hearts coronary flow appears to be
regulated through the tissue energy level ([ATP]free/[ADP]free[Pi]), a
metabolic product of oxygen metabolism by mitochondria, and not by the
tissue oxygen tension.
   2. Mitochondrial oxidative phosphorylation in intact cells and
tissues is dependent on oxygen tension throughout the physiological
range. This allows oxidative phosphorylation to serve as an important
tissue oxygen sensor.
   3. The apparent Km of mitochondrial cytochrome c oxidase for
oxygen is dependent on the pH of the suspending medium,
[ATP]/[ADP][Pi] and the state of reduction of cytochrome c.
   4. When physiological levels of [ATP]/[ADP][Pi], pH and
cytochrome c reduction are used, oxidative phosphorylation by
suspensions of isolated mitochondria has an oxygen dependence similar
to that observed in intact cells.

Partially supported by GM-21524

REFERENCES

Alella, A., Williams, F.L., Bolene-Williams, C. and Katz, L.N., 1955,
    Interrelation between cardiac oxygen consumption and coronary
    blood flow, Am. J. Physiol., 183: 570-582.
Aw, T.Y. and Jones, D.P. 1982, Secondary bioenergetic hypoxia:
    inhibition of sulfation and glucuronidation reactions in isolated
    hepatocytes at low O_2 concentration, J. Biol. Chem., 257;
    8997-9004.

Eckenhoff, J.E., Hafkenschiel, J.H., Laudmesser, C.M. and Harmel, M., 1947, Cardiac oxygen metabolism and control of the coronary circulation, Am. J. Physiol., 149: 634–649.

Erecińska, M., Wilson, D.F. and Nishiki, K., 1978, Homeostatic regulation of cellular energy metabolism: Experimental characterization in vivo and fit to a model., Amer. J. Physiol., 234: C82–C89.

Holian, A., Owen, C.S. and Wilson, D.F., 1977, Control of respiration in isolated mitochondria: Quantitative evaluation of the dependence of respiratory rates on [ATP],[ADP] and [Pi], Arch. Biochem. Biophys., 181: 164–171.

Jones, D.P. and Kennedy, F.G., 1982, Intracellular O_2 gradients in cardiac myocytes. Lack of a role for myoglobin in facilitation of intracellular O_2 diffusion, Biochem. Biophys. Res. Commun., 105: 419–424.

Jones, D.P., and Mason, H.S., 1978, Gradients of O_2 concentration in hepatocytes, J. Biol. Chem. 253: 4874–4880.

Kashiwagura, T., Wilson, D.F. and Erecińska, M., 1984, Oxygen dependence of cellular metabolism: The effect of O_2 tension on gluconeogenesis and urea synthesis in isolated rat hepatocytes, J. Cell. Physiol. in Press.

Longmuir, I.S., 1957, Respiration rate of rat liver cells at low oxygen concentrations, Biochem. J. 65: 378–382.

Neely, J.R., Liebmeister, H., Battersby, E.J. and Morgan, H.E., 1967, Effect of pressure development on oxygen consumption by isolated rat heart, Amer. J. Physiol. 212: 804–814.

Nuutinen, E.M., Nishiki, K., Erecińska, M. and Wilson, D.F., 1982, Role of mitochondrial oxidative phosphorylation in regulation of coronary blood flow, Am. J. Physiol., 243: H159–H169.

Oshino, N., Sugano, T., Oshino, R. and Chance, B., 1974, Mitochondrial function under hypoxic conditions: The steady states of cytochromes $\underline{a} + \underline{a}_3$ and their relation to mitochondrial energy states, Biochim. Biophys. Acta, 368: 298–310.

Peterson, L.C., Nicholls, P. and Degn, H., 1974, The effect of energization on the apparent Michaelis-Menten constant for oxygen in mitochondrial respiration, Biochem.J. 142: 249–252.

Reves, J.G., Erdmann, W., Mardis, M., Karp, R.B., King, M. and Lell, W.A., 1978, Evidence for existence of intramyocardial steal, in "Oxygen transport to Tissue III", I.A. Silver, M. Erecińska and H. Bicher eds. Plenum, New York, p. 755–760.

Sugano, T., Oshino, N.and Chance, B., 1974, Mitochondrial functions under hypoxic conditions: The steady states of cytochrome $\underline{c}$ reduction and of energy metabolism. Biochem. Biophys. Acta, 347: 340–358.

Warburg, O. and Kubowitz, F., 1929, Atmung bei sehr kleinen Sauerstoffdrucken, Biochem. Z., 214: 5–18.

Wilson, D.F., Owen, C.S. and Erecińska, M., Drown, C., and Silver, I.A., 1979a, The oxygen dependence of cellular energy metabolism, Arch. Biochem. Biophys., 195: 485–493.

Wilson, D.F., Erecińska, M., Drown, C. and Silver, I.A., 1977a, Effect of oxygen tension on cellular energetics, Amer. J. Physiol., 233(5): C135-C140.

Wilson, D.F., Owen, C.S. and Erecińska, M., 1979b, Quantitative dependence of mitochondrial oxidative phosphorylation on oxygen concentration: A mathematical model., Arch. Biochem. Biophys., 195: 494-504.

Wilson, D.F., Owen, C.S. and Holian, A., 1977b, Control of mitochondrial respiration: A quantitative evaluation of the roles of cytochrome c and oxygen, Arch. Biochem. Biophys., 182: 749-762.

REGULATION OF MITOCHONDRIAL RESPIRATION IN LIVER

Arthur J. Verhoeven, Carlo W.T. van Roermund,
Peter J.A.M. Plomp, Ronald J.A. Wanders,
Albert K. Groen and Joseph M. Tager

Laboratory of Biochemistry, B.C.P. Jansen Institute
University of Amsterdam, P.O. Box 20151, 1000 HD Amsterdam
(The Netherlands)

INTRODUCTION

In studies on the control of mitochondrial respiration carried out in the past 10 years, particular attention has been focussed on cytochrome c oxidase and the adenine nucleotide translocator as rate-controlling steps. On the basis of the observation that the first two phosphorylation sites of the respiratory chain are in near equilibrium with the extramitochondrial phosphate potential, Wilson and coworkers[1-5] have concluded that regulation of respiration occurs at the cytochrome c oxidase step, the effective rate of this reaction being dependent on the extramitochondrial phosphate potential. According to this model, the adenine nucleotide translocator does not exert significant control on respiration. In contrast, Davis and coworkers[6-8], Kunz and coworkers[9-11], Lemasters and Sowers[12], and our own group[13,14] have concluded that the adenine nucleotide translocator is a rate-controlling step for mitochondrial oxidative phosphorylation. The uncertainty about the precise role of the adenine nucleotide translocator and of the cytochrome c oxidase step in controlling respiration is due to the difficulty of quantifying the contribution of various steps to control of a metabolic pathway such as mitochondrial oxidative phosphorylation. Kacser and Burns[15-17] and Heinrich and Rapoport[18-20] have developed a theoretical framework for quantifying the amount of control that a particular step in a metabolic pathway exerts on flux through that pathway.

USE OF CONTROL ANALYSIS IN STUDYING REGULATION OF METABOLIC FLUXES

In order to quantify the amount of control exerted by a step in a pathway on flux through that pathway, Kacser and Burns[15], and

241

Heinrich and Rapoport[18] proposed the concept of the flux-control coefficient. The flux-control coefficient, formerly known as control strength*, of a step in a metabolic pathway is defined as the fractional change in flux through the pathway induced by a fractional change in the amount of enzyme under consideration. In mathematical terms:

$$C_{E_j}^J = \left(\frac{dJ/J}{dE_j/E_j} \right)_{ss}$$

where J is the flux through the pathway and E_j is the enzyme under consideration.

If the concentrations of the initial substrate and the end product of the pathway are kept constant, the sum of all the flux-control coefficients in the pathway is equal to unity. This relation is called the "summation theorem"[15]. In mathematical terms:

$$C_{E_1}^J + C_{E_2}^J + \dots C_{E_n}^J = 1$$

Note that the summation theorem links the flux-control coefficients of the different enzymes to each other. If under a particular condition the value of one of the flux-control coefficients changes, the value of the flux-control coefficient of at least one other enzyme will also change in order to keep the sum equal to 1. It is clear that the flux-control coefficient of an enzyme is dependent not only on the properties of that enzyme, but also on the properties of all the other enzymes involved in the pathway.

MEASUREMENT OF FLUX-CONTROL COEFFICIENTS

How can one measure the flux-control coefficient of an enzyme or, for that matter, of a transport step in a metabolic pathway? An obvious way to change the activity of an enzyme or of a transport protein is to use a specific inhibitor. For instance, when an irreversible inhibitor is used, i.e. an inhibitor for which the K_I of the enzyme is much lower than the concentration of the enzyme in the pathway, the flux-control coefficient is given by:

$$C_{E_j}^J = - \frac{I_{max}}{J} \cdot \left(\frac{dJ}{dI} \right)_{I=0}$$

where I_{max} refers to the amount of inhibitor required for total inhibition of the enzyme.

---

*Recently agreement was reached between investigators using control analysis upon the use of a new standard terminology for control parameters (see Ref. 21).

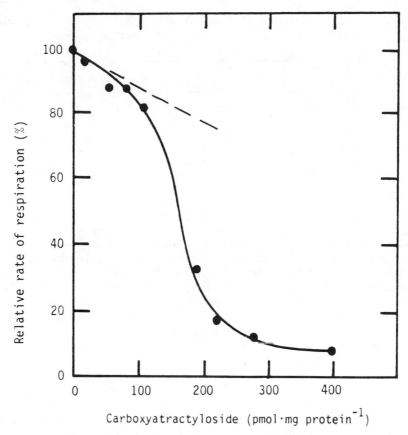

Fig. 1. Determination of the flux-control coefficient of the adenine
nucleotide translocator on respiration in rat-liver mitochondria. Mitochondria (about 1 mg protein/ml) were incubated at 25 °C in an oxygraph vessel equipped with a Clark-
type electrode in a medium containing: 100 mM KCl, 25 mM
Mops/Tris, 1 mM EGTA, 10 mM potassium phosphate, 20 mM
succinate, 2 mM malate, 1 mM ATP, 10 mM $MgCl_2$, 20 mM glucose
and 1 µg rotenone/ml. The final pH was 7.0. After 1 min of
incubation, State-3 respiration was induced by addition of
a saturating amount of hexokinase. Different amounts of carboxyatractyloside were added as indicated in the figure.

THE FLUX-CONTROL COEFFICIENT OF THE ADENINE NUCLEOTIDE TRANSLOCATOR
AND OTHER STEPS ON RESPIRATION IN ISOLATED RAT-LIVER MITOCHONDRIA

We have used carboxyatractyloside as a specific, irreversible
inhibitor in order to measure the flux-control coefficient of the
adenine nucleotide translocator on mitochondrial respiration. Rat-

Table 1. Distribution of control among different steps during
State 3 respiration of rat-liver mitochondria.

Step	Flux-control coefficient (%)
Adenine nucleotide translocator	29 + 5
Proton leak	4 + 1
Dicarboxylate carrier	33 + 4
Cytochrome c oxidase	17 + 1
bc_1-complex	3 + 0.5
Total	86 + 6

Mitochondria were incubated as described in the legend to Fig. 1 in
a medium containing 100 mM KCl, 50 mM Tris/HCl, 1 mM EGTA, 10 mM
potassium phosphate, 20 mM succinate, 2 mM malate, 1 mM ATP, 10 mM
$MgCl_2$, 20 mM glucose and 1 µg rotenone/ml. The final pH was 7.4.
State-3 respiration was induced by addition of a saturating amount
of hexokinase. The flux-control coefficients of the various steps
were determined as described in the text. The values are means +
S.E. of 4 different preparations.

liver mitochondria were incubated with succinate in the presence of
excess ADP and different concentrations of carboxyatractyloside
(Fig. 1). The shape of the curve in Fig. 1 shows that carboxyatractyloside does not behave as an ideal irreversible inhibitor. The
amount of inhibitor needed to fully inhibit all enzyme activity was
therefore derived by extrapolation of the linear part of the inhibition curve to the point of residual respiration in the presence
of excess inhibitor. By measuring also the initial slope of the curve,
the flux-control coefficient of the adenine nucleotide translocator
on respiration could be calculated. The flux-control coefficient of
the adenine nucleotide translocator on oxygen uptake in this experiment was 0.23. That is, 23% of the control on oxygen uptake is
exerted by the adenine nucleotide translocator. Clearly, the adenine
nucleotide translocator is not the *only* step controlling respiration.
Other steps must also contribute to the control of oxygen uptake.

We have used analogous procedures for measuring the flux-control
coefficients of other steps in mitochondrial oxidative phosphorylation[22]. Table 1 shows the distribution of control among different
steps during State-3 respiration of rat-liver mitochondria incubated
in the presence of succinate at pH 7.4. The flux-control coefficient
of the dicarboxylate carrier was estimated using phenylsuccinate and

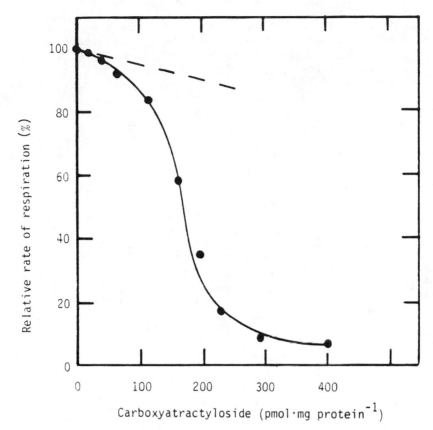

Fig. 2. Determination of the flux-control coefficient of the adenine
nucleotide translocator on respiration in rat-liver mitochondria respiring with glutamate + malate. Mitochondria
were incubated as described in the legend to Fig. 1 in a
medium containing: 100 mM KCl, 25 mM Mops/Tris, 1 mM EGTA,
10 mM potassium phosphate, 10 mM glutamate, 1 mM malate,
1 mM ATP, 10 mM MgCl$_2$ and 20 mM glucose. The final pH was
7.0. State-3 respiration was induced by addition of a saturating amount of hexokinase. Different amounts of carboxyatractyloside were added as indicated in the figure.

that of cytochrome c oxidase using azide. The flux-control coefficient
of the bc_1-complex was estimated using hydroxyquinoline-N-oxide,
assuming that the K_I of the inhibitor is equivalent to the K_D. The
data in Table 1 show that most of the control was exerted by the
adenine nucleotide translocator, the dicarboxylate carrier and cytochrome c oxidase.

Recently, Forman and Wilson[5] have presented data from which they concluded that the adenine nucleotide translocator exerts no control on respiration. They suggested that the discrepancy between their results and the results obtained in our group was due to the high concentration of free Mg^{2+} ions used in our experiments. Another important difference between our experiments and those of the group of Wilson is that we routinely use succinate as respiratory substrate, whereas Wilson and coworkers used glutamate + malate in the experiments referred to. We have therefore compared the flux-control coefficients of the adenine nucleotide translocator on respiration with the two substrates. The flux-control coefficient of the adenine nucleotide translocator was lower with glutamate + malate than with succinate: 10% and 23%, respectively (cf. Figs. 1 and 2). Almost the same value for the flux-control coefficient of the adenine nucleotide translocator with glutamate + malate as respiratory substrate can be calculated from the data of Forman and Wilson[5]. In the presence of a low concentration of free Mg^{2+} ions the values for the flux-control coefficients of the adenine nucleotide translocator obtained with the two substrates were almost the same as those obtained in the presence of a high concentration of free Mg^{2+} ions. The difference in the magnitude of the flux-control coefficients of the adenine nucleotide translocator on respiration with the two different substrates must be due to the fact that different enzyme systems are used to reduce coenzyme Q. Probably the control by the enzyme system responsible for reducing coenzyme Q is higher with glutamate + malate as substrate than with succinate. As indicated above, a decrease in the flux-control coefficient of one step must lead to an increase in the flux-control coefficient of at least one other step.

THE FLUX-CONTROL COEFFICIENT OF THE ADENINE NUCLEOTIDE TRANSLOCATOR IN ISOLATED HEPATOCYTES

It is clear that the value of the flux-control coefficient of the adenine nucleotide translocator is highly dependent on the experimental conditions. Therefore, results obtained with isolated mitochondria cannot be extrapolated directly to the situation in the intact cell. For this reason we have also measured the flux-control coefficient of the adenine nucleotide translocator in intact hepatocytes. The same approach was used as with isolated mitochondria. Rat-liver cells were incubated with lactate + pyruvate and different concentrations of carboxyatractyloside (Fig. 3, Ref. 23). The flux-control coefficient of the adenine nucleotide translocator on oxygen uptake calculated from the inhibitor titration curve is 26%. It is clear that in the intact cell, too, control of mitochondrial oxidative phosphorylation is shared by several steps.

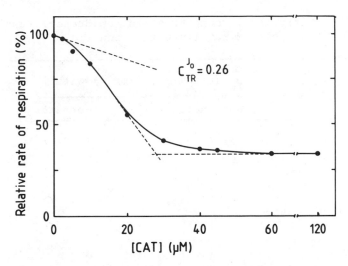

Fig. 3. Determination of the flux-control coefficient of the adenine
nucleotide translocator on mitochondrial respiration in isolated rat-liver cells. The cells (10 mg/ml) were incubated
with 10 mM lactate plus 1 mM pyruvate and different concentrations of carboxyatractyloside (CAT). After 30 min the rate
of oxygen uptake was measured. The flux-control coefficient
of the adenine nucleotide translocator on respiration was
calculated as indicated in the text. The initial slope of the
curve $(dJ/d[CAT]_{out})$ and the value for $([CAT]_{out})_{max}$ were
derived as shown in the figure. The value for J was corrected
for non-mitochondrial respiration. Non-mitochondrial respiration was determined by addition of an excess of antimycin
(70 µM) to the oxygraph vessel and, in the absence of CAT,
accounted for 20 ± 1% (mean ± S.D., n=6) of the rate of
oxygen uptake (from Ref. 23).

SITE OF ACTION OF THE STIMULATION BY HORMONES OF RESPIRATION IN ISOLATED RAT-LIVER MITOCHONDRIA

The conclusion that control of mitochondrial oxidative phosphorylation is shared by several steps is at variance with the conclusions of Wilson and coworkers[1-5]. An essential element in the
approach of Wilson and his group[1-5] is that the first two sites of
the respiratory chain, including the adenine nucleotide translocator,
are in near equilibrium. Wilson and coworkers therefore conclude that
all control of respiration must be exerted by the cytochrome *c* oxidase
step. In recent years, several investigators have shown that treatment
of animals with a number of hormones leads to a stimulation of respiration in liver mitochondria. If the model of Wilson and coworkers
(Refs. 1-5) were correct, the hormones should act on cytochrome *c* oxidase.

Table 2. Effect of hormone treatment on State-3 respiration in isolated rat-liver mitochondria.

Treatment	J_0 (natom·min^{-1}·mg^{-1}) with		Reference
	succinate	TMPD + ascorbate	
Control	144 + 8	208 + 12 (3)	24
Glucagon (6 min)	208 + 11	219 + 21 (3)	
Control	82 + 9	104 + 3	25,26
α-Adrenergic agonists (10-30 min)	112 + 5	108 + 4	
Control	150 + 8	146 + 8	27
Dexamethasone (3 h)	206 + 10	164 + 8	

The values given in the table are, unless indicated otherwise, the mean + S.E. of 6-7 preparations. The effect of α-adrenergic stimulation on succinate oxidation was studied in mitochondria obtained from isolated hepatocytes.

Some data from the literature on the effect of hormone treatment on State-3 respiration in isolated rat-liver mitochondria are summarised in Table 2. Treatment with glucagon, α-adrenergic agonists and dexamethasone stimulate respiration with succinate by about 40%. In contrast, there is no effect of the hormones on respiration with TMPD + ascorbate, suggesting that the activity of cytochrome c oxidase is not affected by these hormones.

We have obtained analogous results with thyroid hormone. When hypothyroid rats were treated with thyroid hormone for 24 h, there was a marked stimulation of succinate oxidation (Table 3). In contrast, there was no significant effect of the hormone treatment on cytochrome c oxidase activity. Of course, the possibility cannot be excluded that the hormones do have an effect on cytochrome c oxidase activity, but that this effect is seen only when succinate is the substrate and not when TMPD + ascorbate is used.

The enzymes that have been postulated to play a role in the stimulation by hormones of State-3 respiration with succinate include succinate dehydrogenase[28-31], the adenine nucleotide translocator[32,33] and the bc_1-complex[27,34]. In view of these uncertainties we have applied control analysis in order to determine which step or steps are activated by hormones. Stimulation by a hormone of the

Table 3. Effect of thyroid hormone treatment of hypothyroid rats
on mitochondrial respiration.

Mitochondria from livers of	Rate of succinate oxidation in State 3 (natom $O \cdot min^{-1} \cdot mg^{-1}$)	Cytochrome c oxidase activity (natom $O \cdot min^{-1} \cdot mg^{-1}$)
Hypothyroid rats	227 ± 4 (12)	615 ± 17 (6)
Hypothyroid rats treated with T_3 for 24 h	338 ± 7 (12)	661 ± 26 (6)

Rats were made hypothyroid by addition of 6-n-propylthiouracil to
the drinking water (0.05% (w/v) for 2-3 weeks).
Liver mitochondria were isolated after a 24-h treatment of the hypothyroid rats with either thyroid hormone (40 μg T_3/100 g body weight)
or vehicle (0.01 M NaOH) only. The rate of succinate oxidation in
State 3 was measured under the conditions described in the legend to
Fig. 1. Cytochrome c oxidase activity was measured in the presence of
0.25% (w/v) Tween-80, 20 μM cytochrome c, 10 mM ascorbate, 1 mM TMPD,
50 mM Tris/HCl and 1 mM EDTA. The final pH was 7.4.

flux through the pathway will lead to a redistribution of control so
that the flux-control coefficients of enzymes which are activated
decrease or remain unchanged. However, an increase in the flux-control
coefficient of an enzyme does not necessarily mean that this step is
not affected by the hormone.

   We have measured the flux-control coefficients of four steps in
oxidative phosphorylation in mitochondria from hypothyroid rats and
from hypothyroid rats treated with thyroid hormone for 24 h. The
flux-control coefficients of the dicarboxylate carrier, the adenine
nucleotide translocator and cytochrome c oxidase were determined as
described above. The flux-control coefficient of the bc_1-complex was
measured using antimycin A, assuming irreversible inhibition[35]. The
results are shown in Table 4. After treatment with the hormone, there
was an increase in the flux-control coefficients of the adenine nucleotide translocator, the dicarboxylate carrier and cytochrome c
oxidase. In contrast, the flux-control coefficient of the bc_1-complex
decreased after hormone treatment. The fact that the bc_1-complex
exerts less control after hormone treatment indicates that it must
have been activated. Indeed, as shown in Fig. 4, the number of antimycin A – binding sites increased from 27 ± 2 pmol/mg protein (n=4)
in the hypothyroid rats to 42 ± 4 pmol/mg protein (n=4) in the hor-
mone-treated rats.

Table 4. Effect of thyroid hormone treatment of hypothyroid rats on distribution of control during State-3 respiration in liver mitochondria.

Step	Flux-control coefficient (%) in mitochondria from	
	hypothyroid rats	T_3-treated rats
Adenine nucleotide translocator	18 ± 4	27 ± 5[*]
Dicarboxylate carrier	21 ± 2	34 ± 4[*]
bc_1-Complex	21 ± 2	14 ± 2[*]
Cytochrome c oxidase	14 ± 0.3	18 ± 0.5[*]
Σ	74 ± 2	93 ± 8[**]

[*] $P < 0.025$ with paired t-test.   [**] $P < 0.05$ with paired t-test.

Hormone treatment of the animals was carried out as described in the legend to Table 3. Incubations for the mitochondria were as described in the legend to Fig. 1. The flux-control coefficients of the various steps were determined as described in the text. The values given are the means ± S.E. of 2-4 experiments.

The data of Table 4 indicate that thyroid hormone must have affected the activity not only of the bc_1-complex, but also of at least one other enzyme. This can be deduced from the fact that the sum of the flux-control coefficients of the steps measured increased significantly after treatment with thyroid hormone. Therefore, the hormone must have had an activating effect on a step or steps not measured in these experiments. One possible candidate is succinate dehydrogenase; most of the hormones studied seem to have a greater effect on succinate oxidation than on the oxidation of NAD-linked substrates[24,26,28].

These findings make physiological sense. Since the control of mitochondrial respiraton is distributed among a number of steps, hormones can exert their effects efficiently by activating more than one step in the pathway.

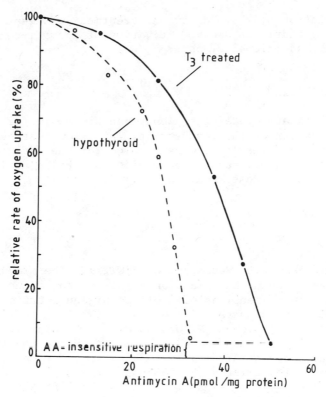

Fig. 4. Effect of thyroid hormone treatment on the inhibition by
antimycin A of State-3 respiration in rat-liver mitochondria.
Rats were treated as described in the legend to Table 4.
Mitochondria were incubated under the conditions described
in the legend to Fig. 1. After 1 min of incubation State-3
respiration was induced by addition of a saturating amount
of hexokinase; different amounts of antimycin A (from a
concentrated solution in ethanol) were added as indicated
in the figure. The number of antimycin A – binding sites was
determined from the minimal amount of inhibitor required to
obtain maximal inhibition of oxygen uptake.

CONCLUSIONS

    Control analysis of mitochondrial oxidative phosphorylation
allows us to draw the following conclusions:
- In isolated mitochondria control of respiration is distributed
  among several steps, including cytochrome c oxidase and the adenine
  nucleotide translocator.
- In the intact cell, too, control of respiration is distributed
  among several steps.

The stimulation by thyroid hormone treatment of respiration in liver mitochondria is due to activation of the bc_1-complex and one or more additional steps.

ACKNOWLEDGEMENTS

The authors are grateful to Wendy van Noppen for her expert help in the preparation of this manuscript. This study was supported by a grant from the Netherlands Organization for the Advancement of Pure Research (Z.W.O.) under the auspices of the Netherlands Foundation for Chemical Research (S.O.N.).

REFERENCES

1. M. Erecińscka, R.L. Veech and D.F. Wilson, Thermodynamic relationships between the oxidation-reduction reactions and the ATP synthesis in suspensions of isolated pigeon heart mitochondria, Arch. Biochem. Biophys. 160: 412-421 (1974).
2. D.F. Wilson, M. Stubbs, N. Oshino and M. Erecińska, Thermodynamic relationships between the mitochondrial oxidation-reduction reactions and cellular ATP levels in ascites tumor cells and perfused rat liver, Biochemistry 13: 5305-5311 (1974).
3. D.F. Wilson, M. Stubbs, R.L. Veech, M. Erecińska and H.A. Krebs, Equilibrium relations between the oxidation-reduction reactions and the adenosine triphosphate synthesis in suspensions of isolated liver cells, Biochem. J. 140: 57-64 (1974).
4. N.G. Forman and D.F. Wilson, Energetics and stoichiometry of oxidative phosphorylation from NADH to cytochrome c in isolated rat liver mitochondria, J. Biol. Chem. 257: 12908-12915 (1982).
5. N.G. Forman and D.F. Wilson, Dependence of mitochondrial oxidative phosphorylation on activity of the adenine nucleotide translocase, J. Biol. Chem. 258: 8649-8655 (1983)
6. E.J. Davis , L. Lumeng and D. Bottoms, On the relationships between the stoichiometry of oxidative phosphorylation and the phosphorylation potential of rat liver mitochondria as functions of respiratory state, FEBS Lett. 39: 9-12 (1974).
7. E.J. Davis and L. Lumeng, Relationships between the phosphorylation potentials generated by liver mitochondria and respiratory state under conditions of adenosine diphosphate control, J. Biol. Chem. 250: 2275-2282 (1975).
8. E.J. Davis and W.I.A. Davis-van Thienen, Control of mitochondrial metabolism by the ATP/ADP ratio, Biochem. Biophys. Res. Commun. 83: 1260-1266 (1978).
9. U. Küster, R. Bohnensack and W. Kunz, Control of oxidative phosphorylation by the extramitochondrial ATP/ADP ratio, Biochim. Biophys. Acta 440: 391-402 (1976).

10. G. Letko, U. Küster, J. Duszyński and W. Kunz, Investigation of the dependence of the intramitochondrial [ATP]/[ADP] ratio on the respiration rate, Biochim. Biophys. Acta 593: 196–203 (1980).

11. W. Kunz, R. Bohnensack, G. Böhme, U. Küster, G. Letko and P. Schönfeld, Relations between extramitochondrial and intramito- chondrial adenine nucleotide systems, Arch. Biochem. Biophys. 209: 219–229 (1981).

12. J.J. Lemasters and A.E. Sowers, Phosphate dependence and atrac- tyloside inhibition of mitochondrial oxidative phosphorylation. The ADP-ATP carrier is rate-limiting. J. Biol. Chem. 254: 1248– 1251 (1979).

13. T.P.M. Akerboom, H. Bookelman and J.M. Tager, Control of ATP transport across the mitochondrial membrane in isolated rat- liver cells, FEBS Lett. 74: 50–54 (1977).

14. R. van der Meer, T.P.M. Akerboom, A.K. Groen and J.M. Tager, Relationship between oxygen uptake of perifused rat-liver cells and the cytosolic phosphorylation state calculated from indicator metabolites and a redetermined equilibrium constant, Eur. J. Biochem. 84: 421–428 (1978).

15. H. Kacser and J.A. Burns, The control of flux, in: "Rate Control of Biological Processes", D.D. Davies, ed., pp. 65–104, Cambridge University Press, London (1973).

16. H. Kacser and J.A. Burns, Molecular democracy: who shares the controls?, Biochem. Soc. Trans. 7: 1149–1161 (1979).

17. H. Kacser and J.A. Burns, The molecular basis of dominance, Genetics 97: 639–666 (1981).

18. R. Heinrich and T.A. Rapoport, A linear steady-state treatment of enzymatic chains. General properties, control and effector strength, Eur. J. Biochem. 42: 89–95 (1974).

19. R. Heinrich and T.A. Rapoport, A linear steady-state treatment of enzymatic chains. Critique of the crossover theorem and a general procedure to identify interactions with an effector, Eur. J. Biochem. 42: 97–105 (1974).

20. R. Heinrich and T.A. Rapoport, Mathematical analysis of multi- enzyme systems. II. Steady state and transient control, Bio- systems 7: 130–136 (1975).

21. H.V. Westerhoff, A.K. Groen, R.J.A. Wanders and J.M. Tager, Modern theories of metabolic control and their applications, Bioscience Rep. (1984) in press.

22. A.K. Groen, R.J.A. Wanders, H.V. Westerhoff, R. van der Meer and J.M. Tager, Quantification of the contribution of various steps to the control of mitochondrial respiration, J. Biol. Chem. 257: 2754–2757 (1982).

23. J. Duszynski, A.K. Groen, R.J.A. Wanders, R.C. Vervoorn and J.M. Tager, Quantification of the role of the adenine nucleotide translocator in the control of mitochondrial respiration in iso- lated rat-liver cells, FEBS Lett. 146: 262–266 (1982).

24. R.K. Yamazaki, Glucagon stimulation of mitochondrial respiration, J. Biol. Chem. 250: 7924–7930 (1975).

25. M.A. Titheradge and R.C. Haynes, The hormonal stimulation of ureogenesis in isolated hepatocytes through increases in mitochondrial ATP production, Arch. Biochem. Biophys. 201: 44-55 (1980).
26. M.A. Titheradge and H.G. Coore, Hormonal regulation of liver mitochondrial pyruvate carrier in relation to gluconeogenesis and lipogenesis, FEBS Lett. 71: 73-78 (1976).
27. E.H. Allan, A.B. Chisholm and M.A. Titheradge, The stimulation of hepatic oxidative phosphorylation following dexamethasone treatment of rats, Biochim. Biophys. Acta 725: 71-76 (1983).
28. V.T. Maddaiah, S. Clejan, A.G. Palekar and P.J. Collipp, Hormones and liver mitochondria: effects of growth hormone and thyroxine on respiration, fluorescence of 1-anilino-8-naphthalene sulfonate and enzyme activities of complex I and II of submitochondrial particles, Arch. Biochem. Biophys. 210: 666-677 (1981).
29. E.A. Siess and O.H. Wieland, Glucagon-induced stimulation of 2-oxoglutarate metabolism in mitochondria from rat liver, FEBS Lett. 93: 301-306 (1978).
30. E.A. Siess and O.H. Wieland, Isolated hepatocytes as a model for the study of stable glucagon effects on mitochondrial respiratory functions, FEBS Lett. 101: 277-281 (1979).
31. M.A. Titheradge and R.C. Haynes, Glucagon treatment stimulates the oxidation of durohydroquinone by rat liver mitochondria, FEBS Lett. 106: 330-334 (1979).
32. B.M. Babior, S. Creagan, S.H. Ingbar and R.S. Kipnes, Stimulation of mitochondrial adenosine diphosphate uptake by thyroid hormones, Proc. Nat. Acad. Sci. USA 70: 98-102 (1973).
33. J. Bryla, E.J. Harris and J.A. Plumb, The stimulatory effect of glucagon and dibutyryl cyclic AMP on ureogenesis and gluconeogenesis in relation to the mitochondrial ATP content, FEBS Lett. 80: 443-448 (1980).
34. A.P. Halestrap, The nature of the stimulation of the respiratory chain of rat liver mitochondria by glucagon pretreatment of animals, Biochem. J. 204: 37-47 (1982).
35. J.A. Berden and E.C. Slater, The allosteric binding of antimycin to cytochrome b in the mitochondrial membrane, Biochim. Biophys. Acta 256: 199-215 (1972).

QUANTITATION OF FLUXES IN THE GLUCONEOGENIC, GLYCOLYTIC, AND
PENTOSE PHOSPHATE PATHWAYS IN ISOLATED RAT HEPATOCYTES: ENERGETIC
CONSIDERATIONS

Jacob J. Blum and Michael S. Rabkin

Department of Physiology
Duke University Medical Center
Durham, N.C. 27710

INTRODUCTION

     For any given substrate mixture and hormonal state, a large
number of factors serve to regulate the flow of metabolites along
the major pathways of carbohydrate metabolism in hepatocytes. In
addition to the amounts of enzymes present, these factors include
the intracellular levels of various effectors such as fructose
2,6-bisphosphate, ADP, ATP, and alanine, among others, and the
phosphorylation states of several key enzymes. Enzyme levels are
subject to long term regulation by dietary and hormonal influences,
while effector levels and the phosphorylation state of regulatory
enzymes are subject to moment-to-moment changes in hormonal states.
While studies on purified enzymes or on tissue homogenates have
contributed enormously to our present understanding of the many
factors that help regulate metabolic fluxes, a more complete understanding of in vivo regulation of intermediary metabolism requires
studies on perfused liver or, in so far as they can be considered
as representative of the intact liver, on isolated hepatocytes.
One approach to the problem of measuring flux patterns along major
pathways of metabolism is to incubate the cells with a suitable
substrate mixture with one substrate in any given experiment being
labeled with ^{14}C, and measure the rate of label accumulation in
products such as glycogen, lipids, etc., under quasi-steady-state
conditions. The theoretical considerations underlying this approach
have been reviewed (Blum and Stein, 1982) and will not be repeated
here. The method was originally developed in studies on the
metabolism of the ciliate Tetrahymena pyriformis, but has been
shown to be applicable to isolated hepatocytes (Crawford and Blum,
1983). In this latter study, hepatocytes isolated from fed rats
were incubated with a mixture of glucose (10 mM), ribose (1 mM),

255

mannose (4 mM), glycerol (3 mM), acetate (1.25 mM), and ethanol
(5 mM). Data on label flow into products during the 0-20 and 20-40
min intervals after the start of the incubation were used in conjunction with a complete model of the gluconeogenic, glycolytic,
and pentose phosphate pathways and a simplified model of the relevant mitochondrial reactions to obtain good estimates of most of
the fluxes in the pathways under investigation. We (Rabkin and
Blum, submitted for publication) have recently completed a study
of the metabolism of hepatocytes isolated from red rats and incubated - in the presence and absence of glucagon - with a mixture
of glucose, ribose, fructose, alanine, and acetate. The metabolic
model used in these studies (Fig. 1) utilized a more comprehensive
representation of the tricarboxylic acid cycle and associated
reactions than that employed by Crawford and Blum (1983). In the
present paper, we shall deal only with the flux pattern in the
"upper" portion of the model, i.e., the flow of metabolites along
the glycolytic, gluconeogenic, and pentose phosphate pathways, and
will focus primarily on "futile" cycling at the glycogen/G6P*,
FDP/F6P, and glucose/G6P substrate cycles, though we shall also
present new information concerning flows through triose phosphate
dehydrogenase.

METHODS

Hepatocytes were prepared according to Wood and Blum (1982)
and were incubated as previously described (Crawford and Blum,
1983) except that the substrate mixture contained glucose (10 mM),
fructose (4 mM), ribose (1 mM), L-alanine (3.5 mM), and acetate
(1.25 mM) with only one substrate labeled in any given flask.
Approximately 42 measurements of label incorporation into metabolic
products such as CO_2, glycogen, glucose, fatty acids, lipid glycerol,
alanine, and glutamate, were made at the end of interval I (0-20
min) and interval II (20-40 min), under quasi-steady-state conditions. This number was well in excess of the approximately 29
independent flux parameters to be estimated, and permitted a
stringent fit to the data. In each experiment paired flasks were
run with and without 0.1 µM glucagon. Metabolic fluxes were estimated as previously described (Blum and Stein, 1982). Statistical
criteria described in Crawford and Blum (1983) showed that the fit
to the data was excellent. These flux values were also in accord
with the observed changes in concentrations of glucose, glycogen,
fructose, alanine, lactate, and urea and with the oxygen consumption

---

*Abbreviations used are: G6P, glucose-6-phosphate; F6P, fructose-
6-phosphate; FDP, fructose 1,6-bisphosphate; DHAP, dihydroxyacetone
phosphate; GAP, glyceraldehyde-3-phosphate; PEP, phosphoenolpyruvate.

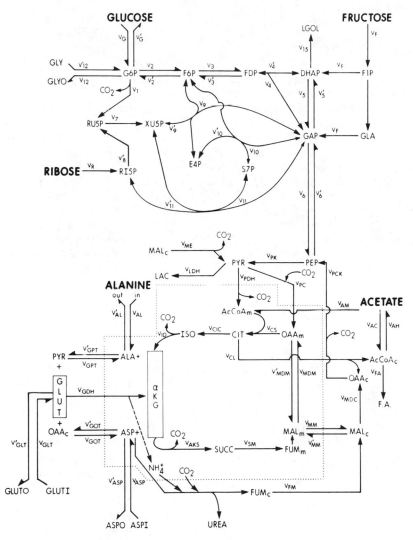

Fig. 1. Metabolic scheme used for analysis of data obtained from studies on hepatocytes from fed rats incubated (in the presence and absence of glucagon) with a substrate mixture containing glucose, ribose, fructose, alanine, and acetate.

in each interval (data not shown). The flux values presented are therefore realistic estimates of the flow of metabolites in the intact hepatocytes under these conditions, within the limits described below.

RESULTS AND DISCUSSION

Figure 2 shows the flux of metabolites for hepatocytes incubated in buffer containing a mixture of glucose, mannose, ribose, glycerol, acetate, and ethanol. Figures 3 and 4 show the flux pattern for hepatocytes incubated with a mixture of glucose, fructose, ribose, alanine and acetate in the absence (Fig. 3) and presence (Fig. 4) of 0.1 M glucagon. In each of these figures the upper and lower numbers of each pair are the flux value (nmole/ 20 min·mg protein) during the first (0-20 min) and second (20-40 min) intervals, respectively. The ranges of these values consistent with a 5% increase in fit parameters are given elsewhere (Rabkin and Blum, submitted). Many of the flux values are determined to within rather narrow limits. While certain unidirectional fluxes (such as V_9 and V_9') are not closely determined, the net flow through the bidirectional flux pair (e.g., V_9-V_9') is, nevertheless, tightly determined.

Flux through Triose Phosphate Isomerase

In the study of Crawford and Blum (1983), the unidirectional fluxes through triose phosphate isomerase were tightly determined and small relative to other fluxes around the DHAP and GAP nodes (Fig. 2). The computer program used to obtain the flux values also computes the specific activities of each carbon atom of each metabolite. It was found that these values of V_5 and V_5' were too low to permit isotopic equilibration of DHAP and GAP. Since equilibration of triose phosphates has been assumed by many investigators in obtaining estimates of futile cycling between F6P and FDP and of pentose cycle activity (see Crawford and Blum, 1982 and references therein), methods based on the assumption of triose phosphate equilibration could have yielded erroneous results had they been used on hepatocytes incubated with the glucose/ mannose/ribose/glycerol/acetate/ethanol mixture. In the 0-20 min interval for hepatocytes incubated with the glucose/ribose/ fructose/alanine/acetate mixture V_5 and V_5' are large enough so that the triose phosphates were close to isotopic equilibrium, both in the presence (Fig. 4) and absence (Fig. 3) of glucagon. In the 20-40 min interval, however, the unidirectional fluxes V_5 and V_5' have decreased sufficiently so that for several of the labeled substrates the triose phosphates are no longer at isotopic equilibrium in both the glucagon-treated and control cells.

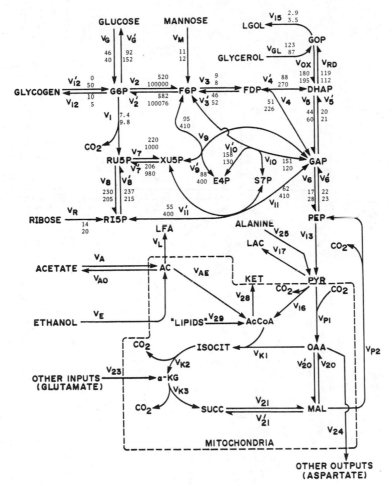

Fig. 2. Metabolic scheme used for analysis of data obtained in
studies on hepatocytes incubated with a substrate mixture containing glucose, ribose, mannose, glycerol,
ethanol, and acetate. Only the flux values (units: nmol/
20 min·mg protein) "above" the level of PEP are shown.
For further details, see Crawford and Blum (1983).

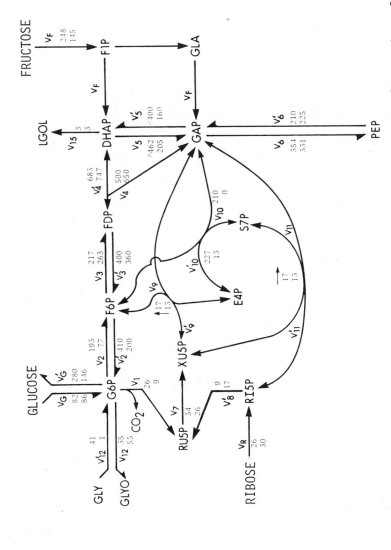

Fig. 3. Upper portion of the metabolic scheme in Fig. 1 with best fit flux values for control hepatocytes (Rabkin and Blum, submitted). The numbers shown are the fluxes, in nmol/20 min·mg protein, during the first (0–20 min) and second (20–40 min) intervals (upper and lower numbers of each pair, respectively).

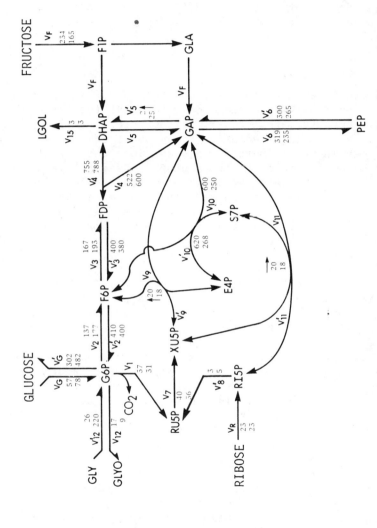

Fig. 4. Upper portion of the metabolic scheme of Fig. 1 with best fit flux values for glucagon-treated hepatocytes. The data used were obtained from paired experiments with the control cells shown in Fig. 3.

261

The direction of net flow between DHAP and GAP is also of
interest. These are most clearly illustrated in Fig. 5. In the
experiments of Crawford and Blum (1983), $V_5 > V_5'$ throughout the 40-
min incubation. In the present studies on control hepatocytes,
net flow across triose phosphate dehydrogenase is also from DHAP
to GAP throughout the incubation. However, in glucagon-treated
hepatocytes the net flow was from GAP to DHAP and increased
markedly in the second interval. Thus both the direction of net
flow and the degree of isotopic equilibration across triose phosphate isomerase can vary markedly depending on experimental
conditions.

Futile Cycling

There are three sites above the level of PEP in the glycolytic
and gluconeogenic pathways where energetically "futile" cycling can
occur. Previous attempts to quantify the rate of futile cycling
in hepatocytes have required assumptions about the rates of isotopic exchange in one or more of the reactions catalyzed by
hexosephosphate isomerase, fructose bisphosphate aldolase, and/or
triose phosphate isomerase, as well as estimates of ^{3}H-isotope
discrimination in some of these reactions and of exchange reactions
catalyzed by transaldolase. The problems associated with these
and related methods (such as the lack of equilibration of the
triose phosphate in the example just described) have been
described in detail by Katz and Rognstad (1976), Hue (1981), and
Crawford and Blum (1982), and a thorough discussion of futile
cycline in hepatocytes is available (Hue, 1982). The only assumptions that underlie the analysis of the data used to obtain the
flux values shown in Figs. 2-4 are that the system is effectively
in the steady state and that the reaction scheme used is an
adequate representation of the glycolytic, gluconeogenic, and pentose phosphate pathways. Insofar as these two assumptions are
valid, the present data automatically provide the information
necessary to quantify futile cycling. Although all the information needed in the following discussion is in Figs. 2, 3, and 4,
it is useful to select the essential features and present them in
more readable form (Figs. 5 and 6).

The Glucose/Glucose-6-Phosphate Cycle

In each of the three studies summarized in Fig. 6, glucose
was released into the medium during both intervals. Net glucose
release was determined by the balance between gluconeogenesis
$(V_2' - V_2)$, glucose uptake (V_G), glycogen synthesis (V_{12}) and degradation (V_{12}'), and flux through glucose-6-phosphate dehydrogenase
(V_1). Net glucose release by hepatocytes incubated in the highly
reducing substrate mixture used by Crawford and Blum (1983) was
less than in the present studies, and glucose output was twice as
high in interval II as in interval I. In the present study

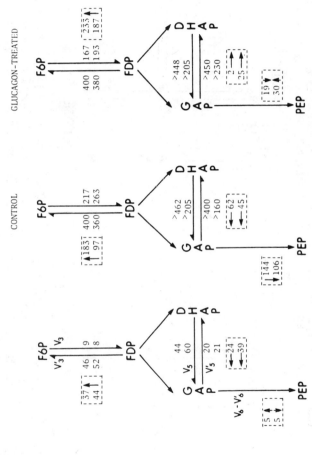

Fig. 5. Metabolic flow patterns at the F6P/FDP substrate cycle and in the lower portion of the Embden–Meyerhof pathway. For further details, see legend to Fig. 6.

263

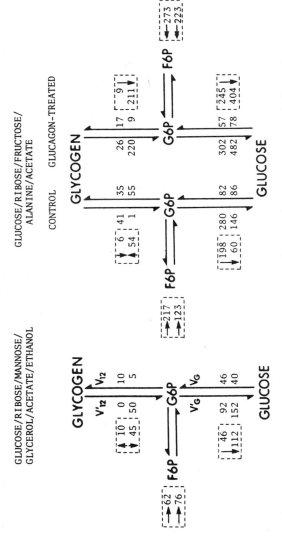

Fig. 6. Metabolic flow patterns at the glycogen/G6P and the glucose/G6P substrate cycles. The upper and lower numbers next to each heavy arrow are the flux values (nmol/20 min·mg protein) for the indicated reactions during the first and second intervals, respectively, for hepatocytes incubated with the substrate mixtures shown. The net flows for each pair of opposing reactions are shown in the appropriately placed dotted squares, with the direction of the net flow indicated by thin arrows.

there was a substantial decrease in net glucose output by the control hepatocytes in interval II, whereas glucagon-treated hepatocytes had higher glucose release in the second interval. It is noteworthy that in the two cases where glucose release was greater from 20-40 min, most of the increase came from an increase in glycogenolysis rather than in gluconeogenesis (cf. Figs. 2, 3, and 4).

In each of the three studies there was little change in flux through glucokinase, V_G, between the first and second intervals (Fig. 6), which is consistent with the sole dependence of glucokinase activity in glucose concentration (Storer and Cornish-Bowden, 1976). Glucose-6-phosphatase activity (V_G') is also believed to be largely determined by the intracellular concentration of its substrate. In the study of Crawford and Blum (1983) G6P levels were not measured. Instead they were computed by using the flux V_G in conjunction with appropriate K_m and V_m values. The intracellular concentrations of G6P so computed agreed with literature values. In the present studies G6P levels were measured and found to change slightly from 0.72±0.26 (S.D.) at t=0 to 0.98±0.26 at the end of 20 min and 0.84±0.17 at the end of 40 min for the control cells. The G6P levels in glucagon-treated cells, however, increased significantly, rising to 2.68±0.94 and 2.20±0.81 at the end of the first and second intervals, respectively. The increase in V_G in the glucagon-treated cells is consistent with their higher level of G6P. In the control cells, however, V_G' decreased in the second interval with no significant decrease in G6P levels. The reason for the decrease in glucose-6-phosphatase activity with time in the control cells is not clear.

Stein and Blum (1978) have defined the futility, F, of a substrate cycle as the reverse flux (i.e., that flux which determines energy "wastage") per unit net flux. Table 1 shows that for the glucose/G6P cycle F decreased 3-fold (from 1.0 to 0.36) during incubation of hepatocytes in the reducing substrate mixture of Crawford and Blum (1983), whereas it increased 3-fold (from 0.41 to 1.4) in control cells incubated with the fructose plus alanine mixture used in the present experiments. Although the addition of glucagon markedly reduced the futility at this substrate cycle, it also increased net flux through the cycle; hence there was hardly any change in the amount of ATP "wasted" throughout each 40-min interval. Under the three conditions so far examined, about 4% of the total ATP produced by the hepatocytes was "wasted" because glucokinase was not regulated.

The Glycogen/G6P Substrate Cycle

In the experiments of Crawford and Blum (1983), the best-fit value for phosphorylase flux (V_{12}') was zero in the first interval, rising to 50 nmol/20 min·mg protein in the second interval

Table 1. ATP Consumption and "Futility" of Three Substrate Cycles

Substrate Cycle	Conditions	Futility Interval I	Futility Interval II	ATP "wasted"/ATP produced (%) Interval I	ATP "wasted"/ATP produced (%) Interval II
Glucose/G6P	a	1.0*	0.36	4.4	3.4
	b	0.41	1.4	4.1	4.6
	c	0.23	0.19	3.0	4.4
Glycogen/G6P	a	0	0.11	0	0.42
	b	5.8	0.02	1.8	0.1
	c	1.9**	0.04	0.9	0.5
F6P/FDP	a	0.2***	0.2	0.85	0.67
	b	1.2	2.7	11	14
	c	0.72	1.0	9	11

[a] glucose/ribose/mannose/glycerol/ethanol/acetate mixture
[b] control cells   fructose mixture
[c] glucagon-treated cells

*F = $V_G/(V_G'-V_G)$; "wasted" ATP = V_G = glucokinase

**F = $V_{12}/(V_{12}'-V_{12})$; "wasted" ATP = V_{12} = glycogen synthase

***F = $V_3/(V_3'-V_3)$; "wasted" ATP = V_3 = phosphofructokinase.

The values used for ATP produced in each interval were calculated from the fit to the entire metabolic scheme for each condition.

(Fig. 2). Since flux V_{12} (glycogen synthase) was 10 and 5 nmol/20 min·mg protein in the first and second intervals, respectively, there was a small net glycogen deposition in interval I followed by a larger net glycogenolysis in interval II. If glycogen synthase was active only during the early portion of the second interval and then only phosphorylase was active for the rest of the interval, F would be zero throughout interval II and no ATP would have been wasted. If, however, the fluxes V_{12} and V_{12}' were at their average value throughout the second interval, then the value of F = 0.11 shown in Table 2 is computed, corresponding to a waste of only about 0.4% of the total cellular ATP production. Thus computations made with either set of assumptions lead to the same conclusion, i.e., there was virtually no futile cycling in either interval at the glycogen/G6P cycle for hepatocytes incubated in the reduced substrate mixture. Hepatocytes incubated in the fructose plus alanine-containing mixture had a high value for F during interval I when net glycogenolysis occurred, but even the worst case computations (i.e., V_{12} and V_{12}' are at the average rates shown in Figs. 3 and 4 throughout each interval) show that less than 2% of the ATP produced would have been wasted (Table 1). In the second interval glycogen synthesis occurred in the virtual absence of any glycogenolysis, and F was practically zero. In the presence of glucagon, F was smaller than in control cells in interval I and negligible in interval II, in both intervals less than 1% of the ATP produced could have been "wasted" at this cycle. Thus in each condition studied at most 2% of the ATP produced was wasted during interval I by the glycogen/G6P cycle, and in interval II less than 0.5% was wasted.

The F6P/FDP Substrate Cycle

Many factors are known to influence phosphofructokinase (PFK) and fructose bisphosphatase (FDPase), two enzymes that play a key role in the regulation of glycolysis and gluconeogenesis in liver (reviewed by Hue, 1982). Prominent among these are the concentrations of F6P (the substrate of PFK), FDP (the substrate for FDPase and an activator of PFK), 6-phosphogluconate (an activator of PFK; Sommercorn and Freedland, 1982), ATP (an inhibitor of PFK as well as one of its subtrates), citrate (an inhibitor of PFK), and, most potent of all, fructose 2,6-bisphosphate, which activates PFK and inhibits FDPase. The intracellular concentration of fructose 2,6-bisphosphate depends on the concentration of its precursor, F6P, and on the activity of the single enzyme (PFK2/FDPase2) which catalyzes the phosphorylation and dephosphorylation of F6P at carbon 2 (Pilkis et al, 1983). Regulation in situ is further complicated by the fact that both PFK and FDPase can be phosphorylated in intact hepatocytes. Glucose induces the phosphorylation of PFK in hepatocytes from fed rats, an action which is enhanced by glucagon but inhibited by alanine (Brand and Soling, 1982). The phosphorylation of muscle PFK appears to decrease its sensitivity to activation by fructose 2,6-bisphosphate (Fod and Kemp, 1982). Glucose increases the level of fructose 2,6-bisphosphate (Hue, 1982). Glucagon also acts on this complex system by causing (via a cAMP-dependent kinase) phosphorylation of PFK2/FDPase2, thereby reducing the rate at which this enzyme forms fructose 2,6-bisphosphate (Hers and Van Schaftingen, 1982). Because of the large number of factors that can affect flux through these two opposing enzymes, it is of particular interest to measure these fluxes in the intact cell. As noted above, previous studies (reviewed by Hers, 1982) have shown that considerable "futile" cycling may occur at these steps, but quantitation has been diffi-cult.

The flux through FDPase exceeded that through PFK for all con-ditions examined (i.e., net gluconeogenesis). Therefore the flux V_3 is "futile". In fed hepatocytes incubated with the reducing substrate mixture used by Crawford and Blum (1983) flux through PFK (V_3) was very small (Fig. 2 and Fig. 5) and F was approximately 0.2 in both intervals (Table 1). Twenty to thirty times as much F6P was converted to FDP per 20 min in hepatocytes incubated in the fructose plus alanine-containing substrate mixture employed in the present studies, both in the absence and presence of glucagon (Fig. 5). This resulted in higher values for F. Flux through PFK increased about 20% during interval II in both the control and glucagon-treated hepatocytes. Since these increases in V_3 were accompanied by relatively smaller decreased in flux V_3', the futility increased still further in the second interval. Thus while each substrate mixture had 10 mM glucose and 1 mM ribose, V_3 was much lower in the substrate mixture containing ethanol and glycerol than it was in the substrate mixture containing alanine and fructose, and the futility correspondingly lower. Further-more, the addition of glucagon to the latter cells caused relatively small changes in the fluxes through PFK and FDPase, resulting in an appreciable - but far from complete - reduction in "futile" cycling. In the reducing substrate mixture, less than 1% of the total ATP produced was consumed at this substrate cycle (Table 1). In the fructose plus alanine-containing mixture, over 9% of the ATP produced was expended at this step. Indeed, in hepatocytes incubated in the absence of glucagon, about 18% of the total ATP produced by the major reactions of intermediary metabo-lism is consumed by the operation of the three "futile" cycles considered here. Surprisingly, glucagon reduced this only slightly.

The Pentose Phosphate Pathway

The substrate mixture employed by Crawford and Blum (1983) allowed a fairly complete specification of the bidirectional fluxes catalyzed by the enzymes of the pentose phosphate pathway. The present studies gave much more information concerning metabolite flows in the mitochondria and associated cytosolic reactions (not presented here; Rabkin and Blum, submitted), and correspondingly less information about bidirectional fluxes in the pentose phosphate pathway. Net fluxes, however, were tightly determined. Net flow into the F6P node via transketolase and transaldolase ($V_9-V_9'+V_{10}-V_{10}$) was 14 and 20 nmoles/20 min·mg in the experiments of Crawford and Blum (1983) in intervals I and II, respectively, 34 and 26 in the control hepatocytes studied here, and 40 and 36 in the glucagon-treated hepatocytes. Although the absolute contribution of the pentose phosphate pathway to F6P formation was roughly half as much in the cells incubated in the reduced substrate mixture as in the fructose plus alanine mixture, the percent contribution to gluconeogenesis was higher in the reducing substrate mixture. This reflects the large rates of gluconeogenesis occurring in the present studies.

Simultaneous Gluconeogenesis and Glycolysis

In the experiments shown in Fig. 2 considerable gluconeogenesis was occurring ($V_2'>V_2$), mostly from the glycerol and ribose in the substrate mixture, and net flow in the lower portion of the Embden–Meyerhof pathway was small: 5 nmol/20 min·mg from GAP to PEP in interval I and the same amount in the opposite direction in interval II, see Fig. 5. In control hepatocytes incubated with the fructose plus alanine-containing substrate mixture, 144 and 106 nmol/20 min·mg protein flowed in the direction GAP to PEP during intervals I and II, respectively. Thus under these conditions there was a large gluconeogenic flux flowing from GAP to glucose at the same time that a large glycolytic flux flowed from GAP to PEP. This is a direct consequence of the large input from fructose via the fructokinase pathway into DHAP and GAP. In the presence of glucagon the glycolytic flow was greatly reduced relative to control cells during the first interval (associated with and possibly caused by a decreased flux through pyruvate kinase), and reversed in the second interval, corresponding to the onset of a net contribution by alanine into gluconeogenesis (not shown).

CONCLUSION

These studies show that the flux patterns in the glycolytic and gluconeogenic pathways differ appreciably between hepatocytes from fed rats incubated with a mixture of glucose/ribose/mannose/ethanol/glycerol/acetate as compared with a mixture of glucose/ribose/fructose/alanine/acetate and that glucagon added to hepatocytes incubated in the latter substrate mixture causes marked changes in the flux pattern as compared with controls. A more detailed discussion of these pathways and their relationships to events occurring beyond the level of P-enolpyruvate (i.e., in the tricarboxylic acid and urea cycles and associated cytosolic reactions) will be presented elsewhere (Rabkin and Blum, submitted).

ACKNOWLEDGEMENT

This work was supported by NIH grant 5 RO1 HD01269.

REFERENCES

Blum, J.J., and Stein, R.B., 1982, On the analysis of metabolic networks, in: "Biological Regulation and Development," Vol. 3A, R.F. Goldberger and K.R. Yamamoto, eds., Plenum Press, New York.

Brand, I.A., and Soling, H.D., 1982, Metabolite-controlled phosphorylation of phosphofructokinase in rat hepatocytes, Eur. J. Biochem., 122:175.

Crawford, J.M., and Blum, J.J., 1982, On the use of trace levels of [1-^{14}C]galactose to estimate cycling between pentose 6-phosphate and fructose diphosphate, Arch. Biochem. Biophys., 216:42.

Crawford, J.M., and Blum, J.J., 1983, Quantitative analysis of flux along the gluconeogenic, glycolytic and pentose phosphate pathways under reducing conditions in hepatocytes isolated from fed rats, Biochem. J., 212:585.

Foe, L.G., and Kemp, R.G., 1982, Properties of phospho and dephospho forms of muscle phosphofructokinase, J. Biol. Chem., 257:6368.

Hers, H.G., and Van Schaftingen, E., 1982, Fructose 2,6 bisphosphate two years after its discovery, Biochem. J., 206:1.

Hue, L., 1981, The role of futile cycles in the regulation of carbohydrate metabolism in the liver, Adv. Enzymol., 52:247.

Hue, L., 1982, Futile cycles and regulation of metabolism, in: "Metabolic Compartmentation," H. Sies, ed., Academic Press, New York.

Katz, J., and Rognstad, R., 1976, Futile cycles in the metabolism of glucose, Curr. Top. Cell. Regul., 10:237.

Pilkis, S.J., Walderhaug, M., Murray, K., Beth, A., Venkataramu, S.D., Pilkis, J., and El-Maghrabi, M.R., 1983, 6-Phosphofructo-2-kinase/fructose 2,6-bisphosphate from rat liver - isolation and identification of a phosphorylated intermediate, J. Biol. Chem., 258:6135.

Sommercorn, J., and Freedland, R.A., 1982, Regulation of hepatic phosphofructokinase by 6-phosphogluconate, J. Biol. Chem., 257:9424.

Stein, R.B., and Blum, J.J., 1978, On the analysis of futile cycles in metabolism, J. Theor. Biol., 72:487.

WHY IS THERE A DELAY IN THE INCREASED OXYGEN CONSUMPTION DURING THE REST-WORK TRANSITION IN SKELETAL MUSCLE?

Richard J. Connett

University of Rochester Medical Center
Department of Physiology, Box 642
Rochester, NY 14642

INTRODUCTION

During the rest-work transition in skeletal muscle it has long been known that the increase in oxidative supply of ATP lags the increase in consumption of ATP. The balance is supplied by muscle stores of phosphocreatine (PCr) and glycolysis leading to accumulation of lactate in the muscle. Several hypotheses have been advanced to account for the lag in increase of $\dot{V}O_2$. These have focused on limits to the delivery of substrates to the mitochondrion:

1) limiting oxygen supply
2) limiting supply of reducing equivalents
3) limiting ADP and/or phosphate (Pi)

With the advent of a new method for rapid freezing of active muscle in situ (1) and measuring the cellular concentration of oxygen (1,2,3), the studies reported here were undertaken to see if one or more of the hypotheses could be eliminated. A well defined autoperfused red muscle (dog gracilis) was used. The muscles were stimulated through the motor nerve without autonomic recruitment. Previous studies under steady-state conditions indicated that at a stimulus frequency of 4/s these muscles work aerobically, i.e. tissue PO_2 is greater than required for $\dot{V}O_2$ $_{max}$ and there is negligible lactate efflux to the blood (1,13). This preparation thus seemed ideal for a study of the coupling of $\dot{V}O_2$ to substrate supply during the transition from rest to aerobic work.

271

METHODS

Probability distributions for intracellular PO_2 were constructed on each frozen muscle using a measurement of myoglobin saturation based on a 4 wavelength cryomicrospectrophotometric technique (16) with a spatial resolution on the order of 2-3 mitochondria. Each measurement was made at the center of a single cell, viewed in cross-section. Sampling took account of both heterogeneity among neighboring cells and among regions separated by 1-2 cm. The overall error of the saturation measurement is <5%. The transform from saturation to PO_2 is based on a measured P_{50} for dog gracilis of 5.3 torr at $37°C$ (16). The transform is most precise below the P_{50}. A thorough description of the $\dot{V}O_2$, Mb saturation, and PO_2 data is available in (2,3).

Phosphocreatine (PCr), creatine, glucose-6-phosphate, and ATP were measured on the sample used for the myoglobin assay. All measurements used specific enzymatic assays based on fluorometric detection of NADH or NADPH. All metabolite values were normalized to the total creatine content of resting muscles (20.8 µmoles/g) to correct for water shifts during isometric contraction. When cellular concentrations were required a value of 0.56 ml H_2O/g wet tissue was used.

RESULTS AND DISCUSSION

Hypothesis 1: Limiting Oxygen Supply

In a previously described series of experiments the $\dot{V}O_2$ and blood flow in response to stimulation at 4/s was measured as a function of time during the rest-work transition (2,3). The increase in blood flow occurred rapidly and reached 80% of its steady-state value within 10 sec (2,3,4). The rise in $\dot{V}O_2$ was exponential with time and could be approximated by the equation:

$$V_t = V_i + V_f (1-10^{-kt}) \tag{1}$$

where: $V_t = \dot{V}O_2$ at time t
$V_i = \dot{V}O_2$ in resting muscles
V_f = steady-state $\dot{V}O_2 - V_i$
$k = 0.0208/s$
and   t = time in sec.

In a series of experiments designed to examine intracellular parameter conditions during the rest-work transition the muscles were rapidly frozen at rest and 5, 10, 15, 30, 60 and 180 sec after the start of stimulation. $\dot{V}O_2$ was not directly determined at times less than 60 sec in this series. Figure 1 shows the estimated $\dot{V}O_2$ using resting and 180 sec determinations from this series and equation 1. Directly measured values for the 60 sec muscles are shown on the curve for comparison with the calculated values.

Tissue PO_2 was measured cryomicrospectrophotometrically in 50 cells in each of 5 muscles at each time point by C. R. Honig and T. E. J. Gayeski (2). The lowest 5th percentile of the PO_2 values in the population of 250 cells at each time is also plotted in Figure 1. This fraction of the population was selected as the smallest fraction of the cells that might have a detectable effect on the measured total $\dot{V}O_2$ if they were oxygen limited. During the period of lowest $\dot{V}O_2$ (0-15 sec) the PO_2 in the lowest 5% of the population is equal to or greater than the resting values. As $\dot{V}O_2$ increases toward steady-state the PO_2 falls. However, even at 30 sec when PO_2 is lowest, it is greater than 2 torr. This is well above the critical PO_2 for oxygen consumption in mitochondria in dog gracilis at $\dot{V}O_{2\ max}$ (for evidence and discussion see ref. 1,2,3 and 5). The pattern of PO_2 change is consistent with a rapid increase

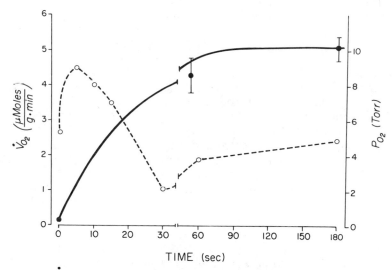

TIME (sec)

Figure 1. $\dot{V}O_2$ and tissue PO_2 during the rest-work transition.

The solid line indicates the time course of $\dot{V}O_2$ during stimulation to twitch at 4/s. The solid points ( ) indicate the mean ± SEM for $\dot{V}O_2$ measured in muscles used for PO_2 and metabolite assay (see text). The lowest 5th percentile of cell PO_2 in the muscle population at each time point (ref. 2) is indicated by the dashed line (0---0).

in blood flow and a slower increase in $\dot{V}O_2$ as seen in this and other studies (4,6). If blood flow is further increased at steady-state by adenosine treatment no further increase in $\dot{V}O_2$ is seen (1). In summary, the absolute values of tissue PO_2 and the temporal pattern during the rest-work transition are inconsistent with an oxygen limit to $\dot{V}O_2$, i.e. hypothesis 1 is not supported.

Hypothesis 2: Limiting Supply of Reducing Equivalent

Samples of the same muscles used for PO_2 and metabolite assays were sent to the Johnson Research Foundation where fluorescence measures of the reduced NAD and Flavin were carried out by Mr. Jeff Olgin under the direction of Dr. J. Haselgrove and Dr. B. Chance. Although these assays do not permit absolute redox values to be obtained, preliminary results (not shown) indicate that the redox potential was almost identical in these muscles at 5, 10, 30, 60 and 180 sec. The 15 sec point showed a large shift toward oxidation. Although these measures are only rough estimates of the redox potential the identity at several time points throughout the rest-work transition suggest that a limit in the availability of reducing equivalents to run oxidative phosphorylation is unlikely to be the cause of the lag in the increase in $\dot{V}O_2$ at the onset of stimulation, i.e. hypothesis 2 is not supported.

Hypothesis 3: Limiting ADP and/or Phosphate

In each of the muscles frozen for tissue PO_2, phosphocreatine (PCr), creatine, glucose-6-phosphate (G-6-P) and ATP were measured. The ATP concentrations at each time point are shown in Figure 2A. As might be expected, the buffer effect of PCr maintains the tissue content of ATP relatively stable throughout the stimulation period. For the first 15 sec of stimulation there is no significant change in [ATP]. Between 15 and 60 sec of stimulation there is a small decrease. Finally, as the muscle reaches steady-state between 1 and 3 min of stimulation there is a slight increase toward but not to resting value.

It is generally accepted that the free cytosolic ADP in muscle cannot be directly measured but is best estimated from enzyme equilibrium calculations. Several studies have indicated that creatine phosphokinase is very close to equilibrium in active muscle tissue, e.g. (8). Therefore we used the measured Cr, PCr and ATP values to estimate the concentrations of cytosolic ADP. The calculations were carried

out as described by McGilvery & Murray (9). It was assumed
that the intracellular pH was 7.0, free [Mg^{2+}] was 1 mM and the
binding and equilibrium constants used were those reported by

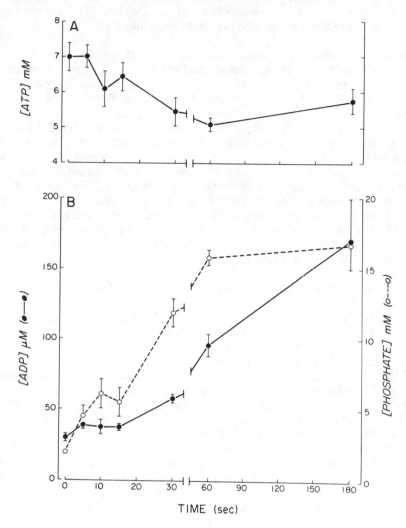

Figure 2. Estimated concentrations of ATP, ADP and phosphate.

The data are expressed as mean ± SEM for 5 muscles at each
time point except rest (10 points) and 3 min (8 points). A.
Directly measured [ATP]. B. ADP and P_i calculated as described
in the text.

Veech and Lawson (7,10). The computations were done for each muscle and the averaged values at each time point are plotted in Fig. 2B. There is a small increase in ADP during the first 5 sec of stimulation. The concentration then stabilizes through 15 seconds of stimulation after which it increases throughout the remainder of the stimulation period.

Tissue phosphate levels were not directly measured. Several studies have been shown using both direct chemical determinations and NMR that phosphate increases in proportion to the fall in PCr with appropriate correction for increases in sugar phosphates. Since the largest change is in G6P, it was used for correction. Although there is some uncertainty concerning the resting phosphate concentrations, values based either on NMR or careful direct analysis range from 0.5 - 3.0 mM. I used 2 mM as determined by NMR in red skeletal muscle (8). The expected range is within the error of the estimates during the rest-work transition and is less than 10% of the values at times greater than 15 sec. Thus this initial value problem is not a major one. The values were calculated from equation 2 for each muscle and the results at each time point averaged and plotted in Figure 2B.

$$P_t = 2 + (PCr_i - PCr_t) + (ATP_i - ATP_t) - (G6P_t - G6P_i) \qquad (2)$$

where: P = phosphate concentration and subscripts i and t refer to resting and time t respectively.

Phosphate increases throughout the first minute of stimulation and then stabilizes as the oxygen consumption reaches steady-state. Results suggest that the only parameters changing in a manner appropriate to regulate the changes in $\dot{V}O_2$ during the rest-work transition are ADP and phosphate. To further examine the quantitative relationship between $\dot{V}O_2$ and these compounds two approaches used in studies on isolated mitochondria were taken. The first of these tests the hypothesis that mitochondrial adenine translocase is limiting to $\dot{V}O_2$ and thus ADP levels ultimately control $\dot{V}O_2$. The second approach relates both ADP and phosphate to $\dot{V}O_2$ via the cytosolic phosphorylation potential.

Translocase Limit

Various studies of the adenine nucleotide translocase reaction have demonstrated that it binds cytosolic ADP with a high affinity and this binding is competitively inhibited by ATP binding. Two approaches can be taken to quantitating this relationship: a full rate equation including the ATP inhibition or, if ATP is high relative to the inhibition constant, a simple rate equation with an apparent Km which includes the effective ATP inhibition (e.g. 11,12). Reported inhibition constants are on the order of 100-800 µM and ATP concentrations in the muscle are relatively stable in the range of 5-7 mM (Figure 2A). Therefore the second approach as expressed in equation 3 was used. Estimates of the gracilis muscle V_{max} based on measured $\dot{V}O_2$ $_{max}$ (1,13) gave a minimal estimate of V_{max} of 40 µMoles ADP/g·min. Estimates of V_{max} based on heart mitochondrial translocase capacity and gracilis muscle mitochondria content gave a value of ᴫ60 µMoles ADP/g·min (13).

$$\dot{V}O_2 = 1/6 \cdot V_{max}/(1 + Km/[ADP]) \tag{3}$$

The fits to the data using V_{max} = 40-60 µMoles ADP/g·min and apparent Km values in the range of 30-60 µM were considered. In order to fit any data point with the $V_{max} \geq$ 40, apparent K_m had to be $\geq$ 40 µM. Figure 3 shows the estimated $\dot{V}O_2$ (solid line) and the translocase rate estimate (0-0) for Km = 50 µM and Vmax = 44 µMoles ADP/g·min. The agreement between the translocase prediction and the muscle $\dot{V}O_2$ is excellent between 30 and 180 sec. This is the region of the largest

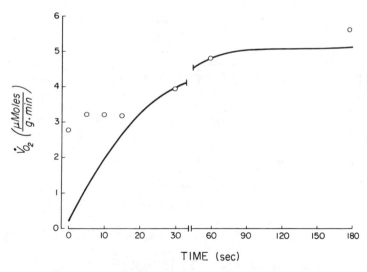

Figure 3. Fit of translocase hypothesis.

The solid line shows measured $\dot{V}O_2$ from Figure 1. The open symbols indicated $\dot{V}O_2$ computed from ADP concentrations and the adenine translocase model as described in the text.

change in ADP (Figure 2) and is consistant with a translocase limit. However, at earlier times, when the ADP levels are lower, the true $\dot{V}O_2$ is much smaller than that predicted from the translocase hypothesis. This is true even at rest when the issues of concentration gradients and transient conditions are unlikely to account for any deviation. Thus I conclude that as the system approaches $\dot{V}O_{2\ max}$ ($\sim70\%$ in this case) the ADP concentration may dominate the control of $\dot{V}O_2$ probably via adenine nucleotide translocase. However, at lower turnover rates factors other than ADP concentration must be involved.

Thermodynamic Approach

From the above analysis it is clear that factors other than a simple change in ADP concentration must be involved in the regulation of $\dot{V}O_2$ during the rest-work transition. The most likely suspect is phosphate. Both equilibrium (14) and non-equilibrium (15) thermodynamic analysis of oxidative phosphorylation suggest that $\dot{V}O_2$ may be linearly related to the

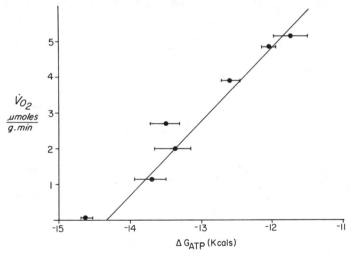

Figure 4. Relationship of measured $\dot{V}O_2$ to ΔG_{ATP}.

ΔG_{ATP} was computed from the data in Figure 2 by the equation:
$$\Delta G_{ATP} = -\{7.0 + 1.42 \log [ATP]/[ATP] [P_i]\}$$

The error bars indicate the range obtained using SEM for each of the concentrations. The line was computed from least squares fit to the 5, 10, 30, 60 and 180 points and has the equation:

$$\dot{V}O_2 = 2.08\ \Delta G_{ATP} + 2.98\ ,\ r^2 = .98$$

free energy of hydrolysis of ATP, especially under the conditions of nearly constant redox potential which appears to exist in these muscles. The thermodynamic approach provides a way of relating the cytosolic concentations of ATP, ADP and phosphate to the $\dot{V}O_2$. Figure 4 shows the relationship between ΔG_{ATP} and $\dot{V}O_2$ during the rest-work transition in dog gracilis muscle. The line was obtained by fitting only those points which had the same redox value as estimated from fluorescence meaurements. The fit is excellent (see equation in figure legend). Those points which are not on the line are the resting and 15 sec points which have different redox potentials as estimated from fluorescence measurements. Although the variation in the data precludes a detailed quantitative analysis from this logarithmic approach it is clear that most of the variation in the $\dot{V}O_2$ throughout the rest-work transition can be accounted for by the change in ΔG_{ATP}. As steady-state is approached this term is dominated by the changes in ADP and is consistent with a translocase-limited operation of the mitochondria. At lower $\dot{V}O_2$ during the early period of the rest-work transition the phosphate term dominates. Thus we are led to conclude that at low rates of energy turnover in these muscles phosphate concentrations may be a primary factor in regulating $\dot{V}O_2$ but as $\dot{V}O_2 {}_{max}$ is approached the delivery of ADP to the phosphorylating sites can become limiting to the rate of oxidative phosphorylation.

In summary, during the rest-work transition to an aerobic steady-state in a red muscle neither oxygen nor carbon substrate limits are responsible for the lag in the increase in $\dot{V}O_2$. The control of $\dot{V}O_2$ can be best described by the cytosolic phosphorylation potential as expressed by ΔG_{ATP}. This term is dominated by phosphate at low rates of energy turnover and by ADP at high rates of turnover. A rate limiting role for mitochondrial adenine nucleotide translocase is consistent with the data at high rates of energy turnover. This is in agreement with the previous suggestion that the maximal oxidative rate in muscle is ultimately limited in most cases by the enzyme capacity rather than the rate of delivery of substrates (13).

REFERENCES

1. Connett, R.J., T.E.J. Gayeski, and C.R. Honig. Lactate accumulation in fully, aerobic, working dog gracilis muscle. Am. J. Physiol. 246: H120-H128, 1984.

2. Honig, C.R., T.E.J. Gayeski, and R.J. Connett. Balance between O_2 availabiity and $\dot{V}O_2$ in rest-work transition as measured by myoglobin saturation in

subcellular volumes. Adv. Exp. Med. Biol. In Press, 1984.

3. Honig, C.R., T.E.J. Gayeski, and R.J. Connett. O_2 transport in the rest-work transition illustrates new functions for myoglobin. Am. J. Physiol. submitted.

4. Honig, C.R., C.L. Odoroff and J.L. Frierson. Capillary recruitment in exercise: rate, extent, uniformity, and relation to blood flow. Am. J. Physiol. 238: H31-42, 1980.

5. Honig, C.R. Hypoxia in skeletal muscle at rest and during the transition to steady work. Microvasc. Res. 13: 377-398, 1972.

6. Piiper, J., D.E. DiPrampero and P. Cerretelli. Oxygen debt and high energy phosphates in gastrocnemius muscle of the dog. Am. J. Physiol. 215: 523-531, 1968.

7. Veech, R.L., J.W. Randolph Lawson, N.W. Cornell, and H.A. Krebs. Cytosolic phosphorylation potential. J. Biol. Chem. 254: 6538-6547, 1979.

8. Kushmerick, M.J. Insight into the energetics of skeletal and smooth muscle by 31-P NMR. 2nd International Congress on Myocardial and Cellular Bioenergetics and Compartmentation, 1984.

9. McGilvery, R.W. and Murray, T.W. Calculated equilibria of phosphocreatine and adenosine phosphates during utilization of high energy phosphate by muscle. J. Biol. Chem. 249: 5845-5850, 1974.

10. Lawson, J.W.R. and R.L. Veech. Effects of pH and free Mg^{2+} on the keg of the creatine kinase reaction and other phosphate hydrolyses and phosphate tranfer reations. J. Biol. Chem. 254: 6538-6547, 1979.

11. Davis, E.J. and L. Lumeng. Relationships between the phosphorylation potentials generated by liver mitochondria and respiratory state under conditions of adenosine diphosphate control. J. Biol. Chem. 250: 2275-2282, 1975.

12. Jacobus, W.E., R.W. Moreadith and K.M. Vandegaer. Mitochondria respiratory control. J. Biol. Chem. 257: 2397-2402, 1982.

13. Connett, R.J., T.E.J. Gayeski and C.R. Honig. Lactate production in a pure red muscle in absence of anoxia: mechanisms and significance. Adv. Exp. Med. Biol. 159: 327-335, 1984.

14. Wilson, D.F., M. Stubbs, N. Oshino and M. Erecinska. Thermodynamic relationships between the mitochondrial oxidation-reduction reactions and cellular ATP levels in a cites tumor cells and perfused rat liver. Biochemistry 13: 5305-5311, 1974.

15. Rothschild, K.J., S.A. Ellias, A. Essig and H. E. Stanley. Nonequilibrium linear behaviour of biological systems. Biophys. J. 30: 209-230, 1980.

16. Gayeski, T.E.J. A Cryogenic Microspectrophotometric Method for Measuring Myoglobin Saturation in Subcellular Volumes; Application to Resting Dog Gracilis Muscle (Ph.D. dissertation). Rochester, NY: Univ. of Rochester, 1981. (Univ. Microfilms, No. DA8224720, Ann Arbor, MI, 1981).

COMPARTMENTATION AND FUNCTIONAL MECHANISMS IN MYOCARDIAL FAILURE AND MYOCARDIAL INFARCTION

R. J. Bing, Y. Sasaki, M. Chemnitius and W. Burger

Huntington Medical Research Institutes
100 Congress Street
Pasadena, CA   91105

INTRODUCTION

Compartmentation is a term denoting confinement in space
(anatomic compartmentation) and function (functional compartmentation). The result of compartmentation is functional specificity
and maintenance of anatomic and functional integrity. Under pathologic conditions, spatial and functional integrity and specificity
are obliterated. The extent and specificity of damage to anatomic
and functional compartmentation depend on the cause of the pathologic
condition. If this cause is well defined, the consequences are
also clearly discernible. However, if there are several poorly
defined causes, the functional changes are diffuse. Myocardial
failure and myocardial infarction are cases in point. In the former,
the causes are not clearly defined and thus changes in structure
and function are poorly outlined. In myocardial infarction, due to
regional ischemia both cause and effect are more easily defined.
It is the purpose of this report to describe changes in compartmentation and specific mechanism in two conditions: myocardial failure
and myocardial infarction.

MYOCARDIAL FAILURE

The difficulty in studying disturbances in intermediary metabolism in myocardial failure is the lack of an experimental model.
Acute failure produced in hearts perfused in vitro or in vivo is
very different from failure occurring from chronic overload.
Therefore early attempts have been made to study the failing human
heart. The early investigations were carried out by means of
coronary sinus catheterization in the middle 1950's.[1] The results

283

revealed no changes in extraction of foodstuffs by the human heart.
It was clear however that balance studies across the heart could
not reveal changes in compartmentation as related to specific
mechanisms. Autopsy analyses of the human heart obtained six hours
after death were also inconclusive, demonstrating a decrease in the
activity of mitochondrial enzymes such as isocitrate dehydrogenase,
and a rise in glyceraldehyde-3-phosphate dehydrogenase.[2] It was
our original idea, that the deficiency in myocardial failure lies
at least partially in the function of contractile proteins.[3] This
finding was supported by the early studies of Kako and Bing who
found diminished contractility of actomyosin bands prepared from
failing human hearts.[4] Early studies on properties of myosin from
failing human hearts showed changes in molecular shape and/or
weight which were thought to be commensurate with denaturation of
proteins.[5]

New light has been shed by Swynghedauw on changes in specific
function of myosin from failing hypertrophied hearts.[6] He found
that a decrease in contractility of the heart is correlated with a
fall in the activity of myosin ATPase. This was due to isoenzymic
reversion to the fetal form of myosin which possesses a low ATPase
activity. Although this finding so far has not been confirmed in
human myocardial failure, it gives credance to the original concept
formulated in 1952, that myocardial failure may be in part due to
malfunction of contractile elements.[3]

Alcohol results in marked loss of compartmentation and specific
function. However only in man does alcohol ingestion result in
cardiomyopathy with loss of contractility. This is a puzzling
finding, since in the experimental animal changes in compartmentation and specific function are pronounced. Thus in rats exposed
to ethanol (30%) for an average of five weeks, several parameters
of contractility (dp/dt_{max}, Vmax, stiffness of series elastic
elements) are remarkably altered[7] and the biochemistry of hearts
of animals exposed to ethanol is also changed.[8]

A possible cause of the loss of contractility in myocardial
failure lies in disturbances in excitation-contraction coupling or,
in more precise terms, in disturbances in Ca^{++} transfer to the
contractile elements.[9] On first glance this does not appear to be
due to decompartmentation; however the loss of specific enzymatic
function in cellular membranes, suggests this possibility. Knowledge of membrane function and Ca^{++} transfer is the fastest growing
area in the field of cardiac metabolism. The time appears right,
after Katz, Carafoli, Tada, Dhalla, Schwartz, Reuter, Mommaerts,
Wollenberger,[10-17] and others have laid the groundwork. From these
studies the role of different membrane systems in the control of
calcium availability has become apparent.[10,13] These membrane
systems, particularly sarcolemma (SL) and sarcoplasmic reticulum
(SR), regulate calcium transport.[17]

A series of enzymes in the SL membrane exist in compartmentalized spaces. The difficulty in defining the role of SL has been due to impurities of the preparation of sarcolemmal vesicles. Carafoli[11] and Tada and Katz[12,18] have described the role of adenylate cyclase, of ($Ca^{++} + Mg^{++}$) ATPase, of cyclic AMP, and of protein kinase and of calmodulin in calcium transport. Most of this work has been carried out on sarcoplasmic reticulum. Heart SL possesses two systems for Ca^{++} transport out of the cell: the Na^+/Ca^{++} exchange and Ca^{++} pumping ATPase.[11] Of particular importance is the finding by St. Louis and Sulakhe[20] that in the presence of oxalate, cAMP-dependent phosphorylation of proteins in SL vesicles stimulates the uptake of Ca^{++}.[20] The ($Ca^{++} + Mg^{++}$) ATPase of SL is regulated by Ca^{++} + calmodulin-and cAMP-dependent phosphorylation.[12] This ATP dependent outward pumping in SL is supplementary to the main mechanism of ejection of Ca^{++} which occurs in exchange for Na^+.[11] The ATP-dependent Ca^{++} transport system accumulates Ca^{++} in SL in the presence of ATP. Thus Ca^{++} binding by sarcolemmal vesicles can be used as an index of Ca^{++} movement. In addition, a slow inward movement occurs which is largely due to Ca^{++} selective ion channels.[12] However this report is not concerned with Ca^{++} transport by this mechanism.

Stimulation of Ca^{++} accumulation by cardiac SR in vitro occurs by preincubation of the SR vesicles with exogenous PK and cyclic AMP and also beta-1-agonists.[12] The effects of beta-1-agonists, which are mediated by adenyl cyclase, protein kinase and Ca^{++} + Mg^{++}-ATPase can therefore be determined in SR by measuring calcium binding. The effect of cAMP-dependent protein kinase results in SR in the phosphorylation of phospholamban (a protein), leading to an increase in calcium uptake and release.[12]

SL vesicles exhibit ATP-dependent Ca^{++} accumulation in the presence of oxalate,[20] indicating the existence of transmembrane Ca^{++} flux. This however may be due to contamination with SR.[12] In SL, phosphorylation occurs by endogenous and exogenous cAMP-protein kinase.[35] Walsh et al[27] observed that SL proteins were phosphorylated in SL vesicles and that phosphorylation increased when the hearts were exposed to epinephrine. Apparently catecholamines lead to PK-catalyzed phosphorylation of SL proteins, which may contribute to the inotropic response. The determination of phosphorylation of SL vesicles represents therefore a possible means of assessing the activity of beta-1-agonists.

We have employed these two parameters, ATP dependent Ca^{++} uptake and phosphorylation by and of SL as indices for changes in specific function occurring in the ischemic failing heart preparations and after beta agonists. Global ischemia was produced in dog hearts in a supported working heart preparation perfused with a fluorocarbon (FC-43) oxygenated in an infant bubble oxygenator with a mixture of 95% O_2 and 5% CO_2 (Fig. 1).[21,22,23] This assures

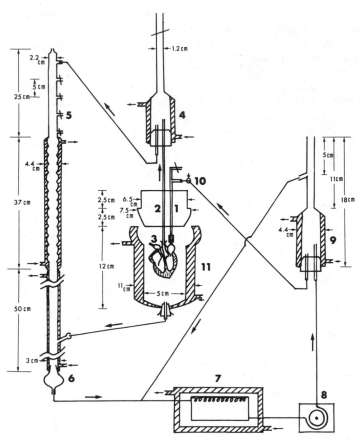

Fig. 1. Schematic representation of the perfusion system for
working heart preparations of larger mammals. Atrial cannula (1), aortic cannula (2), pulmonary artery cannula (3),
aortic pressure chamber (4), condenser with variable afterload settings (5), filter (6), infant bubble oxygenator
(7), roller pump (8), atrial bubble trap (9), three-way
stopcock (10), water jacketed heart chamber (11). The
direction of perfusate flow is indicated by large arrows;
small arrows show water circulation in the jackets (37° C).

survival of larger mammalian hearts because, in contrast to crystalloid perfusates, the use of FC-43 emulsion provides the heart with
an adequate amount of oxygen (5.4 vol% at 760mm Hg as compared to
2.4 vol% at 760mm Hg). The oxygen consumption of the rabbit heart
perfused with FC-43 is 0.35ml O_2/g dry weight/minute. Adequate
oxygenation is also confirmed by biochemical studies involving high
energy phosphates and glycolytic compounds.[22] Failure following
global ischemia was produced by completely arresting inflow and

outflow to and from the heart for periods ranging from 1 to 20 minutes, depending on the hemodynamic conditions. We refer to this preparation as ischemic failing heart preparation. dp/dt, cardiac output, coronary flow and left ventricular pressures were recorded prior to and following these ischemic periods. When dp/dt had fallen to approximately 40% of its control value, perfusion via the supporting Sarns Pump was cut off and the heart was perfused by a syringe with 140ml of cold Krebs-Henseleit solution. The heart was then suspended in 500ml of ice-cold saline solution.

Preparation of SL was carried out according to the method of Jones;[24] ATP dependent Ca^{++} uptake in SL vesicles was determined with the method of Caroni and Carafoli[25] modified by Church and Sen[26] using millipore filtration. Purity of SL vesicles was ascertained by marker enzymes. For SL: K^+-stimulated p-nitrophenyl-phosphatase (and $Na^+ + K^+$-ATPase); for SR: azide insensitive Ca^{++}-activated ATPase; for mitochondria: succinate-cytochrome c-reductase. In addition SL was distinguished by the effect of Na^+ (40mM) in effecting Na^+/Ca^{++} exchange.[25]

Phosphorylation of SL was determined using a procedure similar to that employed for Ca^{++} binding except for the addition of EGTA (2mM), 3-isobutyl-1-methylxanthine (1mM), $[\gamma-^{32}P]$ ATP (2μCi; 50μmoles) and 5'guanylylimidodiphosphate (10^{-6}M). Ouabain and ATP were omitted. After fixed times of incubation ^{32}P incorporation in SL was determined according to the method of St. Louis and Sulakhe.[20]

Preliminary results on Ca^{++} uptake by SL vesicles are illustrated in Fig. 2. Four sets of experiments on calcium uptake were carried out: 1) on SL obtained from beating hearts in situ; 2) on hearts perfused in vitro; 3) on ischemic failing heart preparations; 4) on SL of ischemic failing hearts after the application of TA-064, a beta-1-agonist. In this instance the heart was removed at the height of the positive inotropic effect. TA-064 (10^{-3}M in 1ml of Krebs-Henseleit solution) was injected over a period of 30 seconds into the tubing leading to the left atrium.

The highest degree of Ca^{++} uptake occurred in SL obtained from beating hearts in situ (Fig. 2). SL prepared from hearts perfused in vitro had lower Ca^{++} uptake. The lowest calcium uptake was observed in hearts with global ischemia (Fig. 2). TA-064 when administered to ischemic failing heart preparations, considerably increased Ca^{++} uptake as compared to the ischemic control.

The results demonstrate that in ischemic failing heart preparations, Ca^{++} uptake by SL is markedly reduced and that this reduction can be overcome by the application of a beta-1-agonist. One cannot extrapolate the findings to other types of acute myocardial failure preparations, since it has been shown in this laboratory that acute failing heart preparations differ in their biochemical

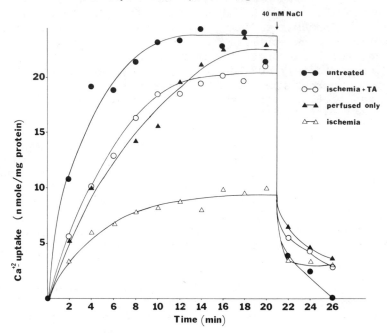

Fig. 2. Ca^{++} uptake by SL plotted against time obtained from hearts removed in situ (untreated), after perfusion in vitro (perfused only), after intermittent global ischemia, (ischemia), and after global ischemia and TA-064 (ischemia + TA). The lowest Ca^{++} uptake occurred in the ischemic failing heart preparations. TA-064 increases Ca^{++} uptake by SL above Ca^{++} uptake in ischemic failing heart preparations.

manifestations.[23] The effect of TA-064 is probably similar to that of calecholamines, caused by beta adrenergic activation of a SL adenylate cyclase with intracellular rise of cAMP.[12]

Fig. 3 demonstrates preliminary data on the effect of TA-064 and of isoproterenol on phosphorylation of sarcolemmal vesicles obtained from non failing heart preparations in vivo. In both instances, an increase in ^{32}P incorporation could be observed. Possibly the beta-1-agonist activates adenylate cyclase and the

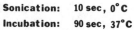

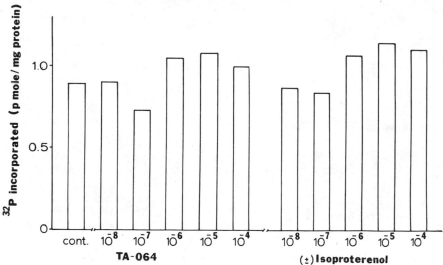

Fig. 3. Phosphorylation by SL expressed as dose response obtained
from hearts perfused in vitro, after the addition of two
beta-1-agonists, TA-064 and isoproterenol. Both agents
increase SL phosphorylation at higher concentrations.

cAMP dependent protein kinase system. Reference was already made
to Walsh who found that two SL proteins were phosphorylated in SL
vesicles from rat hearts perfused with inorganic ^{32}P and that
phosphorylation of these SL membranes increased when the hearts
were exposed to epinephrine.[27] Therefore beta-1-agonists appear to
lead to cAMP dependent phosphorylation of SL proteins and to a
positive inotropic response.

Cardiac SL preparations contain an endogenous cAMP-protein
kinase system. St. Louis and coworkers demonstrated that the addition of exogenous protein kinase further catalyzed the phosphorylation of guinea pig heart sarcolemma.[35] Similar results are shown
in Fig. 4, which illustrates that the addition of cyclic-AMP $(10^{-7}M)$

289

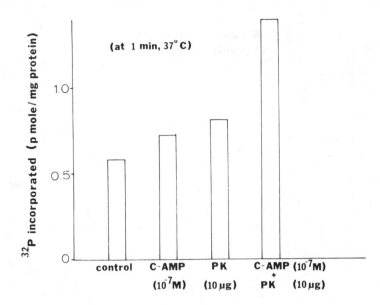

Phosphorylation of Dog Heart SL

Fig. 4. The effect of separate and combined administrations of c-AMP and PK on phosphorylation of SL. The most pronounced effect is seen after combination of both cAMP and PK.

or of protein kinase (10µg) alone or in conjunction increases the degree of phosphorylation of SL vesicles. Fig. 5 illustrates that, similar to the data on Ca^{++} uptake presented in Fig. 2, phosphorylation of SL vesicles from the ischemic heart preparation is markedly reduced. The addition of TA-064 increases phosphorylation almost to the level of SL prepared from SL of perfused but non-ischemic not failing preparations. These data show that a beta-1-agonist can increase phosphorylation by SL vesicles.

MYOCARDIAL INFARCTION

This subject will be discussed primarily to illustrate the difference in response of heart muscle to regional ischemia as

Phosphorylation of Dog Heart SL

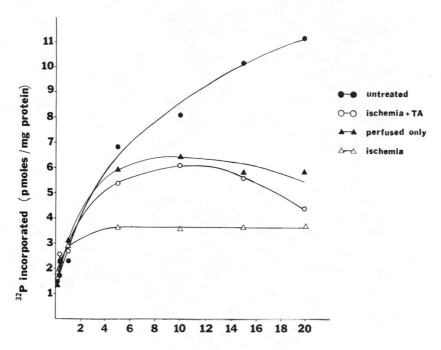

Fig. 5.   Phosphorylation of SL plotted against time.   For further
explanations see Fig. 2.

compared to myocardial failure.   In the former decompartmentation
and loss of specific functions are much more evident as seen in both
structural and functional disturbances.

Fig. 6 illustrates the specific metabolic changes induced by
local ischemia.   They affect the glycolytic pathway, mitochondrial
respiration, fatty acid metabolism and contractile function.
Obviously these changes are the result of diminished blood flow to
the ischemic region.   It is surprising that in the dog with regional
myocardial ischemia of one hour duration, a flow reduction through
the center of the infarct of only 68% was found, reaching 75% after
three hours.[28]   The degree of metabolic changes depends on the
degree and duration of ischemia.   After three hours, subendocardial
ischemia is more pronounced than in other portions of the myocardium.[28]

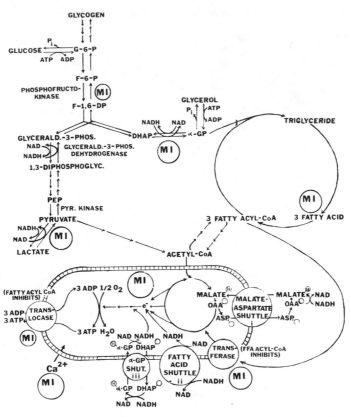

Fig. 6.   Schematic illustration of the effect of myocardial ischemia on various pathways of intermediary cardiac metabolism.

One of the metabolic consequences of this reduction in flow is diminished washout of lactic acid, CO_2 and protons resulting in severe acidosis.[29]   Using nuclear magnetic resonance (NMR), Flaherty and associates have recently demonstrated that the magnitude of intracellular acidosis and the associated increase in inorganic phosphate correlated inversely with recovery of post-ischemic ventricular structure and function.[30]   The increase in proton referred to by Opie, also leads, according to Williams, to consistent prolongation of the proton spin-lattice relaxation time (T_1) in the ischemic region.[31]   Hollis and coworkers had previously shown that it is possible, using Phosphorus-31 NMR spectra, to identify regional myocardial ischemia.[32]   The changes in glycolytic pathways induced by regional myocardial ischemia have been well defined.   There is a pronounced rise in tissue levels of lactic acid, and in α-glycerophosphate, representing diminished washout

292

and decline in the NAD/NADH ratio. The subsequent decreased intra-cellular pH, together with the elevation of free fatty acids, is responsible for the inhibition of phosphofructokinase.

The changes in free fatty acids and Acyl-CoA levels referred to by a number of authors are responsible for inhibition of several enzymes.[33,34] Acyl-CoA accumulation during infarction leads to inhibition of adenosin nucleotide transferase, and inhibits trans-locase, which is responsible for the exchange of extramitochondrial ADP for intramitochondrial ATP.[29]

Regional ischemia leads to a decrease in mitochondrial respira-tion.[28] This is the biochemical equivalent of the severe damage and decompartmentation of mitochondrial structures observed in regional myocardial ischemia.[35] QO_2 values of ischemic mitochondria are significantly depressed, indicating that mitochondrial perform-ance during state III respiration is disturbed.[28] Minor reductions are also noticed in respiratory control indices (RCI) and in the ADP:O ratios.[28] As a result of severe mitochondrial damage both ATP and CP levels are dramatically reduced. Three hours after onset of ischemia the level of ADP is also diminished.[28] It is not surprising that these breakdowns in compartmentation occurring with ischemia, affect myocardial contractility.[28] When ischemic heart muscle fibers are dissected and suspended in 50% glycerol for one week, their contractility is severely impaired as compared to fibers from nonischemic regions as shown by decline in maximal developed tension (P_0), maximal rate of tension development (dp/dt_{max}), and an increase in the t_0 (time from onset of contraction to peaks tension). Velocity of contraction (V_{max}) is also reduced.

SUMMARY

Changes in compartmentation and specific mechanism in acute myocardial failure due to global ischemia and in regional myocardial ischemia in dog hearts are described. Ischemic failure was produced by periodic arrest of flow to supported heart preparations perfused with a fluorocarbon (FC-43). Sarcolemmal vesicles (SL) prepared from ischemic failing heart preparations exhibited diminished Ca^{++} binding and phosphorylation. TA-064, a beta-1-agonist partially abolished the reduction in Ca^{++} binding and phosphorylation of SL vesicles. The addition of cyclic-AMP (cAMP) and of protein kinase (PK) increased phosphorylation of SL vesicles obtained from non failing heart preparations. Combination of cAMP and of PK had the greatest effect. In contrast to myocardial failure, myocardial infarction is known to produce a large variety of specific distur-bances in intermediary cardiac metabolism. Apparently in ischemic failing heart preparations, Ca^{++} binding and phosphorylation by SL are deficient. The results with TA-064 and isoproterenol suggest that phosphorylation of SL may play a role in the positive inotropic effect of beta-1-agonists.

REFERENCES

1. R. J. Bing, Metabolism of the heart, "Harvey Lectures, Series L," Academic Press, New York (1954-1955).
2. R. J. Bing, C. Wu and S. Gudbjarnason, Mechanism of heart failure, Circ. Res. Suppl. II:64-69 (1964).
3. R. J. Bing and M. Taeschler, Cardiac failure and cardiac muscle, Cardiologia 21:283-289 (1952).
4. K. Kako and R. J. Bing, Contractility of actomyosin bands prepared from normal and failing human hearts, J. Clin. Invest. 37:465-470 (1958).
5. M. L. Nebel and R. J. Bing, Contractile proteins of normal and failing human hearts, Arch. Int. Med. 111:190-195 (1963).
6. A. M. Lompre, K. Schwartz, A. D'Albis, G. Lacombe, N. Van Thiem and B. Swynghedauw, Myosin isoenzyme redistribution in chronic heart overload, Nature 282:105-107 (1979).
7. Y. Maruyama, R. J. Bing, J. S. M. Sarma and R. Weishaar, The effect of alcohol on active and passive stiffness, and on isometric contractions of glycerinated heart muscle in rats, Jap. Heart J. 19:513-521 (1978).
8. J. S. M. Sarma, S. Ikeda, R. Fischer, Y. Maruyama, R. Weishaar and R. J. Bing, Biochemical and contractile properties of heart muscle after prolonged alcohol administration, J. Mol. Cell. Cardiol. 8:951-972 (1976).
9. R. J. Bing, Cardiac Metabolism: Its contributions to alcoholic heart disease and myocardial failure, Circulation 58:965-970 (1978).
10. A. M. Katz, Regulation of myocardial contractility 1958-1983: An odyssey, J. Am. Coll. Cardiol. I:42-51 (1983).
11. P. Caroni and E. Carafoli, The Ca^{2+}-pumping ATPase of heart sarcolemma, J. Biol. Chem. 256:3263-3270 (1981).
12. M. Tada and A. M. Katz, Phosphorylation of the sarcoplasmic reticulum and sarcolemma, Ann. Rev. Physiol. 44:401-423 (1982).
13. N. S. Dhalla, P. K. Das and G. P. Sharma, Subcellular basis of cardiac contractile failure, J. Mol. Cell. Cardiol. 10:363-385 (1978).
14. A. Schwartz, L. A. Sordahl, M. L. Entman, J. C. Allen, Y. S. Reddy, M. A. Goldstein, R. J. Luchi and L. E. Wyborny, Abnormal biochemistry in myocardial failure, Am. J. Cardiol. 32:407-422 (1973).
15. H. Reuter, Localization of beta adrenergic receptors, and effects of noradrenaline and cyclic nucleotides on action potentials, ionic currents and tension in mammalian cardiac muscle, J. Physiol. 242:429-451 (1974).
16. W. F. H. Mommaerts, Energetics of muscular contraction, Physiol. Rev. 49:427-508 (1969).

17. A. Wollenberger and H. Will, Protein kinase-catalyzed membrane phosphorylation and its possible relationship to the role of calcium in the adrenergic regulation of cardiac contraction, Life Sciences 22:1159–1178 (1978).

18. M. Tada, M. Inui, M. Yamada, M. Kadoma, T. Kuzuya, H. Abe and S. Kakiuchi, Effects of phospholamban phosphorylation catalyzed by adenosine 3':5'-monophosphate- and calmodulin-dependent protein kinases on calcium transport ATPase of cardiac sarcoplasmic reticulum, J. Mol. Cell. Cardiol. 15: 335–346 (1983).

19. P. Caroni, L. Reinlib and E. Carafoli, Charge movements during the Na^+–Ca^{2+} exchange in heart sarcolemmal vesicles, Proc. Natl. Acad. Sci. USA 77:6354–6358 (1980).

20. P. V. Sulakhe, N. L. Leung and P. J. St. Louis, Stimulation of calcium accumulation in cardiac sarcolemma by protein kinase, Can. J. Biochem. 54:438–445 (1976).

21. R. J. Bing, Cardiac perfusion, past and present, in: "Myocardial Ischemia and Lipid Metabolism (Advances in Myocardiology)," A. M. Katz and F. Ferrari, eds., Plenum Press, New York (1984).

22. J. -M. Chemnitius, W. Burger, M. Montllor and R. J. Bing, A cardiac perfusion model for larger mammalian hearts utilizing a perfluorochemical, J. Mol. Cell. Cardiol. (in press).

23. W. Burger, J. -M. Chemnitius, J. Sugihara, R. Navos and R. J. Bing, The effects of a new cardiotonic drug (TA-064) on normal and failing heart preparations, J. Pharmacol. Exp. Therap. (in press).

24. L. R. Jones, S. W. Maddock and H. R. Besch, Unmasking effect of alamethicin on the (Na^+,K^+)-ATPase, beta-adrenergic receptor-coupled adenylate cyclase, and cAMP-dependent protein kinase activities of cardiac sarcolemmal vesicles, J. Biol. Chem. 255:9971–9980 (1980).

25. P. Caroni and E. Carafoli, An ATP-dependent Ca^{2+}-pumping system in dog heart sarcolemma, Nature 283:765–767 (1980).

26. J. G. Church and A. K. Sen, Regulation of canine heart sarcolemmal Ca^{2+}-pumping ATPase by cyclic GMP, Biochim. Biophys. Acta 728:191–200 (1983).

27. D. A. Walsh, M. S. Clippinger, S. Sivaramakrishnan and T. E. McCullough, Cyclic adenosine monophosphate dependent and independent phosphorylation of sarcolemma membrane proteins in perfused rat heart, Biochemistry 18:871–877 (1979).

28. R. Weishaar, J. S. M. Sarma, Y. Maruyama, R. Fischer and R. J. Bing, Regional blood flow, contractility and metabolism in early myocardial infarction, Cardiology 62:2–20 (1977).

29. L. H. Opie, II. Metabolic regulation in ischemia and hypoxia. Effects of regional ischemia on metabolism of glucose and fatty acids, Circulation Res. 38:52–74 (1976).

30. J. T. Flaherty, M. L. Weisfeldt, B. H. Bulkley, T. J. Gardner, V. L. Gott and W. E. Jacobus, Mechanisms of ischemic myocardial cell damage assessed by phosphorus-31 nuclear

magnetic resonance, Circulation 65:561-571 (1982).

31. E. S. Williams, J. I. Kaplan, F. Thatcher, G. Zimmerman and S. B. Knoebel, Prolongation of proton spin lattice relaxation times in regionally ischemic tissue from dog hearts, J. Nucl. Med. 21:449-453 (1980).

32. D. P. Hollis, R. L. Nunally, W. E. Jacobus and G. J. Taylor, Detection of regional ischemia in perfused beating hearts by phosphorous nuclear magnetic resonance, Biochem. Biophys. Res. Commun. 75:1086-1091 (1977).

33. S. V. Pande and J. F. Mead, Inhibition of enzyme activities by free fatty acids, J. Biol. Chem. 243:6180-6185 (1968).

34. A. L. Shug and E. Shrago, A proposed mechanism for free fatty acid effects on energy metabolism of the heart, J. Lab. Clin. Med. 81:214-218 (1973).

35. P. J. St. Louis and P. V. Sulakhe, Phosphorylation of cardiac sarcolemma by endogenous and exogenous protein kinases, Arch. Biochem. Biophys. 198:227-240 (1979).

ACKNOWLEDGMENTS

This work was supported by grants from The Council for Tobacco Research, U.S.A., Inc. and The Margaret W. and Herbert Hoover, Jr. Foundations, Pasadena, California. Drs. M. Chemnitius and W. Burger are McCollum Fellows in Experimental Cardiology. The authors wish to express their gratitude to Marianne Metz for technical assisttance, to Dr. Philipson from U.C.L.A. for his advice in carrying out these experiments and to Carol Glasser for help in the preparation of the manuscript.

MYOCARDIAL PROTECTION OF HYPERTROPHIED HEARTS BY ADMINISTRATION

OF CARDIOPLEGIA ACCORDING TO REGIONAL MYOCARDIAL TEMPERATURE

G. Görlach[1], H.H. Scheld[1], F. Podzuweit[2], J. Mulch[1]
W. Schaper[2], F.W. Hehrlein[1]

1 Dept. of Cardiovascular Surgery, Justus-Liebig-
University
Klinikstr. 29
D-6300 Giessen, W.-Germany

2 Max-Planck-Institute for Physiological and Clinical
Research, Dept. of Experimental Cardiology
D-6350 Bad Nauheim, West-Germany

INTRODUCTION

Hypertrophied hearts are known to be extremely vulnerable to
ischemia, because of their reduced content of high energy phosphates (1, 2, 3). The reduction of myocardial temperature is one
of the most important factors of myocardial protection during
heart arrest (4, 5). Cardioplegic solutions of different
composition are used in our hospital. To test, which of them are
able to protect hypertrophied hearts in a sufficient amount, we
studied myocardial protection in patients undergoing aortic valve
surgery. According to regional myocardial temperature we inter-
mittently infused cardioplegia so that the temperature of the
heart did not increase above 15°C in any region of the heart.
Myocardial protection was estimated by measuring the high energy
phosphate and lactate content of the myocardium.

METHOD

The study included 61 patients with aortic stenosis,
insufficiency and combined aortic valve disease. The mean age

of the patients was 53,4 years. 15 were women and 46 were men. According to New York Heart Association 45 were in class III and 16 in class IV. The mean left ventricular enddiastolic pressure was 17,54 mm Hg ranging from 4 - 36 mm Hg. The mean left ventricular muscle mass measured 262,54 $\pm$ 38,41 g/m^2. We built up three different groups, which were comparable to each other according to age, sex and hemodynamics (fig. 1). In group 1 we used the Bretschneider (6), in group 2 the Hamburg (7) and in group 3 the St. Thomas (8) cardioplegia.

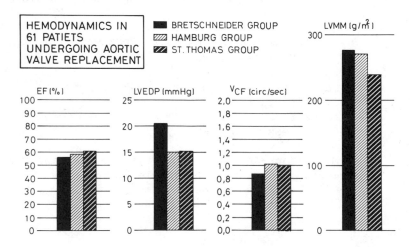

Fig. 1. EF ejection fraction, LVEDP left ventricular end-
        diastolic pressure, VcF velocity of circumferential
        fiber shortening, LVMM left ventricular muscle mass.

Thermistor probes, which we used for continuous measurement of regional myocardial temperature, were placed in the septum, the anterior, the lateral and the posterior wall of the left ventricle. Before aortic cross-clamping the left ventricle was vented. After cross-clamping the aortic root was incised and cardioplegia was infused directly into both coronary ostia. Following an initial infusion of 2000 ml we administered additional cardioplegia if regional myocardial temperature increased above 15°C in one region of the heart or if electrical or mechanical activity of the heart appeared. During heart arrest body temperature was reduced to 28°C.

Myocardial biopsies were taken by a Tru-Cut-Needle[R+] from the left ventricular apex in the region between left anterior descendens and diagonal arteries. The wet weight of the biopsies ranged from 10 to 30 mg. Before ischemia, at the end of the ischemic period and after 10 minutes of reperfusion we took biopsies. They were immediately frozen with liquid nitrogen. Following freeze drying adenosinetriphosphate (ATP), adenosine diphosphate (ADP), creatine phosphate (CP) and lactate were determined by fluorometry.

RESULTS

The control specimen showed no significant difference of ATP, ADP, CP and lactate between the three groups (fig. 2). Only the ATP-level was slightly higher in the St. Thomas group.

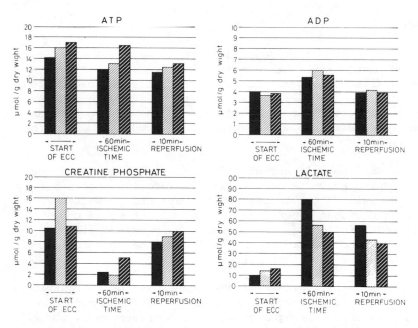

Fig. 2. Metabolites determinded from myocardial biopsies before ischemia, after ischemia and after 10 min. of reperfusion. ATP adenosinetriphosphate, ADP adenosine diphosphate.

+ Travenol GmbH, Munic

The ischemic period measured 60,50 $\pm$ 12,91 minutes in group
1, 60,40 $\pm$ 17,64 min. in group 2 and 59,26 $\pm$ 12,84 min. in group
3. After a mean ischemic time of 60 minutes ranging from 38 to
107 minutes ATP decreased not significantly, while CP fell
clearly and lactate accumulated. Again no significant difference
occured between the three groups (fig. 2). A negative correlation
of r = -0,416 (p $<$ 0,01) existed between ATP and left ventricular muscle mass.

Following 10 minutes of reperfusion CP increased and lactate
decreased, but both metabolites did not reach the control
level. As before the metabolites showed the same behavior in all
groups and significant differences could not be recognized
(fig. 2).

DISCUSSION

Myocardial protection depends on the preservation of high
energy phosphates (9). The increased vulnerability of hypertrophied hearts to ischemia is caused by their reduced content
of high energy phosphates (1, 2, 3). In our study we recognized
a negative correlation between ATP at the end of ischemia and
left ventricular muscle mass, which is in accordance with former
studies (10).

During cardioplegic arrest differences of regional myocardial
temperature are known to occur (11). Therefore we continuously
registered regional myocardial temperature and prevented an
increase of regional myocardial temperature above 15°C by
intermittend infusion of cardioplegia. This method allows a
comparison of the myocardial protection by the three cardioplegias independent of temperature.

Despite a small decrease of ATP there was not a significant
decline of ATP after ischemia. From this results we conclude
that the high energy phosphates were well preserved by the
methods of myocardial protection, which we performed. After
ischemia CP decreased and lactate accumulated. The alterations
of these metabolites were reversible after 10 minutes of reperfusion. But as our results demonstrate 10 minutes of reperfusion were not enough for complete reversal of ischemia.

The metabolites determined in our study behave in the three groups in the same way. From our results we conclude that the three cardioplegias which we used were able to protect hyper-trophied hearts in a sufficient amount during an ischemic period of 60 minutes, if regional myocardial temperature in any region of the heart does not increase above 15°C.

REFERENCES

1. S.R.K. Iyengar, S. Ramchand, E.J.P. Chavette, C.K.S. Iyengar, and K.G. Lynn, Anoxic cardiac arrest. An experimental and clinical study of its effects. Part I, J Thorac Cardiovasc Surg 82:692 (1981)

2. J.D. Sink, G.L. Hellom, W.D. Carrie, R.C. Hill, C.O. Olsen, R.N. Jones and A.S. Wechsler, Response of the hyper-trophied myocardium to ischemia. J Thorac Cardiovasc Surg, 81:865 (1981)

3. R.N. Jones, W.D. Currie, C.O. Olsen, R.B. Peyton, P. van Trigt, and A.S. Wechsler, Recovery of metabolic function in hypertrophied canine hearts following global ischemia. Circulation 62 Suppl 3:80 (1980)

4. G.D. Buckberg, A Proposed Solution to the Cardioplegic Controversy, J Thorac Cardiovasc Surg 77:803 (1979)

5. W.A. Lell, E. Buttner, Myocardial Preservation during Cardiopulmonary Bypass. In: A.J. Kaplan: Cardiac Anesthesia Volume II, pp 525-551, Grune & Stratton, New York (1983)

6. C.J. Preusse, M.M. Gebhard, J.J. Bretschneider, Myocardial equilibration process and myocardial energy turnover during initation of artificial cardiac arrest with cardioplegic solution - reasons for a sufficiently long cardioplegic perfusion. Thorac Cardiovasc Surgeon 29:71 (1981)

7. N. Bleese, V. Döring, P. Valmar, H.J. Krebber, H. Pokar, and G. Rodewald, Clinical Application of Cardioplegia in Aortic-Cross-Clamping Periods Longer than 150 Minutes, Thorac Cardiovasc Surgeon 27:390 (1979)

8. P. Jynge, D.J. Hearse, J. deLeiris, D. Fenvray, M.V. Braim-bridge, Protection of the ischemic myocardium, J Thorac Cardiovasc Surg 76:2 (1978)

9. H.J. Bretschneider, G. Hübner, D. Knoll, B. Lohr, H. Nordeck, and P.G. Spieckermann, Myocardial resistance and bio-chemial basis, J Cardiovasc Surg 16:241 (1975)

10. A.S. Wechsler, Deficiencies of Cardioplegia - hyper-
    trophied Ventricle. A Textbook of Clinical Cardioplegia.
    R.M. Engelmann, S. Levitzky (ed), Futura Publishing
    Company Mount Lisco, New York 1982; 381
11. R.C.J. Chiu, P.E. Blundell, M.J. Scott, S. Cain, The
    importance of Monitoring Intramyocardial Temperature
    during Hypothermic Myocardial Protection. Ann Thorac
    Surg 28:318 (1979)

ABSTRACT

Hypertrophied hearts are known to be extremely vulnerable to
ischemia. During cardioplegic arrest different regional myocardial
temperature are known to occur. We investigated myocardial
protection in 61 patients with aortic valve disease undergoing
aortic valve replacement. Three different cardioplegic solutions
were used. Regional myocardial temperature was continuously
controlled and adjusted to a temperature of not more than $15^{\circ}C$
by intermittend infusion of cardioplegia. Before, after heart
arrest and after 10 minutes of reperfusion we did myocardial
biopsies and determined high energy phosphates and lactate. From
our results we conclude that three cardioplegic solutions were
able to protect hypertrophied hearts adequate during an ischemic
period of 60 minutes if the regional myocardial temperature does
not increase above $15^{\circ}C$.

HEART MYOCYTES AS MODELS OF

THE CELLULAR RESPONSE TO ISCHEMIA

Gerald P. Brierley, William C. Wenger, and
Ruth A. Altschuld

Department of Physiological Chemistry
College of Medicine, Ohio State University
Columbus, Ohio 43210

INTRODUCTION

Isolated adult heart cells (myocytes) with properties
suitable for metabolic studies are now available in a number of
laboratories. These cells are Ca^{2+}-tolerant and show excellent
viability and stability. They also retain the electrical
properties, responsiveness to hormones and the complex
morphological features of heart muscle cells in situ (1-5). Such
myocyte preparations should be of considerable value in defining
the response of heart cells to ischemia. Myocytes offer a unique
opportunity to examine metabolic properties and transport
reactions in ventricular muscle cells in the absence of variables
due to tissue perfusion and without contributions from vascular
cells or other cell types that may be present in intact tissue.
In addition, the myocytes can be subjected to uniform
perturbations in media of well-defined composition, can be
serially sampled to determine the time course of responses, and
are amenable to controlled disruption for compartmental analysis
(6,7).

HYPERCONTRACTURE OF MYOCYTES

Ca^{2+}-tolerant myocytes retain viability and normal
morphology for several hours when incubated aerobically with
substrate (see 7 and 8, for example). These cells deteriorate by
two distinctive pathways when subjected to anaerobic incubation

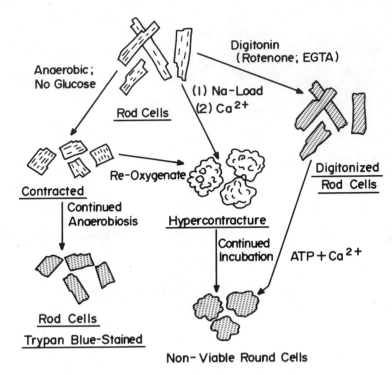

Figure 1 - Interconversion of morphological forms of heart myocytes.

in the absence of glucose (Fig. 1). In the first, the de-energized myocytes lose sarcolemmal integrity on a relatively long time scale as anaerobic incubation is continued. The anaerobic cells become highly contracted (9), but the alignment of the sarcomeres and the overall features of cell morphology are retained. These cells lose cytosol enzymes and take up trypan blue as the sarcolemma loses its integrity (8,10) with further incubation (Fig. 1).

The second pathway for cell deterioration becomes apparent when the anaerobic myocytes are reaerated (7,8). Reaeration produces a gross distortion of cell morphology with the production of round cells with protruding blebs of cytoplasm (Fig. 1; see 11 for micrographs of this cell form). Since the contractile elements of these cells lose their normal alignment and are fused into an amorphous mass, we have designated this process as "hypercontracture." The hypercontracted round cells retain an intact sarcolemma, as indicated by the fact that they exclude succinate and trypan blue, retain cytosol enzymes, and are capable of establishing low Na^+/K^+ ratios and high levels of cellular creatine phosphate (7). These hypercontracted cells lose sarcolemmal integrity rapidly on continued incubation, however, and appear to be very susceptible to mechanical trauma (8).

Hypercontracture of myocytes is also produced in aerobic cells in which intracellular Na^+ has been increased by incubation or washing in the cold (12). These Na^+-loaded myocytes hypercontract when exposed to physiological levels of Ca^{2+} (12) and the morphological forms produced cannot be distinguished from those resulting from reaeration of anaerobic cells (see Fig. 1). It seems likely that the production of these "hypercontracted" cells in vitro is the equivalent of the formation of contraction bands in intact tissue. The aggregated clumps of disorganized actinomyosin seen in contraction band necrosis (13) closely resemble those seen in hypercontracted myocytes. Contraction bands are associated with irreversible processes leading to cell death and it has been postulated that this abnormal contracture may cause rupture of the sarcolemma and the characteristic loss of cellular components seen in situ (13,14). This model shifts emphasis away from currently popular theories of the pathogenesis of ischemic injury which focus on sarcolemmal membrane changes (15, for example) and relegates the sarcolemma to the role of a passive victim of the contracture process.

Contraction bands occur in severely injured myocardial cells following reperfusion of ischemic tissue, when anoxic myocardium is re-oxygenated (the oxygen paradox), and when Ca^{2+} is re-introduced after Ca^{2+}-free perfusion (the Ca paradox) (13). Myocyte hypercontracture is also produced under each of these conditions. The cells hypercontract when re-oxygenated after conditions chosen to simulate ischemia (8), in protocols analogous to the oxygen paradox in situ (7), and when Na^+-loaded myocytes are exposed to Ca^{2+} (12,16), a protocol that retains many of the features of the Ca-paradox in situ (17). The most obvious point of departure between contraction band formation and hypercontracture of myocytes is that the isolated cells retain an intact sarcolemma (7), whereas the process in situ leads to sarcolemmal rupture and enzyme release (17,18). It has been suggested that the same process occurring in attached cells could lead to sarcolemmal rupture in situ, but produce only internal rearrangements in a completely disassociated myocyte (14). This point clearly requires further verification.

MYOCYTES AND THE OXYGEN PARADOX

Myocytes incubated anaerobically in the absence of glucose lose ATP and creatine phosphate (CP) in a relatively short time (7). There is also a parallel decline in the total adenine nucleotide (AN) pool and the lost nucleotide appears as extracellular adenosine and inosine (19). Reaeration of the anaerobic myocytes results in restoration of the adenylate energy charge in these cells (7) with a net resynthesis of small amounts of AN (19). The hypercontracture that accompanies reaeration of these cells is prevented by inclusion of glucose during the anaerobic incubation and by cyanide or dinitrophenol added prior to reaeration (7). It therefore seems likely that the process requires a decrease in high energy phosphate or AN (or both) during the anaerobic incubation and that ATP must be made available from oxidative phosphorylation upon reaeration (7). In each of these respects the hypercontracture of myocytes resembles the phenomenon of "oxygen paradox" in intact heart tissue (14,18). The reaerated cells contain sufficient ATP to restore CP levels to about 70% of control and to re-establish low Na^+/K^+ ratios (7). The presence of 1 mM Ca^{2+} accelerates the loss of myocyte viability during anaerobic incubation and increases the number of cells that go into hypercontracture when re-aerated (7). However, the presence of EGTA during anaerobic incubation and re-aeration does not abolish the contracture. It appears that large numbers of cells have sufficient Ca^{2+} available from intracellular sources to support the hypercontracture process.

It should be noted that the anaerobic cells contract into nearly square forms (7,9). Following re-aeration these forms are seen to relax and contract for several cycles before rounding up in hypercontracture. The restoration of ATP levels in these cells occurs before the hypercontracture process is complete and the bulk of the mitochondria appear to remain competent during and after hypercontracture. It appears, therefore, that the production of ATP by mitochondrial oxidative phosphorylation is contributing to the process of hypercontracture and that the greatly diminished AN pool is probably one of the primary lesions in this type of cellular deterioration. It also appears likely that derangements of intracellular Ca^{2+} metabolism that develop under low-energy conditions may contribute to hypercontracture.

MYOCYTES AND THE CALCIUM PARADOX

Myocytes show low Na^+/K^+ ratios as isolated (16), but gain Na^+ and lose K^+ rapidly when incubated under de-energizing conditions or at low temperature (which inhibits the Na^+-K^+ ATPase). Cells with an elevated Na^+/K^+ ratio are Ca^{2+}-sensitive and hypercontract when exposed to 1 mM Ca^{2+} (Fig. 1). The Ca^{2+}-sensitive cells can be made Ca^{2+}-tolerant by incubation under conditions that restore low Na^+/K^+ ratios (12). The Na^+-loaded myocytes accumulate Ca^{2+} more rapidly than cells with more normal Na^+/K^+ ratios (12) and it appears likely that the additional Ca^{2+} enters the cells in exchange for internal Na^+. The net uptake of Ca^{2+}

is inhibited by H^+ (8) and decreased pH also prevents hypercontracture when Na^+ loaded cells are exposed to Ca^{2+} (2). These observations suggest that an influx of extracellular Ca^{2+} or a dislocation of intracellular Ca^{2+} is responsible for the observed hypercontracture when cells are Na^+-loaded.

The permeability of myocytes to Na^+ (and probably to K^+ as well) is increased as extracellular Ca^{2+} is decreased (16). This effect can be seen as an increased Na^+/K^+ ratio in de-energized cells and also as increased lactate production as extracellular Ca^{2+} is decreased in suspensions of anaerobic myocytes supplemented with glucose (16). The latter cells show high rates of anaerobic glycolysis and maintain nearly normal Na^+/K^+ ratios. Since virtually all of the additional lactate production is abolished by ouabain, it appears that these myocytes expend considerable glycolytic ATP in Na^+-pumping compared to Ca^{2+}-supplemented cells. The lack of significant net uptake of Ca^{2+} under these conditions in Ca^{2+}-supplemented cells suggests that the low internal Na^+ is not simply the result of Na^+/Ca^{2+} exchange (16). It seems possible that Ca^{2+} bound to the sarcolemma may restrict the permeability of the sarcolemma to monovalent cations via as yet undefined pathways (16).

The hypercontracture of myocytes on exposure to Ca^{2+} closely resembles the phenomenon of "Ca^{2+}-paradox" in situ (17,18) in which hearts subjected to Ca^{2+}-free perfusion develop contracture bands and release intracellular enzymes when Ca^{2+} is re-introduced. Either the increased Na^+ content (which would lead to increased Ca^{2+} uptake) or the energy-drain imposed by additional Na-pumping could contribute to hyper-contracture in myocytes (see the discussion in Ref 16). However, it has been established that Na^+-loading in the cold induces Ca^{2+}-dependent hypercontracture and that these cells maintain elevated levels of ATP and CP (16). It therefore appears that Na^+-loading is sufficient to produce hypercontracture when myocytes are exposed to Ca^{2+} and that high-energy phosphate depletion is not an essential component of the reaction under these conditions.

The number of cells that hypercontract upon exposure to Ca^{2+} is a function of the intracellular Na^+ content (Table I). The number of Ca^{2+}-tolerant myocytes decreases from 60% of the total cells to 12% as the internal Na^+ content doubles (Table I). Intracellular Na^+ is not elevated to these levels during Ca^{2+}-paradox protocols in intact hearts (20), so it seems unlikely that contraction band necrosis could depend solely on Ca^{2+} influx by Na^+/Ca^{2+} exchange. However, a massive Ca^{2+} influx as a result of sarcolemmal damage could produce the same response in situ that is promoted by Na^+-loading of the

Table I - Ca^{2+}-Sensitivity of Heart Myocytes as a Function of Intracellular Na^+ Content

Time at 0° (min)	Na^+_i (ngion·mg^{-1})	Ca^{2+}-Tolerant Cells (% Total)
0	148±20	60±2
5	230±15	37±7
10	250±18	31±10
20	270±25	21±4
30	290±20	12±3

Freshly prepared rat heart myocytes were suspended in a nominally Ca^{2+}-free Krebs-Ringer-phosphate buffer at 2 mg protein/ml for the indicated time (see 16 for preparation conditions and the composition of the medium). The cells were re-isolated, the Na^+ content determined (16), and suspended in the same buffer containing Ca^{2+} (1 mM), Ca^{2+}-tolerant cells are defined as those maintaining their rod-shaped morphology and excluding trypan blue after 3 min at 37°. Mean ± SEM (n=4).

myocytes. Ca^{2+}-free perfusion of intact heart tissue causes separation of intercalated disks and cells remain connected only in the area of the gap junctions (13,21). The resumption of contractile activity in these poorly attached cells may lead to physical rupture of the gap junctions with a consequent loss of internal components and massive influx of external Ca^{2+}. Interventions that are most effective in preventing the Ca^{2+} paradox (low temperatures or the addition of the Ca^{2+}-antagonist, diltiazem, during the Ca-free phase) prevent separation of the intercalated disks (13,22). These observations, taken together with those on isolated myocytes, strongly support the suggestion of Ganote that physical membrane damage is the cause of enzyme release in the Ca paradox (13).

DIGITONIN-TREATED MYOCYTES

Treatment of myocytes with digitonin in the appropriate concentration range results in selective lysis of the sarcolemma (6). The digitonin-lysed cells take up trypan blue, are permeable to succinate, AN, and other metabolites, release 90% or more of cytosol proteins, such as myoglobin and lactic dehydrogenase (LDH), and retain mitochondrial enzymes (6). The mitochondria, sarcoplasmic reticulum and myofribils appear normal in electron micrographs of digitonin-lysed cells, but the sarcolemma and T-system are completely disrupted. Small vesicles (apparently derived from the sarcolemma) remain attached to the cell surface by intermediate filaments. Myocytes treated with EGTA and rotenone (to block respiration and ATP formation by the mitochondria) retain their rod-cell configuration when lysed with digitonin (Fig. 1). These digitonin-lysed rod-cells round up in hypercontracture when treated with mM concentrations of both ATP and Ca^{2+} (Fig. 1).

The digitonized cells also retain the rod-cell morphology of untreated myocytes when the digitonin treatment is carried out in Krebs-Ringer-phosphate buffer (16) in the presence of Mg-ATP and EGTA. The number of cells that retain their rod-like configuration under these conditions is a function of the Mg^{2+}-ATP concentration. In a typical experiment, 77% of the cells retained their rod-cell morphology after digitonin-lysis in a medium containing 10 mM Mg-ATP and 0.1 mM EGTA. The percentage of rod cells fell to 36% when the ATP was decreased to 1 mM and to only 21% in a medium containing 0.1 mM ATP. These studies establish that the cells remain rod-shaped and relaxed when the sarcolemma is disrupted in a medium containing high concentrations of Mg-ATP and low level of free Ca^{2+} (pCa of 7.2)

PHASIC CONTRACTION OF MYOCYTES

Freshly prepared rat heart myocytes in which the sarcolemma is intact show low intracellular Na^+/K^+ ratios and do not contract spontaneously when suspended in buffers containing physiological levels of Ca^{2+} (1). Synchronous contractions can be produced in such cells by electrical stimulation, however (23, for example). In contrast, intact myocytes with elevated levels of internal Na^+ show spontaneous phasic contractions, even when suspended in low Ca^{2+} buffers (25μM or less, Ref. 12). This contractile activity of Na^+-loaded myocytes is not inhibited by Ca^{2+}-antagonists, such as verapamil or diltiazem, but is abolished immediately by caffeine (10 mM), a reagent that mobilizes Ca^{2+} from the sarcoplasmic reticulum (see 24 for a recent review).

Removal of the sarcolemma from myocytes by digitonin treatment as described above produces a "chemically-skinned" cardiac cell (see 24). These digitonin-treated myocytes undergo phasic contractions when low levels of Ca^{2+} are added to cells suspended in Krebs-Ringer-phosphate (see 16) containing 10 mM Mg-ATP and 0.1 mM EGTA. The phasic contraction under these conditions is abolished by caffeine (10 mM) and by procaine (10 mM). The frequency of contraction of such digitonin-treated myocytes depends on the calculated pCa of the EGTA-Ca buffers thus established. When the pCa is 7.2, the cells average 10 contractions per minute. At a pCa of 5.2 this increases to 35 contractions per minute. If the free Ca^{2+} is increased to 25 μM or above (pCa of 4.6), the digitonin-treated rod-cells hypercontract into round forms and show loss of sarcomere alignment and disorganization of the myofibrils.

The phasic contraction of digitonin-treated myocytes indicates that both the contractile elements and the sarcoplasmic reticulum retain their functional integrity after lysis of the sarcolemma with digitonin. In addition, the ability to produce hypercontracture in digitonin-treated myocytes by increasing the free Ca^{2+} concentration in the presence of ATP establishes that the sarcolemma has no direct role in the hypercontracture process. The formation of blebs on the myocyte surface prior to hypercontracture could be taken as an indication that sarcolemmal defects contribute directly to the loss of cell alignment. The observation that hypercontracture can be induced in myocytes in which the sarcolemma is completely disrupted is a strong indication that the blebs may be formed by the contractile elements forcing mitochondria and other components outward to distort the sarcolemma. It is possible, of course, that changes in the permeability of the sarcolemma to Ca^{2+} may contribute to the increase in free Ca^{2+} relative to ATP that appears to lead to hypercontracture. Such changes could result from mechanical rupture, as discussed above, or from chemical changes during anoxic incubation. Titration experiments are currently in progress that should define the limiting concentrations of ATP and free Ca^{2+} that permit phasic contractions to be sustained and the exact threshold for the induction of hypercontracture.

RELEASE OF ENZYMES FROM MYOCYTES

The release of enzymes from heart cells to the serum following myocardial infarction provides considerable diagnostic information. Isolated myocytes contain levels of LDH, creatine phosphokinase (CPK), and aspartate aminotransferase (AST), as well as LDH and CPK isoenzyme profiles that are quite comparable to those of intact tissue, and these preparations have been used to examine the factors involved in the release of enzymes from heart cells (10). Myocytes incubated anaerobically in the absence of glucose lose sarcolemmal integrity by the criterion of trypan blue uptake on a fairly long time scale (7,10). Under these conditions there is a gradual loss of LDH, CPK, and AST to the suspending medium. The fraction of the freely soluble cytoplasmic enzymes lost is equivalent to the fraction of the cells made permeable to trypan blue (10). This relationship holds over a wide range of cell viability (17-95% viable by dye exclusion) and suggests that there is simultaneous and complete release of soluble cytoplasmic enzymes as each individual cell sustains sarcolemmal damage and becomes permeable to the dye

310

(10). The alternative possibility that the sarcolemma becomes selectively permeable, first to lower molecular weight components and then to larger enzymes as a function of time of de-energization, is clearly not supported by these data. Adult rat heart myocytes show barely detectable levels of cytosol ATP at times of anaerobic incubation in which most of the cells are still viable by enzyme-release and trypan blue-exclusion criteria (19). A direct relationship between depletion of ATP and loss of sarcolemmal integrity has been noted by others in other cell preparations (25, for example) and is not apparent from our studies. The basis for this discrepancy is not yet clear and requires further investigation.

The mitochondrial isoenzymes of AST (ASTm) and malate dehydrogenase (MDHm) are present in serum following a myocardial infarction, but appear later and in smaller amounts than their cytosol counterparts. Mitochondrial CPK (CPKm) is rarely observed in serum. We have examined the release of these mitochondrial enzymes from rat heart myocytes and from isolated heart mitochondria suspended in media chosen to mimic the intracellular milieu. Under conditions of simulated lactic acidosis the mitochondria swell extensively (see 26) and release $67\pm7\%$ of total CPK_m while digitonin-lysed myocytes (6) release only $7\pm3\%$ of this isoenzyme. Myocytes hypercontracted prior to the enzyme-release protocol released $28\pm7\%$ of CPK_m. These and other data suggest that cell morphology influences the degree of enzyme release by providing a physical constraint on swelling of the mitochondria.

This possibility was explored by treating the myocytes with sufficient digitonin to lyse the outer membrane of the mitochondria, as well as the sarcolemma. This requires 270 µg digitonin·mg^{-1} protein compared to the 17 µg·mg^{-1} necessary to disrupt the sarcolemma. The lower level of digitonin releases no CPK_m from myocytes whereas the higher level results in quantitative release of this isoenzyme in 15 minutes at 4° in Krebs-Ringer-phosphate, pH 7.4. Myocytes incubated anaerobically without glucose for four hours at 37° release $66\pm6\%$ of the matrix enzyme MDH_m when the outer membrane of the mitochondrion is lysed, as opposed to $10\pm3\%$ for control cells. The release of AST_m follows a similar pattern. These results suggest that prolonged anaerobic incubation results in loss of inner membrane integrity and release of matrix enzymes to the intermembrane space. These enzymes (and CPK_m) then appear to be retained in this space by the outer membrane that remains impermeable to these enzymes. Such considerations could possibly explain the delayed and limited release of mitochondrial enzymes to the serum following a myocardial infarction. It should also be noted that CPK_m is readily released from myocytes and mitochondria when the outer membrane of the mitochondrion is lysed in all media of physiological ionic strength (M. Murphy and Wenger, in preparation) and appears bound to the inner membrane only in low ionic strength media, such as sucrose or mannitol (see also 27).

ACKNOWLEDGMENTS

These studies were supported in part by United States Public Health Services Grant HL23166 and by a Grant-in-Aid from the Central Ohio Heart Chapter.

REFERENCES

1. G.P. Brierley, C.M. Hohl, and R.A. Altschuld, 1983, Ion movements in adult rat heart myocytes, in: "Myocardial Injury," J.J. Spitzer, ed., Plenum Pub. Corp., New York, p. 231.

2. J.W. Dow, N.G.L. Harding, and T. Powell, 1981, Isolated cardiac myocytes I. Preparation of adult myocytes and their homology with intact tissue, Cardiovas. Res. 15:483.

3. J.W. Dow, N.G.L. Harding, and T. Powell, 1981, Isolated cardiac myocytes II. Functional aspects of mature cells, Cardiovas. Res. 15:549.

4. B.B. Farmer, M. Mancina, E.S. Williams, and A.M. Watanabe, 1983, Isolation of calcium tolerant myocytes from adult rat hearts: Review of the literature and description of a method, Life Sci. 33:1.

5. R.L. Kao, E.W. Christman, S.L. Luh, J.M. Kraubs, G.F.O. Tylers, and E.H. Williams, 1980, The effects of insulin and anoxia on the metabolism of isolated mature rat cardiac myocytes, Arch. Biochem. Biophys. 203:587.

6. R.A. Altschuld, C. Hohl, A. Ansel, and G.P. Brierley, 1981, Compartmentation of K^+ in isolated rat heart cells, Arch. Biochem. Biophys. 209: 175.

7. C.M. Hohl, A. Ansel, R.A. Altschuld, and G.P. Brierley, 1982, Contracture of isolated rat heart cells on anaerobic to aerobic transition, Am. J. Physiol. 243: H1022.

8. R.A. Altschuld, J.R. Hostetler, and G.P. Brierley, 1981, Response of isolated rat heart cells to hypoxia, re-oxygenation, and acidosis, Circ. Res. 49: 307.

9. R.A. Haworth, D.R. Hunter, and H.A. Berkoff, 1981, Contracture in isolated adult rat heart cells, Circ. Res. 49: 1119.

10. M.P. Murphy, C.M. Hohl, G.P. Brierley, and R.A. Altschuld, 1982, Release of enzymes from adult rat heart myocytes, Circ. Res. 51: 560.

11. M.A. Russo, A. Cittadini, A.M. Dani, G. Inesi, and T. Terranova, 1981, An ultrastructural study of calcium induced degenerative changes in dissociated heart cells, J. Mol. Cell. Cardiol. 13: 265.

12. R.A. Altschuld, L. Gibb, A. Ansel, C. Hohl, F.A. Kruger, and Brierley, G.P., 1980, Calcium tolerance of isolated rat heart cells, J. Mol. Cell. Cardiol. 12: 1383.

13. C.E. Ganote, 1983, Contraction band necrosis and irreversible myocardial injury, J. Mol. Cell. Cardiol. 15:67.

14. C.E. Ganote and J.P. Kaltenbach, 1979, Oxygen-induced enzyme release: early events and a proposed mechanism, J. Mol. Cell. Cardiol. 11: 289.

15. R.B. Jennings and K.A. Reimer, 1981, Lethal myocardial ischemic injury, Am. J. Pathol. 102: 241.

16. C.M. Hohl, R.A. Altschuld, and G.P. Brierley, 1983, Effects of calcium on the permeability of isolated adult rat heart cells to sodium, Arch. Biochem. Biophys. 221:197.

17. P.M. Grinwald and W.G. Naylor, 1981, Calcium entry in the calcium paradox, J. Mol. Cell. Cardiol. 13:867.

18. D.J. Hearse, S.M. Humphrey, and G.R. Bullock, 1978, The oxygen paradox and the calcium paradox: Two facets of the same problem?, J. Mol. Cell Cardiol. 10: 641.

19. T. Geisbuhler, R.A. Altschuld, R.W. Trewyn, A.Z. Ansel, K. Lamka, and G.P. Brierley, 1984, Adenine nucleotide metabolism and compartmentation in isolated adult rat heart cells, Circ. Res. (in press).

20. L.E. Alto and N.S. Dhalla, 1979, Myocardial cation contents during induction of calcium paradox, Am. J. Physiol. 237: H713.

21. M. Ashraf, 1979, Correlative studies on sarcolemmal ultrastructure, permeability, and loss of intracellular enzymes in the isolated heart perfused with calcium-free medium, Am. J. Pathol. 97: 411.

22. M. Ashraf, M. Onda, Y. Hirohata, and A. Schwartz, 1982, Therapeutic effect of diltiazem on myocardial cell injury during the calcium paradox, J. Mol. Cell. Cardiol. 14:323.

23. R.A. Haworth, D.R. Hunter, H.A. Berkoff and R.L. Moss, 1983, Metabolic cost of the stimulated beating of isolated adult rat heart cells in suspension, Circ. Res. 52:342

24. A. Fabiato, 1983, Calcium-induced release of calcium from the cardiac sarcoplasmic reticulum, Am. J. Physiol. 245:C1.

25. J.C. Altona and A. van der Laarse, 1982, Anoxia-induced changes in composition and permeability of sarcolemmal membranes in rat heart cell cultures, Cardiovas. Res. 16: 138.

26. M. Jurkowitz, K.M. Scott, R.A. Altschuld, A.J. Merola, and G.P. Brierley, 1974, Ion transport by heart mitochondria. Retention and loss of energy coupling in aged heart mitochondria, Arch. Biochem. Biophys. 165: 98.

27. T.Y. Lipskaya, V.D. Templ, L.V. Belousova, E.V. Molokova, and I.V. Rybina, 1981, Investigation of the interaction of mitochondrial creatine kinase with the membrane of the mitochondria, Biochimiya (English Translation) 45:877.

BIOLOGIC BASIS FOR LIMITATION OF INFARCT SIZE

Keith A. Reimer and Robert B. Jennings

Department of Pathology
Duke University Medical Center
Durham, North Carolina 27710

INTRODUCTION

The purpose of this chapter is to review several aspects of the biology of acute myocardial ischemic injury, in order to provide a framework within which possible therapies to limit infarct size may be considered.

GENERAL BIOLOGY OF MYOCARDIAL ISCHEMIA, INFARCTION AND REPAIR

Myocardial infarction is a complex dynamic process in which cardiac myocytes undergo necrosis and eventual replacement by scar tissue as a consequence of myocardial ischemia. The major aspects of this dynamic process are summarized in Figure 1. Ischemia has been defined as the reduction in blood flow to a level at which oxygen supply is insufficient (hypoxia) to provide enough energy to support the function of the tissue, i.e. to meet the metabolic demand. Although hypoxia is an important component of ischemia, the reduction in arterial collateral blood flow causes, in addition to hypoxia, a reduction in substrate supply, and accumulation in the tissue of numerous catabolites such as lactate, glycolytic intermediates, $H_2PO_4^-$ and the H^+ ion.[1-4]

The initial consequences of myocardial ischemia include inhibition of oxidative metabolism and reduced contractile function. The loss of contractile function occurs within seconds of the onset and is of obvious importance to the well-being of the experimental animal or patient; moreover, restoration of arterial flow is not followed by prompt restoration of contractile function.[5,6] Nevertheless, it is important to note that the loss of contractile function does not necessarily imply that

315

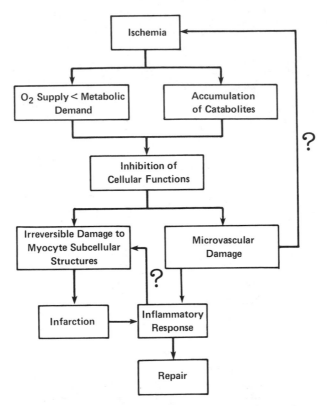

Figure 1.   Myocardial infarction is a complex dynamic process in which
cardiac myocytes undergo necrosis and eventual replacement
by scar tissue as a consequence of myocardial ischemia. The
major aspects of this dynamic process are illustrated on this
schematic diagram (see text for discussion).

the ischemic myocytes have died.   Although dead myocytes are, by
definition, non-contractile, living myocytes also may lose contractility;
thus, contractile failure cannot be used as an absolute indication of
myocyte cell death.

One or more other cellular functions, such as maintenance of ionic
homestasis, is crucial for cell survival. The absence of one or more such
functions must at some point result not simply in the inactivity of the
cellular machinery, but in the destruction of that machinery and the
consequent irreversible damage to the affected myocytes. However, the
precise cause of irreversible injury remains unknown (See below).

The process of infarction may involve more than the direct
consequences of ischemia on the affected myocytes. For example, the
microvasculature also is injured by ischemia.[6-9]   Endothelial damage
occurs and may result in accumulation of granulocytes, platelet

Table 1. Potential Causes of Irreversibility[*]

HEP Depletion
      Cessation of anaerobic glycolysis
      Loss of purine nucleotides
      Catabolism without resynthesis
      Activation of Phospholipases/Proteases

End Product Accumulation (Lactate, H^+, Fatty Acyl Derivatives, Etc.)
      Enzyme denaturation
      Membrane damage

Altered Ionic Gradients and Increased Intracellular Osmolarity
      Cell swelling with membrane disruption
      Calcium overload
          Activation of Phospholipases/Proteases
          Impaired mitochondrial function
          Activation of ATP-ases

[*]The three major categories of change which are associated with the irreversible state and which may be the cause of irreversibility are listed in this table as isolated events even though they often are closely interrelated. For example, activation of proteases or phospholipases may occur because of excess intracellular Ca; the rise in intracellular Ca may occur because of depletion of HEP.

aggregation, microthrombi or intramyocardial hemorrhage. Thus, as the duration of ischemia increases it can, in theory, increase in severity. However, whether such events ever contribute to the death of additional myocytes, even in the setting of reperfusion, remains open to question. In our studies, and in those of some other investigators, these changes have been observed only within the confines of an evolving infarct.[6-8] Most evidence now available supports the concept that endothelial cells undergo ischemic injury more slowly than the highly differentiated myocytes and that severe microvascular damage is a later event occurring in areas in which myocytes already have been lethally injured.

Another aspect of the process of myocardial infarction is the inflammatory response to either injured myocytes or microvasculature (Figure 1). Whereas the inflammatory response is essential for the repair of the infarct, there is evidence that one or more components of the inflammatory process also may cause additional myocyte injury. For example, it is well known that polymorphonuclear neutrophils are rich in a variety of lysosomal proteases and lipases which may be released along with superoxide radicals into the interstitial milieu of an infarct. Some recent evidence suggests that the inflammatory response may cause additional myocyte necrosis.[10]

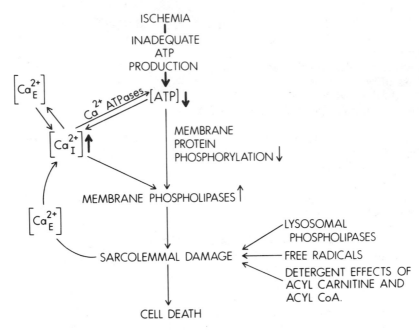

Figure 2. The potential relationships between ATP depletion, Ca^{2+} influx, and sarcolemmal damage, which form the basis for various hypotheses of the events leading to sarcolemmal damage are diagrammed. ATP utilization exceeds the capacity of anaerobic glycolysis to produce high-energy phosphates (HEP). Intracellular Ca^{2+}, Ca^{2+}_I. may increase either because of increased membrane permeability to Ca^{2+} or because of inadequate ATP to support the mechanisms responsible for Ca^{2+} extrusion from the cell or sequestration of Ca^{2+} by the sarcoplasmic reticulum. Possible mechanisms of sarcolemmal damage include activation of endogenous sarcolemmal phospholipases by the increased Ca^{2+}_I or depressed phosphorylation of membrane proteins that ordinarily inhibit the activity of the endogenous phospholipases of the sarcolemma. Lysosomal phospholipase release, free radicals, or the detergent action of acyl carnitine or acyl coenzyme A also are possible causes of sarcolemmal damage in myocardial ischemia. Reproduced from reference 18 with permission of the publisher.

SOME POSSIBLE MECHANISMS OF ISCHEMIC CELL DEATH

Three of the general metabolic consequences of ischemia which could be the eventual cause of irreversible cell injury are listed in Table 1.[11] Each of the general reactions occur and it has been impossible to dissect which, if any, are the important variables in zones of severe ischemia. For example, some of the consequences of severe high energy phosphate depletion include cessation of anaerobic glycolysis, continued

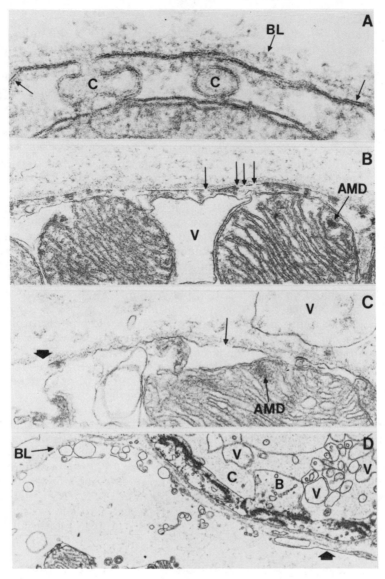

Figure 3.   The effect of episodes of <u>in vivo</u> ischemia on the structure of the sarcomlemma is summarized in this plate. In all four panels, the tissue was fixed similarly using glutaraldehyde and postosmication.   Panel (A) shows sarcolemma of control nonischaemic myocardium.   Several caveolae (C) in various stages of attachment are shown.   The trilaminar structure of the plasmalemma of the sarcolemma is clearly visible (arrows), but where it tilts away from the perpendicular to the section (center of the panel), it appears to widen or becomes indistinct.   A fuzzy coat, the basal lamina (BL) or glocycalyx, 15–35 nm thick, covers the plasmalemma at the cell surface.

(Continued)

Figure 3. Continued

Panel (B) shows a myocyte after 30 min of ischemia. This myocyte demonstrates some of the ultrastructural changes associated with irreversible injury. At this early time interval, only a few ischaemic myocytes exhibit these changes. There are numerous tiny defects in the plasmalemma (arrows), vacuoles (V) in the sarcoplasm and mitochondria are enlarged and exhibit a clear matrix which contains prominent amorphous matrix densities (AMD). Panel (C) shows the changes in the sarcolemma caused by 40 min of ischemia in vivo (without reflow). There is one small (60 nm) gap in the plasmalemma and a larger region where the glycocalyx is generally intact but the plasmalemma is not identifiable (thick arrowhead). The vesicle (V) in the interstitium is typical of fully developed ischemic injury. A large matrix density (AMD) is present in the enlarged mitochondria. Panel (D) is a view of a subsarcolemmal bleb adjacent to a capillary (C) after three hours of severe ischemia in vivo without reflow. The capillary shows blebs (B) of endothelium extending into the lumen and vesicles of swollen endothelium within the lumen. Much of the basal lamina of both the capillary and myocyte is intact. However, the plasmalemma of the sarcolemma is broken up and can be identified as circular profiles under the basal lamina. Intact plasmalemma is present at the thick arrowhead. The most marked damage to the plasmalemma occurs in localized areas of cell swelling. Reproduced from reference 19 with permission of the publisher.

catabolism without resynthesis of enzymes, cofactors or structural components of the cell, and perhaps activation of endogenous proteases or phospholipases. Glycolytic ATP production ceases when sarcoplasmic ATP decreases to very low levels because ATP is required to phosphorylate fructose-6-phosphate to fructose-1,6-diphosphate, an early step in the glycolytic pathway. Sarcoplasmic ATP from anaerobic glycolysis may be critical to support activities such as ionic gradients[12]; thus, exhaustion of ATP supplies from this source probably is the ultimate cause of loss of ionic gradients.

One or more of the many catabolites, including the hydrogen ion, which accumulate in ischemia also may have toxic effects on the cell.[13] Fatty acyl derivatives such as acyl CoA or acyl carnitine may act as detergents and disrupt cell membranes.[14]

Ischemia results in altered ionic transport even before marked loss of tissue ATP has occurred.[15,16] Depressed cell volume regulation together with the accumulation of small molecular weight intracellular catabolites causes cell swelling with possible structural disruption. Increased sarcoplasmic Ca^{2+} also has widespread potential deleterious effects which include activation of various phospholipases and proteases, impaired mitochondrial function, and activation of ATPases which would accelerate the loss the HEP pool.[17]

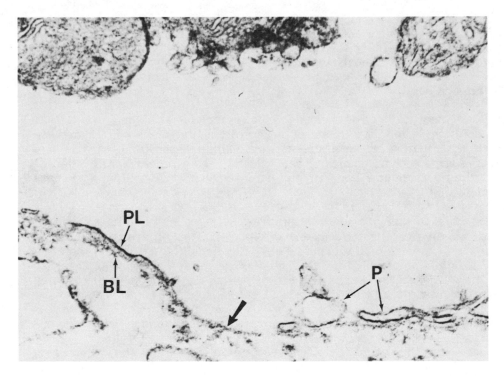

Figure 4.   Sarcolemmal disruption observed in a myocyte from the subendocardial zone of the ischemic region of a dog heart after 40 minutes of coronary occlusion and five minutes of reperfusion. There is a large edematous space (central clear area) separating the sarcolemma from the myofibrillar apparatus of the myocyte. The sarcolemma is composed of a basal lamina (BL) or glycocalyx and a trilaminar unit membrane, the plasmalemma (PL). The basal lamina appears intact but the plasmalemma has been disrupted in some areas (e.g., large arrow) and has reformed as circular profiles (P) in other areas. Reproduced from reference 31 with permission of the publisher.

Several current hypotheses center on sarcolemmal damage as the immediate cause of myocardial ischemic death. The interrelationships among ATP depletion, Ca^{2+} influx and sarcolemmal damage, which form the basis for these hypotheses are illustrated in Figure 2.[18] Sarcoplasmic Ca^{2+} may increase because of increased influx from the extracellular space or sarcoplasmic reticulum, or because insufficient ATP is available to support Ca^{2+} extrusion from the cell or uptake by the sarcoplasmic reticulum.   Increased Ca^{2+} may, in turn, cause accelerated ATP depletion.   Not shown on this diagram is the concept that damage to cytoskeletal supports of the membrane plus swelling induced by the osmolar load of ischemia may break the sarcolemma.[19]

Ultrastructural evidence favors the hypothesis that sarcolemmal damage occurs early and is a lethal event in the ischemic myocyte.[19] Figure 3 illustrates discontinuities in the plasmalemma of ischemic myocytes. These discontinuities become detectable by 30-40 minutes of severe ischemia in vivo and become larger and more numerous with increasing duration of ischemia.

A second line of evidence for sarcolemmal damage is that reperfusion, after 40 minutes of severe ischemia, results in immediate further disruption of the sarcolemma.[20] Figure 4 shows the sarcolemma over a large edematous bleb of sarcoplasm. The glycocalyx still is intact but the plasmalemma is massively disrupted, with reformation into small vesicles.

This further membrane disruption with reperfusion is associated with massive calcium overload and the formation of contraction bands (Figure 5).[4] Some of the excess Ca^{2+} is accumulated by mitochondria in the form of the phosphate; it is visible as crystalline or granular densities in the mitochondrial matrix. The myofibrillar disruption is visible even by light microscopy as contraction-band necrosis.[21] These changes may be induced either by reperfusion, in vivo, or by aerobic or anaerobic incubation of slices of previously ischemic myocardium in a fluid medium.

A third line of evidence for sarcolemmal damage is that, when slices of myocardium, irreversibly injured by ischemia, are incubated in vitro, the tissue cannot restore ion gradients and cannot exclude large molecules, such as inulin, to which the cell membrane is normally impermeable (Figure 6).[19] The inulin diffusible space (IDS) increases dramatically and the slices also lose creatine to the medium.[11] Combined with ultrastructural observations showing cellular but not interstitial edema, the increased IDS is indicative of entry of the large (5000 molecular weight) inulin molecule into the cell water of the myocytes.

The mechanism of disruption of the sarcolemma in irreversible ischemic injury is unknown. Several possible mechanisms of membrane damage are listed in Figure 2.[18] For example, either ATP depletion or Ca^{2+} overload could cause membrane damage through activation of phospholipases.[22] Other potential causes of membrane damage include release and activation of lysosomal phospholipases, production of free radicals,[23] and/or the detergent effects of fatty acyl derivatives.[14]

BASIS FOR INTERVENTION TO LIMIT INFARCT SIZE

As a basis for limiting infarct size, one could intervene at any one of the general steps illustrated in Figure 1. Intervening to improve oxygen supply or to reduce metabolic demand are straightforward from the conceptual point of view. Intervening to directly prevent the specific mechanism of cell death is a very desirable aim as well; however, it will be impossible to achieve until we know the mechanism of ischemic cell

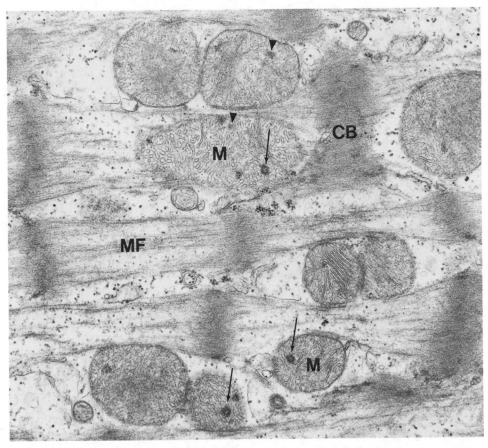

Figure 5.   Ultrastructural features of contraction band necrosis. This illustration shows a cardiac myocyte from the subendocardial zone of the ischemic region of a dog heart after forty minutes of coronary occlusion and ten minutes of reperfusion. The myofibrils (MF) have been completely disrupted with myofibrillar proteins from several adjacent sarcomeres condensed into tangled masses referred to as "contraction bands". There has been massive influx of calcium into the myocyte as evidenced by the annular crystalline mitochondrial (M) densities (arrows) that contain calcium and phosphate.[20,34] These changes, referred to as contraction band necrosis, are characteristic of myocardial cell death associated with ischemia and reperfusion. The arrowheads indicate amorphous matrix densities that are also characteristic of irreversible ischemic cell injury and which can be seen before, as well as after, reperfusion.[31] This illustration is from work reported in reference 32.

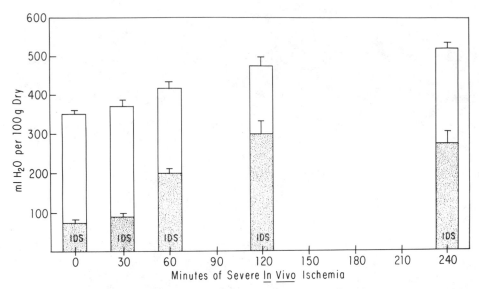

Figure 6. The relationship between total tissue water (TTW) and inulin
diffusible space (IDS), as a function of the period of in vivo
ischaemia, is shown. The TTW is represented by the total
height of the bar and the IDS is represented by the shaded
portions. The brackets are the standard errors of the mean.
These data are plotted from the experiments reported in
reference 33. The IDS and TTW were increased significantly
after ≥ 60 min of ischaemia, but not at 30 min. Reproduced
from reference 19 with permission of the publisher.

death. Thus, developing therapies to intervene at this level only can be
done by trial and error. Such interventions must be selected based on a
best guess of what may be a critical step in the transition to
irreversibility. Conversely, testing certain interventions, to determine
whether they limit ischemic injury, may lead to a better understanding of
the pathogenesis of ischemic cell death.

Simple models of myocardial ischemic injury may be used to
evaluate the role of specific metabolic pathways or organelle function in
the pathogenesis of ischemic injury. Infarction in man, or intact
experimental animals such as dogs, however, is a complex process in
which temporal and spatial considerations add other dimensions to the
biologic basis for limiting infarct size. Occlusion of a coronary artery
produces ischemia throughout the anatomic region supplied by the artery.
However, not all of this anatomic area at risk becomes infarcted. Some
of the subepicardial region is usually spared, especially toward the lateral
edges of the subepicardial ischemic region.[7] This pattern of infarction is
typical in man as well as in dogs.[24] The salvage of parts of the
subepicardium is probably due to the frequent persistence of significant
quantities of collateral blood flow in the subepicardial region. There is an
inverse correlation between infarct size vs. subepicardial collateral flow
in dogs (Figure 7), which indicates that collateral flow is a major
determinant of the transmural extent of infarction.[7]

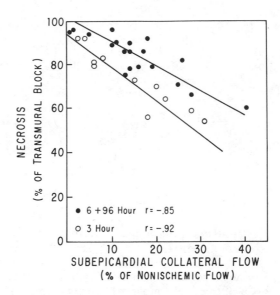

Figure 7.　The relation between transmural necrosis and subepicardial collateral flow is illustrated. Permanent infarcts and infarcts reperfused at 6 hours formed the same line and were combined (closed circles). Infarcts reperfused at 3 hours are indicated by the open circles. In both groups the transmural extent of necrosis was inversely related to subepicardial collateral flow measured at 20 minutes after LCC occlusion. Thus, in each group necrosis could be predicted from early collateral flow. However, the 3-hour line was below the line defined by the 6-hour and permanent infarcts. Thus, reperfusion at 3 hours resulted in less necrosis than expected from the level of collateral flow. Reproduced from reference 7 with permission of the publisher.

　　　Whereas the final infarct size is related in part to the initial area at risk and subepicardial collateral flow, not all of the ischemic myocardium destined for infarction dies simultaneously.[7] This has been demonstrated by reperfusion of ischemic myocardium at various times after the onset of ischemia. Early reperfusion e.g. after 40 minutes of ischemia in circumflex arterial occlusions in the open-chest anesthetized dog, results in subendocardial infarcts, with salvage of the subepicardial region, a result which obviously shows that the damaged subepicardial zone was still viable even though the subendocardial region was irreversibly injured. Reperfusion at three hours resulted in less subepicardial salvage. Thus, there is a transmural progression of ischemic injury with increasing duration of coronary occlusion which is illustrated schematically in Figure 8.[7] The reason for this transmural progression of ischemic injury may be partly related to the gradient of collateral flow.[7,25] However, several investigators have shown that a similar progression of injury occurs even in the absence of coronary flow, perhaps related to intrinsic metabolic

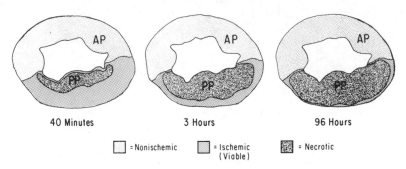

PROGRESSION OF CELL DEATH VS TIME
AFTER LCC OCCLUSION

40 Minutes   3 Hours   96 Hours

☐ = Nonischemic   ☐ = Ischemic   ▨ = Necrotic
(Viable)

Figure 8.   The progression of cell death versus time after LCC occlusion is shown. Necrosis occurs first in the subendocardial myocardium. With longer occlusions, a wavefront of cell death moves from the subendocardial zone across the wall to involve progressively more of the transmural thickness of the ischemic zone. Thus, there is typically a large zone of subepicardial myocardium in the ischemic bed that is salvageable by early reperfusion but that dies in the absence of such an intervention. In contrast, the lateral margins in the subendocardial region of the infarct are established as early as 40 minutes after occlusion and are sharply defined by the anatomical boundaries of the ischemic bed. Reproduced from reference 7 with permission of the publisher.

differences across the wall of the ventricle.[26-29] Nevertheless, the final determinant of whether myocytes live or die is the absolute volume of collateral flow.

The ideal therapy instituted immediately after coronary occlusion might prevent infarction. Because the severely ischemic myocytes die quickly, it is unlikely that this will often be possible clinically; thus, the realistic clinical goal, based on the above temporal and spatial biology of infarction, must be the conversion of a potentially transmural infarct to one which is subendocardial, or at least non-transmural.[30]

In testing an intervention in an experimental model as complex as infarction, it is essential to have control of baseline variables. In the dog heart, the major determinants of infarct size include the size of the vascular area at risk, collateral blood flow, and hemodynamic determinants of metabolic demand.[7] Infarct size can be normalized to area at risk and plotted vs. subepicardial collateral flow.[30] The top curve of Figure 9 shows this relationship for an ideal group of controls. An intervention which limits infarct size should produce a downward shift in the relationship between infarct size and collateral flow when baseline collateral flow (measured before therapy) is used in the analysis (left panel). In addition, an intervention which improves collateral flow should

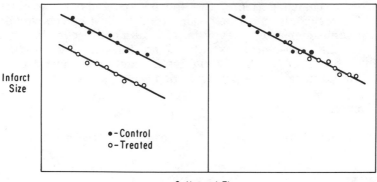

THEORETICAL RESULTS c̄ PROTECTION WHICH IS FLOW
INFORMATION VS. DEPENDENT

Infarct
Size

•-Control
o-Treated

Collateral Flow
(Post Therapy)

Figure 9.   Hypothetical results of an ideal experiment to illustrate how
the relationship between infarct size and collateral blood flow
can be used to evaluate the effects of therapy. With any
therapy that limited infarct size, infarcts would be smaller
than predicted by baseline collateral flows and the regression
of infarct size vs. flow would be shifted downward. With such
an intervention that did not alter collateral blood flow, the
regression line of infarct size vs. flow also would be shifted
downward when a post-treatment measure of flow was used
(left panel).   Conversely, an intervention, which limited
infarct size by improving collateral blood flow, would shift
points to the right along the control regression line when a
post-treatment measure of flow was used (right panel). Thus,
incorporation of collateral flow measurements should
1) permit detection of a positive effect with greater
precision, and 2) provide information about the mechanism of
treatment effect.   Reproduced from reference 30 with
permission of the publisher.

limit infarct size by shifting points down the curve (right hand panel)
when collateral flow, measured after initiation of therapy, is used for the
analysis.   By having control of such baseline variables, it is possible to
detect a positive effect with good precision and to gain general
information about the mechanism of protection (e.g. whether protection
is independent of changes in flow or is related to improved collateral
perfusion).

In summary, consideration of the biologic basis for limitation of
infarct size must include consideration of possible mechanisms of lethal
injury of myocytes but also must include consideration of the possible

contributing role of the microvasculature and the inflammatory response. In applying such information to complex experimental models of infarction or to human patients, the spatial and temporal evolution of myocardial infarction also must be considered. It must be recognized that the realistic achievement of therapy in most clinical circumstances is the limitation of the transmural extent of an infarct. In testing any intervention, control of baseline variables is essential to avoid erroneous conclusions and to improve the precision of the test system.

Acknowledgement

Grant support: Supported in part by NIH grants HL23138 and HL27416.

REFERENCES

1. S. Gudbjarnason, Acute alterations in energetics of ischemic heart muscle. Cardiology 56: 232 (1971,72).
2. S. M. Cobbe, P. A. Poole-Wilson, The time of onset and severity of acidosis in myocardial ischaemia. J. Mol. Cell Cardiol. 12: 745 (1980).
3. K. I. Shine, Ionic events in ischemia and anoxia, Am. J. Pathol. 102: 256 (1981).
4. K. A. Reimer, R. B. Jennings, A. H. Tatum, Pathobiology of acute myocardial ischemia: Metabolic, functional and ultrstructural studies. Am. J. Cardiol. 52: 72A (1983).
5. J. M. Weiner, C. S. Apstein, J. H. Arthur, F. A. Pirzada, W. B. Hood, Jr., Persistence of myocardial injury following brief periods of coronary occlusion. Cardiovasc. Res. 10: 678 (1976).
6. R. A. Kloner, S. G. Ellis, R. Lange, E. Braunwald, Studies of experimental coronary artery reperfusion. Effects on infarct size, myocardial function, biochemistry, ultrastructure and microvascular damage. Circulation 68: I8 (1983).
7. K. A. Reimer, R. B. Jennings. The "Wavefront Phenomenon" of myocardial ischemic cell death. II. Transmural progression of necrosis within the framework of ischemic bed size (myocardium at risk) and collateral flow. Lab. Invest. 40: 633 (1979).
8. M.C. Fishbein, J. Y-Rit, U. Lando, K. Kanmatsuse, J. C. Mercier, W. Ganz, The relationship of vascular injury and myocardial hemorrhage to necrosis after reperfusion. Circulation 62: 1274 (1980).
9. P. F. McDonagh, The role of the coronary microcirculation in myocardial recovery from ischemia. Yale J Biol. Med. 56: 303 (1983).
10. J. L. Romson, B. G. Hook, S. L. Kunkel, G. D. Abrams, M. A. Schork, B. R. Lucchesi, Reduction of the extent of ischemic myocardial injury by neutrophil depletion in the dog. Circulation 67: 1016, 1983.

11. K. A. Reimer, R. B. Jennings, M. L. Hill, Total ischemia in dog hearts in vitro. II. High energy phosphate depletion and associated defects in energy metabolism, cell volume regulation, and sarcolemmal integrity. Circ. Res. 49: 901 (1981).

12. T. F. McDonald, E. G. Hunter, D. P. MacLeod, Adenosinetriphosphate partition in cardiac muscle with respect to transmembrane electrical activity. Pflugers Arch 322: 95 (1971).

13. J. R. Williamson, S. W. Schaffer, C. Ford, B. Safer, Contribution of tissue acidosis to ischemic injury in the perfused rat heart. Circulation 53: I3 (1976).

14. J. R. Neely, D. Feuvray, Metabolic products and myocardial ischemia, Am. J. Pathol. 102: 282 (1981).

15. R. B. Case, Ion alterations during myocardial ischemia, Am. J. Cardiology 56: 245 (1971,72).

16. J. L. Hill, L. S. Gettes, Effect of acute coronary artery occlusion on local myocardial extracellular K+ activity in swine, Circulation 61: 768 (1980).

17. W. G. Nayler, The role of calcium in the ischemic myocardium. Am. J. Pathol. 102: 262 (1981).

18. R. B. Jennings, K. A. Reimer, Lethal myocardial ischemic injury. Am. J. Pathol. 102: 241 (1981).

19. R. B. Jennings, C. Steenbergen, Jr., R. B. Kinney, M. L. Hill, K. A. Reimer, Comparison of the effect of ischaemia and anoxia on the sarcolemma of the dog heart. Eur. Heart J. 4: 123 (1983).

20. R. A. Kloner, C. E. Ganote, D. Whalen, R. B. Jennings, Effect of a transient period of ischemia on myocardial cells: II. Fine structure during the first few minutes of reflow. Am. J. Pathol. 74: 399 (1974).

21. K. A. Reimer, R. B. Jennings, Effects of reperfusion on infarct size —experimemtal studies. Eur. Heart J. in press, 1984.

22. K. R. Chien, R. G. Pfau, J. L. Farber, Ischemic myocardial cell injury. Am. J. Pathol. 97: 505 (1979).

23. P. S. Rao, M. V. Cohen, H. S. Mueller, Production of free radicals and lipid peroxides in early experimental myocardial ischemia. J. Mol. Cell. Cardiol 15: 713 (1983).

24. J. T. Lee, R. E. Ideker, K. A. Reimer, Myocardial infarct size and location in relation to the coronary vascular bed at risk in man. Circulation 64: 526 (1981).

25. S. Koyanagi, C. L. Eastham, D. G. Harrison, M. L. Marcus, Transmural variation in the relationship between myocardial infarct size and risk area. Am. J. Physiol. 242: H867 (1982).

26. R. B. Dunn, D. M. Griggs, Jr., Transmural gradients in ventricular tissue metabolites produced by stopping coronary blood flow in the dog. Circ. Res. 37: 438 (1975).

27. H. Fujiwara, M. Ashraf, S. Sato, R. W. Millard, Transmural cellular damage and blood flow distribution in early ischemia in pig hearts. Circ. Res. 51: 683 (1982).

28.   C. Eng, S. Cho, E. S. Kirk, The wavefront pattern of necrosis occurs despite uniform blood flow conditions. Circulation 66: II-66 (1982) (abstract).

29.   J. E. Lowe, R. G. Cummings, D. H. Adams, E. A. Hull-Ryde, Evidence that ischemic cell death begins in the subendocardium independent of variations in collateral flow or wall tension. Circulation 68: 190 (1983).

30.   K.A. Reimer, R. B. Jennings, Verapamil in two reperfusion models of myocardial infarction: Temporary protection of severely ischemic myocardium without limitation of ultimate infarct size. Lab. Invest. In press, 1984.

31.   R. B. Jennings, C. E. Ganote, K. A. Reimer, Ischemic tissue injury, Am. J. Pathol. 81: 179 (1975).

32.   M. B. Rocco, K. A. Reimer, R. B. Jennings, Failure of calcium chelated blood to prevent reperfusion induced indices of irreversible ischemic injury. Circulation 59 & 60: II216 (1979) (abstract).

33.   R. B. Jennings, H. K. Hawkins, J. E. Lowe, M. L. Hill, S. Klotman, K. A. Reimer, Relation between high energy phosphate and lethal injury in myocardial ischemia in the dog. Am. J. Pathol. 92: 187 (1978).

34.   A. C. Shen and R. B. Jennings, Myocardial calcium and magnesium in acute ischemic injury. Am. J. Pathol. 67: 417–440, 1972.

MITOCHONDRIAL TRANSMEMBRANE PROTON ELECTROCHEMICAL POTENTIAL, DI-
AND TRICARBOXYLATE DISTRIBUTION AND THE POISE OF THE MALATE-
ASPARTATE CYCLE IN THE INTACT MYOCARDIUM

Risto A. Kauppinen, J. Kalervo Hiltunen and
Ilmo E. Hassinen

Department of Medical Biochemistry
University of Oulu
Finland

INTRODUCTION

The unconditional requirement of closed membrane structures
for oxidative energy conversion and conservation in eucaryotes
entails the problem of subcellular compartmentation. Although much
can be deduced from the in vitro characteristics of the permeability properties of the mitochondrial membranes and the behaviour of enzyme systems in vitro, understanding of the regulation
of certain fundamental regulatory phenomena such as mitochondrial
respiration has been awaiting data obtained in intact cells and
tissues. Methodological progress in the field of metabolic compartmentation has brought into focus the subcellular distribution
of effectors and the metabolites related to the tricarboxylic acid
cycle.

A mutual regulation of carbohydrate and lipid metabolism can
be demonstrated, in heart muscle, as exemplified by the glucose-
sparing effect of free fatty acids[1]. This is usually explained by
a fatty acid-induced increase in citrate[2], an allosteric inhibitor
of phosphofructokinase (PFK). However, citrate accumulation occurs
primarily in the mitochondria, and it has been reported that the
activity of the tricarboxylate translocator is low in heart muscle
mitochondria[3]. Also, the transmembrane pH gradient which develops
in isolated mitochondria leads us to anticipate that citrate is
mainly confined to mitochondria.

The free $NADH/NAD^+$ pool in the mitochondrial matrix is at a
lower redox potential than in the cytosol[4], which means that the
mitochondrial disposition of the reducing equivalents arising in

331

the cytosol during aerobic glycolysis is energy-dependent. According to the current view, this is effected by the malate-aspartate cycle, energized by the mitochondrial membrane potential through the mediation of the electrogenic glutamate-aspartate translocator[5]. Previous reports on the subcellular distribution of glutamate and aspartate in the isolated perfused rat liver and isolated hepatocytes are at variance[6,7,8], and do not support equilibrium between the translocator function and the membrane potential or pH, casting doubt on whether there is sufficient energization of the translocator to drive hydrogen transport by the malate aspartate cycle in intact cells.

The present paper summarizes recent work from this laboratory concerning metabolite compartmentation and mitochondrial electric and chemical gradients. These have been measured by tissue fractionation in non-aqueous solvents[9], a method which has proved useful for separating mitochondrial and extramitochondrial spaces in the intact myocardium.

EXPERIMENTAL

Female and male Sprague-Dawley rats were fed ad libitum, anesthetized with pentobarbital and heparinized before excision of the heart as described previously[10]. The isolated heart was perfused in a retrograde manner according to the Langendorff procedure with Krebs-Ringer bicarbonate solution containing 10 mM glucose and equilibrated with O_2/CO_2 (19:1). The cellular ATP consumption was varied by changing the mechanical work output of the heart by lowering the beating frequency to 1.1-1.5 Hz by excision of the sinus node or by arresting the heart in the diastole with hyperpotassemia.

After freeze-clamping, the tissue was freeze-dried at $-55°C$ for 72-96 h and dispersed in a C_7H_{16}/CCl_4 mixture with a rotating-knife homogenizer or sonicator. The homogenate was resolved into fractions enriched with mitochondrial or cytosolic structures by centrifugation at 27000 x g for 2 h in a discontinuous C_7H_6/CCl_4 density gradient[11]. Citrate synthase and phosphoglycerate kinase were used as indicator enzymes for the matrix and extramatrix compartments, respectively. The data reduction was performed as decribed by Elbers et al.[9].

The tissue water spaces were estimated by determining the total tissue water from the wet weight/dry weight ratio, the extracellular water by perfusion with $[^{14}C]$-inulin carboxylic acid and the mitochondrial matrix water by determining the mitochondrial population density in the tissue and the mitochondrial matrix water space in experiments with isolated mitochondria. The mitochondrial matrix water was found to be 1.01

μl/mg tissue protein and the extramatrix water 4.43 μl/mg tissue protein in the beating isolated heart.

Metabolites were assayed enzymatically as described previously[10,11,12].Citrate, 2-oxoglutarate and aspartate measurements employed the alkali-induced NAD^+ fluorescence method to enhance sensitivity. [^3H]-Triphenylmethylphosphonium ($TPMP^+$) cation and [$1-^{14}C$]-propionate were used to probe the mitochondrial membrane potential and transmembrane pH, respectively[13]. The solvent mixture used for the non-aqueous subcellular fractionation did not extract $TPMP^+$ from the lyophilized, powdered tissue[13]. The method has been validated for the other metabolites previously[9].

RESULTS AND DISCUSSION

Mitochondrial energy state

The cytosolic phosphorylation state of the adenine nucleotides can be estimated from the cytosolic creatine, phosphocreatine and inorganic phosphate (P_i) concentrations on the basis of the near-equilibrium of the creatine kinase reaction[14], although the amount of tightly bound ADP in the rat myocardium is high, 0.49 μmol/g wet weight[15]. There are no useful equilibrium reactions in the mitochondrial matrix to provide indicator metabolites for the free ATP/ADP ratio in rat heart, and therefore the mitochondrial total ATP and ADP concentrations are used to calculate the mitochondrial phosphorylation potential.

The cytosolic phosphorylation potential responds, to changes in the workload of the muscle, the G of ATP hydrolysis being −58.8 and −61.4 kJ/mol in the beating and potassium-arrested heart, respectively[11].It is significant that the mitochondrial and cytosolic ATP/ADP ratios change in opposite directions, suggesting that part of the energy charge of the mitochondrial membrane is used for active transport of the adenylates. Although a lower ATP/ADP ratio in the mitochondrion would still be compatible with limitation of mitochondrial respiration at the adenylate translocase level if the adenylate translocator were electrogenic, a lowering of the mitocondrial ATP/ADP ratio concomitantly with a decrease in the ATP consumption argues against this.

From the distribution of the mitochondrial membrane potential probe $TPMP^+$ a of 125 mV can be calculated for the heart beating at 5 Hz[13]. This is also sensitive to the energy expenditure of the muscle, increasing to 150 mV when the frequency of contraction is lowered to 1.5 Hz. The distribution of [^{14}C]propionate gives a pH value of 0.63 (alkaline inside) across the mitochondrial membrane in the heart beating at 5 Hz, the value decreasing to 0.53 upon lowering of the heart rate to 1.5 Hz[13]. Thus it appears

333

that there is a tendency for the energy charge of the membrane to shift from the osmotic to the electric form upon energization. The energetics of proton transport can be best described in terms of the electrochemical potential $\Delta\tilde{\mu}\,H^+ = F \cdot \Delta\Psi + 2.303\ RT\ pH$, which amounts to 15.5 kJ/mol in the heart beating a 5 Hz and increases to 17.1 kJ/mol when the heartbeat is lowered to 1.5 Hz[13] (Table 1).

In conjunction with the data on the phosphorylation state of the adenylate system, the data on the proton gradients can be tested within the context of the chemiosmotic hypothesis. The H^+/ATP stoichiometry in the combined reactions of H^+-ATPase and

Table 1. Protonic and electric mitochondrial transmembrane gradients in isolated perfused rat hearts

Value	Heart rate (Hz)	
	5	1.5
$TPMP^+$ (concentration ratio)[a] mitochondrial/cytosolic	109.2±14.5	283.5±32.2
Propionate (concentration ratio) mitochondrial/cytosolic	4.6±0.6	4.1±1.0
Mitochondrial $\Delta\Psi$ ((mV, negative inside)[b]	125.3±6.6	150.1±3.3
Mitochondrial ΔpH (pH units, alkaline inside)[c]	0.63±0.06	0.53±0.12
Mitochondrial $\Delta\tilde{\mu}_{H^+}$ (kJ/mol)	15.5±0.5	17.1±0.6
ΔG_{ATP_c} (kJ/mol)[d]	55.8±0.5	57.5±0.5
H^+/ATP (molar ratio)	3.6	3.4

[a] $TPMP^+$, triphenylmethylphosphonium cation
[b] Calculated from $\Delta\Psi = (\ln\,[TPMP^+]_m - \ln[TPMP^+]_c)\ RT/F$
[c] Calculated from $\Delta pH = \log[P^-]_m - \log[P^-]_c$ where $[P^-]$ is the propionate concentration
[d] Calculated from the creatine kinase equilibrium.
   $\Delta G = -31.9$ kJ/mol$+RT \cdot \ln([Cr] \cdot [P_i] \cdot 7.06 \cdot 10^{-3}) - RT \cdot \ln[CrP]$ where $[CrP]$, $[Cr]$ and $[P_i]$ are the average tissue concentrations of phosphocreatine, creatine and phosphate.
Data adapted from ref. 13 with permission of the publisher.

adenylate translocator would be $\Delta G_{ATP}/\Delta \tilde{\mu} H^+ = 58.8/15.5 = 3.8$. The reaction of the H^+-ATPase proper is described by the intramitochondrial ΔG_{ATP} and $\Delta \tilde{\mu} H^+$: $48.2/15.5 = 3.1$ in the isolated beating rat heart.

If the adenylate translocator were electrogenic and in close equilibrium with the mitochondrial membrane potential in intact tissue it would obey the equation

$$\Delta \Psi = \frac{RT}{F} \ln \frac{[ATP_m]/[ADP_m]}{[ATP_c]/[ADP_c]}$$

where m and c refer to the concentrations in the matrix and cytosol, respectively. The diffusion potential imposed by the asymmetry of the adenylate distribution becomes 103 mV (negative inside) in the beating heart and 145 mV in the arrested heart, using the adenylate distribution values from ref[11]. These values are close to the actual potential measured by the $TPMP^+$ probe and suggest that the electrogenic adenylate translocator may be in equilibrium in intact tissues.

The notion of near equilibrium of the total reaction sequences of oxidative phosphorylation is strengthened by data obtained from the intact tissue of the isolated perfused heart. Reflectance spectrophotometry of the heart gives a redox potential of +294 mV for cytochrome c and the average tissue concentration of reactants in the glutamate dehydrogenase system -314 mV for the free $NADH/NAD^+$ in the mitochondrial matrix[16]. The free energy change in the reactions between NADH and cytochrome c can be calculated from the equation $\Delta G_{o/r} = nF \cdot E_h$, where E_h is the redox potential difference between the donor and acceptor redox couples and F the Faraday constant. The free energy change in this span of the respiratory chain then becomes -115.8 kJ/2e⁻. If ATP synthesis is energized by the protonic gradients and there are two H^+ pumping sites between NADH and cytochrome c, the efficiency of oxidative phosphorylation would be $2 \cdot G_{ATP}/G_{o/r} = 2 \cdot 58.8/115.8 = 1.0$, i.e. the entropy increase would be zero and the reaction in complete equilibrium. There are certain uncertainties in the estimation of the free $NADH/NAD^+$ ratio of the mitochondrial matrix in intact myocardium. Glutamate dehydrogenase has been shown to be in near equilibrium[17], but the determination of the matrix NH_4^+ concentration must be tempered with reservation brought about by reports that part of the total extractable NH_4^+ in liver cells and mitochondria is bound and released in acid extraction[18], although use of acid extractable NH_4^+ as free NH_4^+ has given redox values which agree well with independent indicator enzyme systems[4]. Isolated perfused rat hearts in a closed circuit develop an extracellular NH_4^+ concentration of 20 µM[19]. If this is taken as the mitochondrial concentration (assuming that the NH_4^+ distribution is determined by the pH which is equal but opposite in polarity at the inner mitochondrial and plasma membranes), the mitochondrial NADH/NAD$^+$ pool is at a potential of -334 mV. This value would increase the ΔG of the redox reactions between NADH and cytochrome c to -121 kJ/2e$^-$ which is still compatible with a near equilibrium of oxidative phosphorylation in this region of the respiratory chain.

Metabolite compartmentation

Glutamate and aspartate. The mitochondrial transmembrane distribution of glutamate in the myocardium follows the pH, the $[glu_m]/[glu_c]$ concentration ratio being 4.0±0.6 in the beating isolated rat heart[10]. The transmembrane gradient of aspartate is steeper and of opposite polarity compared with that of glutamate. There is a large body of evidence to suggest that the glutamate translocator is an electrogenic antiport[20]. If so, the glutamate and aspartate distribution should impose a diffusion potential obeying the equation

$$\Delta\Phi = \frac{RT}{F} \ln \frac{[glu_m]\cdot[asp_c]}{[glu_c]\cdot[asp_m]},$$

which would equal the membrane potential if the translocator were in equilibrium. The diffusion potential of glutamate and aspartate exchange is 102 mV (negative inside) in the beating heart, and a close relation to the membrane potential is indicated by the increase to 123 mV in the heart arrested by hyperpotassemia[10]. Comparison of these diffusion potentials with the mitochondrial membrane potentials estimated by the probe TPMP$^+$ (123 and 150 mV) suggests that the electrogenic glutamate-aspartate translocator is in equilibrium in the myocardium.

The glutamate-aspartate translocator is an essential component of the malate-aspartate cycle[5], which is used for the up-hill transport of reducing equivalents from the cytosolic NADH into mitochondria. The electrogenicity of the translocator can be employed to energize the cycle and to drive the mitochondrial NADH/NAD$^+$ pool to a more reduced state than the cytosolic pool by a potential span approaching the mitochondrial membrane potential. Under standard conditions (perfusion pressure 80 cm H$_2$O, 10 mM glucose) the cytosolic free NADH/NAD$^+$ pool in a Langendorff-perfused heart is at -215 mV[21]. Thus the transmembrane difference between the redox potentials of the free NADH/NAD$^+$ pools is 119 mV when the matrix NH$_4^+$ concentration is taken as 20 µM (see above). This is indeed close to the measured membrane potential of 125 mV. The measured diffusion potential of glutamate-aspartate exchange is 102 mV, but this is perhaps a minimum estimate, because the 11-fold transmembrane gradient and low matrix aspartate concentration impose a certain experimental uncertainty.

Tricarboxylic acid cycle intramediates. The compartmentation of two tricarboxylic acid cycle intermediates has been measured in the isolated perfused heart[12]. Citrate shows a 16-fold concentration gradient across the mitochondrial membrane and its cytosolic concentration is no more than 80 μM in the beating heart, but increases to 220 μM during potassium-induced arrest[12]. Citrate has been considered to be implicated in the feedback regulation of glycolysis by the tricarboxylic acid cycle[2]. The excursions of the cytosolic citrate concentrations are in the low fringe of those effective in the regulation of PFK[22]. The regulation of glycolysis in heart muscle is known in less detail than in the liver, and especially the recently described regulation by fructose-2,6-diphosphate in the liver[23] has not been characterized in the myocardium. The activity of the tricarboxylate translocator is low in heart muscle mitochondria[3] but the maximum activity reported is in excess of that needed for the transitions observed in transmembrane distribution[12].

2-Oxoglutarate is also mainly mitochondrial in the myocardium. The 14-fold concentration gradient[12] across the mitochondrial inner membrane is equal to that anticipated, provided that the distribution of weak acids permeating the membrane only in undissociated form obeys the equation

$$\Delta pH = \frac{1}{n} \log \frac{[A_m]}{[A_c]} ,$$

where n is the number of dissociable protons and subscripts m and c refer to the matrix and cytosolic compartments, respectively.

CONCLUSIONS

Data gathered from experiments on isolated perfused rat hearts allow a generalized picture to emerge of the state of mitochondrial membrane transport phenomena in intact tissues. The concept of equilibrium networks in oxidative metabolism, as advanced during the last 15 years, emphasizes that a redox gap exists between the cytosolic and mitochondrial matrix compartments of the cell. This has been considered to be mainly due to the equilibrium constants of enzyme reactions working as linkers and the fixed concentrations of key metabolites which are distributed evenly[24]. Later work has demonstrated considerable concentration gradients for metabolites, maintained most probably by the mitochondrial energy charge in the form of protonic and electric gradients.

The data presented here indicate that in intact tissue a metabolic equilibrium network extends along definite stretches of the mitochondrial respiratory chain and across the mitochondrial membranes (Fig. 1).

The two proximal proton pumping sites of the respiratory chain are in near equilibrium with the extramitochondrial adenylate phosphorylation state. The electrogenic adenylate translocator is in equilibtium with the membrane potential indicating that the translocator is used in building up the extramitochondrial phosphorylation potential.

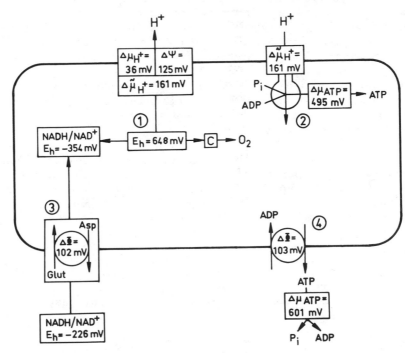

Fig. 1.   Equilibrium network between transmembrane redox and diffusion potentials, intra- and extramitochondrial
phosphorylation potentials and redox potential spans in
the respiratory chain in the mitochondrion of the isolated rat heart perfused with Krebs-Ringer bicarbonate
solution containing 10 mM glucose.
Symbols: $\Delta\tilde{\mu}_{H^+}$ = 2.303 RT· pH/F; $\Delta\Psi$, membrane potential;

$$\Delta\tilde{\mu}_{H^+} = \Delta\mu_{H^+} + \Delta\Psi; \ \Delta\mu_{ATP} = \Delta G_{ATP}/F;$$
$$\Delta\Phi = \frac{RT}{F} \ln \frac{[A]_m/[B]_m}{[A]_c/[B]_c},$$

where A and B are compounds transported in electrogenic
antiport and subscripts m and c refer to the matrix and
cytosolic compartments, respectively.
1, respiratory chain; 2, H^+-ATPase; 3, malate-aspartate
cycle and glutamate-aspartate translocator; 4, ATP-ADP
translocator.
Data adapted from refs. 10,11,12 and 13 with permission of
the publishers.

It is also important to recall in this context that although a large body of data has been accumulated in favour of a coupling of adenylate translocation with membrane potential[25], this has recently been challenged and attributed to preferential binding of ADP in the mitochondrial matrix[26]. The electrogenic glutamate-aspartate translocase is also in equilibrium with the membrane potential, suggesting that this is also the driving force in the hydrogen pumping of into the mitochondria, because the redox potential difference between the mitochondrial and cytosolic free $NADH/NAD^+$ pools is within experimental limits equal to the membrane potential and diffusion potential of glutamate-aspartate exchange (Fig. 1), an essential component of the malate-aspartate cycle. Compared with other tissues such as the liver[4], the redox potential of the mitochondrial free $NADH/NAD^+$ pool in the heart muscle is remarkably negative. Probably as a consequence of this, the phosphorylation potential of the adenylates is higher in the heart than in the liver. The high mitochondrial free $NADH/NAD^+$ ratio in the heart muscle may not be due to a different mechanism or to the efficiency of hydrogen transfer into the mitochondria, since the transmembrane NAD^+ redox potential difference is practically the same in the liver and the heart muscle. It may merely be due to a different set point of the mitochondrial NADH-producing reactions.

The magnitude of the proton electrochemical potential across the mitochondrial membrane in the intact myocardium[13] is shown to be sufficient to drive ADP phosphorylation if one uses the H^+/ATP stoichiometries reported for ATP synthesis in isolated mitochondria[27,29].

Acknowledgements

Supported by grants from the Medical Research Council of the Academy of Finland and under a contract with the Finnish Life Insurance Companies.

REFERENCES

1. E. A. Newsholme and C. Start, "Regulation in Metabolism", Wiley, London (1973).
2. P. B. Garland, P.J. Randle, and E. A. Newsholme, Citrate as an intermediary in the inhibition of phosphofructokinase in rat heart muscle by fatty acids, ketone bodies, pyruvate, diabetes and starvation, Nature 200:169 (1963).
3. S. Cheema-Dhadli, B. H. Robinson, and M. L. Halperin, Properties of the citrate transporter in rat heart: implications for regulation of glycolysis by cytosolic citrate, Can. J. Biochem. 54:561 (1975).

4. D. H. Williamson, P. Lund, and H. A. Krebs, The redox state of free nicotinamide-adenine dinucleotide in the cytoplasm and mitochondria of rat liver, Biochem. J. 103:514 (1967).

5. B. Safer, C. M. Smith, and J. R. Williamson, Control of the transport of reducing equivalents across the mitochondrial membrane in perfused rat heart, J. Mol. Cell. Cardiol. 2:111 (1981).

6. E. A. Siess, D. G. Brocks, and O. H. Wieland, Distribution of metabolites between the cytosolic and mitochondrial compartments of hepatocytes isolated from fed rats, Hoppe-Seyler's Z. Physiol. Chem. 359:785 (1978).

7. M. E. Tischler, D. Friedrichs, K. Coll, and J. R. Williamson, Pyridine nucleotide distributions and enzyme mass action ratios in hepatocytes from fed and starved rats, Arch. Biochem. Biophys. 184:222 (1977).

8. S. Soboll, R. Elbers, R. Scholz, and H.-W. Heldt, Subcellular distribution of di- and tricarboxylates and pH gradients in perfused rat liver, Hoppe-Seyler's Z. Physiol. Chem. 361:67 (1980).

9. R. Elbers, H. W. Heldt, P. Schmucker, S. Soboll, and H. Wiese, Measurement of the ATP/ADP ratio in mitochondria and in the extramitochondrial compartment by fractionation of freeze-stopped liver tissue in non-aqueous media, Hoppe-Seyler's Z. Physiol. Chem. 355:378, (1974).

10. R. A. Kauppinen, J. K. Hiltunen, and I. E. Hassinen, Mitochondrial membrane potential, transmembrane difference in the NAD$^+$ redox potential and the equilibrium of the glutamate-aspartate translocase in the isolated perfused rat heart, Biochim. Biophys. Acta 725:425 (1983).

11. R. A. Kauppinen, J. K. Hiltunen, and I. E. Hassinen, Subcellular distribution of phosphagens in isolated perfused rat heart, FEBS Lett. 112:273 (1980).

12. R. A. Kauppinen, J. K. Hiltunen, and I. E. Hassinen, Compartmentation of citrate in relation to the regulation of glycolysis and the mitochondrial transmembrane proton electrochemical potential gradient in isolated perfused rat heart, Biochim. Biophys. Acta 681:286 (1982).

13. R. Kauppinen, Proton electrochemical potential of the inner mitochondrial membrane in isolated perfused rat hearts, as measured by exogenous probes, Biochim. Biophys. Acta 725:131 (1983).

14. R. W. McGilvery and T. W. Murray, Calculated equilibria of phosphocreatine and adenosine phosphates during utilization of high energy phosphate by muscle, J. Biol. Chem. 249:5845 (1974).

15. J. K. Hiltunen and I. E. Hassinen, Energy-linked regulation of glucose and pyruvate oxidation in isolated perfused rat heart. Role of pyruvate dehydrogenase, Biochim. Biophys. Acta 440:377 (1976).

16. I. E. Hassinen and K. Hiltunen, Respiratory control in iso

lated perfused rat heart. Role of the equilibrium relations between the mitochondrial electron carriers and the
adenylate system, Biochim. Biophys. Acta 408:319 (1975).

17. E. M. Nuutinen, J. K. Hiltunen, and I. E. Hassinen, The glu
tamate dehydrogenase system and the redox state of
mitochondrial free nicotinamide adenine dinucleotide in
myocardium, FEBS Lett. 128:356 (1981).

18. R. J. A. Wanders, J. B. Hoek and J. M. Tager, Origin of the
ammonia found in protein-free extracts of rat liver
mitochondria and rat hepatocytes, Eur. J. Biochem. 110:197
(1980).

19. T. Takala, J. K. Hiltunen, and I. E. Hassinen, The mechanism
of ammonia production and the effect of mechanical work
load on proteolysis and amino acid catabolism in isolated
perfused rat heart, Biochem. J. 192:285 (1980).

20. K. F. LaNoue and A. C. Schoolwerth, Metabolite transport in
mitochondria, Ann. Rev. Biochem. 48:87 (1979).

21. E. M. Nuutinen, Subcellular origin of the surface
fluorescence of reduced nicotinamide nucleotides in the
isolated perfused rat heart, Basic. Res. Cardiol. 79:49
(1984).

22. T. -F. Wu and E. J. Davis, Regulation of glycolytic flux in
an energetically controlled cell-free system: The effects
of adenine nucleotide ratios, inorganic phosphate, pH and
citrate, Arch. Biochem. Biophys. 209:85 (1981).

23. L. Hue, Role of fructose 2,6-bisphosphate in the regulation
of glycolysis, Biochem. Soc. Transact. 11:246 (1983).

24. H. A. Krebs and R. L. Veech, Pyridine nucleotide interrela
tions, in: "The Energy Level and Metabolic Control in
Mitochondria", S. Papa, J. M. Tager, E. Quagliariello, and
E. C. Slater, ed., Adriatica Editrice, Bari (1969).

25. P. V. Vignais, Molecular and physiological aspects of adenine
nucleotide transport in mitochondria, Biochim. Biophys.
Acta 496:1 (1976).

26. D. F. Wilson, M. Erecinska, and V. L. Schramm, Evaluation of
the relationship between the intra- and extramitochondrial
[ATP]/[ADP] ratios using phosphoenolpyruvate car-
boxylkinase, J. Biol. Chem. 258:10464 (1983).

27. A. Alexandre, B. Reynafarje, and A. L. Lehninger, Stoichio
metry of vectorial H^+ movements coupled to electron
transport and to ATP synthesis in mitochondria, Proc.
Natl. Acad. Sci. U.S.A. 75:5296 (1978).

28. G. F. Azzone, T. Pozzan, and S. Massari, Proton electrochemi
cal gradient and phosphate potential in mitochondria,
Biochim. Biophys. Acta 501:307 (1978).

SARCOMERE LENGTH-TENSION RELATIONSHIP IN TOAD ATRIOVENTRICULAR

PACEMAKER: LENGTH DEPENDENT ACTIVATION

José R. López and David Lea

Laboratorio de Biofísica del Músculo, Centro de
Biofísica y Bioquímica, Instituto Venezolano de
Investigaciones Científicas IVIC, Apartado 1827
Caracas 1010A, Venezuela

The relationship between cardiac sarcomere length and force
generation has been extensively studied over the years (1,2,3,4).
However, the experimental results remain incomplete and the conclusions somehow contradictory.

While in skeletal muscle the dependence of force generation
on muscle length is related to two independent factors: i) the
amount of overlapping of contractile filaments (5) and ii) the
degree of activation of the contractile system (6,7,8,9,10), about
cardiac muscle less specific information is available (11,12).

The present study was undertaken to characterize the length
tension curve in spontaneously beating atrioventricular pacemakers
and extend previous studies, with particular reference to the
question of the role of the activation factor on the relationship
between force generation and sarcomere length.

METHODS

Experiments were carried out using spontaneously regularly
beating atrioventricular pacemakers (A.V.), dissected from the
hearts of the tropical toad Leptodactylus insularis. After deca-
pitation of the animals, the hearts were removed, and pinned in a
dissecting dish filled with normal Ringer solution. The atrium
was separated from the ventricle following the atrioventricular
sulcus, and by careful dissection the atrioventricular node lying
beneath the endocardium, around the atrioventricular valve was
identified. By further dissection, spontaneously beating atrioventricular pacemakers, were isolated. They showed an elliptical

343

shape with a length of about 7 mm, and thickness ranged between 140–160 µm.

Once dissected the pacemakers were transferred to an experimental chamber and mounted horizontally with one end held by a fine stainless steel wire hook fixed to the bottom of the chamber. The other end was attached to a fine glass hook mounted on the lever of a force transducer (RCA 5734 or Cambridge Technology-400). The position of the force transducer could be adjusted to give the desired resting length of the AV preparations. The signal from the force transducer was monitored on a chart recorder (Gould-Brush M22).

Solutions

The normal Ringer solution had the following composition in (mM): NaCl 115, KCL 2.5, $CaCl_2$ 1.8, $MgCl_2$ 1.8, glucose 5, Tris buffer 5, adjusted to pH 7.8. The $[Ca^{2+}]_E$ was modified in the bathing solution from 1.8 mM in normal Ringer to 3.6, 5, 10, 15 mM to obtain high-calcium solution. In order to block the pacemaker contractile activity, a low calcium solution was prepared in which $CaCl_2$ was omitted and EGTA 1.8 mM was added. Fixative solutions was prepared with 1% (V/V) of glutaraldehyde in addition to the constituents of the normal Ringer.

All the experiments were carried out at room temperature (20–22°C).

Determination of striation spacing

Striation spacing at rest was determined with an ordinary light microscope with a 40X water-immersion objetive (N.A. 0.75) and verified later with the aids of a transmission electron microscope. The overall pacemaker length was measured through a Wild stereo microscope. The striation spacing below optimum length for force was calculated from the distance between the ends of the pacemaker at 1.9 µm, after the setting for such spacing was determined by light microscope.

The mechanical properties of this preparation remained relatively stable for many hours, and reproducible length-tension curves could be obtained.

Electron microscopy study

At the end of each experiment the bathing solution of the experimental chamber was quickly replaced by low calcium Ringer in order to block the spontaneous activity of the pacemakers cell, and then with glutaraldehyde Ringer(1% V/V) solution, previous

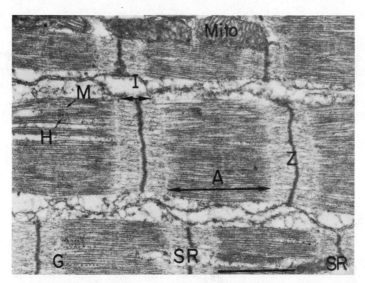

Fig. 1. Low magnification electron micrograph of atrioventricular pacemaker. The myofilaments are arranged in two groups which alternate to produce the cross-striated pattern. It can be observed the A, I, H bands, the Z and M lines. Note the presence of sarcoplasmic reticulum (SR), and large mitochondria (Mito). There are dense granules of glycogen (G) in the mioplasm. Resting sarcomere length 1.9 µm. Calibration bar 1 µm.

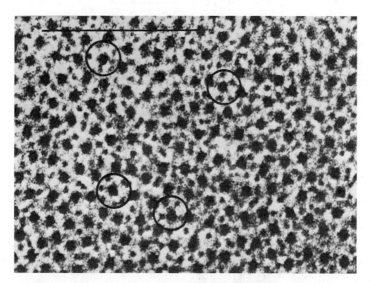

Fig. 2. Transverse section of AV pacemaker through the A band. The disordered array of the myofilaments can be observed. Calibration bar 0.25 µm.

345

determination of the striation spacing. After fixation for 1 hour, the AV preparation was removed from the experimental chamber and postfixed in osmium tetroxide (1%) for an additional hour. Subsequent to a progressive dehydration with alcohol, the AV pacemakers were embedded in Epon 812, and then cut on a Sorvall MT2 ultramicrotome in longitudinal and transverse planes. Sections were suspended on 300 mesh copper grids, stained with uranyl acetate followed by lead citrate, and examined via a Siemens Elmiskop 101 Electron Microscope. Final observations and measurements were made from photographs enlarged up to X40,000.

RESULTS

Atrioventricular pacemaker structure

The electron microscopy study of the atrioventricular pacemakers reveal that the ultrastructure of these cells is similar to those described for working myocardium (13) and skeletal muscle (17). However, the fact that the contractile activity of this conduction tissue is much less prominent than in working myocardium is reflected in a lower degree of organization.

At least 10 longitudinal sections from different portions of each pacemaker were examined. The most relevant ultrastructural aspects found were the following: the myofibrils were longitudinally divided into sarcomeres showing the usual bands of striated cardiac and skeletal muscle (13,14,15,16,17). The orientation of myofibrils was in the majority of the sections observed in a single axis; however, in a few sections it could be observed oriented in random fashion. The Z line was distinguished by its relatively marked density and appeared to be less straight than in myocardium or skeletal muscle fibers. The longitudinal distance between two adjacent Z lines was of 1.92 μm at rest, which defines the length of a sarcomere. A value for sarcomere length of 2.05 and 1.89 μm has been reported by Winegrad (18) in atrial trabeculae and ventricular strips at rest. Extending from each Z line toward the center of the sarcomere was observed the I band, composed of slender filaments with a longitudinal orientation. The A band was identified occupying most of the sarcomere, with a central band referred as H band, which was dissected by a narrow, darkly stained M line (Fig. 1). Thus examination of longitudinal sections indicate that the AV pacemaker fibers, like skeletal muscle and working myocardium (14,16,17) has a double array of filaments. The thin filaments appear to extend from the level of the Z line through the I band and into the A band. The thick filaments traverse the central portion of the sarcomere including both A bands, the H band, and the centrally located M line. The examination of transverse sections confirms this interpretation. Sections through the A band disclose a somewhat dis-

346

ordered array of thin filaments in relation to thick filament (Fig. 2) while at the level of Z lines or I bands showed a single array of thin filaments.

No significant differences could be detected in the contractile response of pacemakers which were oxigenated and those which were not.

Length tension relationship

The length tension curve was determined by changing the length of the AV pacemaker preparation, and recording several responses (spontaneous twitching) at each length. The contractile force associated with the spontaneous beating was recorded at sarcomere lengths between 1.4-2.2 μm (all values corrected for shrinkage). The A.V. pacemakers were allowed to equilibrate (at each length) before data were collected. They were never shortened below a sarcomere length 1.3 μm or streched over 2.2 μm. The data shows that the maximum force was obtained at a sarcomere length of 2.2 μm (L.max). At lengths below 2.2 μm, the contractile force decreased along a curvelinear mode, declining to zero at sarcomere lengths of about 1.3-1.4 μm. The following values for relative tension were found as % of L.max: 80% at 2.1 μm, 65% at 2.0 μm, 51% at 1.9 μm, 40% at 1.8 μm, 22% at 1.6 μm, 14% at 1.4 μm. Fig. 3, shows the actual force records obtained from an AV pacemaker whose length was changed over a complete curve (1.5-2.1 μm) from longest to shortest and back to longest again. It can be observed the relation between peak developed tension and sarcomere length. In Fig. 4, are presented the results from several experiments which were plotted to show how the twitch force related to the spontaneous beating, varies with the striation spacing. The dashed curve represents a summary of the data obtained by Gordon et al., (5) and the solid line interconnects the data points (mean $\pm$ SD) at each striation spacing. It is immediately obvious that the tension decreases as the sarcomere lengths was reduced from the optimum values. Resting tension increased rapidly when the sarcomeres lengthened beyond 2.2 μm. Stretching beyond 2.2-2.3 μm were not attempted in these series of experiments because they produced substantial deleterious of the muscle preparation.

Length dependent activation

Length tension curves were obtained following an experimental protocol identical to the one described previously, but in the presence of different calcium concentrations in the bathing solution. The $[Ca^{2+}]_E$ was changed from 1.8 mM to 3.6, 5, 10, and 15 mM, and the entire curve was explored. When the $[Ca^{2+}]_E$ was increased, the twitch force amplitude associated to the spontaneous beating was increased at all lengths, but the potentiation was length dependent, being the degree of enhancement not the same at

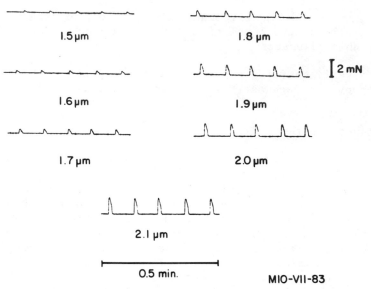

Fig. 3. Experimental records of twitch responses at different sarcomere lengths. The Av pacemaker was held at each length for about 5 beats. The order in which the responses were elicited was the following: 1.9, 1.5, 2.0, 1.8, 1.6, 2.1 and 1.7 μm. All the responses were obtained from the same AV preparation.

all the lengths. Twitch force was markedly increased at short lengths but not at long lengths. Fig. 5 shows the relative effect of the high extracellular calcium concentrations (3.8,5,10 and 15 mM) on force development at different muscle lengths. It is obvious that the degree of potentiation was inversely related to muscle length independently of $[Ca^{2+}]_E$ present in the bathing media. Potentiation of twitch force was greatest at 1.4 μm, and it became gradually less as the pacemaker was stretched to 2.2 μm.

Stretch induced change in frequency

The isolated pacemakers generally beat spontaneously at a frequency which was constant for each preparation. They usually showed an intrinsic rate that ranged from 5 to 24 beats/min, for long periods of time (up to 6-8 hrs) and as long as the length of the muscle was held constant. However, in the majority of the pacemakers studied, the frequency of discharge was increased when the muscle preparation was stretched (from 1.4-2.2 μm) whereas

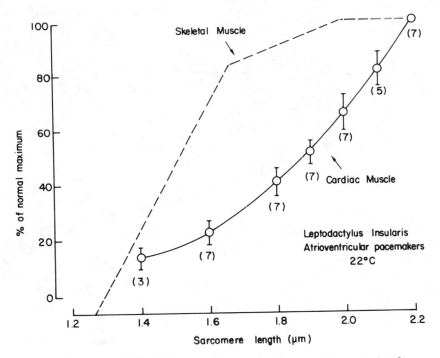

Fig. 4. Length tension data from single atrioventricular pacemakers. Tension production was measured at different sarcomere
length and has been expressed as a percentage of L.max (2.2 μm).
The dashed curve represents part of the sarcomere length-tension
relation described by Gordon et al., 1966 in skeletal muscle.
Each point is the average (± SDM) of several responses obtained
from (3-7) pacemakers.

release of stretching resulted in a slowing of the beating rate.
This phenomenon was more marked at lengths (2.5-2.6 μm) which were
not explored systematically. The percent increase over intrinsic
rate varied from one preparation to another, but in general was in
the order of 15-20%. The speed with which the stretch was applied
influenced the response remarkably. Thus, a single quick stretch
generally produced a greater increase in the beating rate than a
stepwise stretch.

DISCUSSION

This study demonstrates for the first time that the AV pacemaker cells, isolated from the tropical toad Leptodactylus insularis, can be clearly defined ultrastructuraly as working myocardium (13,14,15), even thought its basic function is as conducting
tissue.

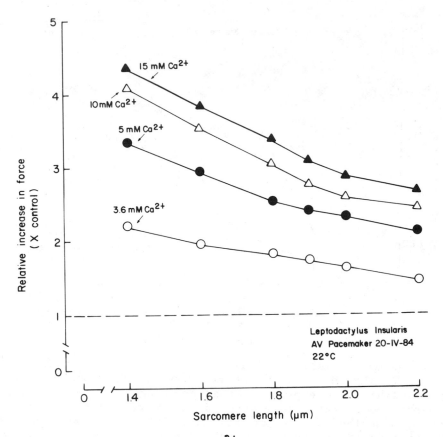

Fig. 5. The effects of high $[Ca^{2+}]_E$ on the twitch force at different muscle lengths. The ratio of the response in high calcium to control force has been plotted for 3.6 mM Ca^{2+} (open circles), 5 mM Ca^{2+} (filled circles), 10 mM Ca^{2+} (open triangles), and 15 mM Ca^{2+} (filled triangles). All the responses were obtained from the same pacemaker at 22°c.

The results indicate that the ascending limb of the sarcomere length relation, obtained in AV pacemaker, reproduce some of the features of the length-tension relation described by Gordon et al (5). However, we did not find a clear plateau over a range of sarcomere lengths extending from about 2.0 to 2.2 μm, which can be associated with the increase of resting tension in this segment of the curve.

In relation to the importance of the activation factor in the generation of force at short sarcomere length through changes in $[Ca^{2+}]_E$ the results clearly indicate that alterations of calcium concentrations in the extracellular medium did not induce proportional changes on developed tension at all muscle lengths. The fact, that the enhancement in force generation was considerable more evident at short than at long muscle lenghts, indicates that the ascending limb of the length-tension curve can not simply be explained on the basis of variation in the amount of overlap between the contractile filaments (5), and that other factors, like level of activation appears to play an important role in determining the relation between force and length in this segment of the curve, as it has been showed in skeletal curve (6,8,9).

The increase in rate beats of the atrioventricular pacemaker associated with stretch observed in this study agrees very well with previous reports obtained from the in situ dog heart study (19). These observations suggest that the phenomenon of acceleration and deceleration associated with stretch and release respectively, are the result of reaction within the node itself. This modification in frequency of discharge might be related to some change in the resting potential (depolarization) observed in other cardiac preparations (20).

CONCLUSION

The results of our experiments in AV pacemakers, as well as the results obtained by others in different preparations of cardiac muscle (11,12) and skeletal muscle (6,7,8,9,10) suggest that at least two independent mechanisms are involved in the relation between force and sarcomere length.

a.- A length dependence of the interaction between two sets of filaments.

b.- A length dependence related to the degree of activation.

ACKNOWLEDGEMENTS

We are grateful to Mrs. Isabel Otaegui for her secretarial assistance and Mrs. Dhuwya Palma for the illustrations. The technical assistance of Mr. Gustavo Cordovez and Mrs. Nancy Linares is gratefully acknowledged.

This research was supported by grants from Consejo Nacional de Investigaciones Científicas y Tecnológicas de Venezuela (CONICIT) S1-1277 and Muscular Dystrophy Association (M.D.A.).

REFERENCES

1.- Sonnenblick E.H. Force velocity relations in mammalian heart muscle. Am. J. Physiol. 202:931-939, 1962.

2.- Nilsson E. Influence of muscle length on the mechanical properties of myocardial contraction. Acta Physiol. Scand. 85:1-23, 1972.

3.- Pollack G.H., and Huntsman Ll. Sarcomere length-active force relations in living mammalian cardiac muscle. Am. J. Physiol. 227:383-389, 1974.

4.- Julian F., and Sollins M.R. Sarcomere length tension relations in living rat papillary muscle. Circulation Research. 37:299-308, 1975.

5.- Gordon A.M., Huxley, A.F., Julian F.G. The variation in isometric tension with sarcomere length in vertebrate muscle fibres. J. Physiol. 184:170-192, 1966.

6.- Rüdel R., and Taylor S.R. Striated muscle fibers: Facilitation of contraction at short lengths by caffeine. Science 172:387-388, 1971.

7.- Schoenberg M., and Podolsky R. Length-force relation of calcium activated muscle fibers. Science 176:52-54, 1972.

8.- López J.R., Waneck L., and Taylor J.R. Skeletal muscle: Length-dependent effects of potentiating agents. Science 214:79-82, 1981.

9.- Taylor S.R., López J.R., Griffiths P.J., Trube G., and Cecchi G. Calcium in excitation-contraction coupling of frog skeletal muscle. Can. J. Physiol. Pharmacol. 60:489-502, 1982.

10.- Sugi H., Ohta T. and Tameyasu T. Development of the maximum isometric force at short sarcomere lengths in calcium activated muscle myofibrils. Experientia 39:147-148, 1983.

11.- Allen D.G., Jewell B.R., and Murray J.W. The contribution of activation processes to the length-tension relation of cardiac muscle. Nature 248:606-607, 1974.

12.- Huntsman L.L., and Stewart D.K. Length dependent calcium inotropism in cat papillary muscle. Circ. Res. 40:366-371, 1972.

13.- Staley N.A., and Benson E.S. The ultrastructure of mammalian cardiac muscle. J. Biophys. Biochem. Cytol. 9:325-351, 1961.

14.- Sommer J.R., and Johnson E.A. Cardiac muscle. A comparative ultrastructural study with special reference to frog and chicken hearts. Z. Zelifursch. 98:437-468, 1969.

15.- Sommer J.R., and Johnson E.A. Cardiac muscle. A comparative study of purkinge fibers and ventricular fibers. J. Cell. Biol. 36:497-526, 1968.

16.- Huxley H.E. Structural basis of muscular contraction. Proc. R. Soc. Lond (Biol) 178:131-149, 1971.

17.- Huxley H.E. The contractile structure of cardiac and skeletal muscle. Circulation 24:328-335, 1961.

18.- Winegrad S. Resting sarcomere length-tension relation in living frog heart. J. Gen. Physiol. 64:343-355, 1974.

19.- Brooks C., McC., Lu H.H., Lange G., Mangi R., Shaw R.B., and Geoly K. Effects on localized stretch of the sino-atrial node region of the dog heart. Am. J. Physiol. 211:1197-1202, 1966.

20.- Deck K.A. Dehnungsversuche an der spezifischen Herz-muskulatur. Arch. Ges. Physiol. 278:13-14, 1963.

MYOCARDIAL ACIDOSIS AND THE MITIGATION OF TISSUE ATP DEPLETION

IN ISCHEMIC CARDIAC MUSCLE: THE ROLE OF THE MITOCHONDRIAL ATPase*

William Rouslin

Pharmacology and Cell Biophysics
University of Cincinnati College of Medicine
Cincinnati, OH

INTRODUCTION

A number of reports have now appeared demonstrating a marked inhibition of the mitochondrial oligomycin-sensitive ATPase as the result of the interruption of blood flow (ischemia) in a number of tissues including liver,[1,2] kidney,[3,4] skeletal muscle[5] and cardiac muscle.[6-9] By and large, the ATPase inhibition observed in ischemic tissues appears to be reversible if blood flow is resumed early enough,[2,4,6,9] suggesting that this inhibition represents a regulatory response of the oligomycin-sensitive ATPase complex to one or more metabolic alterations within the ischemic cells.

Upon the interruption of blood flow to cardiac muscle there is a rapid depletion of tissue oxygen[10] and a consequent cessation of mitochondrial electron flow. In response, glycolytic flux increases rapidly and dramatically[10-12] and, together with the block to proton removal imposed by the lack of blood flow, quickly precipitates a severe cell acidosis.[13,14] In the studies reported here, a direct link is demonstrated between this rapid drop in cell pH and the inhibition of the mitochondrial oligomycin-sensitive ATPase which occurs concomitantly in ischemic cardiac muscle. Moreover, we show that the ATPase inhibition is reversible both in situ upon reperfusion of the ischemic myocardium, and in vitro upon the state 4 re-energization of isolated mitochondria. We also show that pre-perfusion of heart muscle with oligomycin (to inhibit the mitochondrial ATPase) caused a nearly

*Supported by NIH grants HL 22619-04S1 (IVB) and HL30926-01A1

355

90% decrease in the net rate of tissue ATP depletion during a subsequent autolytic (in vitro ischemic) interval during which tissue pH was held constant.

Our results suggest that the protonic inhibition of the mitochondrial ATPase plays a major role in slowing tissue ATP depletion in ischemic heart muscle cells, and that the underlying mechanism of this protonic inhibition appears to be the reversible association of the ATPase inhibitor protein of Pullman and Monroy[15] with the mitochondrial ATPase.

METHODS

Production of In vivo Ischemic Myocardium

Regionally ischemic myocardium was produced in open chest, anesthetized dogs by occluding the left circumflex coronary artery as described earlier.[8,9]

Production of Pretreated Myocardium: the Femoral-Left Circumflex Coronary Arterial Shunt Model

Mongrel dogs of either sex weighing 25–35 kg were anesthetized with sodium pentobarbital (30 mg/kg), intubated and placed on a Harvard respirator. During subsequent surgical procedure, room air supplemented with 95% O_2, 5% CO_2 was administered under positive pressure. Each animal was placed in a left lateral position, electrocardiographic leads attached to the limbs and the femoral arteries and veins exposed on both sides. A Tygon catheter was advanced through the left femoral artery to the thoracic aorta, secured in place and connected to a Statham P23ID transducer for the measurement of blood pressure. The left femoral vein was cannulated for intravenous infusions. An arterial cannula was inserted through the right femoral artery up to the abdominal aorta for later connection to an extracorporeal, femoral-left circumflex coronary arterial shunt tube.

A left thoracotomy was performed through the fourth intercostal space, the pericardium opened and the heart suspended in a pericardial cradle. The proximal 1.5 cm of the left circumflex coronary artery was exposed in preparation for its later cannulation and connection to the extracorporeal shunt tube. A pursestring suture was placed in the right atrial appendage, the animal was heparinized (10,000 units) and a minimum of two min allowed for its circulation. A polyethylene nasal cannula was then inserted through the right atrial pursestring into the coronary sinus and the pursestring tightened to secure the coronary sinus cannula (drain tube) in place. A ligature was then placed just distal to the coronary sinus ostium which when tightened later would actuate the removal of coronary venous blood (and buffer) from the animal through the drain tube into a graduated cylinder. This arrangement prevented the infusion of reservoir buffer into the systemic circulation and also allowed the maintenance of systemic blood volume during the buffer perfusion interval. The ligature just distal to the coronary sinus ostium was left untightened so that blood continued to flow around rather than through the coronary sinus drain tube until the time of reservoir buffer perfusion. A polyethylene (shunt) tube was placed through a Sarns model 3500 roller pump, primed with heparinized saline, then connected at one end to the right femoral arterial cannula and pumped full with blood from the right femoral artery. The portion of the left circumflex coronary artery which had been exposed earlier was ligated proximally, an incision made just distal to the ligation and the output end of the pumped shunt tube from the right femoral artery inserted into the left circumflex artery 8 to 10 mm. The pumped shunt tube was then secured and the rate of blood pumping (from the right femoral artery to the L. circumflex coronary artery) increased until shunt perfusion pressure, measured with a second Statham transducer connected just proximal to the perfusion cannula, equalled systolic arterial pressure (typically just in excess of 100 mm Hg). At this point, blood to the left circumflex coronary distribution area of the left ventricle (approx. 40 g of myocardial mass) was being supplied via the pumped, extracorporeal shunt tube from the right femoral artery. Coronary circulation to the remainder of the heart was minimally altered as indicated by the electrocardiogram.

During a 10 min stabilization period, a one liter, jacketed perfusate buffer reservoir, maintained at 37° and bubbled with 95% O_2, 5% CO_2, was connected by means of a clamped polyethylene tube to a pre-existing inlet port in the pumped shunt tube. The reservoir contained a modified Krebs-bicarbonate buffer medium in which the NaCl was omitted and replaced by 200 mM HEPES-NaOH. The buffer solution contained 4.7 mM KCl, 2.5 mM $CaCl_2$, 1.2 mM $MgSO_4$, 1.2 mM KH_2PO_4, 0.5 mM EDTA, 25 mM $NaHCO_3$, 10 mM glucose and 200 mM HEPES-NaOH where the final pH of the medium was adjusted to 7.5 and the final concentration of Na^+ was approx. 118 mM. When present, oligomycin was at a final concentration of 10 µM.

At the conclusion of the stabilization period, the blood carrying cannula from the right femoral artery was clamped shut and, simultaneously, the buffer carrying tube from the reservoir was opened. Also at this time, the coronary sinus ligature was tightened, allowing the blood-buffer mixture entering the sinus to be drained off by gravity into a graduated cylinder. Buffer perfusion pressure was monitored and maintained equal to systolic arterial pressure by regulating the shunt tube pump. Pump speed had to be increased approximately three-fold to maintain shunt-line pressure equal to arterial pressure upon switching from blood

to buffer, primarily due to the low viscosity of the perfusate
buffer relative to blood. During the time required to perfuse one
liter of buffer (typically 6 min), the buffer-perfused left circumflex coronary distribution area of the left ventricle was
blanched and thus distinctly demarcated from adjacent blood-
perfused myocardium.

A few seconds prior to the exhaustion of the perfusate
buffer, 5 ml of a 10% (w/v) solution of patent blue violet dye in
distilled water was injected into the left atrium, a procedure
which clearly demarcated adjacent blood perfused myocardium (dyed)
from shunt-line perfused myocardium (undyed). In the so-called
blood pre-perfused samples (Figs. 9 and 10), this dye marking procedure was carried out directly after an extended (16 min) stabilization period without an intervening 6 min buffer perfusion
interval. The whole heart was then immediately removed from the
animal and placed into saline, care being taken to interrupt
shunt-line pressure and coronary arterial blood pressure at the
same moment thereby maintaining the original margins of the shunt-

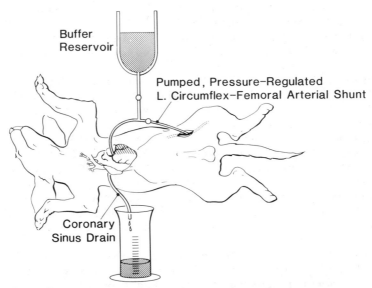

Fig. 1.   Femoral-left circumflex coronary arterial shunt model.
          The model, schematically diagrammed here, allowed the
          pre-perfusion of the L. circumflex coronary distribution
          area of the canine left ventricle (the hash-marked zone)
          with buffers and inhibitors so as to control conditions
          under which a subsequent tissue autolysis (in vitro
          ischemia) occurred.

line perfused area of the left ventricle after removal of the
heart from the animal. The essential features of the femoral-left
circumflex arterial shunt model are schematically depicted in
Fig. 1.

Production of Autolyzed Myocardium and the Measurement of Tissue pH

Autolyzed myocardium was produced as described earlier[8],[9]
using transmural blocks of left ventricle from unoccluded hearts
(Figs. 3 and 4) and, occasionally (Fig. 2), using transmural
samples from the non-ischemic regions of occluded hearts.
Additionally, autolysis was carried out using pretreated myocardial samples (Figs. 7-10). The shunt-line perfused, left circumflex coronary distribution area of the left ventricle weighing
approx. 40 g (depicted in Fig. 1 as the hash-marked area of the
posterior left ventricle) was dissected from the remainder of the
heart excluding a surrounding zone of undyed myocardium approx.
1 cm in width (to avoid inclusion of any incompletely pretreated
tissue). Autolysis of these variously derived transmural samples
of canine left ventricle was then carried out by placing them in
sealed Ziploc plastic bags from which air bubbles adjacent to the
tissue surfaces were expressed. These were immersed in a circulating water bath at 37°C. The whole process of myocardial
dissection and sampling was completed in one min or less.

Tissue pH was measured continuously in regionally ischemic
and in transmural autolyzing samples using a model MI-411B microcombination pH probe (Microelectrodes, Inc., Londonderry, N.H.)
impaled into the mid-myocardium. The electrode was coupled to a
recording pH meter.

Mitochondrial Isolation and In Vitro Incubation

Mitochondria were isolated from control and autolyzed myocardial samples using a Polytron homogenization procedure as
described earlier.[8],[9] In vitro incubation of control mitochondria
(Fig. 5) were carried out as follows. One tenth ml aliquots of
mitochondria at approx. 40 mg protein/ml were added to 0.9 ml of
media equilibrated to 37°C containing 200 mM maleate-KOH buffer at
the pH values indicated, 1.0 mM EGTA and 1.0 µM FCCP. The incubations were stopped after 10 min by the readjustment of the medium
pH to 7.2 with Tris base, centrifugation and resuspension of the
mitochondria in 1.0 ml of 10 mM Tris-Cl, pH 7.8. Each sample was
then sonicated a total of 45s and 50 µl used for each ATPase
assay.

For the experiments depicted in Fig. 6, Panels A and B, the
incubation media also contained 6 mM succinate and 2.5 mM sodium
phosphate. In Fig. 6, Panel A, control mitochondria were incubated with shaking in air at pH 6.27 for the times indicated. In

Panel B, mitochondria from 20 min autolyzed myocardium were incubated with shaking in air at pH 7.2 for the times indicated, and FCCP was added to a final concentration of 1 μM at each time point (upper trace of Panel B only). This final FCCP addition served to stop the ATPase activity reactivation at the level reached at the time of its addition, preserving that activity level for later assay. At the conclusion of the experiments depicted in Fig. 6, all of the mitochondrial samples were centrifuged and resuspended in 1.0 ml of 10 mM Tris-Cl, pH 7.8. Each sample was then sonicated a total of 45 s and 50 ml used for each ATPase assay.

Assays

Mitochondrial ATPase was assayed by a modification of the method of Tzagoloff et al.[16] The 1.0 ml reaction mixture contained 50 μmol Tris-HCl, pH 7.8, 10 μmol $MgCl_2$ and 50 μl sonicated mitochondria. The reaction was started by the addition of 10 μmol ATP-Tris, run for 5 min at 30°C, and stopped by the addition of 1 ml 10% trichloroacetic acid. After protein removal, inorganic phosphate was determined (against a zero time blank) according to the method of Bonting et al.[17] Protein was assayed by the method of Lowry et al.[18]

Tissue ATP content was measured in autolyzed samples that were removed from the Ziploc bags at the times indicated in Figs. 8 and 10. At the times indicated, the samples were frozen rapidly by imersion in liquid nitrogen, then broken into approx. one g pieces which were weighed and then lyophilized overnight. The frozen-dried tissue samples were then powdered finely and the powder extracted with 6% trichloroacetic acid. Aliquots of the acid extracts were then analyzed enzymatically for ATP content using Sigma Chemical Co. ATP assay kits as described in Sigma Chemical Co. Technical Bulletin No. 366-UV.

RESULTS

Fig. 2 presents representative tissue pH traces produced by impaling a microcombination pH electrode into left ventricular midmyocardium during (upper trace) left circumflex coronary artery occlusion and (lower trace) zero flow autolysis in sealed plastic bags at 37°C. The sample used for the autolysis trace came from the nonischemic region of the very same heart from which the upper pH trace was obtained. Both the rate and extent of the pH drop in the zero flow model are in close agreement with those observed in globally ischemic rat hearts by ^{31}P nuclear magnetic resonance.[13]

The data in Fig. 3 show the timecourses of the decrease in mitochondrial ATPase activity in the two models which reflect closely the rates of tissue pH change in each model shown in Fig. 2.

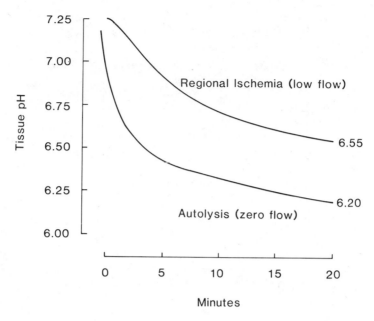

Fig. 2. Tissue pH in regional ischemia and in in vitro autolysis. pH was recorded continuously using a microcombination pH electrode impaled into left ventricular midmyocardium during left circumflex coronary artery occlusion in an anesthetized dog (upper trace) and during the autolysis of a sample taken from the nonischemic region of the same heart in a sealed Ziploc plastic bag at 37°C (lower trace).

The control ATPase specific activity for the low flow regional ischemia timecourse was 1.05 ± 0.06 µmol/min/mg (n=8); that for the zero flow autolysis time course was 1.03 ± 0.05 µmol/min/mg (n=8).

Fig. 4 presents percent of control specific activity averages of four separate autolysis timecourse experiments plotted against a representative tissue pH curve as measured with the microcombination electrode. While most of the tissue pH and specific activity decreases had already occurred by 5 min of autolysis, a relatively linear relationship between the two parameters was revealed with increasing time of autolysis. The control ATPase specific activity for this study was the same as that reported above for the zero flow autolysis timecourse study, i.e., 1.03 ± 0.05 µmol/min/mg.

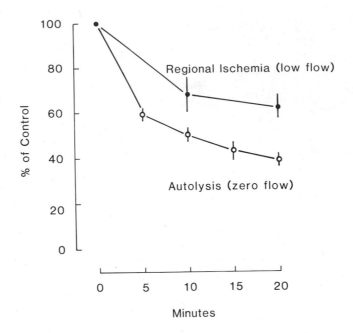

Fig. 3. Oligomycin-sensitive ATPase activity. ATPase activity
was measured in sonicated mitochondria prepared from
regionally ischemic (●) and autolyzed (○) myocardial
samples taken at the times indicated. All data are
averages ±S.E.M. of four determinations.

This same relationship was again demonstrated in the in vitro
incubation experiment depicted in Fig. 5. Here, treatments of
isolated mitochondria under nonenergizing conditions at the different pH values shown produced nearly identical degrees of ATPase
inhibition to those observed after their exposure in situ to very
similar pH values in acidotic autolyzing tissue samples (Fig. 4).

The data in Fig. 5 suggest that, under the non-energizing
conditions which prevail in ischemic myocardium, a drop in pH
alone can cause the ATPase inhibition observed in this study both
in situ and in vitro in isolated mitochondria. Moreover, these
data suggest that our tissue pH measurements actually reflected
closely the intracellular pH to which mitochondria were exposed
in normally perfused, ischemic, and autolyzing myocardium. We
thus, in effect, had used the mitochondrial ATPase as an intracellular pH indicator.

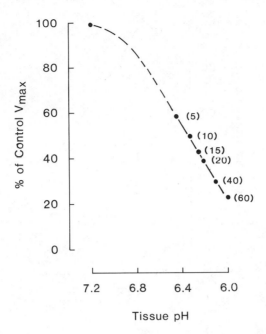

Fig. 4. Per cent of control specific activity of oligomycin-
sensitive ATPase versus tissue pH during myocardial autolysis. All specific activity values are averages of four
separate determinations. Tissue pH was determining using
a microcombination pH electrode as described in the
legend to Fig. 2 and under "Methods." The pH values were
taken from a representative 60-min tracing. The numbers
in parentheses are minutes of autolysis.

The rapidity of the onset of the ATPase inhibition observed
during regional ischemia or autolysis (Fig. 3) suggested to us
that we were witnessing a reversible regulatory phenomenon. We
therefore designed experiments to demonstrate the possible reversal of the ATPase inhibition in situ during the reperfusion of
ischemic tissue. In these experiments, tissue pH was monitored in
our left circumflex occlusion model during 15 min of occlusion,
enough to produce a substantial drop in both tissue pH (Fig. 2)
and in ATPase activity (Fig. 3), followed by 15 min of reperfusion. Upon reperfusion, tissue pH rebounded rapidly at first
returning to normal in 10 min or less. Interestingly, the specific activity of the oligomycin-sensitive ATPase also returned to
normal in mitochondria isolated from the reperfused area (9). The
ATPase inhibition was thus a fully reversible phenomenon in vivo.

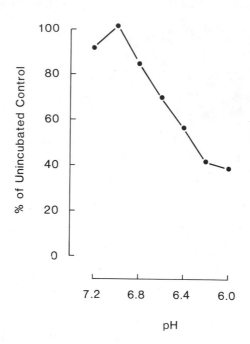

Fig. 5. Per cent of unincubated control oligomycin-sensitive
ATPase activity versus pH in isolated mitochondria.
Control mitochondria were incubated under nonenergizing
conditions for 10 min at 37°C. Following the incubation,
the mitochondria were resuspended in fresh medium, sonicated and assayed for ATPase activity.

Fig. 6 presents experiments with isolated control mitochondria (A) and with mitochondria isolated from 20 min autolyzed
myocardium (B). In the experiment depicted in Panel A with
control mitochondria, ATPase inactivation by incubation at pH 6.27
occurred only under nonenergizing conditions produced by the
dissipation of the trans-inner membrane proton gradient by the
addition of the proton ionophore, FCCP. The inactivation was
virtually complete within the first minute. The experiment
depicted in Panel B with mitochondria from 20 min autolyzed
myocardium shows that reactivation in state 4 at pH 7.2 required
the development and maintenance of a transmembrane proton gradient. The mere removal of the acidotic environment in the presence of a proton ionophore did not reverse the ATPase inhibition.
The reactivation of the ATPase in the absence of FCCP was rapid,
and the intermediate reactivation states obtained at 1, 2, 5, and

10 min of incubation were obtained by the addition of FCCP at the time points indicated. Thus, the addition of a proton ionophore during reactivation served to "freeze" the ATPase activity at the degree of reactivation attained at the time of proton gradient dissipation. The ATPase reactivation shown in Panel B appears to be an in vitro analog of the in vivo process which occurs during the reperfusion of ischemic myocardium.[9]

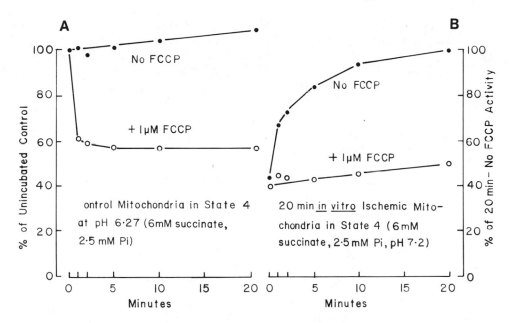

Fig. 6. Oligomycin-sensitive ATPase activity. ATPase activity was measured in control mitochondria during their aeration at pH 6.27 (37°C) in a medium containing 200 mM maleate-KOH, 1 mM EGTA, 6 mM succinate and 2.5 mM sodium phosphate minus (state 4) and plus 1 µM FCCP (A) and in mitochondria from 20 min autolyzed myocardium aerated at pH 7.2 (37°C) in the same medium minus (state 4) and plus 1 µM FCCP (B).

Fig. 7 presents representative tissue pH timecourses for autolyzing myocardial samples which had been pre-perfused with a Krebs-bicarbonate medium modified to include 200 mM HEPES buffer and also HEPES buffer plus 10 µM oligomycin. In this figure and in the autolysis timecourse figures that follow (Figs. 8, 9 and 10), data are presented for the 5 to 20 min autolytic interval

only. The 0 to 5 min interval has been omitted because, in all of
the protocols used in this study, tissue pH dropped rapidly during
the first 5 min of the autolytic process from initial values of
approx. 7.50 and 7.25 for HEPES- and blood pre-perfused tissue,
respectively. In that an important aspect of the design of the
experiments presented in Figs. 7 and 8 was the elimination of
tissue pH as a significant contributor to differences in rates of
tissue ATP depletion, the only data presented are those obtained
from an autolytic interval where there was no significant tissue
pH differential or rapid pH change. The same experimental design
focus also applied to the experiments presented in Figs. 9 and 10
except that there, the effect of a relatively stable tissue pH
differential of approx. 0.6 units was examined.

Fig. 7 shows that there was no significant tissue pH differential between the HEPES and HEPES plus oligomycin protocols.
In both, a relatively mild acidosis developed producing an average
tissue pH for the 5 to 20 min autolytic interval of approx. 6.84.

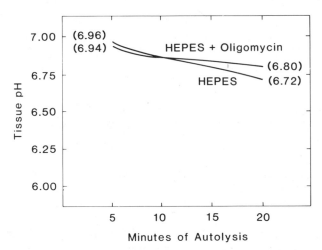

Fig. 7.   Tissue pH timecourses during myocardial autolysis. The
          pH traces were obtained using a microcombination pH probe
          impaled into midmyocardium during autolysis. The muscle
          had been pretreated prior to autolysis with 1 l of a
          modified Krebs-bicarbonate medium containing either 200
          mM HEPES, pH 7.5, or HEPES plus 10 µM oligomycin.

The data presented in Fig. 8 show that pre-perfusion with 10 µM
oligomycin produced a nearly 90% reduction in the net rate of
tissue ATP depletion. In the 15 min autolytic interval examined,
tissue ATP dropped by 3.00 µmoles/g wet weight of tissue in the
HEPES pretreated samples, but only by 0.37 µmoles/g wet weight in
the HEPES plus oligomycin treated tissue.

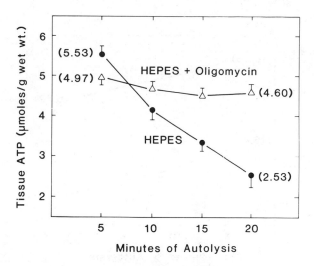

Fig. 8.   Tissue ATP content during myocardial autolysis. Rapidly
frozen tissue samples were analyzed enzymatically for ATP
content as described under "Methods."   The muscle had
been pretreated as described in the legend to Fig. 7.
The data are averages ±S.E.M. of eight determinations.

Fig. 9 presents representative tissue pH timecourses for
autolyzing myocardial samples which had been pre-perfused with the
Krebs-bicarbonate medium containing HEPES, and with blood. As
explained under "Methods," the blood perfused samples were treated
identically to the other samples except that the 6 min buffer perfusion step was replaced by a 6 min extension of the stabilization
period.   It may be seen that HEPES pretreatment greatly mitigated
the severity of the tissue acidosis which developed (in the blood
perfused tissue) suggesting that, while blood is a good buffer of
tissue pH, the HEPES containing perfusate employed here was still
more effective in absorbing protons produced by the ischemic
cells.   A similar effect of HEPES pretreatment of isolated rat
hearts has been reported previously by Garlick et al.[13]   As shown
in Fig. 9, HEPES pretreatment produced an average tissue pH of
approx. 6.84 for the autolytic interval studied whereas blood pre-
perfused muscle exhibited an average pH of approx. 6.22 for the
same autolytic interval.   There was thus approx. a 0.6 pH unit
differential produced between the two protocols.

Fig. 10 shows that the low tissue pH exhibited by autolyzing,
blood pre-perfused myocardium was accompanied by a greatly reduced
net rate of tissue ATP depletion.   Thus, while the HEPES
pretreated tissue lost 3.00 µmoles of ATP/g wet weight of tissue

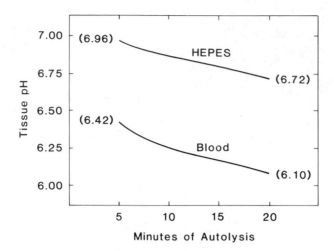

Fig. 9.   Tissue pH timecourses during myocardial autolysis.   The
          pH traces were obtained using a microcombination pH probe
          impaled into midmyocardium during autlysis.   The muscle
          had been pretreated prior to autolysis with 1 1 of a
          modified Krebs-bicarbonate medium containing 200 mM
          HEPES, pH 7.5, or with blood.

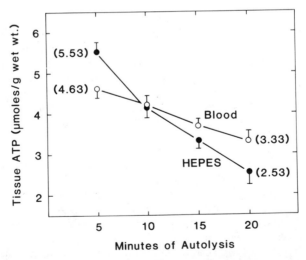

Fig. 10.   Tissue ATP content during myocardial autolysis.   Rapidly
           frozen tissue samples were analyzed enzymatically for
           ATP content.   The muscle had been pretreated as
           described in the legend to Fig. 9.   The data are
           averages ±S.E.M. of eight determinations.

during the 15 min autolytic interval examined, the more acidic blood perfused muscle lost only 1.30 µmoles of ATP/g wet weight. The degree of the pH-dependence of the net rate of tissue ATP depletion observed in this study is indeed quite close to that predicted by both the in situ and in vitro mitochondrial ATPase pH-inhibition profiles shown above (Figs. 2 and 3) and reported earlier.[9]

DISCUSSION

A central finding of the present study is that reduced pH alone appears to be able to cause an inhibition of the ATPase of nonenergized mitochondria either in situ in ischemic and auto-lyzing cardiac muscle or in vitro in isolated cardiac mitochon-dria. The main hypothesis which emerged during the course of the work reported here is that we were actually observing the rever-sible inhibition of the mitochondrial ATPase by its natural pro-tein inhibitor[15] in ischemic and autolyzing cardiac muscle. Indeed, our results are consistent with findings from several laboratories on conditions which regulate mitochondrial ATPase activity by means of the reversible association of the ATPase inhibitor protein. Compelling evidence in support of this mecha-nism is presented in Fig. 6. A number of workers have now reported that the dissociation of the inhibitor from the enzyme is promoted by substrate oxidation and the concomitant generation of a trans-inner membrane electrochemical gradient.[19,20] Indeed, the FCCP-sensitive reactivation of the ATPase reported here in Fig. 6B is remarkably like the FCCP-sensitive, parallel ATPase reactiva-tion and inhibitor protein release reported by Schwerzmann and Pedersen (Fig. 6 of Ref. 20).

The experiment depicted in Fig. 6B suggests that the mere elevation of matrix pH back to 7.2 is not sufficient to reactivate the enzyme. If the alleviation of matrix acidosis were sufficient to accomplish this, then the sustained inhibition observed at pH 7.2 in the presence of FCCP would not have occurred. In agreement with the observations of others,[19,20] active proton pumping is apparently required to reverse the inhibition. On the other hand, the experiment depicted in Fig. 6A shows that, in agreement with Horstman and Racker,[21] a mere drop in pH is sufficient to initiate the inhibition, provided that the proton gradient is dissipated.

A number of workers have shown that the natural ATPase inhi-bitor is unidirectional in its action in that it blocks ATP hydro-lysis under nonenergizing conditions, but does not prevent ATP synthesis during substrate oxidation[20,22] even at reduced pH (Fig. 6A). The unidirectional nature of the inhibitor suggests a pivo-tal role for the reversible inhibition of the ATPase in ischemic cells. Upon the rapid depletion of tissue oxygen, the cessation of mitochondrial electron flow, and the drop in cell pH which

369

characterize the onset of an ischemic episode, a major, immediate problem is the conservation of cell ATP levels for the maintenance of ion gradients and cell membrane integrity.[23,24] Low cell ATP levels have been suggested by a number of workers to be an important correlate and possibly a direct cause of the transition from reversible to irreversible cell injury.[25] To the extent to which a continued, dissipative ATP hydrolysis might be mediated by the nonenergized mitochondrial ATPase, the problem would be greatly exacerbated, resulting in a rapid rate of irreversible cell injury and death.

The mitochondrial oligomycin-sensitive ATPase comprises approximately 90% of the total of all of the ATP hydrolyzing activities of ischemic cardiac muscle.** As such it has enormous potential as a contributor to tissue ATP hydrolysis when not driven in the direction of ATP synthesis. Indeed the data presented in Fig. 8 suggest that nearly 90% of the net rate of tissue ATP depletion observed in buffered autolyzing cardiac muscle can be blocked by oligomycin. Also, Haworth et al.[26] have reported that oligomycin treatment of isolated rat heart cells delayed the onset of contracture by 55%, suggesting to these workers that the mitochondrial ATPase constitutes a significant drain on energy reserves in ischemic heart muscle cells.

While the mitochondrial ATPase has great ATP destroying potential under the non-energizing conditions which prevail in ischemic cardiac muscle cells, only a small fraction of this ATP hydrolyzing activity is ordinarily expressed in ischemic myocardium[8,9] due primarily to the severe acidosis which develops rapidly in blood pre-perfused muscle.[8,9,13,14] Thus, while tissue acidosis is generally regarded as a potentially destructive condition in itself, it may actually constitute a "beneficial" development at least transiently, early in the ischemic process, before cell ATP levels have fallen to critically low values. This would appear to be so primarily because of the inhibitory effects that low cell pH has upon the ATP utilizing systems in heart

---

** Whole canine heart muscle homogenates were assayed for the percent of their total ATPase activity which was attributable to the mitochondrial ATPase, i.e., which could be inhibited by oligomycin. The total homogenate ATPase activity was measured in a medium containing 100 mM NaCl, 10 mM KCl, 1 mM $CaCl_2$, 10 mM $MgCl_2$, 10 mM Na_2ATP, 0.5% (w/v) bovine serum albumin and 20 mM MOPS-NaOH, pH 7.3 in the absence and presence of 2 μM oligomycin. The percent of the total homogenate ATPase activity attributable to the mitochondrial enzyme was 89.9 ± 1.2 (n=4).

muscle cells, including the actomyosin contractile apparatus[27] and the non-energized mitochondrial ATPase.[9] In support of this concept and in agreement with the present study, Bing et al.[28] have reported the development of a precocious contracture in hypoxic rat cardiac muscle brought about by a pretreatment which elevated the pH of the hypoxic muscle. Protective effects of mild acidosis have also been reported by Nayler et al.[29] on hypoxic rabbit hearts and by Acosta and Li[30] on rat myocardial cells deprived of oxygen and glucose.

While glycolysis contributes very little to total cell ATP production in normally perfused heart muscle, its rate increases dramatically upon the cessation of oxidative phosphorylation[10-12] and, in doing so, becomes a major contributor to the maintenance of tissue ATP levels in ischemic cardiac muscle.[12] Thus, glycolysis appears to contribute to the maintenance of cell ATP levels in ischemic cells in two separate ways. First, it produces ATP by substrate-level phosphorylation and second, it participates in the production of the cell acidosis which causes a protonic inhibition of ATP hydrolysis by several ATP hydrolyzing enzymes including the actomyosin system[27] and the undriven mitochondrial ATP synthetase.[9]

While the underlying mechanism of the protonic inhibition of the mitochondrial ATPase suggested by our work[9] remains to be demonstrated directly, the results of our studies continue to suggest that the reversible inhibition of the mitochondrial ATPase observed by us[7-9] and by others[1-6] in ischemic tissues may be mediated by the reversible association of the ATPase inhibitor protein of Pullman and Monroy[15] with the mitochondrial ATPase. The potential significance of this particular mechanism for regulating ATP levels in muscle cells undergoing metabolic state transitions appears not to have been recognized previously.

ACKNOWLEDGMENTS

I thank David A. Ciochetty, Christine A. Trenkamp, Norbert J. Berberich and John L. Erickson for their competent technical assistance, Gwen Kraft for help in preparing the figures, and Liz Wendelmoot and Robin Wright for typing the manuscript.

REFERENCES

1. S. Mittnacht, Jr., S. C. Sherman, and J. L. Farber, Reversal of ischemic mitochondrial dysfunction, J. Biol. Chem. 254:9871-9878 (1979).
2. L. Mela, L. V. Bacalzo, Jr., and L. D. Miller, Defective oxidative metabolism of rat liver mitochondria in hemorrhagic and endotoxin shock, Am. J. Physiol. 220:571-577 (1971).

3. M. T. Vogt, and E. Farber, On the molecular pathology of ischemic renal death. Reversible and irreversible cellular and mitochondrial metabolic alterations, Am. J. Pathol. 53:1-26 (1968).

4. W. J. Mergner, S.-H. Chang, L. Marzella, M. W. Kahng, and B. Trump, Studies on the pathogenesis of ischemic cell injury. VIII. ATPase of rat kidney mitochondria, Lab. Invest. 40:686-694 (1979).

5. A. Kohama, W. A. Boyd, C. M. Ballinger, and I. Ueda, Adenosine triphosphatase activities of subcellular fractions of normal and ischemic muscles, J. Surg. Res. 11:297-302 (1971).

6. D. V. Godin, J. M. Tuchek, and M. Moore, Membrane alterations in acute myocardial ischemia, Can. J. Biochem. 58:777-786 (1980).

7. W. Rouslin, and R. W. Millard, Mitochondrial inner membrane enzyme defects in porcine myocardial ischemia, Am. J. Physiol. 240:H308-H313 (1981).

8. W. Rouslin, Mitochondrial complexes I, II, III, IV and V in myocardial ischemia and autolysis, Am. J. Physiol. 244:H743-H748 (1983).

9. W. Rouslin, Protonic inhibition of the mitochondrial oligomycin-sensitive adenosine 5'-triphosphatase in ischemic and autolyzing cardiac muscle. Possible mechanism for the mitigation of ATP hydrolysis under nonenergizing conditions, J. Biol. Chem. 258:9657-9661 (1983).

10. W. Kubler, and P. G. Spiekermann, Regulation of glycolysis in the ischemic and the anoxic myocardium, J. Mol. Cell. Cardiol. 1:351-377 (1970).

11. J. R. Neely, J. T. Whitmer, and M. Rovetto, Effect of coronary blood flow on glycolytic flux and intracellular pH in isolated rat hearts, Circ. Res. 37:733-741 (1975).

12. A. J. Doorey, and W. M. Barry, The effects of inhibition of oxidative phosphorylation and glycolysis on contractility and high-energy phosphate content in cultured chick heart cells, Circ. Res. 53:192-201 (1983).

13. P. B. Garlick, G. K. Radda, and P. J. Seeley, Studies on acidosis in the ischemic heart by phosphorus nuclear magnetic resonance, Biochem. J. 184:547-554 (1979).

14. S. M. Cobbe, and P. A. Poole-Wilson, The time of onset and severity of acidosis in myocardial ischemia, J. Mol. Cell. Cardiol. 12:745-760 (1980).

15. M. E. Pullman, and G. C. Monroy, A naturally occurring inhibitor of mitochondrial adenosine triphosphatase, J. Biol. Chem. 238:3762-3769 (1963).

16. A. Tzagoloff, K. H. Byington, and D. H. MacLennan, Studies on the mitochondrial adenosine triphosphatase. II. The isolation and characterization of an oligomycin-sensitive adenosine triphosphatase from bovine heart mitochondria, J. Biol. Chem. 243:2405-2412 (1968).

17. S. L. Bonting, K. A. Simon, and N. A. Hawkins, Studies on sodium-potassium-activated adenosine triphosphatase. I. Quantitative distribution in several tissues of the cat, Arch. Biochem. Biophys. 95:416-423 (1961).

18. O. H. Lowry, N. J. Rosebrough, A. L. Farr, and R. J. Randall, Protein measurement with the Folin phenol reagent, J. Biol. Chem. 193:265-275 (1951).

19. R. J. Van de Stadt, B. L. De Boer, and K. Van Dam, The interaction between the mitochondrial ATPase (F_1) and the ATPase inhibitor, Biochim. Biophys. Acta 292:338-349 (1973).

20. K. Schwertzmann, and P. L. Pedersen, Proton-adenosinetriphosphatase complex of rat liver mitochondria: effect of energy state on its interaction with the adenosinetriphosphatase inhibitory peptide, Biochemistry 20:6305-6311 (1981).

21. L. L. Horstman, and E. Racker, Partial resolution of the enzymes catalyzing oxidative phosphorylation. XXII. Interaction between mitochondrial adenosine triphosphatase inhibitor and mitochondrial adenosine triphosphatase, J. Biol. Chem. 245:1336-1344 (1970).

22. K. Asami, K. Juntti, and L. Ernster, Possible regulatory function of a mitochondrial ATPase inhibitor in respiratory chain-linked energy transfer, Biochim. Biophys. Acta 205:307-311 (1970).

23. Y. Gazitt, I. Ohad, and A. Loyter, Changes in phospholipid susceptibility toward phospholipase induced by ATP depletion in avian and amphibian erythrocyte membranes, Biochim. Biophys. Acta 382:65-72 (1975).

24. T. J. C. Higgins, P. J. Bailey, and D. Allsopp, The influence of ATP depletion on the action of phospholipase c on cardiac myocyte membrane phospholipids, J. Mol. Cell. Cardiol. 13:1027-1030 (1981).

25. R. B. Jennings, H. K. Hawkins, J. E. Lowe, M. L. Hill, S. Klotman, and K. A. Reimer, Relation between high energy phosphate and lethal injury in myocardial ischemia in the dog, Am. J. Pathol. 92:187-214 (1978).

26. R. A. Haworth, D. R. Hunter, and H. A. Berkoff, Contracture in isolated adult rat heart cells. Role of Ca^{2+}, ATP and compartmentation. Circ. Res. 49:1119-1128 (1981).

27. A. M. Katz, Effects of ischemia on the contractile processes of heart muscle, Am. J. Cardiol. 32:456-460 (1973).

28. O. H. L. Bing, W. W. Brooks, and J. V. Messer, Heart muscle viability following hypoxia: protective effect of acidosis, Science 180:1292-1298 (1973).

29. W. G. Nayler, R. Ferrari, P. A. Poole-Wilson, and C. E. Yepez. A protective effect of a mild acidosis on hypoxic heart muscle, J. Mol. Cell. Cardiol. 11:1053-1071 (1979).

30. D. Acosta, and C. P. Li, Actions of extracellular acidosis on primary cultures of rat myocardial cells deprived of oxygen and glucose, J. Mol. Cell. Cardiol. 12:1459-1463 (1980).

VASCULAR METABOLISM AND ENERGETICS

Richard J. Paul, Ronald M. Lynch and Joseph M. Krisanda

University of Cincinnati
College of Medicine
Department of Physiology & Biophysics
Cincinnati, OH 45267-0576

INTRODUCTION

The coordination of energy metabolism with energy utilization is crucial to all cells. The matching of ATP utilization with ATP synthesis is particularly critical to normal vascular function because the amount of its preformed phosphagen {ATP plus phosphocreatine (PCr)} is small relative to the rates of utilization concomitant with contraction. The oft cited, but still useful example indicative of this situation is the fact that the preformed phosphagen store would be exhausted before the peak of an isometric contraction is obtained.

Figure 1 shows the time course of an isometric contraction in hog carotid artery and the phosphagen content at various stages (Krisanda & Paul, 1983c). Coordination of ATP synthesis with its utilization is so efficient that no change in the phosphagen pool can be detected in spite of a utilization rate which would exhaust the preformed pool by within 60 seconds. In vascular energy metabolism the flux of ATP through intermediary metabolism thus plays the major role in meeting the immediate contractile energy requirements. This is a different strategy than employed by skeletal muscle in which contractile ATP requirements are met via a large pool of PCr, the resynthesis of which occurs generally after the contractile event. In the past decade much attention in vascular energetics has thus focused on the relations between the rates of intermediary metabolism and the various mechanical and ionic events altered during stimulation in vascular smooth muscle (VSM). This brief review will focus on two aspects of these studies which we feel are likely to be major areas of VSM research in the next decade: a) vascular energy metabolism appears to be functionally, if not structurally compartmentalized; and b) the rate of cross bridge cycling by the contractile apparatus appears to be modulated by intracellular Ca^{2+} in a manner which is independent of force generation—this has renewed interest in a major question in VSM energe-

375

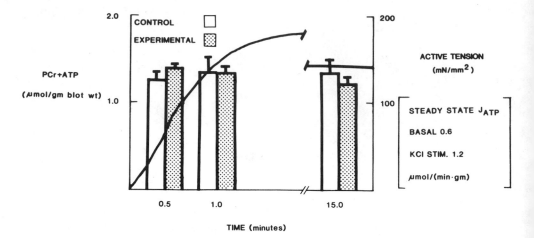

Figure 1. *Tissue phosphagen content (ATP + PCr) as a function of time after initiation of contraction with added KCl at 37°C. Tissue phosphagen is expressed as μmol/g tissue blot weight (mean ± SEM). The time course of isometric tension (solid line) is expressed in mN/mm². Data represent values collected from control and experimental tissues (n= 4-6) frozen by immersion in freon cooled in liquid N₂ at 0, 0.5, 1, and 15 minutes after initiation of contraction and extracted in methanol-EDTA. Inset (lower righthand corner) gives basal and steady state rates of ATP hydrolysis (J_{ATP}) in μmol/min·g determined from measurements of intermediary metabolism. From Krisanda and Paul (1983) Am. J. Physiol. 244:C385-C390 (with permission).*

tics: what mechanisms underlie the high economy of tension maintenance in smooth muscle compared to skeletal muscle?

Functional Compartmentation of VSM Energy Metabolism

In terms of ATP synthesis VSM is primarily dependent on oxidative phosphorylation (Paul, 1980). However, even under fully oxygenated conditions, VSM is characterized by substantial lactate production. While relatively small in terms of ATP production (<30%), aerobic lactate production can account for over 90% of the glucose entering the cell. This inefficient use of glucose by VSM has been an enigma to students of vascular metabolism, particularly as this phenomenon is a characteristic of a very small number of cell types, such as tumor cell lines (Racker, 1977).

Further impetus to the study of this unusual glycolytic component has come from evidence suggesting that an increase in glycolytic metabolism relative to oxidative metabolism is associated with disease states such as hypertension and atherosclerosis (Daly, 1976; Morrison et al., 1972).

Recent evidence has shown that oxidative metabolism and aerobic glycolysis can be varied independently depending on experimental conditions. For example both added KCl (80mM) and ouabain (10^{-5}M) contract porcine coronary arteries and increase the rate of oxygen consumption (J_{O_2}). However, the rate of lactate production (J_{lac}) is increased by added KCl whereas it is inhibited in the presence of ouabain (Paul, Bauer & Pease, 1979; Paul, 1983a). Along similar lines, isoproterenol added to a KCl-induced contracture relaxes isometric force and J_{O_2} returns to baseline but J_{lac} remains at maximally elevated rates (Paul, 1983c). Similar dissociation of oxidative metabolism and lactate production has been reported for porcine carotid artery (Glück and Paul, 1977; Peterson, 1982), rat portal vein (Hellstrand, Jorup and Lydrup, 1983), rat aorta (Kutchai and Geddis, 1982) and for non-vascular smooth muscle (Casteels and Wuytack, 1975; Rubanyi et al., 1982). The independence of these metabolic components suggested that trivial explanations such as the lack of oxidative capacity or local anoxia could not explain the large component of aerobic lactate production observed in smooth muscle. The independence of J_{O_2} and J_{lac} also suggested that the ATP provided by these pathways may be responding to the demands of different ATP utilizing processes. It has been shown for a wide variety of vascular smooth muscle types that in the steady state J_{O_2} is correlated with the level of active isometric force (see Paul, 1980; Hellstrand and Paul, 1982). Recent work (to be discussed below) places some restrictions on this observation, but in general this result has stood the test of time.

Aerobic lactate production on the other hand, while correlated with force under many situations (Peterson and Paul, 1974) appears to be more strongly related to Na-K transport. A critical experiment pointing to this conclusion is the study of the effects of ouabain (Paul et al., 1979), an inhibitor of the Na-K ATPase. Ouabain increases isometric force in most vascular preparations and J_{O_2} measured in porcine coronary and carotid arteries increases in parallel. J_{lac}, however, is inhibited by ouabain. Stimulation of Na-K transport with added KCl on the other hand, increases J_{lac} and as the depolarization also elicits a contraction, P_0 and J_{O_2} are increased.

Table 1 summarizes the results of a variety of experiments in which the metabolic responses to altering contractile and Na-K transport conditions were studied. The correlations between J_{O_2} and force and that of J_{lac} and Na-K transport can be seen under a variety of conditions. These results appear to be qualitatively similar for a wide range of vascular smooth muscles including both tonic muscles (Paul, 1983a) and the phasic rat portal vein (Hellstrand et al., 1983) although less than the complete

TABLE 1: Changes in Contractile, Metabolic and Na-K Transport Parameters from Basal Levels in Porcine Carotid Artery

CONDITIONS	ISOMETRIC FORCE	OXYGEN CONSUMPTION	LACTATE PRODUCTION	Na-K TRANSPORT	PHOSPHORYLASE a ACTIVITY	GLUCOSE UPTAKE
(Changes with Respect to Basal, Unstimulated Conditions)						
KCL (80 mM)	↑	↑	↑	↑	↑	↑
KCL+ Isoproterenol	↓	↓	↑	↑	↑	
Ouabain (10^{-5}M)	↑	↑	↓	↓	↑	—
Na$^+$-free (K+ substitution)	↑	↑	↓	↓		—
K$^+$-free	↑	↑	↓	↓		

separability of J_{lac} and J_{O_2} is observed in the latter. Rat aorta in our laboratory appeared to be an exception in that K$^+$-free and ouabain both stimulated total J_{lac} (Paul, 1983a; Garwitz and Paul, unpublished observations). However, lactate production from exogenous glucose (see below) has been reported to be inhibited by ouabain and stimulated by gramicidin in this tissue (Kutchai and Geddis,1982) which is compatible with the proposed functional coupling. Thus, while one must always use caution when generalizing about vascular smooth muscle, evidence is accumulating which suggests that the functional correlations described here may indeed reflect a general pattern.

The functional compartmentation observed in vascular smooth muscle raises many questions about the organization of cellular metabolism. Of particular interest is whether it is a reflection of a structural compartmentation or some less tightly coupled diffusional compartmentation, wherein the proximity of ATP utilizing processes to oxidative or glycolytic sources determines the functional coupling. Models for the close association of transport and glycolytic enzymes in the erythrocyte membrane (Parker and Hoffman, 1967; Mercer and Dunham, 1981) and sarcoplasmic reticulum (Entman et al., 1977) have been proposed.

One approach that we have employed to further our understanding of this functional compartmentation has been to identify the control points for carbohydrate catabolism in VSM. Glycogen phosphorylase, a key regulatory enzyme in glycogenolysis, has been shown to be an integral part of a large enzyme complex known as the "glycogen particle" which is associated with the sarcoplasmic reticulum in skeletal muscle. Similar types of structures have been postulated for the erythrocyte plasmalemma. Our attention focused initially on the activity of this enzyme in order to test the hypothesis that it is a control point for aerobic glycolysis and hence Na-K ATPase activity in VSM. As indicated by the direction of changes summarized in Table 1, phosphorylase activity is not necessarily correlated with J_{lac} (Paul, 1983c). For example, when J_{lac} is inhibited in the presence of ouabain phosphorylase activity is found to be increased. Thus phosphorylase is unlikely to be closely involved in the regulation of aerobic glycolysis in VSM.

Studies of the control of glycolysis proved to be of particular significance in that they have indicated the existence of a glucose transport system which may be regulated in VSM. Under resting conditions the intracellular glucose concentration in porcine carotid artery is zero (Lynch and Paul, 1983), indicating that glucose entry into the cell is the rate limiting step for glucose utilization. This also is true for bovine mesenteric artery and guinea pig taenia coli (Arnqvist, 1977) but not apparently for rabbit aorta (Yalcin and Winegrad, 1963). One might anticipate that the inhibition of J_{lac} by ouabain reflects an inhibition of glucose transport. Recent experiments (Lynch and Paul, 1982) utilizing 3-0-methyl glucose as a measure of glucose uptake have shown that glucose transport, however, is not affected by ouabain. Furthermore, under these conditions intracellular glucose content increases. These observations indicate that inhibition of Na-K transport by ouabain is coupled with a direct inhibition of glycolysis rather than glucose transport. Stimulation of Na-K transport with added KCl on the other hand leads to an increase in J_{lac} while intracellular glucose remains zero. Under these conditions glucose uptake is increased which implies that glucose transport must be regulated (Lynch and Paul, 1983).

To place these experiments in perspective, identification of the substrate source(s) for the aerobic production of lactate was essential. Either glucose uptake or glycogen breakdown measured during a KCl contracture would be sufficient to account for most of the lactate produced. Studies on the metabolic fate of exogenous glucose (Lynch and Paul, 1983) have indicated that under resting conditions glucose is the sole source of aerobic lactate production. Furthermore, in spite of a substantial breakdown of glycogen during a KCl-induced contracture exogenous glucose remains the sole substrate for aerobic lactate production. Thus glycogenolysis and glycolysis operate within separate compartments in this VSM. Preliminary evidence indicates that the glycosyl units from glycogen are oxidized during a KCl contracture. Therefore although VSM is reported

COMPARTMENTATION OF
CARBOHYDRATE METABOLISM

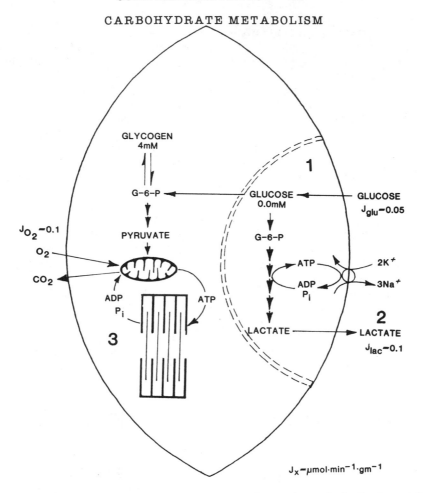

Figure 2. *Schematic representation of carbohydrate utiliza-tion by vascular smooth muscle. (1) Glucose is the sole sub-strate for aerobic lactate production in unstimulated and high K^+ depolarized porcine carotid arteries. Since glucose transport is rate limiting for its utilization, transport must be regulated under conditions were carbohydrate utilization is increased. (2) Aerobic glycolysis can account for 95% of glucose uptake. Alter-ations in aerobic glycolysis independent of oxidative metabolism indicate a functional compartmentation of carbohydrate metabol-ism. (3) Actomyosin interaction (force generation) exhibits a linear relationship to oxygen consumption. Glucosyl units der-ived from glycogen during treatment with high K^+ appear to be used exclusively as an oxidative substrate in coordination with tension generation. The rates are approximate values expressed as $\mu mol/min \cdot g$.*

to utilize free fatty acids as the primary oxidative substrate under resting conditions (Chace and Odessey, 1981), it appears to also utilize glycogen under the increased energy demands concomitant with contracture. In this respect, VSM may exhibit a substrate mobilization pattern similar to that of skeletal muscle (McGilvery, 1974). Our results on the energy metabolism of VSM are schematically summarized in Fig. 2.

Three types of findings are of particular interest: (1) The ATP requirements for the actomyosin ATPase and Na-K ATPase are met by oxidative phosphorylation and aerobic glycolysis respectively; (2) This functional compartmentation reflects a distinct biochemical compartmentation in that glycogenolysis and glycolysis operate via separate enzymatic pools; (3) glucose transport is rate limiting for glycolysis and hence a mechanism for regulating glucose transport must be present in VSM. The last point may be of particular significance to certain vascular disease states in which both Na-K transport (Garwitz and Jones, 1982; Jones, 1973) and carbohydrate metabolism (Daly, 1972; Morrison et al., 1976) are known to be altered.

Vascular Smooth Muscle Energetics

One of the most striking characteristics of VSM is the low rate of ATP hydrolysis required for maintenance of force relative to that of skeletal muscle. The tension cost of porcine carotid artery may be up to 2000-fold less than that of mammalian skeletal muscle. This makes vascular muscle ideally suited for its role in maintenance of vessel caliber in the regulation of circulation. The mechanisms underlying this economy of VSM operation have intrigued muscle physiologists for over 100 years, particularly as the major components of the VSM contractile apparatus, actin and myosin, are grossly similar to those of skeletal muscle. Three major types of hypotheses have been put forth (see Rüegg, 1971): (1) structural factors, such as longer effective sarcomeres in smooth relative to skeletal muscle (Paul & Rüegg, 1978); (2) lower inherent actomyosin ATPase, such as that related to inherent differences in actin-myosin binding (Krisanda and Murphy, 1980; Greene et al., 1983) and (3) modification of the cross bridge cycle rate by special mechanisms associated with "catch" (see Rüegg, 1971) or "latch" states (Murphy et al., 1983).

Although structural differences are evident (Ashton, Somlyo and Somlyo, 1975) most estimates of their effect on the tension cost are less than 10-fold (Paul, 1980). Differences in the ATPase of the isolated actomyosin can be substantial, up to two orders of magnitude have been reported (Marston and Taylor, 1980). While it is difficult to directly relate the actomyosin ATPase of the isolated proteins to the activity in the intact, structured smooth muscle, comparison of the tension-dependent ATPase in living porcine carotid artery to that estimated from isolated actomyosin agree quite closely (Glück and Paul, 1977). Recent attention has been focused on the role of factors which may directly modulate the cross bridge cycle. Dillon et al. (1981) reported that the speed at which porcine carotid artery could shorten declined with the duration following stimulation in spite of the maintenance of constant isometric force. The time course of this decline in shortening speed paralleled that of the phosphorylation state of the myosin light chain ($MLC-P_i$). It was speculated that myosin phosphorylation increased the cross bridge cycle rate as indicated by the changes in shortening velocity and postulated that such changes could also be reflected in the measurements of the rate of ATP utilization. A role for myosin phosphorylation in the regulation of skeletal muscle energetics has also been proposed (Crow and Kushmerick, 1982). However, a relation between $MLC-P_i$ and energy utilization has been questioned in both smooth (Butler and Siegman, 1983) and skeletal (Butler et al., 1983) muscle.

In order to evaluate the role of cross bridge cycle alterations in the overall economy of VSM, the time course of ATP utilization was studied. As indicated in the introduction, because the phosphagen content in VSM is maintained in a steady state from as early as 30 seconds after initiation of contraction, the rate of O_2 consumption can be used as a direct measure of the tissue ATP utilization. The conversion of J_{O_2} to J_{ATP} requires assumption of a stoichiometric ratio. In rat portal vein, the ratio between phosphagen breakdown and oxygen consumption agrees with the theoretically maximal P:O ratio of 3 (Hellstrand and Paul, 1983). It is of interest to note that this is not the case for amphibian skeletal muscle (Paul, 1983b; Kushmerick and Paul, 1976).

As shown in Fig. 3, the rate of O_2 consumption in porcine carotid artery declines from a maximum during the maintenance of constant levels of isometric force. This is also true for rat portal vein (Hellstrand and Paul, 1983). The rate of unloaded shortening velocity (V_{us}), also shown in Fig. 3, exhibits a similar, though not identical, time course. In addition, we have shown that the activity of phosphorylase also shows a similar biphasic time course (Paul, 1983d; Galvas et al., 1981). Thus while isometric force is increasing or constant, J_{ATP}, V_{us} and phosphorylase activity all decrease in the range of 2-4 fold. Whether relations between these correlated parameters exist is conjectural. Murphy et al. (1983) have suggested that shortening velocity and $MLC-P_i$ changes may be related to changes in intracellular Ca^{2+} with time. This hypothesis is supported by recent studies using aequorin to measure the time course of intracellular Ca^{2+} concentration in vascular smooth muscle (Morgan & Morgan, 1982).

Using "chemically skinned" VSM preparations in which the myofibrillar Ca^{2+} concentration can be fixed by the level in the bathing solution, it was shown that unloaded shortening velocity was maintained at relatively constant levels once the maximum speed was obtained (Paul et al., 1983). This was in contrast to the biphasic response observed in living VSM (Krisanda and Paul, 1983a). In addition both isometric force and velocity were Ca^{2+} dependent in the skinned fiber preparation. Interestingly, velocity could be increased after isometric force had reached a maximal

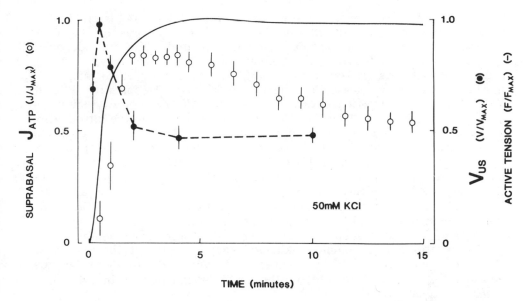

Figure 3. Time course of suprabasal ATP utilization (J_{ATP}), unloaded shortening velocity (V_{us}) and active isometric tension for porcine carotid artery strips stimulated with 50 mM KCl. The steady state J_{ATP} was 0.51 µmol ATP/ min·g (n=11). The steady state V_{us} was 0.008 ± 0.002 muscle lengths/ second (n=10). Maximum active isometric tension was 170 ± 9 mN/mm² (n=11). Data is represented as mean ± SEM. Standard error bars for tension were not included for figure clarity. The tension data did not vary by more that 5% of the mean.

value. ATPase activity in "chemically skinned" taenia coli (Güth and Junge, 1982) was also Ca^{2+} dependent and, similar to V_{us}, could be increased by increasing Ca^{2+} following saturation of the isometric force response. These results suggested that cross bridge cycle rate can be altered independent of isometric force, i.e. that Ca^{2+} controls not only the number of cross bridges but also the kinetics of the cross bridge cycle. Thus a lowering of intracellular Ca^{2+} during an isometric contraction could decrease V_{us} without appreciably changing isometric force if the dependence on Ca^{2+} in the living preparation is similar to that observed in the "chemically skinned" fibers.

In living smooth muscle, the level of intracellular Ca^{2+} is difficult to know with certainty, but it can be altered by changes in the Ca^{2+} concentration of the physiological salt solution used. The dependence of velocity in living VSM on extracellular Ca^{2+} is controversial, although recent experiments (Krisanda and Paul, 1983b; Arner, 1983) support a marked dependency. Based on the observations in "chemically skinned" VSM, a nonlinear relation between force and ATPase activity might be anticipated at high Ca^{++} levels. However, as alluded to in the introduction J_{ATP} is linearly related to force in many VSM (Paul, 1980), though the tension–cost has been reported to be dependent on the mode of stimulation (Hellstrand, 1977; Peterson, 1982). Therefore experiments at high extracellular Ca^{2+} concentrations were conducted to investigate whether the J_{ATP} could be altered independent of isometric force (Krisanda and Paul, 1983b). The ratio of J_{ATP} to force in living porcine carotid artery (tension cost) was found to be constant up to 1.6 mM Ca^{2+}_{o} but increased by a factor of 3 at Ca^{2+}_{o} between 1.6 and 7.5 mM. These experiments confirm the observations in "chemically skinned" VSM and support the hypothesis that Ca^{2+} controls both the number and cycle rate of cross bridges. Whether this effect is mediated by the Ca^{2+}-dependent myosin light chain kinase remains to be clarified.

The magnitude of the modulation of velocity or J_{ATP} is reported to be in the range of 2-4. Therefore, we do not believe that it is the major determinant of the overall high economy of VSM which we feel more likely to be related to intrinsic differences in the actomyosin ATPase. The ability of VSM to trade velocity for lower tension cost would be of substantial physiological significance.

ACKNOWLEDGEMENTS

We should like to acknowledge the excellent technical assitance of Glen Doerman and Christopher Kuettner and the word processing skills of Anita Tolle.

This work was supported by Grants AHA 78-1080, USPHS 23240, 22619. R.J.P is presently an Established Investigator of the Americam Heart Association.

REFERENCES

Arner, A. Force-velocity relation in chemically skinned rat portal vein: effects of Ca^{2+} and Mg^{2+}. Pflügers Arch. European J. Physiol. 397:6-12, 1983.

Arnqvist, H.J. Glucose transport and metabolism in smooth muscle; action of insulin and diabetes. In: The Biochemistry of Smooth Muscle, N.L. Stephens (ed.) Baltimore: Univ. Park, 1977.

Ashton, F.T., A.V. Somlyo, and A.P. Somlyo. The contractile apparatus of vascular smooth muscle: intermediate high voltage stereo electron microscopy. J. Mol. Biol. 98:17-29, 1975.

Butler, T.M. and M.J. Siegman. Chemical energy usage and myosin light chain phosphorylation in mammalian smooth muscle. Federation Proc. 42:57-61, 1983.

Butler, T.M., M.J. Siegman, S.V. Mooers, and R.J. Barsotti. Myosin light chain phosphorylation does not modulate cross-bridge cycling rate in mouse skeletal muscle. Science 220:1167-1169, 1983.

Casteels, R. and F. Wuytack. Aerobic and anaerobic metabolism in smooth muscle cells of taenia coli in relation to active ion transport. J. Physiol. (Lond.) 250:203-220, 1975.

Chace, K.V. and R. Odessy. The utilization by rabbit aorta of carbohydrates, fatty acids, ketone bodies and amino acids as substrates for energy production. Circ. Res. 48(6):850-858, 1981.

Crow, M.T., and M.J. Kushmerick. Myosin light chain phosphorylation is associated with a decrease in the energy cost for contraction in fast twitch mouse muscle. J. Biol. Chem. 257:2121-2124, 1982.

Daly, M.M. Effect of age and hypertension on utilization of glucose by rat aorta. Am. J. Physiol. 230:30-33, 1976.

Dillon, P.F., M.O. Aksoy, S.P. Driska, and R.A. Murphy. Myosin phosphorylation and the cross-bridge cycle in arterial smooth muscle. Science 211:495-497, 1981.

Entman, M.L., E.P. Bornet, W.B. Van Winkle, M.A. Goldstein and A. Schwartz. Association of glycogenolysis with cardiac sarcoplasmic reticulum: II. Effect of glycogen depletion, deoxycholate solubilization and cardiac ischemia: evidence for a phosphorylase kinase membrane complex. J. Mol. Cell. Cardiol. 9:515-528, 1977.

Galvas, P., C. Kuettner, J. DiSalvo, and R.J. Paul. Temporal relations among active isometric force (P_0), cAMP-dependent protein kinase (cPKs) and phosphorylase in bovine coronary arteries (Abstract). Physiologist 24:119, 1981.

Garwitz, E.T. and A.W. Jones. Altered ion transport and its reversal in aldosterone hypertensive rat. Am. J. Physiol. 243(Heart Circ. Physiol. 12):H927-H933, 1982.

Glück, E.V., and R.J. Paul. The aerobic metabolism of porcine carotid artery and its relationship to isometric force: energy cost of isometric contraction. Pflügers Arch. European J. Physiol. 370:9-18, 1977.

Greene, L.E., J.R. Sellers, E. Eisenberg, and R.S. Adelstein. Binding of gizzard smooth muscle myosin subfragment, to actin in the presence and absence of adenosine 5'-triphosphate. Biochemistry 22:530-535, 1983.

Güth, K. and Junge, J. Low Ca^{++} impedes cross-bridge detachment in chemically skinned taenia coli. Nature 300:775-776, 1982.

Hellstrand, P., Oxygen consumption and lactate production of the rat portal vein in relation to contractile activity. Acta Physiol. Scand. 100:91-106, 1977.

Hellstrand, P., C. Jorup and M.L. Lydrup, O_2 consumption, aerobic glycolysis and tissue phosphagen content during activation of the Na^+/K^+ pump in rat portal vein. 1983 (In Press).

Hellstrand, P. and R.J. Paul. Phosphagen content, breakdown during contraction, and O_2 consumption in rat portal vein. Am. J. Physiol. 244:C250–C258, 1983.

Hellstrand, P. and R.J. Paul. Vascular smooth muscle: relation between energy metabolism and mechanics. In: Crass, M.F. III and Barnes, C.D. (eds.) <u>Vascular Smooth Muscle: Metabolism, Ionic and Contractile Mechanisms</u>, Academic Press, Inc., New York, pp. 1–36, 1982.

Jones, A.W. Altered ion transport in vascular smooth muscle from spontaneously hypertensive rats. Circ. Res. 23(5):563–571, 1973.

Krisanda, J.M., and R.A. Murphy. Tight binding of arterial myosin to skeletal F–actin. J. Biol. Chem. 255:10771–10776, 1980.

Krisanda, J.M. and R.J. Paul. Energetics of isometric contraction in porcine carotid artery. Am. J. Physiol., 1983a (in press).

Krisanda, J.M. and R.J. Paul. Is the economy of tension maintenance in vascular smooth muscle (VSM) independent of force or $(Ca^{2+})_o$? (Abstract) Federation Proc. 42:1633, 1983b.

Krisanda, J.M. and R.J. Paul. Phosphagen and metabolic content during contraction in porcine carotid artery. Am. J. Physiol. 244:C385–C390, 1983c.

Kushmerick, M.J. and R.J. Paul. Relationship between initial chemical reactions and oxidative recovery metabolism for single isometric contractions of frog sartorius at 0°C. J. Physiol. London 254:711–727, 1976.

Kutchai, H. and L.M. Geddis. Control of glycolytic rate in rat aorta (Abstract) Federation Proc. 41:450, 1982.

Lynch, R.M. and R.J. Paul. Metabolic compartmentation in vascular smooth muscle: effect of ouabain on glucose transport and catabolism. Fed. Proc. 41(4):983, 1982.

Lynch, R.M. and R.J. Paul. Compartmentation of glycolytic and glycogenolytic metabolism in vascular smooth muscle. (Abstract) Federation Proc. 42(3):647, 1983.

Marston, S.B. and E.W. Taylor. Comparison of the myosin and actomyosin ATPase mechanisms of the four types of vertebrate muscles. J. Mol. Biol. 139:573–600, 1980.

McGilvery, R.W. The use of fuels for muscular work. In. Metabolic Adaptation to Prolonged Physical Exercise (ed.) H. Howald, and J. Poortmans, Birkhauser Velag Basal, 1975.

Mercer, R.W. and P.B. Dunham. Membrane–bound ATP fuels the Na/K pump: studies on membrane-bound glycolytic enzymes on inside-out vesicles from human red blood cell membranes. J. Gen. Physiol. 78:547–568, 1981.

Morgan, J.P. and K.G. Morgan. Vascular smooth muscle: the first recorded Ca^{2+} transients. Pflügers Arch. European J. Physiol. 395:75–77, 1982.

Morrison, E.S., R.F. Scott, M. Kroms and J. Frick. Glucose degradation in normal and atherosclerotic aortic intima-media. Atherosclerosis 16:175–184, 1972.

Murphy, R.A., M.O. Aksoy, D.F. Dillon, W.T. Gerthotter, and K.E. Kamm. The role of myosin light chain phosphorylation in regulation of the cross bridge cycle. Federation Proc. 42:51-56, 1983.

Parker, J.C. and J.F. Hoffman. The role of membrane phosphoglycerate kinase in the control of glycolytic rate by active cation transport in human red blood cells. J. Gen. Physiol. 50:893-916, 1967.

Paul, R.J. Chemical energetics of vascular smooth muscle. In: Handbook of Physiology, edited by D.F. Bohr, H.V. Sparks & A.R. Somlyo. Maryland: American Physiological Society, 1980, vol. II, Sec. 2, p. 201-235.

Paul, R.J. Functional compartmentation of oxidative and glycolytic metabolism in vascular smooth muscle. Am. J. Physiol. 244(Cell Physiol. 13):C399-C409, 1983a.

Paul, R.J. Physical and biochemical energy balance during an isometric tetanus and steady state recovery in frog sartorium at 0°C. J. Gen. Physiol. 81:337-354, 1983b.

Paul, R.J. The effects of isoproterenol and ouabain on oxygen consumption, lactate production, and the activities of phosphorylase in coronary artery smooth muscle. Circ. Res. 52:683-690, 1983c.

Paul, R.J. Coordination of metabolism and contractility in vascular smooth muscle. Federation Proc. 42:62-66, 1983d.

Paul, R.J., M. Bauer and W. Pease. Vascular smooth muscle: aerobic glycolysis linked to Na-K transport processes. Science 206:1414-1416, 1979.

Paul, R.J., G. Doerman, C. Zeugner, and J.C. Rüegg. The dependence of unloaded shortening velocity on Ca^{++}, calmodulin, and duration of contraction in "chemically skinned" smooth muscle. Circ. Res., 53:342-351, 1983.

Paul, R.J. and J.C. Rüegg. Biochemistry of vascular smooth muscle: energy metabolism and proteins of the contractile apparatus. In: Microcirculation, edited by B.M. Altura and G. Kaley. Baltimore: Univ. Park, 1978, vol. II, p. 41-82.

Peterson, J.W. Effect of histamine on the energy metabolism of K^+-depolarized hog carotid artery. Circ. Res. 50:848-855, 1982.

Peterson, J.W. and R.J. Paul. Aerobic glycolysis in vascular smooth muscle: relation to isometric tension. Biochim. Biophys. Acta 357:167-176, 1974.

Racker, E. Why do tumor cells have a high aerobic glycolysis? J. Cell Physiol. 89:697-700, 1977.

Rubanyi, G., A. Toth and A.G.B. Kovach. Distinct effect of contraction and ion transport on NADH fluorescence and lactate production in uterine smooth muscle. Acta Physiol. Acad. Sci. Hung. 59(1):45-58, 1982.

Rüegg, J.C. Smooth muscle tone. Physiol. Rev. 51:201-248, 1971.

Yalcin, S. and A.I. Winegrad. Defect in glucose metabolism in aortic tissue from alloxan diabetic rabbits. Am. J. Physiol. 205(6):1253-1259, 1963.

MYOCARDIAL GLUTAMATE DEHYDROGENASE ACTIVITY

Huey G. McDaniel, and Ronald L. Jenkins

Veterans Administration Medical Center
University of Alabama School of Medicine
Birmingham, Alabama

INTRODUCTION

Glutamic dehydrogenase (GDH) has not been thought to play an important role in cardiac metabolism in the past. Aspartate aminotransferase was shown to mediate glutamate utilization by mitochondria and there was thought to be little GDH activity in heart mitochondria.[1] However, the studies of Godinot et al showed that this enzyme could be purified from pig heart mitochondria and had different properties from the enzyme of beef liver mito- chondria.[2] Takala et al showed that the perfused rat heart pro- duced ammonia and this appeared to come from GDH rather than the purine nucleotide cycle.[3] Ammonia production was stimulated when the perfused heart was working. Studies using pig heart mitochon- dria indicated that glutamate was oxidized via glutamate dehydroge- nase when the mitochondria were oxidizing certain substrates.[4] Studies by Nuutinen et al showed that rat heart mitochondria readily formed ammonia from glutamate.[5]

We have subsequently isolated and characterized glutamic dehydrogenase from rat heart mitochondria.[6,7] We have shown that rat heart also contains cytosolic glutamic dehydrogenase activity which is different from the mitochondrial enzyme.[8] This report deals with the metabolic role of glutamic dehydrogenase in heart and further definition of some of the physical differences in cytosolic and mitochondrial GDH activity.

METHODS AND MATERIALS

Rat hearts were homogenized with nargase and the mitochondria were isolated as previously described.[6] Washed mitochondria, equivalent to 5.0 mg protein were incubated at 30°C, pH 7.2, in 3.11 ml of media containing glutamate, 20 mM; Tris-HCl 15 mM, KH_2PO_4, 15 mM; KCl, 85 mM; MgCl, 4 mM; and either pyruvate, malate or octanoate, 4.0 mM. The rate of oxygen uptake was monitored by a Yellow Springs Instrument system following the addition of ADP, 2.5 mM, to spur state III respiration. As oxygen was depleted, reactions were stopped with 2.0 ml of cold 6% perchloric acid. Proteins were removed by centrifugation and the perchloric acid was neutralized with 7.0 N potassium hydroxide in the cold. Potassium perchlorate percipitate was then removed by centrifugation and the various metabolites were analyzed.

Ammonia was measured enzymatically by the reductive amination reaction of glutamic dehydrogenase. Appropriate blanks were run to correct for ammonia contamination of the reagents. Alpha-keto-gluterate and glutamate were also determined with glutamic dehydro-genase.[10] Aspartate was measured enzymatically.[11] Alanine was measured using a Beckman Amino Acid Analyzer. ATP was measured by bioluminescence with the Liciferase-Luciferin reaction in a LKB luminometer. GTP was similarly measured following concentration by lyophilization, separation by ascending chromatography on cellulose in a n-propanol/ammonia/water system and conversion to ATP by nucleotide diphosphate kinase.[12]

Glutamic dehydrogenase from homogenized and sonicated rat heart and liver mitochondria was fractionated in ammonium sulfate.[6] The 40-60% pellets were reconstituted in tris EDTA pH 7.6 and gel filtration was performed with a Bio Gel A 1.5 M column (1.7 cm x 57 cm) at a 6 cm/hr flow rate. The buffer solution contained tris-HCl, 50 mM; pH 7.6, ADP, 1.0 mM; and ammonium sulfate, 0 to 400 mM. The column was calibrated with standard protein from Bio Gel which was the same in 0 and 400 mM ammonium salfate.

RESULTS

Rat heart mitochondrial GDH gave a series of peaks on Bio Gel A 1.5 M at low ammonium sulfate concentrations. There was a major peak at 240,000 Daltons, a minor peak at 305,000 Daltons and a series of larger molecular weight species.[6] When ammonium sulfate concentration of the column buffer was increased to 400 mM the mitochondrial GDH activity eluted as a single major 240,000 Dalton peak (Fig. 1).

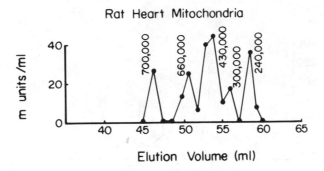

Rat Heart Mitochondria

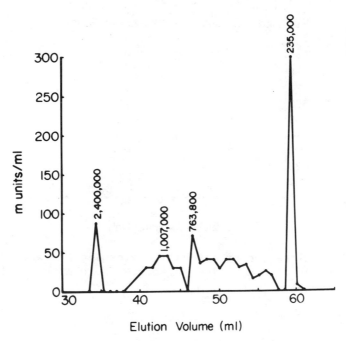

Rat Heart Mitochondria 0.4 Ammonium Sulfate

Fig. 1   Gel filtration of rat heart mitochondria GDH with and
without .4 M ammonium sulfate. The column was 1.7 cm x
57 cm. Bio Gel A 1.5 M.

When rat heart cytosolic GDH was subjected to gel filtration
under very low ammonium sulfate levels, the smaller molecular
species had apparent molecular weight of 242,000 and 332,000
Daltons (Fig. 2). Larger molecular species were also present.
With 400 mM ammonium sulfate there was a major peak at 340,000
Daltons and a minor peak at 1,180,000 Daltons.[8]

391

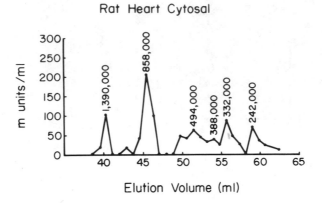

Rat Heart Cytosal

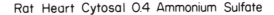

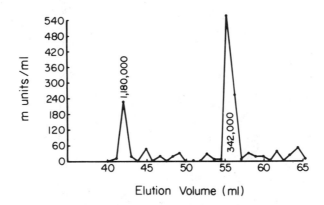

Rat Heart Cytosal 0.4 Ammonium Sulfate

Fig. 2   Gel filtration of rat heart cytosolic GDH with and
without .4 M ammonium sulfate. The column was 1.7 cm x
57 cm Bio Gel A 1.5 M.

When rat liver mitochondrial GDH was subjected to gel filtration under low ammonium sulfate levels a 230,000 Dalton peak, a
305,000 Dalton peak, and several larger polymer peaks eluted.
With 400 and 800 mM ammonium sulfate multiple peaks still disappeared. When the ammonium sulfate was increased to 1,200 mM only a
single peak eluted, which corresponded to a 50,000 Dalton molecular
weight (Fig. 3). This smaller molecular weight fraction was very
unstable and lost most of its activity overnight.

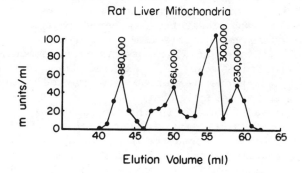

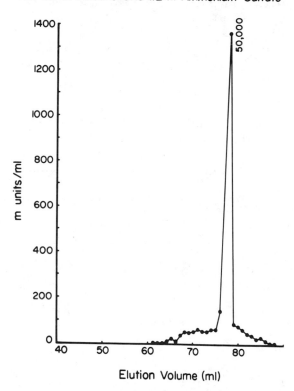

Fig. 3   Gel filtration of rat liver mitochondria GDH with and
           without 1.2 M ammonium sulfate. The column was 1.7 cm x
           57 cm Bio Gel A 1.5 M.

In order to define the function of GDH we incubated rat heart mitochondria with glutamate and various substrates. When glutamate and malate were the two substrates presented to the mitochondria in state III respiration very little ammonia was formed (Table 1). In the presence of pyruvate and glutamate however, ammonia production was greatly increased (Table 1). Alanine formation was also increased while aspartate formation was markedly decreased. Aspartate is badly underestimated in these studies because glutamate, malate and pyruvate in the incubation medium prevented the enzymatic assay from going to completion. Most of the glutamate utilization not accounted for by aspartate, alanine and ammonia is due to unmeasured aspartate. In the presence of octanoic acid, glutamate utilization fell to 25% of the value with either malate or pyruvate. Ammonia formation fell but accounted for a larger percent of glutamate utilization than with malate (Table 1). These studies were with state III respiration. State IV respiration with glutamate and pyruvate led to the active formation of ammonia (Table 1).

Table 1. Mean levels of glutamate (nM ± SEM) utilized and levels of alpha-glutarate, aspartate, alanine and ammonia (nM ± SEM) produced by respiring rat heart mitochondria.

| Substrates | State III | | | State IV |
	Glutamate & Malate	Glutamate & Pyruvate	Glutamate & Octanoate	Glutamate & Pyruvate
Glutamate Utilized	2,002 ± 271	2,334 ± 329	506 ± 115	2,112
α–Keto–glutarate Content	463 ± 148	2,416 ± 201	216 ± 111	1,798
Aspartate Content	675 ± 22	55 ± 7	161 ± 26	195
Alanine Content	307 ± 103	694 ± 203	320 ± 90	1,172
Ammonia Content	40 ± 17	764 ± 99	71 ± 15	778

Table 2. Mean levels of oxygen utilized and ATP & GTP produced by respiring rat heart myoctye mitochondria.

| Substrates | State III | | | State IV |
	Glutamate & Malate	Glutamate & Pyruvate	Glutamate & Octanoate	Glutamate & Pyruvate
nAO_2 Utilized	1,388 ± 18	1,388 ± 6	1,379 ± 27	388
nAO_2/min/mg Protein	134	102	75	6.7
Respiratory Control	7.3	4.8	2.0	---
ATP mM ± SEM	2.30 ± .81	.65 ± .19	.47 ± .02	.20
GTP (nM) ± SEM	1.12 ± .12	.79 ± .54	3.09 ± .90	2.86

Oxygen utilization and ATP and GTP content varied with each substrate (Table 2). Oxygen utilization rate was greatest with malate and least with octanoic acid. The respiratory control and ADP to oxygen ratio indicated that the mitochondria were tightly coupled. Total oxygen utilization in the state III studies was similar with all three substrates because it was allowed to proceed to the same point. ATP content was much greater in the presence of malate. GTP content was greatest in the presence of octanoic acid and least in the presence of pyruvate during state III respiration (Table 2).

DISCUSSION

The conversion of glutamate to alpha-ketoglutarate is a key metabolic reaction which interrelates amino acid and carbohydrate metabolism. In one direction it fixes ammonia (conserving nitrogen), forming the important amino acid glutamate. In the other direction it provides alpha-ketoglutarate, a citric acid cycle component, and ammonia, which easily exits the organelle or cellular site of formation. The need of each organ for this bidirectional reaction is varied. The liver converts amine groups via glutamate and the urea cycle into urea, a nitrogenous end-product excreted in the urine. In the kidney ammonia is formed from glutamate and neutralizes anions in the urine. The alpha-ketoglutarate formed is utilized for energy metabolism by the kidney.

In the heart there is a need for nitrogen conservation because of the constant turn over of ATP. This conservation is evidenced by the fact that the heart does not ordinarily release ammonia.[14] (Under certain circumstances the perfused heart releases ammonia). There is also a need to be able to generate energy from carbohydrates and lipids efficiently and rapidly for myocardial performance. By contrast, skeletal muscle has periods of quiescence between periods of contraction with ATP breakdown. Therefore, it can theoretically afford to be less conserving with nitrogen. This is evidenced by the fact that skeletal muscle releases ammonia (from purines) during contraction in a linear relation to the amount of work performed. The brain primarily uses carbohydrates for energy formation.

Because of the interaction of glutamate with nucleotides, it has been postulated that GDH is regulated by small effector molecules that alter its physical and kinetic properties.[15] Changes in th level of nucleotides or other small effector molecules were thought to regulate the direction and activity of this bidirectional reaction. The other means of regulation was by changes in the level of substrates.[15] Conversion of alpha-ketoglutarate to glutamate operates with NADP(H) while conversion of glutamate to alpha-ketoglutarate uses NAD(H).[4,15]

There have been sporadic reportings of the existence of GDH isoenzymes. The first of these reports employed gel electrophoresis, showing that mammalian tissue contained several GDH isoenzymes.[16] They found different levels of each isoenzyme in different organs. Others have reported GDH activity in liver nuclei with different kinetic properties from liver mitochondrial GDH.[17] Neurons were also reported to contain extramitochondria GDH.[18] GDH purified from pig heart was reported to have different kinetic properties from beef liver GDH.[2] Complicating the issue has been the fact that phospholipids, especially cardiolipin, at low levels bind and inhibit GDH activity.[19]

We have purified GDH from rat heart mitochondria and have shown that its subunit and monomer molecular weight are 20 to 25% smaller than rat liver mitochondrial GDH.[6] This difference was unchanged when the protease inhibitor phenylmethylsulfonyl fluoride (PMSF) was present and when rat heart and liver mitochondria were extracted together.[6] Therefore, it occured in vivo and was not due to degradation of heart mitochondrial GDH during preparation of the enzyme.

What is the function of heart mitochondrial GDH? Borst reported that mitochondrial oxidation of glutamate occurred via transamination.[20] Because of the abundance of alanine and aspartate aminotransferases, it has been thought that myocardial glutamate oxidation occurred by these two reactions. However, it was noted that epinephrine and myocardial work results in ammonia formation by the isolated perfused heart.[3,21] Adenine nucleotide levels were not decreased in the working heart so that the ammonia did not come from nucleotide deamination.[3] The authors postulated that GDH activity was increased in the working heart. Our studies have indicated that GDH activity in heart mitochondria depends upon the substrates being oxidized. In the presence of malate GDH activity was minimal. Only approximately 5% of the glutamate oxidized was accounted for by ammonia formation. In the presence of pyruvate, ammonia formation accounted for about 30% of glutamate oxidation. In the presence of octanoic acid, ammonia accounted for about 15% of the glutamate oxidized. Younes et al also showed significant ammonia production by pig heart mitochondria in the presence of pyruvate.[4]

We propose that glutamate oxidation in heart mitochondria depends upon the amount of oxaloacetate present (Fig. 4). When excess malate was available there was an abundant supply of oxalo-acetate for exchange with glutamate in the aspartate aminotrans-ferase reaction. When there was an excess of pyruvate or fatty acids, the excess of acetyl-CoA led to lower oxaloacetate levels. This happened because of the amount of citrate synthetase present in the heart and the higher affinity of citrate synthetase for oxaloacetate than aspartate aminotransferase. GTP content was in a concentration of 10^{-4} M, if one assumes a water content of 2 µl per mg of mitochondrial protein. There was certainly an excess of GTP over that required for GDH inhibition. However, the amount of free nucleotide not bound to protein was probably two orders of magnitude less. What is the advantage of having a GDH which differs from liver GDH? The advantage probably lies in the fact that phosphate releases GTP inhibition of heart mitochondrial GDH much better than it does liver GDH. Thus, any fall in ATP would lead to an increase in ADP and inorganic phosphate which would release GTP inhibition of heart mitochondrial GDH.

Our studies of rat heart GDH showed a significant amount of GDH in the cytosolic fraction which was not due to mitochondrial contamination. If cytosolic GDH operated with NAD(H) it would lead to glutamate breakdown which is an unfavorable reaction because of the need to maintain glutamate levels. However, if cytosolic GDH operated with the NADP(H) system it would lead to glutamate for-mation. Incubation of cytosolic GDH under in vivo conditions leads to glutamate formation. Thus, cytosolic GDH may function to capture ammonia, thereby, conserving nitrogen for the heart. This is probably a very important mechanism for maintaining purine and amino acid pools in the heart.

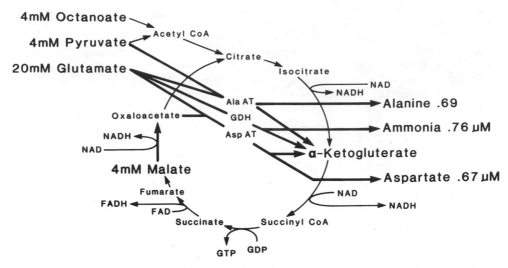

Fig. 4   Aspartate aminotransferase, alanine aminotransferase, glutamic dehydrogenase and the citric acid cycle with substrates incubated with isolated rat heart mitochondria.

In summary, GDH activity in the heart consists of a cytoplasmic isoenzyme that recycles ammonia back into glutamate, thereby conserving nitrogen. The mitochondria have a GDH isoenzyme that is regulated by oxaloacetate levels. In vitro inhibition by GTP is released by phosphate. Both of these isoenzymes play important roles in myocardial metabolism.

REFERENCES

1.   K. LaNone and J. Williamson, Control of the malate-aspartate shuttle in rat heart mitochondria, in: "Colloquium on Bioenergetics and Energy Transduction in Respiration and Photo-synthesis," E. Quagliariello, S. Papa and C. Rossi, eds., Adriatica Editrice, Bari (1972).
2.   C. Godinot and D. Gautheron, Regulation of pig heart mitochondrial glutamate dehydrogenase by nucleotides and phosphate: Comparison with pig heart and beef liver purified enzymes, FEBS Letters. 13:235 (1971).
3.   T. Takala, J. Hiltunen, and I. Hassinen, The mechanism of ammonia production and the effect of mechanical work load on proteolysis and amino acid catabolism in isolated perfused rat heart, Biochem. J. 192:285 (1980).

4. A. Younes, R. Durand, Y. Briand, and D. Gautheron, Interaction des oxydation du pyruvate et du glutamate au niveau des mitochondries de coeur de porc, Bull. Soc. Clin. Biol. 52:811(1970).

5. E. Nuutinen, J. Hiltunen, and I. Hassinen, The glutamate dehydrogenase system and the redox state of mitochondrial free nicotinamide adenine dinucleotide in myocardium, FEBS Letters. 128:356 (1981).

6. H. McDaniel, M. Yeh, R. Jenkins, and A. Razzaque, Glutamic dehydrogenase from rat heart mitochondria, I. Purification and physical properties including molecular weight determination. J. Mol. Cell. Cardiol. 16:295 (1984).

7. H. McDaniel, R. Jenkins, M. Yeh, and A. Razzaque, Glutamic dehydrogenase from rat heart mitochondria, II. Kinetic characteristics, J. Mol. Cell. Cardiol. 16:303 (1984).

8. H. McDaniel, M. Yeh, R. Jenkins, B. Freeman, and J. Simmons, Glutamic dehydrogenase activity in rat heart: demonstration of two forms of enzyme activity, Am. J. Physiol. 246:H483 (1984).

9. F. Wallheim, H. Bergmeyer, and I. Gutmann, Ammonials, in: "Methoden der Enzymatischen Analyse," H. Bergemeyer, ed., Verlag Chemie, Weinheim (1974).

10. E. Bernt and H. Bergmeyer, L-Glutamat, in: "Methoden der Enzymatischen Analyse," H. Bergmeyer, ed., Verlag Chemie, Weinheim (1974).

11. H. Bergmeyer, E. Bernt, H. Mollering, and E. Pfleider, L-Aspartat und L-asparagin, in: "Methoden der Enzymatischen Analyse," H. Bergmeyer, ed., Verlag Chemie, Weinheim (1974).

12. H. Bergmeyer, Nucleosiddiphosphat-kinase, in: "Methoden der Enzymatischen Analyse," H. Bergmeyer ed., Verlag Chemie, Weinheim (1974).

13. H. Mangold, Nucleinsauren und nucleotide, in: Dunnschiectchromatographie," E. Stahl, ed., Springer-Verlag, Berlin (1967).

14. H. McDaniel, W. Rogers, R. Russell, and C. Rackley, Effect of glucose-insulin-potassium during pacing, Circulation 58:132 (1978).

15. B. Goldin and C. Frieden, Glutamic dehydrogenase, in: "Current Topics in Cellular Regulation," B. Horecker and E. Stadtman, eds., Academic Press, New York (1971).

16. H. Helm, L-Glutamate dehydrogenase isoenzymes, Nature. 194:773 (1962).

17. G. DiPrisco and H. Strecker, Glutamate dehydrogenase of nuclear and extra-nuclear compartments of Chang's liver cells, Eur. J. Biochem. 12:483 (1970).

18. T. Kato and O. Lawry, Distribution of enzymes between nucleus and cytoplasm of single nerve cell bodies, J. Biol. Chem. 248:2044 (1973).

19. J. Julliard and D. Gautheron, Regulatory effects of mitochondrial lipids on glutamate dehydrogenase, FEBS Letters 25:343 (1972).

20. P. Borst, The pathway of glutamate oxidation by mitochondria isolated from different tissues, Biochim. Biophys. Acta. 57:256 (1962).

21. E. Davis and J. Bremer, Studies with isolated surviving rat hearts, Interdependence of free amino acids and citric acid cycle intermediates, Eur. J. Biochem. 38:86 (1973).

LONG TERM MODEL FOR EVALUATION OF MYOCARDIAL METABOLIC RECOVERY

FOLLOWING GLOBAL ISCHEMIA

John St. Cyr, Herbert Ward, Jolene Kriett,
David Alyono, Stanley Einzig, Richard Bianco,
Robert Anderson and John Foker

Department of Surgery, University of Minnesota
Minneapolis, Minnesota 55455

ABSTRACT

Myocardial ATP levels remain depressed following significant periods of ischemia (Isc) despite reperfusion (Rpf). Neither the rate of in vivo ATP return following global Isc nor the factors which influence recovery have been defined. In order to determine the time course to complete the return of ATP levels and evaluate methods of enhancing recovery of ATP levels, we have devised a chronic canine model of global Isc. In this model serial ventricular biopsies can be taken in the awake animal over several days without reoperation which allows an investigation of the recovery of the myocardium following a uniform global insult to be performed.

Recovery of ATP levels has been shown to depend, at least in part, on the availability of precursors and the activity of the ATP regenerating enzymes. Because complete recovery of ATP levels takes days, short term (hours) models have limitations. Previous attempts at enhancing ATP recovery following Isc have been only partially successful because either the degree of depression was not great or the period of observation was short, resulting in incomplete return. To identify the best precursor choice, we previously measured the activity of the AMP regenerating enzymes, adenosine kinase (AdK) (adenosine → AMP) and adenine phosphoribosyl transferase (APRT) (adenine → AMP). Because APRT activity was 20 fold higher than AdK with similar Km values for substrates, it appeared that adenine (A) is preferred to adenosine for AMP regeneration in the dog's myocardium. The formation of 5-phospho-ribosyl 1-pyrophosphate (PRPP) may also be rate limiting and,

401

therefore, the effect of ribose (R) on ATP recovery was also evaluated. Recovery of ATP levels was assessed in three groups: (1) normal saline (NS), (2) A (20 mM) in normal saline (A/NS) or (3) A with R (80 mM) in normal saline (A/R) were infused (1.0 ml/min) into the right atrium of dogs for 48 hours following Isc. In all groups, ATP levels fell to between 46-60% of pre-Isc levels during Isc. In the NS dogs, ATP levels continued to fall slightly to 46% pre-Isc levels during the first four hours of Rpf after Isc. By 24 hours no appreciable recovery had occurred and the measured ATP was only 51% of the pre-Isc value. Even by seven days, ATP had not returned fully, and by extrapolation, complete recovery required 9.9±1.4 days. Treated dogs showed, however, that ATP recovery could be significantly enhanced. In the A/NS treated group, the ATP levels rebounded to 69% of pre-Isc values during the first four hours of Rpf following Isc but recovery leveled off during the next 20 hours. Recovery in the A/R treated group rose to 60% of pre-Isc values after four hours of Rpf and continued to improve thereafter. Recovery was virtually complete by 24 hours (96%). The calculated mean recovery rate for the first 24 hours in each group: (NS) 0.04±0.33 nmoles/mg wet wt/day, (A/NS) 0.41±0.55 nmoles/mg wet wt/day and (A/R) 2.44±0.38 nmoles/mg wet wt/day. Our results reveal that (1) This long term model allows serial myocardial sampling in the awake state for investigation of recovery from Isc. (2) ATP recovery following a significant global Isc insult is slow. (3) Precursor availability is an important limiting factor in recovery. (4) Recovery time can be greatly shortened with ATP precursor infusion even when started after Isc. (5) Although A alone initially enhanced ATP recovery, the addition of R provided a more rapid complete return suggesting PRPP formation is also rate limiting.

INTRODUCTION

The recovery of myocardial ATP levels following Isc has been the object of considerable investigation. The observation that ATP levels do not promptly recover with Rpf was first made by Benson (1). Despite the work in this area, long term studies defining the recovery of myocardial ATP levels and evaluating methods of enhancing its return following global Isc have not been reported. Consequently, we have devised a chronic model in which the recovery of the myocardium in the intact animal can be serially assessed.

Many theories have been advanced to explain the reason for the prolonged recovery time of myocardial ATP levels following Isc. Although the subcellular basis for this has yet to be established, it appears that the loss of ATP precursors, at least in part, limits recovery (1,2,3). The loss of ATP precursors through enzymatic degradation and coronary sinus washout has been documented and this has led to many attempts to enhance ATP recovery by the infusion of various precursors. Adenosine, inosine, AICAR-riboside and ribose are some of the precursors that have been used to increase recovery of ATP levels following Isc or the infusion of catecholamines (3-13). Although the results of these studies have been promising, they have been of short duration and it remains to be determined whether ATP recovery can be significantly enhanced and full recovery achieved in the intact animal following global Isc.

The development of a long term intact animal model has allowed us to evaluate the recovery rates of myocardial ATP levels following global Isc. The purpose of this study was to validate this model and use it to compare the ability of adenine, with and without ribose, to enhance the recovery of post-Isc ATP levels.

METHODS

Experimental Procedure

Sixteen conditioned dogs weighing 25-30 kg were anesthetized intravenously with sodium pentothal (12.5 mg/kg) and ventilated with a Harvard respirator with supplemental oxygen provided to maintain a PaO_2 of at least 100 mmHg. Anesthesia was maintained with nitrous oxide and halothane. Temperatures were monitored continuously with an esophageal temperature probe (Electromedics). A right thoracotomy was performed through the fifth intercostal space and the aorta cannulated through the internal mammary artery for arterial pressure monitoring and blood sampling. Blood pressures were measured with Statham P23Db strain gauges and recorded along with lead II ECG tracings on a Beckman Dynagraph 8 channel recorder. Blood gases were measured with an Instrumentation Laboratories Model 326 Blood Gas Analyzer. Hemoglobin was measured using a Coulter Electronics Hemoglobinometer. All instruments were calibrated at the beginning, middle, and end of each experiment. Silastic catheters were placed in the left atrial appendage for pressure monitoring and microsphere injection, the right atrial appendage for saline or drug infusion, and the coronary sinus for blood withdrawal. Catheter positions were confirmed at the completion of each study.

After anticoagulating with heparin (250 units·kg^{-1}), the animals were placed on total cardiopulmonary bypass (CPB) at normothermia (37°C) using standard techniques (3). The arterial perfusion was retrograde from the left femoral artery and the venous drainage from the superior and inferior vena cava via the right atrium. The azygos vein was ligated. Shiley, Model S100A, bubble oxygenators were used. Mean aortic pressure was maintained at 60-80 mmHg by adjusting pump flow to approximately 100 ml·kg^{-1}·min using a Biotronics electromagnetic flow transducer in the arterial infusion line.

After beginning CPB, the dogs were allowed to stabilize for 5-10 min. Septal biopsies (using a 4 mm bronchial biopsy forceps inserted through a right ventriculotomy) were performed for measurement of adenine nucleotide levels. Global myocardial Isc was then produced by crossclamping the ascending aorta at normothermia (37°C) with total arrest occurring within 5-7 min. While the aorta was clamped, a custom designed silastic catheter (1/4 inch internal diameter, 3/8 inch external diameter) with a teflon felt sewing ring was sutured into the right ventricular free wall (Figure 1). Following a 20 min warm Isc period, another septal biopsy was obtained and the aortic crossclamp was removed. Adenine (A) in normal saline (A/NS), A (20 mM) and ribose (R) (80 mM) in normal saline (A/R) or a normal saline (NS) (0.9%) infusion (1 ml/min) alone was started at the beginning of reperfusion via the right atrial catheter. Defibrillation was accomplished with 5-10 watt-sec of direct current after 20 min of Rpf and 10 min later the dogs were weaned from CPB. Heparin reversal was accomplished with protamine sulfate (50-100 mg). The dogs were supported for an additional 60 min off CPB, the biopsy cannula brought through the lateral chest wall, and the chest incision closed. During this time, lactated Ringer's solution and/or whole blood was infused to maintain a left atrial pressure of 5-8 mmHg and a hematocrit of 30-40%.

The infusion of either A/NS, A/R or NS into the right atrium was continued for 48 hours following the end of Isc. Repeat septal biopsies were performed at 4 hours, 1, 2, 3, 5, and 7 days post-Isc. Biopsies were taken sequentially from the apex of the septum toward the base of the septum to avoid re-biopsy of the same area. Simultaneous aortic and coronary sinus blood samples were obtained at 24 hours of infusion for determination of A levels.

Nucleotide and Nucleoside Assays

Biopsies for adenine nucleotides and nucleosides were frozen within 1 sec in liquid nitrogen cooled 2 methylbutane. Blood samples were centrifuged and the plasma mixed with equal parts of 2M perchloric acid. The tissue was extracted within 24 hours in 7.1% perchloric acid, homogenized and centrifuged at 1000 x g. The supernatant was neutralized (pH 7.2) with 2N KOH, 0.4M imidazole and 0.4 M KCl for myocardial biopsies and saturated KOH for blood samples, centrifuged to remove potassium percholate, and stored at -70°C. ATP was assayed spectrophotometrically in a two-step, coupled enzymatic system using hexokinase and glucose-6-phosphate dehydrogenase in which the reduction of NADP at E_{340} was followed (14). The assay for ADP and AMP utilized the oxidation of NADH in the coupled enzymatic system of lactate dehydrogenase and pyruvate kinase (15).

Purine nucleoside levels were determined by injecting 20 ul of the extract onto an Ultrasphere ODS (5 um particle size) column

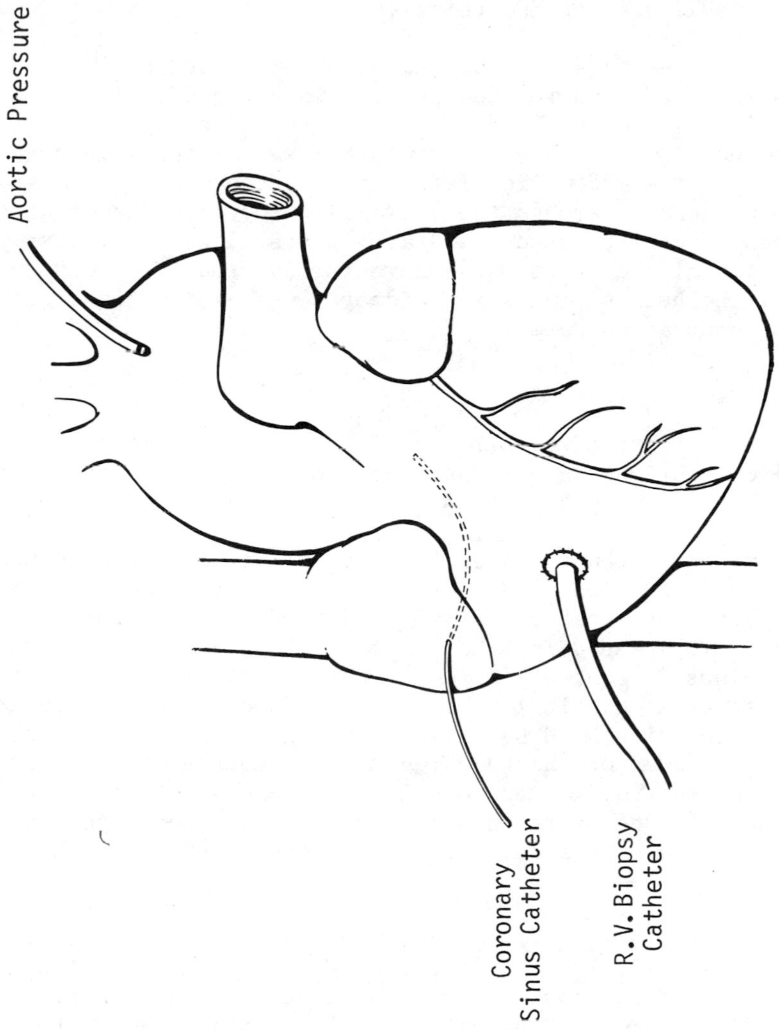

Aortic Pressure

Coronary Sinus Catheter

R.V. Biopsy Catheter

FIGURE 1

(Beckman) and developed with a linear gradient of 0.01 M KH_2PO_4, pH 5.6 (buffer A) and 70% methanol in water (buffer B); gradient 0-32% B in A over 32 minutes; ambient temperature; flow rate 1.0 ml/min in a Beckman Model 334 Gradient Liquid Chromatograph (HPLC) (16). UV absorbance was measured on a Hitachi Model 100-10 spectrophotometer at 254 nm and peak dimensions analyzed with a Hewlett-Packard 3390A Integrator. Peaks were identified by retention times, radiolabeling and relative absorbance at 280/254 nm.

At each biopsy time period, paired arterial and coronary sinus blood samples were drawn for measurement of pH, pCO_2, pO_2 and % saturation. Radionuclide labeled 15±5 microspheres (^{141}Ce, ^{85}Sr, ^{95}Nb, ^{46}Sc and ^{125}I, 3M Co., St. Paul, MN) were infused into the left atrium via the indwelling left atrial catheter and a reference sample was withdrawn through the indwelling aortic catheter at the time periods of control study, and at 4 hours, 1, 3 and 7 days post myocardial global Isc. After the seventh day study, the dog was sacrificed, the hearts, lungs and kidneys were excised and positions of all instrumentation were verified.

Calculations

Adenine extraction was calculated by taking the mean of the individual extractions using: (Arterial Adenine - Coronary Sinus Adenine)/(Arterial Adenine) x 100.

Arterial and coronary sinus O_2 contents were calculated using the following expression: O_2 content (ml $O_2 \cdot$ml blood^{-1}) = (hgb x 1.36 x percent O_2 saturation) + (pO$_2$ x 0.00003). Myocardial oxygen consumption (MVO$_2$) was calculated from: MVO$_2$ = (arterial O_2 content - coronary sinus O_2 content) x (mean left ventricular blood flow), and expressed as ml $O_2 \cdot$min$^{-1} \cdot$g LV. Systemic and coronary vascular resistance were calculated by dividing the mean aortic blood pressure by the cardiac index or the weighted-average left ventricular blood flow respectively. Stroke volume index was defined as the cardiac index divided by the heart rate. Index of cardiac effort was defined as the peak aortic systolic pressure times the heart rate.

Radionuclide labeled "15" microspheres were used to measure tissue blood flow (17,18). On the average 0.9 million spheres suspended in 0.05% polysorbate 80 in isotonic saline were dispersed by ultrasonic treatment (Bransonic 220 Ultrasonic cleaner) for 15 min and injected into the left atrium over 10-15 sec with 10 ml of saline (13). The isotopic order was randomized. Tissue sampling techniques, sample preparation, counting procedures and calculation of blood flows have previously been described (13).

Statistics

Differences within the animal group were evaluated by multi-variage analysis (MANOVA) on the differences from baseline (19). When the p value by MANOVA was less than 0.05, univariate analysis was performed. Student's paired t-test was used to compare pre- and post-Isc ATP levels. Mean recovery time for the parameter measured is defined as the mean slope of the lines fitted to the observed points by the method of least squares. Values represent mean ± S.E.

RESULTS

Using this model, the long term recovery from Isc can be investigated by serial biopsies. The biopsy technique of sampling the endocardial septum through the cannula in the closed-chested dog was compared with our standard left ventricular transmural drill procedure in open-chested animals. Nearly simultaneous biopsies (n=20 pairs) were taken with excellent correlation (coefficient of variation = 12% and r = 0.95).

Previous work in this laboratory has suggested that A would be preferred to adenosine for AMP regeneration in the dog myocardium when adequate R is available to produce PRPP (11). Without A infusion A was not detectable in myocardial tissue (less than 0.02 nmoles/mg wet wt) or serum (less than 1.0 uM) when collected from control animals. During infusion, the mean myocardial tissue A level in treated animals was 0.19±0.07 nmoles/mg wet wt and the mean serum A levels in the ascending aorta and coronary sinus were 18.3±1.3 mcg and 11.0±1.6 mcg, respectively. The calculated extraction of A by the myocardium was 38%.

Adenine nucleotide (ATP, ADP, AMP) levels in myocardial tissue are presented in Table I. As can be seen in the control (NS) dogs, ATP levels continued to fall during the first four hours of Rpf and the eventual recovery from this global insult was prolonged. The mean recovery rate for ATP levels was 0.04±0.33 nmoles/mg wet wt/day and the projected complete recovery time was 9.9±1.4 days. In the A/NS infusion group, the continued fall with Rpf was reversed and the ATP levels rose to 69% of pre-Isc levels at 4 hours of Rpf and maintained this recovery percentage during the next 20 hour period of infusion. The addition of R provided a more sustained recovery. In the treated A/R group, ATP levels rose sharply within the first 4 hours of Rpf and continued. Recovery was virtually complete (96%) by 24 hours. The mean recovery rate for ATP levels during A/R infusion was 2.44±.38 nmoles/mg wet wt/day. (See Table II for mean recovery rates). ATP levels remained high for the entire infusion period of A plus R.

TABLE I: ATP LEVELS (nmoles·mg^{-1} wet wt) AND % RECOVERY IN TREATED AND CONTROL ANIMALS

ATP Levels	Pre-Isc	20 min	% Rec	4 hrs	% Rec	24 hrs	% Rec
NS (n=7)	5.06±0.18	2.54±0.16	50	2.33±0.19	46	2.58±0.26	51
A/NS (n=4)	5.61±0.71	3.37±0.63	60	3.88±0.60*	69	3.78±0.12*	67
A/R (n=9)	4.67±0.30	2.08±0.24	46	2.82±0.26	60	4.46±0.33*	96

* p < .01
Isc = ischemia
NS = normal saline controls
A/R = adenine-ribose
A   = adenine

TABLE II: MEAN ATP RECOVERY RATES (nmoles·mg wet wt^{-1} day)

	Group	N	0-4 hrs	0-24 hrs
1)	NS	(7)	-1.24±.99	.04±.33
2)	A/NS	(4)	3.09±5.21	.41±.55
3)	A/R	(9)	4.23±1.76*	2.44±.38*+

* p < .05 (A/R vs NS)
+ p < .05 (A/NS vs A/R)

Energy charge, which reflects the degree to which adenine nucleotides are charged, was calculated from the following expression: EC = (ATP) + 1/2 (ADP)/(ATP) + (ADP) + (AMP). The energy charge ratio fell approximately 18% in the control (NS) group, approximately 16% in the A/NS group and approximately 22% in the A/R group at 20 minutes of normothermic global Isc. Following the Isc insult, the energy charge ratio gradually returned to its pre-Isc value in the control group by seven days. In the treated groups, the energy charge ratio returned to its relative pre-Isc value by 24 hours in the A/R dogs. The energy charge in the A/NS dogs also paralleled the return of ATP levels.

Hemodynamic parameters, myocardial and renal blood flow and myocardial oxygen consumption were assessed in all groups. No differences were found between control and treated dogs when comparing these parameters, although there were differences found within groups. Sinus tachycardia was present in all dogs following the normothermic global Isc insult on CPB. Mean aortic pressure and left ventricular end-diastolic pressure remained stable in all groups throughout the entire study, whereas cardiac index and stroke volume index decreased in all groups at the initial post-Isc phase but recovered at a rapid rate. Renal blood flow was decreased in all groups at four hours post-Isc, but was back to control flows at 24 hours and thereafter. Following the Isc insult to the end of the entire study, left ventricular blood flow remained elevated with decreased coronary vascular resistance in all groups. The left ventricular endocardial/epicardial blood flow ratios remained stable in the groups throughout the entire study. No changes in myocardial oxygen consumption was found between control and treated dogs or within each group itself.

DISCUSSION

The metabolic recovery of the myocardium from a moderately severe Isc insult takes considerable time. Many studies have demonstrated that myocardial ATP levels do not return promptly with Rpf and have not begun to recover four hours later (1,3). Recovery of ATP levels in the Isc area following 15 min of coronary occlusion was only 75% complete after three days and full return required one week (20). We have found almost 10 days were required for complete return following 20 min of normothermic global Isc. These observations reveal that long term models are needed to investigate the recovery of the post-Isc myocardium.

The availability of a chronic model will prove valuable in the investigation of several basic questions. A model using global rather than regional Isc has additional advantages. Using global Isc allows the investigation of the metabolism of the myocardium involving both its recovery and circulatory support. A global insult is relatively uniform with little contribution from collateral vessels. This, in turn, minimizes myocardial sampling errors. In this model, we have established the validity of sampling the septum through the right ventricle as being metabolically representative of the left ventricular free wall. Additionally, this technique can be used for daily sampling in the awake animal without the need for repeated anesthesia or reoperation.

Results of numerous short term studies have shown that ATP recovery can be augmented, at least initially, by the infusion of ATP precursors in the post-Isc period. The optimum combination of ATP precursors for infusion, however, has not yet been determined. Clearly, de novo adenine nucleotide synthesis is very slow. What is unknown is the number of rate limiting steps that are present. Moreover, circumventing one rate limiting step by an appropriate precursor may only unmask a lesser limiting reaction in another arm of these complex pathways (Figure 2). It is possible, for example, that the best combination may utilize both the purine base and R.

Previous work in our laboratory has found that A appears to be favored over adenosine as an ATP precursor for the following reasons: A comparison of AMP regenerating enzymes in canine myocardium at the end of Isc and during Rpf revealed APRT levels were appreciably higher than AdK levels throughout Isc and Rpf. AdK levels were found to be low (35±0.8 pmole/min/mg protein) and did not change with Isc or Rpf. APRT levels were 20 fold higher throughout Isc and Rpf. The Km of AdK for adenosine and APRT for A were both found to be 10 uM. Moreover, from a physiological standpoint A does not appear to have the adverse property of decreasing renal blood flow. Therefore, it appears that A is preferred over adenosine for AMP regeneration in the canine myocardium.

Other workers have provided evidence that the production of PRPP from glucose is limited by the activity of glucose-6-dehydrogenase (21). The administration of R allows this rate limiting step to be circumvented and thereby enhancing the recovery of ATP levels. The value of this approach has been demonstrated in several short term studies (10-12).

410

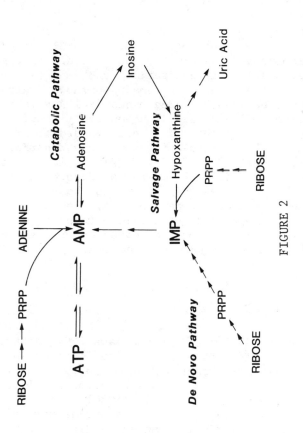

FIGURE 2

411

The combination of both ATP precursors, A and R, produced a sharp rise in ATP levels within the first four hours of Rpf and virtually complete recovery (96%) within 24 hours. This was a substantial increase over the control group, in which ATP return was much slower, taking a calculated 9.9 days for complete recovery. The A group demonstrated a quicker ATP recovery rate than control, but less than the A/R group. These findings clearly indicate that supplying ATP precursors hastens complete ATP recovery in the intact animal after global myocardial Isc. Nevertheless, further information is needed. Currently we are assessing the role of R alone in enhancing ATP recovery. The optimum composition and length of infusion need to be determined in order to maximize the potential effect.

This chronic model of recovery from global Isc has been adapted to also provide information on recovery of function. Despite a great deal of investigation, the important relationship between ATP levels and function remains unknown. Although the relationship between measured myocardial ATP levels and cardiac function following Isc is undoubtedly complex, several points have been established: (1) Both myocardial ATP levels and cardiac function are depressed for a prolonged period following a moderate Isc insult (9,20,22,23). (2) A temporal relationship exists between myocardial ATP levels and diastolic compliance (22,23). (3) Finally, as this study has shown in the intact animal, complete recovery of depressed ATP levels following myocardial Isc can be quickly achieved with precursor infusion. We are currently investing the consequences of enhanced ATP recovery on the return of cardiac function.

REFERENCES

1. E.S. Benson, G.T. Evans, B.E. Hallaway, C. Phibbs, E.F. Freier, Myocardial creatine phosphate and nucleotides in anoxic cardiac arrest and recovery, Amer J Physiol 201: 687-93 (1961).
2. R.M. Berne, The role of adenosine in the regulation of coronary blood flow, Circ Res 47: 807-13 (1980).
3. J.E. Foker, S. Einzig, T. Wang, Adenosine metabolism and myocardial preservation, J Thorac Cardiovasc Surg 80:506-16 (1980).
4. W. Isselhard, D.H. Hinzen, E. Geppert, W. Maurer, Effect of substrate supply on post-asphyctic restoration of adenine nucleotides in rabbit hearts in vivo, Pflugers Arch 320: 195-209 (1970).
5. D.F. DeWitt, K.E. Jochim, D.M. Behrendt, Nucleoside degradation and function impairment during cardioplegia: Amelioration by inosine, Circ 67: I:171-78 (1983).

6. O.A. Smiseth, Inosine infusion in dogs with acute ischoemic left ventricular failure: favourable effects on myocardial performance and metabolism, Cardiovasc Res 17: 19209 (1983).
7. H.B. Ward, T. Wang, S. Einzig, R.W. Bianco, J.E. Foker, Enhanced regeneration of postischemia myocardial adenosine triphosphate concentrations, Surg Forum XXXII:254-6 (1981).
8. C. Nienaber, M. Mauser, W. Schaper, Stimulation of myocardial adenine nucleotide synthesis by postischemic reperfusion with direct purine precursor AICAR* comparison with ribose. (*5-amino-4-imidzole-carboxamide-riboside). J Amer Coll Cardiol, 1(2):667 (1983).
9. R.L. Sabina, K.H. Kernstine, R.L. Boyd, E.W. Holmes, J.L. Swain, Metabolism of 5-amino-4-imidazolecarboxamide riboside in cardiac and skeletal muscle: Effects on purine nucleotide synthesis, J Biol Chem 257:10178-83 (1982).
10. M.K. Pasque, T.L. Spray, G.L. Pellom, P. Van Trigt, R.B. Peyton, W.D. Currie, A.S. Wechsler, Ribose-enhanced myocardial recovery following ischemia in the isolated working rat heart, J Thorac Cardiovasc Surg 83: 390-8 (1982).
11. H.B. Ward, T. Wang, S. Einzig, R.W. Bianco, J.E. Foker, Prevention of ATP catabolism during myocardial ischemia: A preliminary report. J Surg Res 34: 292-7 (1983).
12. H.G. Zimmer, Normalization of depressed heart function in rats by ribose, Science 220: 81-2 (1983).
13. H.B. Ward, S. Einzig, T. Wang, R.W. Bianco, J.E. Foker, Comparison of catecholamine effects on myocardial metabolism and regional blood flow during and after cardiopulmonary bypass, J Thorac Cardiovasc Surg 87: 3: 452-465 (1984).
14. W. Lamprecht, P. Stein, F. Heinz, H. Weisser, in: Methods of enzymatic analysis, H.U. Bergmeyer, ed., Academic Press, Inc., New York (1974).
15. D. Jaworek, W. Gruber, H.U. Bergmeyer, Adenosine-5'-diphosphate and adenosine-5'-monophosphate, in: Methods of enzymatic analysis, H.U. Bergmeyer, ed., Academic Press, Inc., New York (1974).
16. H.K. Webster, J.M. Whaun, Application of simultaneous UV-radioactivity high-performance liquid chromatography to the study of intermediary metabolism. I. Purine nucleotides, nucleosides and bases, J Chromatograph 209: 283-92 (1981).
17. M.A. Heymann, B.D. Payne, J.I. Hoffman, A.M.Rudolph, Blood flow measurements with radionuclide-labeled particles, Progress in Cardiovasc Diseases 20: 55 (1977).
18. P.M. Consigny, Acute and chronic microsphere loss from canine left ventricular myocardium, Amer J Physiol 242: H393-404 (1982).
19. S. Wallenstein, C.L. Zucker, J.L. Fleiss, Some statistical methods useful in circulation research. Circ Res 47: 1-9 (1980).
20. R.A. Kloner, L.W.V. DeBoer, J.R. Darsee, J.S. Ingwall, E. Braunwald, Recovery from prolonged abnormalities of canine myocardium salvaged from ischemic necrosis by coronary reperfusion. Proc Natl Acad Sci USA 78: 7151-6 (1981).

21. H.G. Zimmer, H. Ibel, U. Suchner, H. Schad, Ribose Intervention in the cardiac pentose phosphate pathway is not species-specific, Science 223: 712-714 (1984).

22. H.B. Ward, J.M. Kriett, S. Einzig, R.W. Bianco, R.W. Anderson, J.E. Foker, Adenine nucleotides and cardiac function following global myocardial ischemia, Surg Forum XXXIV: 264-6 (1983).

23. J.M. Kriett, H.B. Ward, R.W. Bianco, S. Einzig, D. Alyono, R.W. Anderson, J.E. Foker, Recovery of adenine nucleotides and cardiac function following ischemia, Circ 68(III): 389 (1983).

THE EFFECT OF REPERFUSION AND STREPTOKINASE ON ISCHEMIC MYOCARDIUM
SERUM CREATINE KINASE ACTIVITY, MM SUBTYPES AND MYOCARDIAL BLOOD
FLOW

Judy Mickelson, C. Jeffrey Carlson, Bianka Emilson, and
Elliot Rapaport

Medical Service, San Francisco General Hospital and the
Cardiovascular Research Institute, University of
California, San Francisco, CA

INTRODUCTION

The amount of myocardium irreversibly damaged after coronary
artery occlusion is of prognostic significance.[1-4] Attempts to
limit the extent of damage using streptokinase have been effective
in reestablishing blood flow to ischemic myocardium.[5-11] We were
interested in the effect streptokinase has on ischemic myocardium
distal to an occlusion when reperfusion occurs and the extent to
which streptokinase affects myocardial reperfusion. We measured
serum creatine kinase and its MM subtypes. These measurements are
simple but indirect means of assessing infarct size that can be
used clinically.[4-12] However, when reperfusion occurs, serial
serum creatine kinase activity is altered.[10,13-15] We obtained
more direct measurements of ischemia and subsequent reperfusion
using radiolabeled microspheres to determine myocardial blood
flow.[16,17]

METHOD

Thirteen mongrel dogs of either sex, weighing 16-23 kg, which
were previously trained to rest quietly in a Povlov sling, were
anesthetized with pentobarbital sodium, 25 mg/kg, endotracheally
intubated, and ventilated with a volume respirator (Harvard
Apparatus Co.). A left thoracotomy and pericardiotomy were performed. The left circumflex coronary artery was exposed and a cuff
occluder (In Vivo Metrics) was positioned around the artery 3-5 cm
from the origin but proximal to the first obtuse marginal branch.
Two epicardial pacing wires were sutured to the surface of the left
ventricle in the area supplied by the left circumflex coronary

artery. These were used to monitor electrocardiographic changes
and arrhythmias during the study. A silastic catheter was introduced into the left atrium and sutured in position for injecting
radiolabeled microspheres, sampling blood, and infusing medications.
These wires and catheter were externalized. The pericardium was
loosely closed and a left thorocostomy tube was positioned and
externalized. The chest was closed and the dog was allowed to
recover. Each dog was given procaine penicillin, 600,000 units,
and streptomycin, 1 g, intramuscularly immediately before surgery
and for the first 4 days after the surgery. Seven days after
surgery, using thiopental sodium anesthesia, a catheter was introduced into the carotid artery and advanced into the ascending aorta
for obtaining reference blood flows for the microsphere myocardial
blood flow determinations and for monitoring pressure during the
study. The study was performed within 2 days.

PROTOCOL

The awake chronically instrumented dogs underwent baseline
electrocardiographic and aortic phasic pressure recording
(Electronics for Medicine DR 12 optical recorder); blood sampling
for creatine kinase (3 ml); and myocardial blood flow determinations. Immediately before inflating the coronary artery cuff
occluder, the dog was mildly sedated with intravenous valium, 2 mg,
and morphine sulfate, 1.5 mg. Then lidocaine, 2 mg/kg bolus, was
administered and the cuff was inflated. To minimize discomfort,
valium, 1-2 mg, and morphine sulfate, 1-2 mg, were administered as
needed each hour. Lidocaine, 1 mg/kg bolus, was given every 15 min
as needed for arrhythmias. The coronary artery cuff occluder
remained inflated for either 2, 3, 5, or 24 h. The electrocardiogram showed acute ST segment elevation in the epicardial leads
during all studies except the 3-h occlusions.

One-half hour before release of the cuff occluder, myocardial
blood flow determinations were repeated and a 1-h continuous
infusion of either streptokinase, 6,000 IU/kg in 10 ml saline, or
saline, 10 ml, was begun (infusion pump model No.600-900, Harvard
Appartus Co.). With permanent coronary artery occlusion, myocardial
blood flow was determined and streptokinase or saline was infused
during the third hour. Blood samples (3 ml) were collected at $\frac{1}{2}$-
to 1-h intervals and an equal volume of saline was administered as
replacement. Twenty-four hours after coronary artery occlusion,
the final myocardial blood flow determinations were obtained. A
lethal dose of pentobarbital sodium was then infused.

The heart was immediately excised, rinsed in saline, and
weighed. The septum and left ventricle were dissected free,

weighed, flattened, and fixed in 10% buffered formalin. These
tissues were divided into three layers of equal thickness:
endocardium, midmyocardium, and epicardium. The papillary muscles
were separated and each of the three layers of the left ventricular
free wall was divided into three segments both from apex to base
and anterior to posterior yielding nine equal segments. Each of
the three layers of the septum was divided into three segments from
apex to base and two segments from anterior to posterior yielding
six equal segments. The segments were weighed and placed in vials
for radionuclide counting.

Thirteen dogs underwent instrumentation, but only 10 underwent
coronary artery occlusion and release. Two of the studies ended
when the dogs had ventricular fibrillation after coronary artery
occlusion but before streptokinase or saline infusion or release of
the occlusion. One dog died after the carotid artery catheter was
placed, the day before the study. Three of the 10 dogs died of
arrhythmias less than 24 h after permanent coronary artery occlusion
(15, 18, and 20 h later). They had saline infusions. Both dogs
that underwent 3-h occlusion did not have infarctions as determined
by electrocardiographic changes, creatine kinase activity curves,
and myocardial blood flow. One dog was given streptokinase and the
other saline.

CREATINE KINASE

The MM isozyme of creatine kinase contains at least three
subtypes that can be separated by isoelectric focusing.[18-20] In
this report MM subtypes are named according to the greatest mobility
away from the cathode toward the anode during separation: M_1, M_2,
M_3. M_x, and M_y, found in some tissues in small amounts, migrate
ahead of M_1 yielding a sequence M_y, M_x, M_1, M_2, and M_3. The subtypes are of interest clinically because the normally predominant
subtype in human and dog serum is M_1, whereas the predominant subtype in human and dog heart is M_3 (Table 1). Hence the initial
increase in serum creatine kinase activity after myocardial infarction is composed chiefly of M_3. This subtype is converted to M_2
and then M_1 in the serum.[21-25] The ratio of subtypes, in particular
$M_3:M_1$, changes predictably in serum after infarction.[21]

Creatine kinase activity was assayed spectrophotometrically at
25°C by the coupled enzyme system of Rosalki[26] using A-Gent CK-NAC
(Abbott Laboratories) or Statzyme CPK-n-1 (Worthington Diagnostics).
Enzyme activity was expressed in International Units/liter. One
International Unit is the amount of enzyme activity that will
transfer the phosphate from creatine phosphate at a rate of
1 μmole/min.

Table 1. Serum and Myocardial Creatine Kinase MM Subtypes
in Human and Dog Tissues[a]

| MM Subtype | pI | Serum | | Myocardium | | |
| | | Human (n=8) | Dog (n=8) | Human (n=2) | Dog (n=8) | |
					Normal	Infarction
M_3	6.88	18+4	12+7	63	34+15[b]	33+13[b]
M_2	6.70	30+4	21+9	30	18+10	18+ 9
M_1	6.45	47+8	58+9	5	22+ 8[c]	17+ 8[c]
M_x	6.25	5+5	9+8	2	4+ 7	7+ 7
M_y	6.20	0	0	0	5+ 7	3+ 5

[a]Data are mean + 1 SD.

[b]Subtype band migrating between M_3 and M_2 called 'A'
(reference 22) identified in normal (8+6%) and infarcted
(11+6%) canine myocardium.

[c]Subtype band migrating between M_2 and M_1 called 'B'
(reference 22) identified in normal (8+6%) and infarcted
(10+9%) canine myocardium.

M_3, M_2, M_1, M_x, and M_y subtypes were separated by isoelectric
focusing and their activity expressed relative to the total
creatine kinase activity because there was not detectable MB or BB
isozyme[27] in dog serum or myocardium. Neutralized isoagarose 1-mm
thin gel (Isogel, FMC Corporation) on a flatbed electrophoresis
system (Pharmacia Fine Chemicals) and carrier ampholytes with a pH
range from 5 to 8 (LKB) was used for the isoelectric focusing. The
gel-ampholyte film was prefocused with 100 volts at 7°C for 10 min.
One- to 5-µl samples were applied with the aid of a mask, and the
film was focused at 7.5 watts constant power using ferritin as a
guide for completion of focusing, which usually required 30 to
45 min. Sodium hydroxide was used for the cathode and either
glutamic acid, aspartic acid, or HEPES was used for the anode.
The coupled enzyme assay of Rosalki using A-Gent CK-NAC was utilized
to identify subtypes on the gel, and they were measured for relative
activity by fluorometric scanning (Turner Instruments). The ratio
of M_3:M_1 subtypes was obtained by multiplying the total creatine
kinase activity (International Units/liter) by the subtype percentage, and dividing these two activities to calculate the ratio.

RESULTS

The myocardial area of interest was defined anatomically as the segments at risk for infarction according to the distribution of the left circumflex coronary artery: the posterior papillary muscle, three segments posteriorly (apex, mid, and base), and two middle segments (apex and mid) including three layers (epicardium, mid-myocardium, and endocardium) for each segment. Control myocardial segments were those outside the risk zone and in which the first blood flow determination was <1 SD below the mean of all the segments (Table 2). This definition was used to exclude damage during the preparative surgery.

Table 2. Control Myocardial Blood Flow Determinations[a]

Study[b]	Baseline[c]	Occlusion[d]	Reperfusion[e]
Dog 1 2 h CAO NS	1.10+0.20	1.50+0.30	1.20+0.50
Dog 5 3 h CAO NS	0.96+0.20	0.90+0.16	0.97+0.13
Dog 6 5 h CAO NS	0.82+0.15	1.20+0.20	0.93+0.15
Dog 7 2 h CAO SK	0.93+0.12	1.03+0.30	1.30+0.15
Dog 8 24 h CAO NS	1.24+0.20	0.96+0.20	---
Dog 9 3 h CAO SK	0.83+0.09	0.85+0.14	0.82+0.19
Dog 10 24 h CAO NS	1.20+0.50	1.24+0.20	---
Dog 11 5 h CAO SK	1.33+0.20	1.35+0.30	1.56+0.38
Dog 12 24 h CAO SK	0.96+0.13	1.32+0.30	1.50+0.30
Dog 13 24 h CAO NS	1.10+0.20	1.00+0.15	---

[a] Data are mean $\pm$ 1 SD.

[b] Hours of occlusion (CAO) and infusion with saline (NS) or streptokinase (SK).

[c] Baseline studies include all myocardial segments and were performed in the resting state before any medications.

[d] Studies were determined ½ h before release of the occlusion or during the third hour when occlusion was permanent (24 h).

[e] Studies were performed ½ h before death, and for studies with permanent (24 h) occlusion the cuff was still inflated.

Segments were considered ischemic if the second blood flow
determined during occlusion was >1 SD below control myocardial
segments. Segments were considered reperfused if the second blood
flow determination was low but returned to control blood flow levels
during the third blood flow determination. Myocardial segments
were considered infarcted if the third blood flow determination was
>1 SD below control (Table 3).

To evaluate the effect of streptokinase on reperfusion of
myocardium at risk, the variation between individual infarct sizes
must be considered. The weight of the myocardial segments that
became ischemic and then either reperfused or infarcted were placed
in a ratio, reperfused myocardium:infarcted myocardium. This ratio
of reperfusion to infarction was greater when streptokinase was
infused than when saline was infused.

The total serum creatine kinase activity increased in a biphasic manner when coronary artery occlusion was released (Table 4).
The first total creatine kinase peak occurred about 5 h after
release of the coronary artery occlusion. This peak was higher in
the studies when streptokinase was infused than when saline was
infused. The weight of myocardial segments reperfused and the ratio
were greater after streptokinase than after saline. The second
total creatine kinase peak occurred 12–18 h after release of
coronary artery occlusion. This second peak was higher than the
first peak when saline was infused. Also the weight of myocardial
segments infarcted was greater after saline than after streptokinase.

Table 3. Myocardial Blood Flow after Coronary Artery
Occlusion and Reperfusion with Streptokinase (SK)
or Saline (NS) in Dogs

| | 2 h | | 5 h | | 24 h | |
Occlusion Time	NS	SK	NS	SK	NS	SK
Ischemic area (g)	11.9	16.6	23.3	20.9	27.0	14.1
Reperfused area (g)	4.9	12.0	8.3	20.9	a	7.0
Infarcted area (g)	7.0	4.6	15.0	2.3	a	7.1
Ratio of reperfused to infarcted area	0.7	2.6	0.5	8:1	a	1.0

[a]Dogs died before the third determinations.

Table 4. Serum Creatine Kinase Activity after Coronary Artery Occlusion and Reperfusion with Streptokinase (SK) or Saline (NS) in Dogs

Occlusion Time	2 h		5 h		24 h	
	NS	SK	NS	SK	NS	SK
Peak CK (IU/L)						
1st:2nd	589:1186	807:650	596:932	1900:1300	-:728	-:1200
Time to peak (h)	5:20½	5:19½	3:20½	6½:17½	-:17½	-:17½
Peak subtype (IU/L)						
Ratio M_3:M_1	0.88	0.40	0.60	1.40	0.68	1.20
Time to peak (h)	3.60	1.60	3.40	2.20	7.00	10.00

When coronary artery occlusion was permanent, the total serum creatine kinase activity increased in a uniphasic manner. The total creatine kinase peak occurred with a similar time interval as the second total creatine kinase peak after coronary artery occlusion and release. The three studies involving permanent occlusion and saline infusion were not completed because the dogs died before 24 h and the third myocardial blood flow determination was not carried out. Myocardial segments that may have been reperfused or infarcted could not be determined.

The ratio of serum MM creatine kinase subtypes $M_3:M_1$ had only one peak that occurred earlier when streptokinase was infused than when saline was infused and preceded the total serum creatine kinase peak by several hours. The ratio was high when the eventual total creatine kinase peak was high. The high total serum creatine kinase may be related to a large area of ischemia with some reperfusion or a small area of ischemia with marked reperfusion; both situations might allow a bolus of M_3 to enter the serum.

DISCUSSION

The myocardial blood flow determinations from this preliminary study suggest that streptokinase allows reperfusion of a greater area of ischemic myocardium than simple mechanical release of coronary artery occlusion. This may be related to lysis of micro-thrombi, alterations in peripheral vascular or microvascular resistances, changes in ventricular loading conditions, or local inflammatory responses. This is clinically relevant because intracoronary drugs are used both before and after coronary angioplasty, the clinical correlate of mechanical release of occlusion.

Reperfusion of large areas of myocardium soon after ischemic events is reflected in early high total serum creatine kinase activity. The final total creatine kinase released from tissue into the serum depends on effective perfusion of the infarcted tissue, the degree of ischemia and related collateral blood flow, and local degradation, lymphatic transport, and lymphatic degradation of creatine kinase.

In this study the total serum creatine kinase activity reflected the amount of ischemic myocardium. The curve is biphasic when reperfusion occurs. The first peak appears proportional to the amount of myocardium in which reperfusion actually occurred. Thus, the total serum creatine kinase activity may not accurately reflect infarct size but a combination of infarct and reperfused ischemic myocardium. Ischemia is reflected earliest by an increase in the MM creatine kinase subtype ratio of $M_3:M_1$. This ratio's increase and peak precede the serum creatine kinase activity peak by several hours. The ratio is important clinically, if it does not peak and fall, there is ongoing release of M_3 from myocardium suggesting continued ischemic damage.

In conclusion, after mechanical release of coronary artery occlusion, streptokinase may cause reflow of a larger area of ischemic myocardium than reperfusion alone. This may allow salvage of some ischemic myocardium and limitation of infarct size.

REFERENCES

1. B. E. Sobel, G. F. Bresnahan, W. E. Shell, and R. D. Yoder, Estimation of infarct size in man and its relation to prognosis, Circulation 46:640 (1972).
2. D. Mathey, W. Bleifeld, P. Hanrath, and S. Effert, Attempt to quantitate relation between cardiac function and infarct size in acute myocardial infarction, Br Heart J 36:271 (1974).
3. W. E. Shell and B. E. Sobel, Biochemical markers of ischemic injury. Circulation 53 (Suppl I):I-98 (1976).
4. R. M. Norris, R. M. L. Whitlock, C. Barratt-Boyes, and C. W. Small, Clinical measurement of myocardial infarct size. Modification of a method for the estimation of total creatine phosphokinase release after myocardial infarction, Circulation 51:614 (1975).
5. M. J. Cowley, A. Hastillo, G. W. Vetrovec, and M. L. Hess, Effects of intracoronary streptokinase in acute myocardial infarction, Am Heart J 102:1149 (1981).
6. G. Lee, J. Giddens, P. Krieg, A. Dajee, M. Suzuki, J. A. Kozina, R. M. Ideka, A. N. DeMaria, and D. T. Mason, Experimental reversal of acute coronary thrombotic occlusion and myocardial injury in animals utilizing streptokinase, Am Heart J 102:1139 (1981).
7. P. Rentrop, H. Blanke, K. R. Karsch, W. Rutsch, M. Schartl, W. Merx, R. Dörr, D. Mathey, and K. Kuck, Changes in left ventricular function after intracoronary streptokinase, Am Heart J 102:1188 (1981).
8. L. A. Reduto, G. C. Freund, J. M. Gaeta, R. W. Smalling, B. Lewis, and K. L. Gould, Coronary artery reperfusion in acute myocardial infarction: beneficial effects of intracoronary streptokinase on left ventricular salvage and performance, Am Heart J 102:1168 (1981).
9. D. G. Mathey, K.-H. Kuck, V. Tilsner, H.-J. Krebber, and W. Bleifeld, Nonsurgical coronary artery recanalization in acute transmural myocardial infarction, Circulation 63:489 (1981).

10. W. Merx, R. Dörr, P. Rentrop, H. Blanke, K. R. Karsch, D. G. Mathey, P. Kremer, W. Rutsch, and H. Schmutzler, Evaluation of the effectiveness of intracoronary streptokinase infusion in acute myocardial infarction: postprocedure management and hospital course in 204 patients, Am Heart J 102:1181 (1981).

11. European Cooperative Study Group for Streptokinase Treatment in Acute Myocardial Infarction, Streptokinase in acute myocardial infarction, N Engl J Med 301:797 (1979).

12. B. E. Sobel, Applications and limitations of estimation of infarct size from serial changes in plasma creatine phosphokinase activity, Acta Med Scand 199 (Suppl 587):151 (1976).

13. K. A. Reimer, J. E. Lowe, M. M. Rasmussen, and R. B. Jennings, The wavefront phenomenon of ischemic cell death. 1. Myocardial infarct size vs duration of coronary occlusion in dogs, Circulation 56:786 (1977).

14. W. E. Shell, J. K. Kjekshus, and B. E. Sobel, Quantitative assessment of the extent of myocardial infarction in the conscious dog by means of analysis of serial changes in serum creatine phosphokinase activity, J Clin Invest 50: 2614 (1971).

15. P. R. Maroko, J. K. Kjekshus, B. E. Sobel, T. Watanabe, J. W. Covell, J. Ross, and E. Braunwald, Factors influencing infarct size following experimental coronary artery occlusion, Circulation 43:67 (1971).

16. G. D. Buckberg, J. C. Luck, D. B. Payne, J. I. E. Hoffman, J. P. Archie, and D. E. Fixler, Some sources of error in measuring regional blood flow with radioactive microspheres, J Appl Physiol 31:598 (1971).

17. M. A. Heymann, B. D. Payne, J. I. E. Hoffman, and A. M. Rudolph, Blood flow measurements with radionuclide-labeled particles, Prog Cardiovasc Dis 20:55 (1977).

18. R. A. Wevers, H. P. Olthuis, J. C. C. Van Niel, M. G. M. Van Wilgenberg, and J. B. J. Soons, A study on the dimeric structure of creatine kinase (EC 2.7.3.2), Clin Chim Acta 75:377 (1977).

19. R. A. Wevers, R. J. Wolters, and J. B. J. Soons, Isoelectric focusing and hybridisation experiments on creatine kinase (EC 2.7.3.2), Clin Chim Acta 78:271 (1977).

20. R. A. Wevers, M. Delsing, J. A. G. Klein Gebbink, and J. B. J. Soons, Post-synthetic changes in creatine kinase isozymes (EC 2.7.3.2), Clin Chim Acta 86:323 (1978).

21. R. L. Morelli, C. J. Carlson, B. Emilson, D. Abendschein, and E. Rapaport, Serum creatine kinase MM isoenzyme sub-bands after acute myocardial infarction, Circulation 67:1283 (1983).

22. D. Abendschein, R. L. Morelli, C. J. Carlson, B. Emilson, and E. Rapaport, Creatine kinase MM isoenzyme subtype transformation after coronary artery occlusion in dogs, Circulation 64 (Suppl IV):IV-153 (1981).

23. J.-P. Chapelle and C. Heusghem, Further heterogeneity demon-
    strated for serum creatine kinase isoenzyme MM, Clin Chem
    26:457 (1980).
24. W. G. Yasmineh, M. K. Yamada, and J. N. Cohn, Postsynthetic
    variants of creatine kinase MM, J Lab Clin Med 98:109 (1981).
25. H. Falter, L. Michelutti, A. Mazzuchin, and W. Whiston, Studies
    on the sub-banding of creatine kinase MM and the 'CK
    conversion factor,' Clin Biochem 14:3 (1981).
26. S. B. Rosalki, An improved procedure for serum creatine
    phosphokinase determination, J Lab Clin Med 69:696 (1967).
27. F. R. Elevitch, "Fluorametric Methods in Clinical Chemistry,"
    Little Brown & Company, Boston (1973).

ACKNOWLEDGMENT

Supported in part by the American Heart Association grant-in-
aid No. 81-982. Dr. Mickelson was a trainee on grant No. HL-07912
from the National Heart, Lung and Blood Institute.

POST-CONTRACTURE REPERFUSION:

EFFECT OF ELEVATED POTASSIUM AND VERAPAMIL

Stanley B. Digerness, William G. Tracy, Nona F. Andrews
and John W. Kirklin

Department of Surgery
University of Alabama in Birmingham
Birmingham, Alabama

INTRODUCTION

We have previously reported that ischemic contracture in the
isolated rat heart can be reversed and functional recovery significantly improved by reperfusing for a brief period of time with
elevated potassium cardioplegic solution, before returning to
normal potassium levels [1]. Similarly, Lazar et al[2] observed
that reperfusing an ischemic dog heart with secondary blood cardioplegia resulted in reversal of ischemic damage. Presumably, this
allows a return to aerobic metabolism and the re-synthesis of high-
energy phosphates without the drain on energy reserves caused by
beating. However, we have found that reperfusion must occur soon
after the peak of contracture (within 1 to 3 min), or recovery will
be poor.

We have repeatedly observed, as have others[3,4], that contracture is followed by regions of hypoperfusion, usually confined
to the subendocardium. This brings up the possibility that contracture in some way limits reflow, possibly through compression of
capillaries, or through direct endothelial damage, resulting in
blockage of the vessels. Verapamil, a calcium antagonist and
coronary vasodilator, might improve flow to those regions of hypoperfusion, and thus improve functional recovery. The following
study was undertaken to determine if the presence of verapamil in
the reperfusion high-potassium buffer can be beneficial following
ischemic contracture.

METHODS AND MATERIALS

Perfused Heart Model

Fed male Sprague-Dawley rats, weighing between 285 and 388 g
were used in this study. Animals were given 300 units heparin intraperitoneally, followed by 18 mg pentobarbital 10 min later,
also intraperitoneally. The hearts were quickly removed, plunged
into ice-cold buffer, then the aorta was cannulated, and perfusion
begun with oxygenated buffer at a perfusion pressure of 100 cm H_2O.
Excess tissue was trimmed away, an opening was made in the left
atrium, and a vent consisting of a short piece of 0.046 inch vinyl
tubing was inserted through the LV wall near the apex.

A needle thermistor probe (Webster Laboratories) was inserted
into the right ventricle through the pulmonary artery. A pacing
lead was attached to the right atrial appendage. The other pole
of the pacer was immersed in the buffer reservoir.

A modification of the isovolumic model of Fallen et al [5]
was used to estimate mechanical function. This model uses a water-
filled balloon placed in the left ventricular cavity. The balloon
schematic is shown in Figure 1.

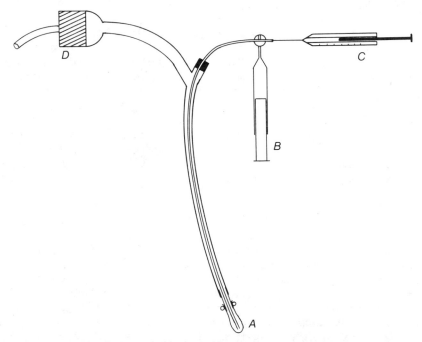

Figure 1. Balloon inflation apparatus. A; latex balloon,
B; reservior, C; microliter syringe, D; pressure transducer.

Latex was obtained from Killian Latex Co. and balloons of approximately twice the internal volume of the left ventricle were made by dipping aluminum forms into the latex and drying in an oven for approximately twenty minutes at 100°C. The balloon and accompanying apparatus were filled with boiled water to eliminate bubble formation. The reservoir syringe provided gross adjustments of balloon volume, and a microliter syringe (Hamilton Co.) provided precise control of balloon volume. The eyelets shown allowed fastening the balloon to the mitral annulus, and the internal teflon tube allowed the insertion of the balloon into the ventricle. Signals from the pressure transducer led to a recorder and differentiator. This isovolumic model allows us to estimate both systolic and diastolic function. Typically, we inflate the balloon in 3 increments of 0.01 ml each, simultaneously recording changes in systolic and diastolic pressure and dP/dt. We are careful to stay on the ascending portion of the pressure-volume curve, and find that this does not cause damage to the heart.

The teflon tube down the center of the balloon and the fact that the shank of the balloon was sutured at the mitral annulus prevented the balloon from herniating out of the left ventricular cavity, yet fluid collecting around the balloon was freely vented and thus did not impart pressure of its own against the balloon. The aortic valve was competent at all times. An incompetent valve was immediately made obvious by the torrential flow through the heart, thus excluding it from the study.

Perfusate Composition

The perfusion fluid was Krebs-Henseleit buffer, having a content of, (mM) Na (143), K (5.9), Mg (1.2), Ca (2.5), Cl (127.7), HCO_3 (25), SO_4 (1.2), and HPO_4 (1.2). This was gassed with 95% oxygen, 5% carbon dioxide, to give a PO_2 of greater than 600 mmHg and a pH of 7.4. Hydrostatic perfusion pressure was kept constant at 100 cm H_2O at all times. To arrest the heart, this buffer was modified by increasing the potassium concentration to 30 mEq/L and lowering the sodium correspondingly to maintain osmolarity. This buffer was gassed in a separate reservoir with 95% oxygen, 5% carbon dioxide. A third buffer had 2 mg/L verapamil in addition to the elevated potassium, and this was also oxygenated.

Groups

Each of eighteen rats were randomly assigned to one of three groups. Group I served as the untreated control group, Group II was reperfused for 5 min with high-potassium buffer, then normal buffer, and Group III was reperfused for 5 min with potassium and verapamil, then normal buffer. All hearts received 23 min of normothermic ischemia and 30 min of reperfusion.

429

Perfusion Sequence

The sequence was as follows: after cannulation of the heart and insertion of the balloon and thermistor probe, the heart rates were measured. Typically, rates ranged from 230 to 340 beats per minute. If endogenous rates were less than 300/min, the hearts were paced at 300. If endogenous rates were greater than 300, the hearts were not paced in the pre-ischemic period but were paced during post-ischemic measurements at the pre-ischemic rate. Pre-ischemic function was determined by inflating the balloon with the microliter syringe, recording developed pressure, dP/dt and end diastolic pressure at each increment. This relationship between end diastolic pressure and balloon volume, is known as the "distensibility slope", by the method of Apstein et al [6]. For an undamaged heart,this slope is near zero, but increases with the degree of damage. At the completion of the functional assay, the balloon volume was returned to baseline, and coronary flow was measured by collecting all effluent that dripped from the heart for a set time interval. The pacer was then turned off.

Total ischemia was instituted by stopping all flow to the heart and immersing it in buffer kept at 37°C. The thermistor placed in the right ventricle allowed us to monitor temperature during the entire period of ischemia. Actual myocardial temperatures varied from 37.0 to 37.4 C. After approximately 15 to 20 minutes of ischemia, the baseline was observed to rise rapidly, and within 2 to 3 minutes, plateau. This was the contracture phenomenon.

After 23 min of ischemia, reperfusion was begun with either normal buffer (Group I) or modified buffer (Groups II and III). After 5 min of reperfusion with modified buffer, hearts in Group II and III were returned to normal buffer for an additional 25 min. Coronary flow was collected continuously, divided into the first and second 5 min of reperfusion, and the final 20 min. In addition to volume determination, the coronary effluents were analyzed for lactate dehydrogenase content by standard enzymatic techniques. From this the total loss of this substance was calculated for each heart.

After 30 min of reperfusion, function was again measured exactly as pre-ischemically, pacing if necessary. Also, coronary flow was again measured. Thus, post-ischemic function was expressed as a percent of pre-ischemic function, each heart serving as its own control.

Finally, the balloon and temperature probe were removed and the hearts were perfused with 10 ml of sodium fluorescein in Krebs-Henseleit buffer. They were then taken off the perfusion cannula, cut transversely into 3 sections and photographed under UV light.

The % of non-reperfused tissue was determined by tracing enlarged photographs of the sections with a planimeter.

The developed pressure and dP/dt signals were analyzed with a microcomputer system. On command, the computer took one second of data, picking the maximum and minimum values of developed pressure, and the maximum positive and negative values of dP/dt. An average of these was then determined and printed out.

During ischemia, the computer sampled the developed pressure channel every second and looked for a consistent rise in pressure in the balloon. When this was found, the total elapsed time from the beginning of ischemia was determined, and printed out. The point of maximum contracture was determined similarly.

Statistics

Measured values within each group were averaged and expressed as the mean and standard error. Unpaired t-tests were used to compare Groups II and III to Group I. For intergroup differences, data were subjected to analysis of variance, then to the Tukey-Kramer procedure [7]. A p value of 0.05 or less was considered significant, and a p value of 0.01 or less was considered highly significant.

RESULTS

Initial Conditions

There were no differences between the three groups in terms of initial developed pressure, dP/dt or end diastolic pressure slope. Likewise, there were no differences in coronary flows, and lactate dehydrogenase release during the intial period was undetactable.

Ischemia

All hearts in each group developed contracture, as evidenced by a rise in left ventricular balloon pressure (Fig. 2). There was no difference between groups in the mean time to the onset of contracture, but individual times to onset within groups varied from 14.0 to 20.7 min.

Reperfusion

After 23 min of normothermic ischemia, reperfusion at 37°C was begun. Hearts in Group I started beating immediately, but within 1 to 2 min had stopped, with a dramatic rise in end diastolic tension. During the reperfusion period tension relaxed somewhat, and a small amount of beating, mostly right ventricular, returned (Figure 2).

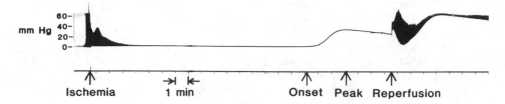

Figure 2. Typical recording of ischemia and contracture in Group I, reperfusion with normal Krebs-Henseleit buffer.

Hearts in Group II did not beat during the 5 min of high potassium reperfusion. Balloon pressure rapidly dropped, then rapidly rose, and gradually relaxed over the remaining 25 min of reperfusion. Beating gradually resumed, but more rapidly than in Group II, except in two of the six hearts, upon reperfusion, balloon pressure declined and stayed down for the remainder of the reperfusion period. Beating and developed pressure returned very rapidly in those two hearts.

Post-ischemic coronary flow was increased slightly but not significantly in Group III compared to the other groups (Table 1). This slightly greater flow persisted throughout the full 30 min reperfusion period, even though verapamil was present only during the first 5 min.

As shown in Table 2, LDH release was significantly less in the first 10 min in both Groups II and III, compared to Group I.

Functional Recovery

Systolic recovery measured after 30 min of reperfusion was uniformly poor in hearts in Group I, with developed pressure recoveries ranging from 6.2 to 40.7%, and a mean of 25.7%. This poor recovery was also seen in both positive and negative dP/dt. Likewise, the increase in end diastolic pressure slopes indicated uniform increases in stiffness of the left ventricles.

Recoveries of developed pressure in Group II ranged from 27.7 to 64.9%, with a mean of 45.0%. This was significantly better than group I (p=0.034). Recovery of positive dP/dt was approaching significance (p=0.060), and negative dP/dt was significantly improved (p=0.034) compared to Group I. The increase in end diastolic pressure slope was insignificantly less.

Recovery of both systolic and diastolic function was more variable in Group III than in the other two groups. Developed pressure recovered anywhere from 5.3 to 106.3%. As a result, it was not possible to demonstrate significant improvement over the other two groups.

Reperfusion Areas

In a comparison of the percent of myocardium reperfused, there was an indication of better perfusion in Groups II and III, but the differences were insignificant (Table 4).

Correlations

After observing that hearts in Group III which developed contracture first had the poorest recovery, we looked for a correlation between the peak-to-reperfusion time interval and recovery of developed pressure. Only in Group III was there found a strong negative correlation (r= -0.964). That is, the earlier a heart developed contracture, the longer the post-contracture interval, and the poorer the recovery. Also in this group, a strong positive correlation (r=0.934) was found between percent reperfused and recovery of developed pressure.

DISCUSSION

The isolated perfused rat heart can be a useful model for investigating the effects of ischemia on mechanical function and correlating this with biochemical observations. It also allows the evaluation of interventions such as pharmaceuticals and reperfusion techniques. In this study it was used to evaluate the possible benefit of adding a calcium antagonist to the reperfusion medium which already contained elevated potassium.

Contracture has often been observed with prolonged ischemia [8,9]. Recovery of mechanical function is characteristically poor following contracture [10,11], although early reperfusion with elevated potassium buffer can bring about relaxation and improve recovery [1].

The addition of agents such as calcium antagonists to the perfusion medium before ischemia has been shown to be beneficial, but no benefit is derived if added to the post-ischemic reperfusion medium [12]. The reason for this remains unclear, but contracture-induced regional hypoperfusion may well be a factor. Certainly, if there is little or no flow to a region such as the subendocardium, the addition of any pharmaceutical agent to the reperfusate will do no good, however beneficial the agent may be. How, then does one improve flow to these hypo-perfused regions? It would be helpful to know the reason for impaired flow, whether edema-induced compression of vessels or direct capillary plugging possibly from endothelial sloughing.

The present study demonstrates that verapamil can produce only a slight increase in coronary flow during the reperfusion period, and can likewise slightly increase the percent of tissue being reperfused. Enzyme release in the reperfusion period, probably reflecting cellular necrosis, is not significantly lessened by the addition of verapamil, probably because the ischemic damage is already too severe to be reversed.

Functional recovery is improved by reperfusing with elevated potassium, but the addition of verapamil did not add further protection. Here again, the variability within the verapamil group prevented the demonstration of significant improvement. The strong negative correlation between the length of time from con-- tracture to reperfusion and the functional recovery was interesting. This seems to indicate that following the development of contracture, cellular damage is hastened, and there is a limited time period in which one can affect an improvement in functional recovery.

The authors are indebted to Mrs. Carolyn Ingram for the preparation of this manuscript.

Supported in part by Ischemic Heart Disease SCOR HL 17667, from the National Institutes of Health.

TABLE 1. Coronary flow upon reperfusion after 23 minutes of normothermic ischemia.

ml

Group	N	First 5 min	First 10 min	Total 30 min
I	6	51.0 + 3.30	106.5 + 5.99	303 + 20.2
II	6	51.6 + 2.92	104.6 + 5.86	308 + 17.0
III	6	57.5 + 7.39	115.6 + 14.32	321 + 43.7

Mean ± SE
Group I: Normal Krebs-Henseleit reperfusion, 30 min, Group II: 5 min elevated potassium reperfusion, 25 min normal reperfusion, Group III: 5 min elevated potassium + verapamil reperfusion, then 25 min normal reperfusion.

434

TABLE 2. Post ischemic LDH release.

Units

Group	N	First 5 min	First 10 min	Total 30 min
I	6	3.24 + 0.339	7.31 + 0.635	21.94 + 2.044
II	6	1.34 + 0.204**	3.79 + 0.560**	15.31 + 1.879*
III	6	1.53 + 0.297**	3.43 + 0.740**	14.95 + 2.61

Mean ± SE

* = P < 0.05, ** = P < 0.01, compared to Group I.

TABLE 3. Post-ischemic function after 30 minutes of reperfusion.

% Recovery, compared to pre-ischemia

Group	N	Developed Pressure	+dP/dt	-dP/dt	EDP Slope Increase mmHg/0.01 ml
I	6	25.7 + 5.00	21.2 + 4.76	22.3 + 4.84	20.0 + 1.22
II	6	45.0 + 6.03*	35.8 + 4.99	40.3 + 5.54*	17.1 + 1.69
III	6	47.6 + 15.79	44.4 + 15.02	47.7 + 16.59	15.7 + 5.20

Mean ± SE
* = P < 0.05, compared to Group I, 2-sample t-test.

TABLE 4. Percent of left ventricle reperfused after ischemia and reperfusion.

Group	N	% Reperfused
I	5	72.6 + 6.12
II	5	81.8 + 3.75
III	5	84.2 + 5.28

Mean + SE

REFERENCES

1. S.B. Digerness, W.G. Tracy, N.F. Andrews, B. Bowdoin,
   J.W. Kirklin, Reversal of myocardial ischemic contracture
   and the relationship to functional recovery and tissue
   calcium, Circulation Suppl. II 68:34 (1983).

2. H.L. Lazar, G.D. Buckberg, A.J. Manganaro, R.P. Foglia,
   H. Becker, D.G. Mulder, J.V. Moloney, Reversal of ischemic
   damage with secondary blood cardioplegia, J. Thorac.
   Cardiovasc. Surg. 78: 688 (1979).

3. K. Alanen, T.J. Nevalainen, J. Lipasti, Ischemic contracture
   and myocardial perfusion in isolated rat heart, Virchows
   Arch (Pathol Anat). 385: 143 (1980).

4. S.M. Humphrey, J.B. Gravin, P. B Herdson, The relationship
   of ischemic contracture to vascular reperfusion in the
   isolated rat heart, J. Mol. Cell. Cardiol. 12: 1397 (1980).

5. E. L. Fallen, W.C. Elliot, R. Gorlin, Apparatus for study
   of ventricular function and metabolism in the isolated
   perfused rat heart. J. Appl. Physiol. 22: 836 (1967).

6. C.S. Apstein, M. Mueller, W.B. Hood, Ventricular contracture
   and compliance changes with global ischemia and reperfusion,
   and their effect on coronary resistance in the rat. Circ.
   Res. 41: 206 (1977).

7. R.R. Sokal, F. J. Rohlf, "Biometry" Freeman, San Francisco
   (1981).

8. D.J. Hearse, P.B. Garlick, S.M. Humphrey, Ischemic contracture
   of the myocardium: mechanisms and prevention. Am. J.
   Cardiol. 39: 986 (1977).

9. D.C. Macgregor, G. J. Wilson, S. Tanaka, D. E. Holnes,
   W. Lixfield, M.D. Silver, L.J. Rubis, W. Goldstein,
   J. Gunstensen, Ischemic contracture of the left ventricle.
   Production and prevention. J. Thorac. Cardiovasc. Surg.
   70: 945 (1975).

10. O.H.L. Bing, M.C. Fishbein, Mechanical and structural
    correlates of contracture induced by metabolic blockade
    in cardiac muscle from the rat. Circ. Res. 45: 298 (1979).

11. P.D. Henry, R. Shuchleib, J. Davis, E.S. Weiss, B. E. Sobel, Myocardial contracture and accumulation of mitochondrial calcium in ischemic rabbit hearts. <u>Am J. Physiol.</u> 233: H677 (1977).

12. J. A. Watts, C.D. Koch, K.F. Lanoue, Effects of Ca^{++} antagonism on energy metabolism: Ca^{++} and heart function after ischemia. Am J. Physiol. 238: H909 (1980).

ULTRASTRUCTURE OF THE HUMAN MYOCARDIUM AFTER INTERMITTENT

ISCHEMIA COMPARED TO CARDIOPLEGIA

G. Görlach[1], H.H. Scheld[1], J. Mulch[1], J. Schaper[2]
F.W. Hehrlein[1]

1 Dept. of Cardiovascular Surgery, Justus-Liebig-
University
Klinikstr. 29
D-6300 Giessen, W.-Germany

2 Max-Planck-Institute for Physiological and Clinical
Research, Dept. of Experimental Cardiology
D-6350 Bad Nauheim, W.-Germany

INTRODUCTION

Despite of many reports about the detrimental effects of
intermittend ischemia induced by ventricular fibrillation as a
method of myocardial protection this method is still used during
coronary surgery (1, 2, 3, 4, 5, 6). The proponents of this
method argue that the duration of ischemia is shorter than
during cardioplegic arrest (7) and that this method is as safe
as cardioplegic arrest (8, 9). In our study we compared myocardial
protection due to cardioplegic arrest and intermittend ischemia
during coronary surgery. The quality of myocardial protection
was estimated by electronmicroscopic studies of myocardial biopsies
taken from patients during coronary surgery.

METHOD

Out of a group of 120 patients with coronary heart disease
undergoing coronary surgery we built up three groups, in which
we used different methods of myocardial protection. All patients
gave us their informed consent to perform the study. In group 1
intermittend aortic cross-clamping with induced ventricular

fibrillation was used, while in the other groups we used cardioplegic arrest with crystalloid cardioplegia. Bretschneider solution (BR) (10) was administered in group 2 and in group 3 St. Thomas solution (ST) (11) was used.

Each group consisted of 40 patients which had a coronary three vessel disease, a stenosis of the left anterior descendens and a diagonal artery of 75 - 90 %, normal ejection fraction, normal left ventricular enddiastolic pressure and normal anterior wall motion during rest. The left ventricle and the right atrium were vented during aortic cross-clamping. The posterior wall of the left ventricle was isolated with cold gauze and the heart topically cooled with cold solution during ischemia. Myocardial temperature was measured in the septum. In group 1 ventricular fibrillation was induced by electric current after aortic cross-clamping and the body temperature was reduced to 31°C (table 1). Myocardial temperature measured 30°C. First we did the distal anastomoses and after the performance of each anastomosis we defibrillated the heart and reperfused the myocardium for 10 minutes. The mean aortic cross-clamping period for one anastomosis was 10 minutes ranging from 6 to 20 minutes. Mean total cross-clamping period measured 75 $\pm$ 21 minutes. The number of coronary anastomoses ranged from 2 to 6 (mean 4).

Table 1.

AORTO CORONARY VEIN BYPASS: MYOCARDIAL PRESERVATION - CARDIOPLEGIA VS INTERMITTENT ISCHEMIA

CARDIOPLEGIA	INTERMITTENT ISCHEMIA
1. HYPOTHERMIC EXTRACORPOREAL CIRCULATION (T REKTUM 28° C)	1. HYPOTHERMIC EXTRACORPOREAL CIRCULATION (T REKTUM 31° C)
2. LEFT VENTRICLE AND RIGHT ATRIUM VENTED	2. LEFT VENTRICLE VENTED
3. CROSS-CLAMPING OF THE AORTA AND THE PULMONARY TRUNC	3. FIBRILLATION OF THE HEART
4. PERFUSION OF THE CORONARY ARTERY SYSTEM WITH ICE COLD CARDIOPLEGIC SOLUTION	4. CROSS-CLAMPING OF THE AORTA
5. MEASUREMENT OF MYOCARDIAL TEMPERATURE	5. MEASUREMENT OF MYOCARDIAL TEMPERATURE
6. ISOLATION OF THE POSTERIOR WALL	6. ISOLATION OF THE POSTERIOR WALL
7. TOPICAL COOLING WITH CARDIOPLEGIC SOLUTION	7. TOPICAL COOLING WITH RINGER'S SOLUTION

After aortic cross-clamping in group 2 and 3 two litres of cardioplegia, which had a temperature of 4°C were infused into the
aortic root. If the myocardial temperature measured in the septum
increased above 15°C we administered additional cardioplegia.
All coronary artery anastomoses were done during one period of
cardiac arrest. The average number of bypass was 4 ranging from
2 to 6 and the duration of cardiac arrest ranged from 20 - 105
minutes (mean 61 ± 15 minutes). Before cross-clamping and before
release of the clamp at the end of the ischemic period we took
myocardial biopsies with a TRU-CUT-NEEDLE[R+] from the apex of
the left ventricle in the region between left anterior descendens and dioganal arteries. We only took biopsies from
myocardial regions which showed normal myocardium. The biopsies
were immediately fixed in 3% glutaraldehyd in 0,1 cacodylate
puffer at pH 7,4. Afterwards the biopsies were prepared for
electron microscopic study as described elsewhere (12).

   A semiquantitative evaluation of ultrastructural changes
was performed according to a specially developed scoring system
(13) (fig. 1, table 2). This scoring system is based on experimental studies of the reversibility of global ischemia of the
isolated canine heart.

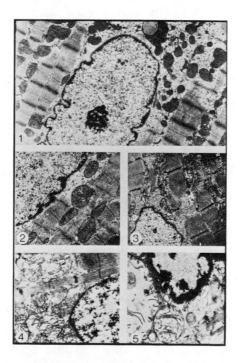

Fig. 1. Shows the different degree of ultrastructural damage,
        1 normal, 2 slight, 3 moderate, 4 severe.

+ Travenol Laboratories, Munic

441

Table 2.

Scoring of the Most Typical Ultrastructural Symptoms Leading to the Classification of Different Degrees of Ischemic Injury versus Normal Myocardial Cells. Irreversible Injury Is Indicated by the Presence of Flocculent Densities in the Mitochondrial Matrix

State of the Myocardium	ULTRASTRUCTURE							
	Mitochondria				Nuclei		Myofilaments	
Normal or Degree of Ischemic Injury	Normal Granules + or −	Flocculent Densities + or −	Matrix Light grading	Cristae Broken grading	Light grading	Pycnotic grading	Contracted or Relaxed	Contracture Bands + or −
normal	+	−	−	−	−	−	contr.	+/−
slight	−	−	+	+	−	−	contr.	+/−
moderate	−	−	++	++	+	+	contr.	+
severe	−	−	+++	+++	+	+	contr.	+
irreversible	−	+	+++	+++	++	++	rel.	++

RESULTS

Control Biopsies

The biopsies taken before ischemia showed in the chronically ischemic myocardium predominantly cellular degeneration and atrophy with replacement of myocardial tissue by fibrosis. Therefore the extracellular space increases. The myocardial cells were of irregular shape showing fingerlike protrusions into the extracellular space (fig. 2).

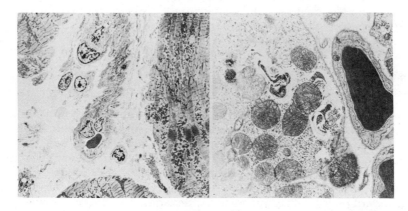

Fig. 2. Electron microscopic picture of control biopsy

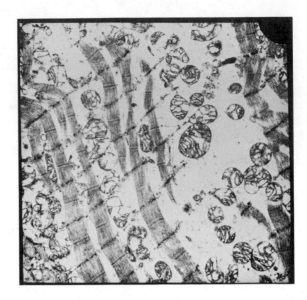

Fig. 3. Presents severe ultrastructural damage after intermittend ischemia

Intermittent Ischemia

Unexpectedly severe damage of myocardial tissue occured after
intermittent ischemia. Myocytes and capillary endothelium showed
an excessive intracellular edema unrelated to duration of
ischemia (fig. 3, table 3). 37,5% of the biopsies showed moderate
and 62,5% showed severe ultrastructural damage according to our
scoring system (table 4). Normal, slight and irreversible degree
of damage were not to be seen.

Cardioplegic Arrest

The biopsies demonstrated subcellular ischemia of moderate
degree, which increased with duration of cardiac arrest (fig. 4,
table 3). Between the two cardioplegic groups there was no
significant difference. Only 2,5% showed severe ultrastructural
damage in group 2, while in group 3 5,0% had severe damage
(table 4). 60% in group 2 and 47,5% in group 3 demonstrated only
a slight degree of ultrastructural damage. Moderate damage was
found in 37,5% in group 2 and in 47,5% in group 3.

Table 3.

DEGREE OF ULTRASTRUCTURAL DAMAGE IN RELATION TO

DURATION OF ISCHEMIA

DEGREE OF DAMAGE	BR	ST	JJ	BR	ST	JJ	BR	ST	JJ
SLIGHT	2	3		22	16				
MODERATE			4	11	14	11	4	5	
SEVERE			5			17	1	2	3
ISCHEMIC TIME (MIN.)		$<$ 40			40 - 60			$>$ 60	

LEGEND: BR: BRETSCHNEIDER,   ST: ST. THOMAS,   JJ: INTERMITTEND ISCHEMIA,   MIN.: MINUTES

Table 4.

AORTOCORONARY VEIN BYPASS

SEMIQUANTITATIVE EVALUATION OF ULTRASTRUCTURAL DAMAGE

DEGREE OF ISCHEMIC INJURY	CARDIOPLEGIA		INTERMITTEND ISCHEMIA
	BRETSCHNEIDER	ST. THOMAS	
SLIGHT	60,0 %	47,5 %	0
MODERATE	37,5 %	47,5 %	37,5 %
SEVERE	2,5 %	5,0 %	62,5 %

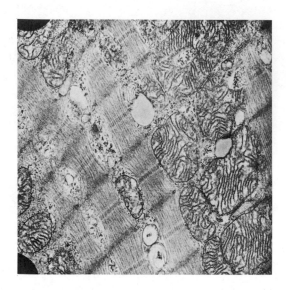

Fig. 4. Typical ultrastructure following cardioplegic arrest.

The perioperative mortality in the three groups was 0% and no complications related to the performance of myocardial biopsies occured. Perioperative myocardial infarction was seen two times in group 1 and three times in group 2 and 3 together but the difference was not statistically significant.

DISCUSSION

Despite short ischemic intervals intermittent ischemia with induced ventricular fibrillation presents not a safe method for myocardial protection. During ventricular fibrillation myocardial oxygen consumption increases to an enormous amount compared to the cardioplegic arrested heart (14). Intermittent periods of reperfusions are not always able to compensate for ischemia (15). Nevertheless repeated reperfusions are known to have detrimental effects to the myocardium (16). Therefore the results of our study are not surprising. While cardioplegia can not completely prevent ischemic alterations of the myocardium, intermittent ischemia cause most times severe ultrastructural alterations. Severe ultrastructural alterations are only rarely registered in the cardioplegic group and may be caused by in-homogenity of distribution of the cardioplegic solution beyond coronary stenosis.

According to our scoring system irreversible damage did not occur, but the scoring system is based on experiments with normal isolated perfused hearts, which did not perform work and which were reperfused up to 120 minutes. The conditions in our study were not comparable and ultrastructural damage of severe degree may not be reversible in our study group. Following intermittent ischemia occuring severe damage may cause fibrosis to a later time and compromise myocardial function. Further investigations will have to proof this hypothesis. As a con-sequence of our results intermittend ischemia should no longer be used for myocardial protection in coronary surgery.

REFERENCES

1. S.J. Phillips, R.H. Zeff, C. Kongtahworn, L.A. Iannone, T.M Brown and D.F. Gordon, Anoxic hypothermic cardioplegia compared to intermittent anoxic fibrillatory cardiac arrest. Clinical and metabolic experience with 1080 patients, Ann Surg 190:80 (1979)
2. E. Hjelms and E. Steiness, Myocardial protection in coronary artery bypass surgery. A study comparing cold cardioplegia and intermittent aortic cross clamping, J Cardiovasc Surg 23:403 (1982)
3. W.R. Chitwood Jr., R.C. Hill, J.D. Sink and A.S. Wechsler, Diastolic ventricular properties in patients during coronary revascularization. Intermittent ischemic arrest versus cardioplegia, J Thorac Cardiovasc Surg 85:595 (1983)
4. H. Vejlstedt, K. Andersen, B. Husum, B.F. Hansen, T. Palm and J. Arnbjerg, Myocardial preservation during anoxic arrest, J Thorac Cardiovasc Surg 16:175 (1982)
5. M.G. Adappa, L.B. Jacobson, R. Hetzer, J.D. Hill, B. Kamm and W.J. Kerth, Cold hyperkalemic cardiac arrest versus inter-mittent aortic cross-clamping and topical hypothermia for coronary bypass surgery, J Thorac Cardiovasc Surg 75:171 (1978)
6. D.M. Folette, D.G. Mulder, J.V. Malony Jr. and G.D. Buckberg, Advantages of blood cardioplegia over continuous coronary perfusion or intermittent ischemia, J Thorac Cardiovasc Surg 76:604 (1978)

7. A. Reikram, G. Semb, S. Landaas, K. Midtb and E. Sivertssen, Comparison of five different operative procedures: cold chemical cardioplegia versus intermittent cross-clamping of the aorta, Scand J Thorac Cardiovasc Surg 16:169 (1982)

8. H.E. Wilson, M.L. Dalton, R.J. Kiphart, and W.M. Allison, Increased safety of aorto-coronary artery bypass surgery with induced ventricular fibrillation to avoid anoxia, J Thorac Cardiovasc Surg 64:193 (1972)

9. J.L. Cox, R.W. Anderson, H.J. Pass, W.D. Currie, C.R. Roc, E. Mikat, A.S. Wechsler, and D.C. Sabiston, The safety of induced ventricular fibrillation during cardiopulmonary bypass in non hypertrophied hearts, J Thorac Cardiovasc Surg 74:423 (1977)

10. C.J. Preusse, M.M. Gebhard, and H.J. Bretschneider, Myocardial equilibration process and myocardial energy turnover during initiation of artificial cardiac arrest with cardioplegic solution - reasons for a sufficiently long cardioplegic perfusion, Thorac Cardiovasc Surgeon 29:71 (1981)

11. P. Jynge, D.J. Hearse, J. deLeiris, D. Fenvray and M.V. Braimbridge, Protection of the ischemic myocardium, J Thorac Cardiovasc Surg 76:2 (1978)

12. J. Schaper and W. Schaper, Ultrastructural correlations of reduced cardiac function in human heart disease, Eur Heart J 4 (Suppl A):35 (1983)

13. J. Schaper, Die Ultrastruktur des Myocards bei Ischämie, Habilitationsschrift, Justus-Liebig-Universität Gießen (1980)

14. C.E. Hottenrot, B. Towers, J.J. Kurkji, J.F. Maloney and G.D. Buckberg, The kazard of ventricular fibrillation in hypertrophied ventricles during cardiopulmonary bypass, J Thorac Cardiovasc Surg 66:742 (1973)

15. S. Levitzky, R.L. Wright, S.R. Nodem, C. Holland, K. Roper, R. Engelman and H. Feinberg, Does intermittent coronary perfusion offer greater myocardial protection than continuous aortic cross-clamping? Surgery 82:51 (1977)

16. H.J. Smith, K.M. Kent and S.E. Epstein, Contractile damage from reperfusion after transient ischemia in the dog, J Thorac Cardiovasc Surg 75:452 (1978)

17. G.D. Buckberg, J.R. Brazier, R.L. Nelson, S.M. Goldstein, D.H. McConnel and N. Cooper, Studies of the effects of hypothermia an regional myocardial blood flow and metabolism during cardiopulmonary bypass. 1. The adequately perfused beating, fibrillating and arrested heart, J Thorac Cardiovasc Surg 73:84 (1977)

ABSTRACT

    A lot of reports informed about the detrimental effects of
intermittent ischemia nevertheless this method is still used
during coronary surgery. We investigated the myocardial protection
due to cardioplegic arrest compared to intermittent ischemia in
120 patients undergoing coronary surgery. In all patients we
took myocardial biopsies from the left ventricle before and
after ischemia. Electron microscopic studies of all biopsies were
performed and the degree of ultrastructural alteration was
determined. The ischemic period in the cardioplegic group was
61 + 15 minutes and in the group with intermittent ischemia the
total ischemic time was 45 + 21 minutes. After ischemia the
myocardium showed most time only damage of moderate or light
degree, while after intermittent ischemia the most biopsies
showed severe ultrastructural damage. From our results we
conclude, that intermittent ischemia is unable to protect the
myocardium in a sufficient amount and should therefore no longer
be used as a method of myocardial protection.

CELLULAR INJURY IN PHOSPHATE DEPLETION: PATHOGENESIS AND MECHANISMS IN THE MYOCARDIUM

N. Brautbar

Department of Medicine and Department of Pharmacology and Nutrition
University of Southern California School of Medicine
2025 Zonal Ave., Los Angeles, Ca 90033

Phosphate depletion is commonly associated with proximal muscle weakness, muscle pain, impaired resting membrane potential (1) and mild elevation of creatine phosphokinase and aldolase (1). Phosphorus depletion in experimental animals has been shown to cause severe muscle weakness and creatinuria (2). Fuller and associates (1) examined the effect of phosphate depletion and repletion on skeletal muscle in the dog; they found that resting muscle membrane potential and muscle content of potassium and total phosphorus fell, while muscle sodium, chloride and water content rose with phosphate depletion. All these abnormalities returned to, or towards, normal with phosphate repletion. Further studies by the same group of investigators demonstrated that overt rhabdomyolysis may be precipitated by the superimposition of severe hypophsophatemia on pre-existing subclinical myopathy (3). In addition, a rise in creatine phosphokinase occurs in patients who develop acute fall in the serum levels of phosphorus (4). The observation that myopathic symptoms develop only in severe hypophosphatemia (4), and that acute hypophosphatemia may be associated with acute rhabdomyolysis suggest that both serum and cellular inorganic phosphorus levels play an important role in the myopathy.

These clinical and experimental observations suggest that skeletal myopathy of phosphate depletion may be at least in part the result of abnormalities in cellular inorganic phosphorus turnover and impaired functional integrity of cell membrane.

This manuscript reviews several studies performed in our laboratory and designed to examine the effects of phosphate depletion on cellular energy metabolism.

The contractile properties of the heart are the result of the interaction of a complex system of intracellular filaments which lie longitudinally in the cell and consist of alternating arrays of thick and thin filaments. The process of contraction requires energy in the form of high energy terminal phosphate grouping of adenosine triphosphate (ATP). Lying alongside of the myofibrils are the mitochondria, which are the intracellular site of ATP production. The mitochondrion is a compartment separated from the cytosol by a membrane which has an inner membrane and outer membrane. The mitochondrial membrane is permeable to some ions and metabolites, and less so to others; therefore, an active mechanism for maintaining intramitochondrial concentration of ions, pH and electric potential is necessary. This energy is derived from the degradation and synthesis of mitochondrial ATP. The ATP produced via oxidative phosphorylation is not able to diffuse effectively from the mitochondrial space to the myofibrils or sarcoplasmic reticulum. Therefore, a mechanism to overcome this is provided by the creatine phsophate shuttle (5).

The current concept of cellular bioenergetics is based on microcompartmentation and ability to utilize spedivid enzymes in energy production, transport and utilization. Three steps are recognized: Step I: Energy production: Energy is produced in the mitochondria via oxidative phosphorylation in the form of ATP. Step II: Energy transport: The energy in the form of ATP is converted to diffusible energy in the form of creatine phosphate. This step is catalyzed via the mitochondrial isoenzymes of creatine kinase. The creatine phosphate then diffuses to the various cellular sites: Sarcoplasmic reticulum, myofibril (5, 7, 8). Step III: Energy in the form of creatine phosphate is tuilized at the myofibrillar site via the myofibrillar isoenzymes of creatine kinase (5, 7). The ADP released after muscle contraction is re-phosphorylated to ATP, and creatine is released to diffuse back to the mitochondrial site for re-phosphorylation. Thus, creatine and the creatine kinase isoenzymes form a shuttle: The creatine phosphate shuttle (5).

The sarcoplasmic reticulum and sarcolemmal membrane play a major role in keeping the cell membrane system and its compartments intact. We have examined in this study aerobic and anaerobic energy production and cellular bioenergetics and the biochemical integrity of the cell membrane.

METHODS

    150-200 g Sprague-Dawley rats were studied after 4, 8, and 12
weeks of selective phosphorus depletion produced by dietary phosphorus restriction.   The animals were fed rat chow conaining 0.025%
phosphorus. Another group of weight- and age-matched, pair-fed
rats received diets containing 0.35% phosphorus and served as
controls. On the day of experiments, rats were anesthetized,
intubated and respirated.

I.   Aerobic energy production

    A biopsy was taken from the left ventricle, utilizing freeze
clamping liquid nitrogen techniques (9) and blood was collected for
the measurement of serum inorganic phosphorus. The myocardial
samples were then analyzed for high energy nucleotides as described
by us previously (9).

    Mitochondria and myofibrils were isolated utilizing standard
methods described previously from our laboratory (9, 10). Substrate oxidation ratio and ADP/O ratios were determined polarographically by means of a Clark oxygen electrode (Gilson Electronics, Middleton, WI).

II.   Anaerobic energy and carbohydrates

    Liquid nitrogen myocardial biopsies were examined for glycogen
utilizing enzymatic methods (10) and glucose-6-phosphate using the
Bessman ashomatic analyzer.

III.   Biochemical integrity of cellular membrane - phospholipid and
lipid synthesis

    Phospholipis precursors

    Samples were also processed for evaluation of acid extractable
phospholipid precursors and glycerol, as well as acid extractable
tissue phospholipids. Myocardial samples were extracted with acid
as described above, and the following phospholipid precursors were
examined wtilizing the Bessman ashomatic phosphorus analyzer:
phosphocholine (PC), phosphoethanolamine (GPE), and cytidine triphosphate (CTP). Glycerol phosphate was measured utilizing enzymatic methods (11).

Fatty acid oxidation

Mitochondria were isolated as described above, and fatty acid oxidation was measured utilizing the Clark electrode.

Long chain fatty acids

Activated fatty acids palmitoil co-enzyme-A was purchased from Sigma (Sigma Biochemicals, St. Louis, Mo.). 50 ul of 2 mM carnitine and 30 ul of 0.1 mM palmytoil co-enzyme-A were added consecutively to the incubation chamber, and oxygen consumption was recorded.

Short chain fatty acids

Beta-hydroxy-butyric acid was obtained from Sigma. The same medium was used for short chain fatty acids. 100 ul mitochondria were added to the incubation oxygraph vessel and 50 ul of 0.4 mM of beta-hydroxy-butyric acid added. This acid was used to examine short chain fatty acid oxidation.

RESULTS

I. Bioenergetics

A. Aerobic energy production

The effects of various durations of phosphate depletion on the serum concentration of phosphorus, body weight and on the intracellular concentration of inorganic phosphorus, adenine nucleotides and creatine phosphate and creatine of myocardium are shown in Table I. Dietary phosphate restriction was associated with a significant ($p < 0.01$) and marked decrement in serum concentration of phosphorus with the levels being lowest after 12 weeks of PD. A significant ($p < 0.01$) reduction in the myocardial concentration of inorganic phosphorus was evident after 4 weeks of phosphate depletion and remained low thereafter. There was a significant ($p < 0.01$) and direct correlation between serum levels of phosphorus and the concentration of inorganic phosphorus in myocardium.

The myocardial concentrations of ATP and ADP in phosphate depleted rats were significantly ($p < 0.01$) lower than those in control animals only after 12 weeks of PD. There was no correlation between the concentrations of these nucleotides and the serum levels of phosphorus or the cellular concentration of inorganic

454

TABLE 1. Effect of 4, 8 and 12 Weeks Of Dietary Phosphate Restriction On The Concentration Of Serum Phosphorus And On Intracellular Concentration Of Inorganic Phosphorus, Adenine Nucleotide And Creatine Phosphate In The Myocardium

| | | Serum Phosphorus (mg/dl) | INTRACELLULAR CONCENTRATION (micromole/gram protein) | | | | | Phosphorylation Potential (M-1) |
			Inorganic Phosphorus	ATP	ADP	AMP	Creatine Phosphate	
CONTROL	n=8	8.5±0.1	28.0±3.5	23.2±1.6	6.0±0.7	1.2±0.1	33.0±1.0	1400±195
4 WEEK PD	n=8	5.8±0.5*	13.6±1.4*	23.8±1.4	6.3±0.3	0.8±0.1	28.7±1.5	3128±295*
CONTROL	n=4	9.2±0.7	25.6±1.8	22.3±3.2	5.2±1.0	1.1±0.5	30.6±1.8	1654±260
8 WEEK PD	n=6	4.5±0.3*	13.2±1.5*	20.1±4.4	6.5±0.9	1.0±0.1	21.0±1.9*	2380±315*
CONTROL	n=4	7.6±0.3	32.0±2.5	27.0±1.1	7.9±0.6	1.3±0.3	32.3±1.3	1071±210
12 WEEK PD	n=7	3.4±0.1*	10.9±1.0*	14.6±1.3*	4.8±0.3*	0.9±0.1	21.7±2.1*	3290±610*

Data are presented as mean ± S.E.

* indicate significant difference from control at $p < 0.01$.

PD = phosphate depletion; ATP = adenosine triphosphate; ADP = adenosine deiphosphate; AMP = adenosine monophosphate.

phosphorus. Phosphorylation potential was signficantly increased at 4 weeks of PD and remained elevated throughout the study (Table I).

The myocardial concentration of creatine phosphate displayed a decrease after 4 weeks of PD but the decrements were statistically signficant (p < 0.01) after 8 and 12 weeks. There were significant (p < 0.01) and direct correlations between the myocardial concentration of creatine phosphate and both myocardial inorganic phosphorus (Figure 1) and serum levels of phosphorus.

Oxygen consumption per unit time was significantly (p < 0.05) reduced both after 8 weeks (94.0 ± 10 vs 65.0 ± 4.0 nmol oxygen/mg protein/min) and 12 weeks (114.0 ± 9.2 vs 82.0 ± 8.0 nmol oxygen/mg protein/min) of PD. Energy charge was unchanged in all stages of PD, and phosphorylation potential calculated according to

$$[ATP]/[ATP][P_i]$$

was significantly elevated at 4 weeks of PD and remained elevated throughout the study (Table I).

B. Mitochondrial energy transport

The activity of creatine phosphokinase was significantly reduced after 4 weeks of phosphate depletion (1.7 ± 0.12 vs 0.50 ± 0.10 IU/mg protein) and fell further after 12 weeks of phosphate depletion. The addition of creatine to state 4 respiring mitochondria signficiantly enhanced oxygen consumption in mitochondria from control but not from phosphate depleted animals as expressed by the ratio of oxygen consumption with and without creatine.

C. Myofibrillar energy utilization

There was also a significant and marked decline in the activity of myofibrillar creatine phosphokinase which became apparent within 4 weeks of phosphate depletion and remained reduced throughout the study.

Total extractable creatine phosphokinase after 4 weeks of phosphate depletion was 2.9 ± 0.5 IU/mg protein, a value significantly lower (p < 0.01) than normal (10.0 ± 0.9 IU/mg protein). There was a significant direct correlation (p < 0.01) between total extractable creatine phosphokinase and serum phosphorus levels (y =

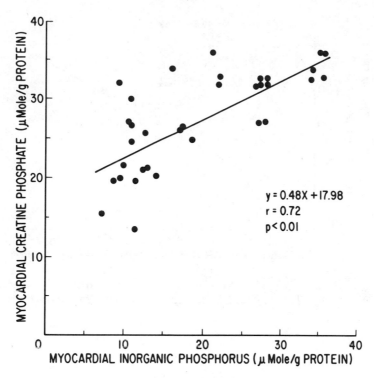

Figure 1:   Correlation between myocardial cellular creatine phosphate and inorganic phosphorus during 4, 8 and 12 weeks of phosphate depletion.

1.7x - 2.3; r = 0.73, n = 10, where y = total extractable creatine phosphokinase and x = serum inorganic phosphorus).

2.   Carbohydrate metabolism and anerobic energy production

The effects of phosphate depletion on carbohydrate pathways of the myocardium are given in Table II. A decrease in glucose-6-phosphate concentration which represents mainly glucose-6-phosphate became evident at 8 weeks of PD (1.5 ± 0.33 vs 3.8 ± 0.6 umol/g protein) and remained low thereafter (p < 0.01). Glycogen content was also sigificantly reduced both at 8 weeks (22.0 ± 2.9 vs 61.6 ±

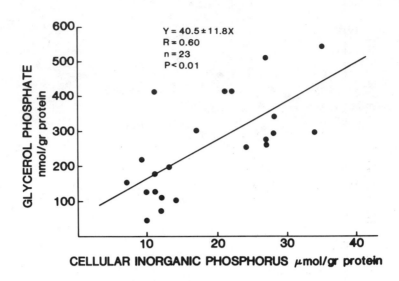

Figure 2: Correlation between cellular inorganic phosphorus (umol/gr protein) and glycerol phosphate (nmol/gr protein); p<0.01.

1.8 ug/mg protein, p < 0.01) and at 12 weeks (32.0 ± 3.1 vs 63.0 ± 4.4 ug;mg protein, p < 0.05) of PD. There was a highly significant correlation between cellular inorganic phosphorus and glucose-6-phosphate content (p < 0.01).

3. Biochemical integrity of cellular membrane - phospholipid synthesis and fatty acid oxidation

At 4 weeks the levels of glycerol phosphoethanolamine and glycerol phosphocholine (1.5 ± 0.33 umole/g protein) were significantly (p < 0.01) lower than in control rats (2.6 ± 0.30 umole/g protein) and remained low at 8 and 12 weeks. In contrast, the levels of phosphocholine and phosphoethanolamine were reduced only at 4 weeks (1.1 ± 0.06 vs 2.0 ± 0.21 umole/g protein). There was a marked fall in the concentration of cytidine triphosphate and glycerol phosphate in phosphate depletion (Table II). The changes in glycerol phosphate were highly correlated with the changes in cellular inorganic phosphorus (Figure 2).

TABLE 2. Effects of Phosphate Depletion on Myocardial Cellular Phospholipid Metabolism and Carbohydrate Pathways#

	Glycerol P (umol/g protein)	Glucose 6-P (umol/g protein)	Glycogen (ug/mg protein)	CTP (nmol/g protein)
NP 4 W	325.0±36.0	5.0±0.9	62.0±9.0	330±40
LP 4 W	270.0±46.0**	5.2±0.5		340±23
8-12 W NP	405.0±51.0	3.8±0.6	62.2±3.1	403±41
8-12 W LP	119.0±12.0*	1.35±0.2*	27.0±3.0*	288±31*

Results are expressed as mean± S.E. of 8-12 rats.
* $p < 0.01$
** $p < 0.05$
NP = normal phosphate diet
LP = low phosphate diet
Glycerol P = glycerol phosphate
Glucose 6-P = glucose-6-phosphate
CTP = cytidine triphosphate

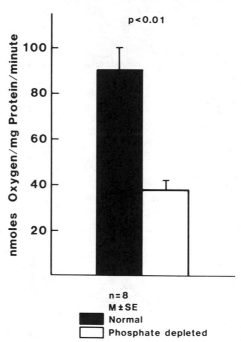

**OXIDATION OF
LONG CHAIN FATTY ACIDS
PALMITOL-COENZYME-A**

Figure 3. Oxidation of long chain fatty acids: QO_2 nmol oxygen/mg protein/min. (normal, solid bar; phosphate depleted, open bar).

After 8-12 weeks of PD, there was a significant fall in the content of phosphatidylcholine from 57.2 ± 1.6 to 29.3 ± 4.1 per cent phospholipid phosphorus ($p < 0.01$), and phosphatidylethanolamine from 39.2 ± 3.0 to 24.0 ± 4.0 percent phospholipid phosphorus ($p < 0.05$). The ratio of phosphatidylcholine to phosphatidylethanolamine was significantly altered with PD from 1.58 ± 0.05 to 1.25 ± 0.09 ($p < 0.01$). No changes were observed in phosphatidylinositol and diphosphatidylglycerol. There was also a significant fall in total phospholipid phosphorus from 8700 ± 680 to 5900 ± 570 nmoles/gram protein ($p < 0.01$).

Mitochondrial oxidation of long chain fatty acids was markedly reduced in 8-12 weeks of phosphate depletion. Mitochondria from phosphate depleted rats demonstrated a marked reduction in the ability to oxidize long chain activated fatty acids (89.7 ± 11.3 vs 37.2 ± 4.1 nMole O_2/mg protein/min, $p < 0.01$) (Figure 3). Respiratory control rate and ADP:O ratios were not different, indicating intact coupled mitochondria.

To further evaluate whether the impaired fatty acid oxidation is the result of reduced mitochondrial acetylcarnitine transferase activity, we examined short chain fatty acid oxidation. There was a marked reduction in the ability of mitochondria from phosphate depleted rats to oxidize short chain fatty acids (38.35 ± 2.11 vs 9.3 ± 3.12 nMol O_2/mg protein/min ($p < 0.01$) (Figure 4).

DISCUSSION

The results of our study show that dietary phosphate restriction is associated with impairments in myocardial cellular bioenergetics, aerobic and anaerobic energy metabolism, and in the biochemical integrity of the cellular membrane.

There were reductions in the cellular concentrations of inorganic phosphorus, ATP and ADP, acid extractable phospholipid precursors, hexose-6-phosphate and glycogen. In addition, the concentrations of creatine, creatine phosphate and the activity of mitochondrial myofibrilar and total extractable creatine phosphokinase were also reduced.

The decrease in the concentration of inorganic phosphorus of the myocardium is, at least partly, due to the marked fall in the concentration of inorganic phosphorus in serum; indeed, there was a direct and significant correlation between these two parameters. The demonstration in our study that creatine phosphate of the rat myocardium is reduced during phosphate depletion indicates that the

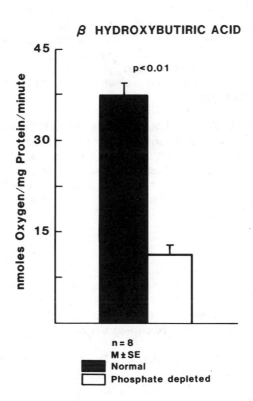

Figure 4. Oxidation of short chain fatty acids: QO_2, nmol oxygen/mg protein/min. (normal, solid bar; phosphate depleted, open bar).

transfer of energy from the mitochondria to the contractile apparatus (the creatine phosphate energy shuttle) is impaired.

The changes in cellular inorganic phospharus may influence the cell via several mechanisms:

1. **The phosphorylation state of the cell-ATP:** The supply of inorganic phosphorus in the cytosol plays a major regulatory role in mitochondrial respiration, glycolysis, and oxidative ATP synthesis. The relationship between energy supplying and energy utilizing processes in the intact cell is the net energy state of the cell, and is represented by the phosphorylation potential, which is the ratio of cytosolic ATP/ADP x P_i. From this equation it is clear that any condition which will increase the ratio will signal the mitochondria and will slow respiration and oxidative phosphorylation. Indeed, the phosphorylation potential in the phosphate depleted rats was markedly elevated, and mitochondrial respiration and oxygen consumption were reduced. It is therefore possible to suggest a mechanism whereby the extremely sensitive phosphorylation potential is immediately altered by the changes in cytosolic inorganic phosphorus.

2. **Adenine nucleotide pool - AMP deaminase de-inhibition:** Cytosolic inorganic phosphorus content is an important regulator of the overall adenine nucleotide pool size. A marked reduction in intracellular phosphorus content results in accelerated degradation of AMP via the deinhibition of AMP deaminase and, in turn, a reduction in the total adenine nucleotide pool. This mechanism may play a role in cell injury only in situations where hypophosphatemia develops rapidly and there is intracellular "trapping" of free inorganic phosphorus, such as: acute hyperalimentation, or fructose administration. Indeed, our data here do not support such a mechanism since AMP and IMP levels in phosphate depletion were not different from those of normal controls.

3. **Creatine phosphate shuttle:** The decrease in the concentration of creatine phosphate occurred after 8 weeks of phosphate depletion and was preceeded by reduced activity of mitochondrial creatine phosphokinase. These observations suggest that the alteration in the activity of this enzyme, at least partly, is responsible for the reduction in the content of creatine phosphate.

The activity of mitochondrial creatine phosphokinase, as well as that of the myofibrils, was markedly reduced. Thus, it appears that PD affects the activity of these isoenzymes present at various locations in the myocardial cells. The decrease in intracellular concentration of inorganic phosphorus could be a critical factor regulating the activity of the enzyme either via enzyme synthesis or its phosphorylation. A decrease in intracellular concentration of inorganic phosphorus could, therefore, result in reduced activity of the enzyme. Indeed, the changes in cellular creatine phosphokinase activity were correlated with the reduction in serum phosphorus levels. This, and the observation that creatine phosphate levels were correlated with the myocardial inorganic phosphorus, suggest that inorganic phosphorus may regulate creatine phosphokinase activity. The reduction in the activity of the creatine phosphokinase isoenzymes may play a critical role in the cardiomyopathy of phosphate depletion.

4. Carbohydrate metabolism: The fall in glucose-6-phosphate concentration and the reduced levels of glycogen are compatible with reduced glycolysis, glucose phosphorylation, and reduced glycogen synthesis. Indeed, decreased glucose uptake as well as insulin resistance have been reported in hypophosphatemic patients (12) and rats (13). Increased glucose-6-phosphate utilization could also be present and contribute to its reduced cellular content. Our data do not support or refute this possibility. However, the metabolic pathway of glucose-6-phosphate is facilitated by phosphofructokinase. This enzyme is sensitive to the cellular concentration of inorganic phosphorus and is inhibited when the latter is low. It is reasonable to suggest that in phosphate depletion the activity of this enzyme is reduced, and therefore increased utilization of glucose-6-phosphate does not occur.

The reduced cellular levels of glycogen are consistent with impaired glucose phosphorylation and glycogen synthesis, but the possibility of increased glycogen breakdown cannot be ruled out. Indeed, Horl et al (14) have reported both decreased glycogen synthesis and increased glycogen breakdown in the myocardium of phosphate depleted rabbits.

5. Lipid metabolism - membrane integrity: Most of the energy for myocardial contraction is derived from the oxidation of fatty acids. The finding of reduced oxidation of both long and short chain fatty acids suggests the presence of impairments at various steps of the mitochondrial processes responsible for the oxidation of fatty acids. The transport and oxidation of long chain fatty acids requires intact activity of acetylcarnitine transferase of the outer and inner mitochondrial membrane, adequate carnitine content, and sufficient acetyl-CoA (15, 16). Therefore, a defect in any of these steps could account for the reduced oxidation of long chain fatty acids. In contrast, short chain fatty acids enter mitochondria freely and independently of the activity of the acetyl

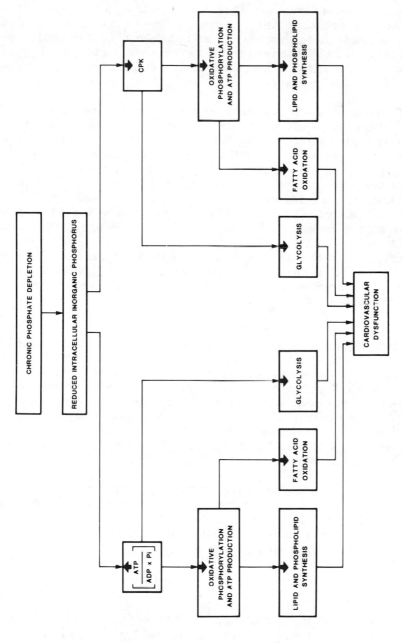

Figure 5: Proposed chain of events leading to intracellular phosphorus store depletion and cellular injury in phosphate depletion.

carnitine transferase or carnitine (16). Therefore, impaired oxidation of short chain fatty acids should indicate depletion of acetyl-CoA. The observation that Co-A synthesis requires ATP for its synthesis, and that the levels of the latter are reduced in phosphate depletion is, moreover, compatible with the notion of an intramitochondrial impairment in fatty acid oxidation. Such a derangement could also be responsible for the impaired oxidation of the long chain fatty acids.

Several lines of evidence suggest an abnormality of cell membrane integrity in phosphate depletion. The derangement in cell membrane integrity may be due to abnormalities in phospholipid biosynthesis. Indeed, the findings of reduced phosphatidylcholine (PC), phosphatidylethanolamine (PE) and total phospholipid phosphorus in the myocardium of phosphate depleted rats demonstrate impaired biochemical integrity of the cell membrane. Furthermore, the observation of altered ratios of PC/PE is compatible with altered membrane phospholipid abnormality and possibly function.

Since all of the abnormalities described in our study were preceeded by a fall in cellular inorganic phosphorus and creatine phosphokinase isoenzymes, we propose the following cellular mechanism to mediate the skeletal myopathy of phosphate depletion (Figure 5).

Prolonged hypophosphatemia causes a reduction in intracellular inorganic phosphorus stores, and this, in turn, reduces the activity of the creatine phosphokinase isoenzymes. Since creatine phosphokinase plays a major regulatory role in mitochondrial respiration, energy transport, and myofibrillar energy utilization, phosphate depletion would result in impairment in all these steps. The reduction in creatine phosphokinase activity also impairs phospholipid synthesis, and, in turn, cellular membrane functional integrity will be impaired.

Since phosphate depletion is not an isolated metabolic abnormality and is associated with hypomagnesemia and hypercalcemia, it is not possible to rule out some effects of intracellular megnesium depletion or calcium overload in addition to the reduction of intracellular inorganic phosphorus stores.

REFERENCES

1. T. J. Fuller, N. W. Carter, C. Barcenas, J. P. Knochel, Reversible changes of the muscle cell in experimental phosphorus deficiency. J. Clin. Invest. 57:1019 (1976).
2. H. Schneider, and H. Steenbock, A low phosphate diet and the

response of rats to vitamin D. J. Biol. Chem. 128:159 (1939).

3. J. P. Knochel, C. Barcenas, J. R. Cotton, Hypophosphatemia and rhabdomyolysis. J. Clin. Invest. 62:1240 (1978).

4. J. P. Knochel, Hypophosphatemia. West. J. Med. 134:15 (1981).

5. S. Bessman, P. Gegan, Transport of energy in muscle: the phosphoryl creatine shuttle. Science 211:448 (1981).

6. M. Mahler, Progressive loss of mitochondrial creatine phospho-kinase activity in muscular dystrophy. Biochem. Biophys. Res. Comm. 88:895-906 (1979).

7. V. Saks, N. Lipin, V. Sharnov, E. Chagov, The localization of the MM isoenzyme of creatine kinase on the surface membrane of myocardial cells and its functional coupling to ouabain inhibited (Na,K) ATPase. Biochim. Biophys. ACTA 465:550 (1970).

8. S. Bessman, P. Gegen, W. Yeng, W., and S. Viitanen, Inti-mate coupling of creatine phosphokinase and myofibril-lar adenosinetriphosphatase. Biochem Biophys. Res. Comm. 96:1414 (1980).

9. N. Brautbar, R. Baczynski, C. Carpenter, S. Moser, P. Geiger, P. Finander and S. G. Massry, Impaired energy metabolism in rat myocardium during phosphate depletion. Am. J. Physiol. 242:F669-704 (1982).

10. N. Brautbar, C. Carpenter, R. Baczynski, R. Kohen, and S. G. Massry, Impaired energy metabolism in skeletal mus-cle during phosphate depletion. Kid. Intern. 24:53-57 (1983).

11. N. Brautbar, J. Tabernero-Romo, J. Coats, S. Massry, Effects of phosphate depletion on lipid metabolism. Kid. Int. (in press).

12. R. A. DeFronzo, and R. Lang,   Hypophosphatemia and glucose intolerance: Evidence for tissue insensitivity to insulin. New Engl. J. Med. 303:1259-1263 (1980).

13. J. L. Davis, S. B. Lewis, T. A. Schultz, R. A. Kaplan, and J. D. Wallin, Acute and chronic phosphate depletion as a modulator of glucose uptake in rat skeletal muscle. Life Science 24:629-632 (1979).

14. W. H. Horl, W. Kreusser, A. Heidland, and E. Ritz, Abnor-malities of glycogen metabolism in cardiomyopathy of phos-phorus   depletion, in: Phosphate and Mineralis in Health and Disease.   Editors, S.G. Massry, E. Ritz and H. Jahn, pp 343-350, Plenum   Press, New York, (1980).

15. C. L. Hoppel,   Carnitine palmitoyl transferase and transport of fatty acids, in: The Enzymes of Biological Membranes. Vol. 2. Editors: A. Martonosi, Plenum Press, New York, pp 119-143, (1976).

16. E. P. Brass, and C. L. Hoppel, Carnitine metabolism in the fasting rat. J. Biol. Chem. 253:2688-2693 (1978).

DIABETES MELLITUS AND HYPOTHYROIDISM INDUCE CHANGES IN MYOSIN
ISOENZYME DISTRIBUTION IN THE RAT HEART - DO ALTERATIONS IN FUEL
FLUX MEDIATE THESE CHANGES?

Wolfgang H. Dillmann

Department of Medicine
University of California, San Diego
San Diego, CA.

The different pathophysiological mechanisms which influence
the formation of specific cardiac proteins are only incompletely
understood. Changes in the level of specific cardiac proteins
could result for example, from alterations in the hormonal milieu,
changes in cardiac substrate consumption, alterations in the level
of high energy phosphates and other mechanisms. Recent investigations have shown that the level of one specific group of proteins
in the rat heart ventricle, the isozymes of myosin, are markedly
influenced by insulin lack,[1,2] and hypothyroidism. [3,4] The existence of three myosin isoenzymes in the rat ventricle (myosin V_1,
V_2, V_3) has recently been well documented.[3-5] In normal rat
hearts myosin V_1, which has the highest Ca^{++}-activated myosin
ATPase activity, predominates, whereas in hypothyroid or diabetic
rats myosin V_3, which has the lowest myosin ATPase activity, becomes the predominant form.[1-4] The hypothyroidism and diabetes-
induced myosin V_3 predominance results in a decrease in Ca^{++}-
activated myosin ATPase activity. A very close correlation between
the activity of this enzyme and the maximal velocity of muscle
contraction is well established.[6,7] In addition a very close correlation exists between high levels of V_1 isomyosin and the maximal
speed of contraction of rat papillary muscle.[8] Administration of
physiological doses of thyroid hormone to hypothyroid rats and of
insulin to diabetic rats reverts the myosin isoenzyme distribution
to the normal pattern.[1,2,4]

The isoforms of myosin are distinguished by the form of myosin
heavy chains which they contain. Myosin V_1 is constituted of two
myosin heavy chain-alpha (MHC-α), myosin V_2 of one MHC-α and one
MHC-β, and myosin V3 of two MHC-β. Changes in the predominance

469

of MHC-α and MHC-β are accompanied by alterations in the corresponding specific mRNA.[9,10] It appears likely that the two forms of myosin heavy chain are products of different genes which are differentially expressed in the rat ventricle.

The hormone lack induced changes in myosin isoenzyme distribution could be mediated by alterations in substrate consumption. It has, for example, been well established that in the heart of diabetic rats a marked increase in fatty acid consumption and a marked decrease in glucose consumption occurs.[11] Glycolysis is decreased in the heart of hypothyroid animals.[12] We wanted to determine if changes in the level of specific cardiac proteins occur when the consumption of fatty acids or glucose is altered in the absence of corresponding changes in insulin or thyroid hormone levels. The distribution of myosin isoenzymes in the rat heart is used as a parameter to investigate the interrelationship between alterations in thyroid hormone or insulin levels and changes in substrate consumption.

To determine if changes in cardiac substrate consumption influence myosin isoenzyme distribution we placed diabetic rats on a fructose diet and quantitated ventricular myosin isoenzyme distribution.[13] Unlike glucose, fructose can be phosphorylated and metabolized to trioses in the absence of insulin,[14] and could thus serve as a carbohydrate fuel for cardiac muscle. An effect of fructose on the Ca^{++}-activated myosin ATPase activity and myosin isoenzyme distribution in the heart of insulin-deficient rats may thus point to an influence of cardiac metabolites on cardiac protein formation.

To determine the influence of fructose feeding on myosin isoenzyme distribution in diabetic rats the following experiments were performed. Male Sprague-Dawley rats between 6 and 8 weeks of age were made diabetic by i.v. administration of 65 mg streptozotocin/kg body weight (BW) and maintained in a diabetic state for 4 weeks. Blood glucose was determined 4 days and 4 weeks after streptozotocin administration and was 124±18 mg/dl in control animals, 427±38 mg/dl in animals treated with 65 mg streptozotocin/kg BW. Control and diabetic animals were then divided into groups of 4 animals each and maintained for an additional 4 weeks on either a regular diet (diet A), a glucose diet (diet B), or fructose diets (diets C, D, E and F). Diet A was in a block form and consisted of 47% complex carbohydrate, 24% protein, 4% fat and 3.6% fiber. Diet B contained 60% glucose, 20% casein, 14% fiber, 4% salt mix, and 2% vitamin mix. In diet C glucose was replaced by 60% fructose, tﾑe other ingredients remaining the same.

After 4 weeks on the different diets, animals were killed by exsanguination and ventricles were immediately frozen in liquid nitrogen and stored at -80°C for 2-8 days. Myosin was purified from rat ventricles as previously described,[15,16] and the Ca^{++}-activated ATPase activity of myosin was determined.[15,16] The release of inorganic phosphate from ATP was determined by the method of Fiske and Subbarow.[17] Protein concentrations were determined by a Biuret method.[18] Myosin isoenzymes were separated in cylindrical gel tubes by pyrophosphate polyacrylamide gel electrophoresis as described by Hoh et al.[2], except that 2 mM cysteine was added to the running buffer of Hoh et al. (20 mM $M_2Na_2P_4$, 10% glycerol, pH 8.8). After electrophoresis proteins were stained in a solution containing 0.05% Coomassie blue, 20% methanol, and 10% acetic acid. Gels were destained in 10% methanol and 10% acetic acid. The amount of each isoenzyme was determined by densitometric scanning as previously described,[15] and is expressed as percent of total myosin.

Blood was collected in heparin from the tail vein and plasma obtained by centrifugation was immediately frozen at -80°C. Plasma T_4 was analyzed by competitive protein binding assay[19] and T_3 by radioimmunoassay.[20] Plasma insulin was determined by a solid phase RAI using the micromedic system. Plasma glucose was determined at the beginning and at the end of the experimental periods by the glucose oxidase method. Fructose levels were determined by the enzymatic method described by Bernt and Bergmeyer.[21]

Diabetic rats fed 60% fructose for 4 weeks showed a significant increase in Ca^{++}-activated myosin ATPase activity. The magnitude of the increase was quite consistent and ranged from 20-30% (Ca^{++}-myosin ATPase diabetic regular diet 0.553±0.065 μmol Pi/mg protein. min S.D., diabetic 60% fructose diet 0.661±0.078 μmol Pi/mg protein. min S.D.). In contrast, administration of diet in which fructose was replaced by 60% glucose did not lead to an increase in Ca^{++}-activated myosin ATPase activity (Ca^{++}-myosin ATPase diabetic regular diet 0.593±0.097 versus 0.586±0.074 in diabetic 60% glucose diet). Feeding normal rats a high fructose or high glucose diet did not influence Ca^{++}-activated myosin ATPase activity.

We determined myosin isoenzyme distribution in aliquots of the same hearts which were used for Ca^{++}-activated myosin ATPase activities. In control animals myosin V_1 predominates and can be precisely determined. The minor components V_2 and V_3 are more difficult to quantitate, but V_2 represents approximately 19±4% and V_3 13±5% of the total myosin. Myosin V_1 predominance increased from 18 to 37% predominance in diabetic animals on the fructose diet with a concomitant decrease in V_3 predominance. Providing diabetic rats with 60% glucose in their diet or placing normal rats on the high fructose diet did not influence myosin isoenzyme distribution.

Feeding diabetic animals a fructose or glucose diet led to a further decrease in weight gain and increased hyperglycemia, but did not modify insulin or thyroid hormone levels. Fructose feeding may therefore have led to further deterioration of the general metabolic state of the animals. Previous reports have shown that the decreased T_4 or T_3 levels of diabetic animals are not primarily responsible for the change in myosin isoenzyme distribution.[15] Fructose feeding of diabetic rats did not elevate insulin levels. Similar findings were previously reported by Kaiser et al.[22] In diabetic animals on a fructose diet, fructose levels were 14 ± 5 mg/dl, whereas no fructose was detectable in the blood of normal rats or diabetic rats fed a regular diet. Urinary ketone levels determined by the sodium nitro-prusside method were weakly positive in the different groups of diabetic animals, and negative in the control rats.

The results of these studies show that fructose feeding of diabetic rats increases cardiac Ca^{++}-activated myosin ATPase activity and changes ventricular myosin isoenzyme distribution by increasing myosin V_1 predominance. The specific effects of fructose on cardiac myosin occur without concomitant improvement in the general metabolic status of the animals, and changes in insulin, T_4 or T_3 levels. Thus, the effect of fructose feeding on Ca^{++}-activated myosin ATPase activity and increased myosin V_1 predominance in rats mimics those of insulin administration. These changes occur in the absence of alterations in insulin levels. It is therefore possible that fructose mediates the increase in myosin ATPase activity and changes myosin isoenzyme distribution through alteration in cardiac metabolism. Insulin administration and fructose feeding may induce similar specific changes in the metabolism of the diabetic heart, which lead to the effects on myosin ATPase activity and myosin iso-enzyme distribution.

The routes through which fructose feeding influences Ca^{++}-activated myosin ATPase activity and myosin isoenzyme distribution are currently unclear, but known alterations in fuel flux in diabetic hearts and established metabolic effects of insulin and fructose can provide the basis for speculation concerning the routes of fructose action. In normal hearts more than 70% of all high energy phosphate is derived from fatty acid breakdown through β-oxidation and 30% is provided by glycolysis, whereas in diabetic hearts fatty acid break-down through β-oxidation is markedly increased and glycolytic flux contributes to high energy phosphate formation in a very minor fashion.[11,23] Fructose can enter the glycolytic pathway in the absence of insulin, the enzymes which play a major role in fructose metabolism (fructose 1-phosphate kinase and fructose diphosphate aldolase) are insulin-independent and present in muscle tissue.[24] Fructose could therefore serve as an alternate carbohydrate fuel for the diabetic heart and, for example, rectify a decrease in the flux through the glycolytic pathway which results from the lack of insulin. The concentration of a specific glycolytic metabolite may increase in the hearts of fructose-fed rats and could influence myosin isoenzyme formation. In addition, the increase in β-oxidation which prevails in the diabetic heart inhibits the glycolytic flux,

472

whereas insulin administration inhibits β-oxidation, increases the activity of the tricarbocyclic acid cycle and stimulates cardiac glycolysis.[23] It is interesting to note that a marked decrease in β-oxidation and increased flux through the tricarbocyclic cycle has been observed in the rat liver after fructose administration.[25] The findings described above indicate that changes in glycolytic flux may influence myosin isoenzyme predominance.

We then determined if interventions which can alter fatty acid oxidation may have a similar effect. An increase in fatty acid oxidation occurs in the heart in diabetes mellitus. To evaluate if decreased fatty acid consumption of the diabetic hearts can result in changes in myosin isoenzyme distribution, the effect of methyl palmoxirate was then determined in diabetic rats. The fatty acid analogue methyl palmoxirate has been reported to inhibit oxidation of long chain fatty acids in vivo in a variety of species and in vitro using isolated hepatocytes, kidney cortex, adipose tissue, hemidiaphragm muscle and rat hearts.[26-30] As a result of this inhibition glucose oxidation has been reported to be accelerated in heart and in smooth and skeletal muscle.[27,30,31]

Diabetes mellitus was induced in rats as described above. Hypothyroidism was induced by surgical thyroidectomy and by placing animals on 0.1% propylthiouracil in the drinking water. The thyroidectomized animals were used 4-6 weeks after surgery when they stopped gaining weight. Food intake and body weight were determined twice a week for the duration of the experiment. Control, diabetic and hypothyroid animals were then divided into the following groups of animals. 1) Control rats, untreated. 2) Control rats receiving 25 mg methyl palmoxirate/kg BW/day for 4 weeks. The drug was administered by gavage in 0.5 ml of 5% vehicle tragacant once a day at 9:00-10:00 h. 3) Diabetic rats, untreated. 4) Diabetic rats receiving after 4 weeks of diabetes 25 mg methyl palmoxirate/kg BW/day for an additional 4 weeks. The drug was administered as described above. 5) Diabetic rats receiving 5 mg methyl palmoxirate/kg BW/day for 4 weeks as described above. 6) Diabetic rats receiving the vehicle tragacant for 4 weeks. 7) Diabetic rats receiving 2 units protamine zinc insulin/100 g BW s.c. per day for 4 weeks. 8) Hypothyroid rats receiving 25 mg methyl palmoxirate/kg BW/day for 4 weeks. 9) Hypothryoid rats receiving the vehicle tragacanth for 4 weeks. Methyl palmoxirate was a generous gift of Dr. G. Tutwiler, McNeil Pharmaceutical Company, Spring House, Pennsylvania. Blood was obtained from the tail vein 4 and 24 h after the administration of methyl palmoxirate.

After 4 weeks on methyl palmoxirate animals were killed by exsanguination. A time course of 4 weeks was chosen because preliminary studies indicated that after this time the maximal change in Ca^{++}-activated myosin ATPase activity and myosin isoenzyme distribution was established (data not shown). Administration of methyl palmoxirate for 4 days did not lead to a change in Ca^{++}-activated myosin ATPase activity (Ca^{++}-myosin ATPase activity in diabetic + vehicle tragacant 0.65±0.025 umol pI/mg protein.min versus 0.62±0.04 umol Pi/mg protein.min in hearts from diabetic + 25 mg methyl palmoxirate/kg BW/day). Body weights and heart weights were determined, cardiac ventricles were immediately frozen in liquid nitrogen and stored at -80°C for 2-8 days. Myosin was purified and separated and Ca^{++}-activated myosin ATPase was determined as described above.

The specific activity of Ca^{++}-activated myosin ATPase was determined in normal rats, untreated diabetic rats and diabetic rats treated with 25 mg methyl palmoxirate/kg BW p.o./day. In addition diabetic rats were treated with the vehicle tragacanth and 2 units of protamine zinc insulin/100 g BW/day. Diabetic rats receiving methyl palmoxirate for 4 weeks showed a significant increase in Ca^{++}-activated myosin ATPase activity (Ca^{++}-myosin ATPase diabetic + Vehicle tragacanth 0.609±0.05 versus 0.912±0.06 umol Pi/mg protein. min in diabetic + 25 mg methyl palmoxirate, and 0.766±0.05 in diabetic + 5 mg methyl palmoxirate rats). A dose of 5 mg methyl palmoxirate led to a 34% increase and 25 mg methyl palmoxirate increased Ca^{++}-activated myosin ATPase activity by 66%. The methyl palmoxirate-induced increase in myosin ATPase activity followed therefore a rough dose response relationship. The level of myosin ATPase activity was similar in untreated diabetic rats and diabetic rats which received the vehicle tragacanth. A dose of 2 units protamine zinc insulin increased myosin ATPase activity significantly but could not completely normalize the enzyme levels in this experiment. In contrast, administration of 25 mg methyl palmoxirate/kg BW/day to hypothyroid animals for 4 weeks did not result in a change in Ca^{++}-activated myosin ATPase activity (Tx + methyl palmoxirate 0.59±0.03 umol Pi/mg protein.min, Tx + vehicle tragacanth 0.60±0.04 umol Pi/mg protein.min). Administration of a physiological dose of 0.3 ug T3/kg BW/day to hypothyroid rats could normalize Ca^{++}-activated myosin ATPase activity (Tx + T3 0.98±0.7 umol Pi/mg protein.min). Administration of 25 mg methyl palmoxirate to normal rats did not lead to a change in Ca^{++}-activated myosin ATPase activity.

We determined myosin isoenzyme distribution in aliquots of the same hearts which we used for Ca^{++}-activated myosin ATPase activities. In control animals myosin V_1 predominates (70-80% of total myosin) and can be precisely determined, but the minor components V_2 and V_3 are difficult to quantitate. We noted some variation in the isoenzyme distribution in normal rats. In some animals myosin V_2 and V_3 were not clearly detectable. Administration of 25 mg/kg methyl palmoxirate to normal rats had no influence on myosin isoenzyme distribution.

In diabetic animals myosin V3 predominates and represents 66% of total myosin. Methyl palmoxirate administration had a marked influence on myosin isoenzyme distribution in diabetic rats. Administration of 25 mg/kg methyl palmoxirate to diabetic rats led to a myosin isoenzyme distribution pattern which is characterized by myosin V_1 predominance (diabetic rats myosin V_1 19±7 versus 58±6 in diabetic + methyl palmoxirate). However, the myosin isoenzyme distribution is not returned completely to the normal pattern. In diabetic rats treated with 5 mg/kg methyl palmoxirate a significant diminution of myosin V3 levels occurs (diabetic rats myosin V_3 68±9 versus myosin V3 29±3 of total myosin in diabetic + 5 mg methyl palmoxirate). In all experiments, methyl palmoxirate-induced changes in myosin ATPase activity and myosin isoenzyme distribution correlated well with each other.

It is of particular interest that the methyl palmoxirate-induced increase in myosin ATPase activity and alteration in myosin isoenzyme levels occurs in the absence of changes in insulin or thyroid hormone levels (diabetic rats insulin uU/ml 6±3, diabetic + 25 mg methyl palmoxirate 7±2 uU/ml). Administration of 25 mg/kg methyl palmoxirate to diabetic rats decreased blood glucose levels by 30% 4 h after administration of the drug in comparison to vehicle tragacant treated diabetic animals. In contrast, glucose levels 24 h after administrtion of 25 mg/kg methyl palmoxirate were not significantly lowered. Administration of 5 mg/kg methyl palmoxirate or the vehicle tragacanth did not lower blood glucose values significantly at either time point, though under other experimental protocols and bleeding times others have reported this dose to lower blood glucose.[29,30]

The results of these studies show that administration of the fatty acid oxidation inhibitor methyl palmoxirate to diabetic rats increases cardiac Ca^{++}-activated myosin ATPase activity and changes ventricular myosin isoenzyme distribution by increasing myosin V_1 predominance. The effect of methyl palmoxirate showed a rough dose-response relationship with 25 mg methyl palmoxirate/kg BW/day inducing a significantly larger increase in myosin ATPase activity and myosin isoenzyme distribution than the effect observed after 5 mg methyl palmoxirate. The specific effects of methyl palmoxirate on cardiac myosin occur without concomitant changes in insulin, T_4 or T_3 levels and the effect of the drug is therefore not simply mediated through alterations in the levels of these hormones which are known to influence cardiac myosin isoenzyme formation.

The routes through which methyl palmoxirate influences Ca^{++}-activated myosin ATPase activity and myosin isoenzyme distribution are currently unclear, but known alterations in fuel flux in diabetic hearts and established metabolic effects of insulin and methyl palmoxirate can provide the basis for speculation concerning the routes of methyl palmoxirate action. In normal hearts more than 70% of all high energy phosphate is derived from fatty acid breakdown through β-oxidation and 30% is provided by glycolysis, whereas in diabetic hearts fatty acid breakdown through β-oxidation is markedly increased and glycolytic flux contributes to high energy phosphate formation in a very minor fashion.[32]

Methyl palmoxirate is a potent inhibitor of the carnitine dependent transport of long chain fatty acid into the mitochondria.[28] A coenzyme A ester formed from the drug has been shown to be an active-site-directed irreversible inhibitor of carnitine palmityol transferase 1,[33,34] an enzyme thought to be the rate-limiting step for long chain fatty acid oxidation. Addition of methyl palmoxirate has been shown to inhibit fatty acid oxidation and stimulate glycolysis in a variety of tissues,[30] including heart,[27] and leads in several animal species to an inhibition of gluconeogenesis and a marked lowering of plasma glucose and ketones.[26,27,28,30,33] It has been postulated that the products of fatty acid oxidation, like citrate, inhibit glycolysis.[35] Increased β-oxidation may therefore be an important factor for the decreased glucose utilization which occurs in diabetes mellitus. Administration of methyl palmoxirate to diabetic rats therefore decreases cardiac β-oxidation and probably increases glycolytic flux, and stimulates pyruvate dehydrogenase.[35,27,28,30] Similar metabolic alterations will result from insulin administration.[36] One could therefore speculate that methyl palmoxirate and insulin-induced increases in Ca^{++}-activated myosin ATPase and myosin isoenzyme distribution result from similar specific changes in the metabolism of the heart, and are related to decreased β-oxidation and/or tte increased glycolytic flux. Administration of methyl palmoxirate to normal or hypothyroid rats did not change Ca^{++}-activated myosin ATPase activity or myosin isoenzyme distribution. Thus methyl palmoxirate does not act independently of the specific metabolic disturbances which occur in diabetic rats. It is ineresting to note that T_3 administration leads to an increase in fatty acid consumption.[37]

The effect of methyl palmoxirate administration on myosin V_1 predominance in diabetic rat hearts together with our findings that placing diabetic rats on a 60% fructose diet also increases ventricular V_1 predominance may indicate that changes in cardiac substrate consumption can influence cardiac myosin isoenzyme formation. These findings may provide a stimulus for more detailed examination of the general relationship between alterations in cardiac metabolism and the formation of specific contractile proteins.

REFERENCES

1. W.H. Dillmann, Diabetes Mellitus Induces Changes in Cardiac Myosin of the Rat. Diabetes 29:579 (1980).

2.   A. Malhotra, S. Penpargkul, F.S. Fein, E.H. Sonnenblick, J. Scheuer, The Effect of Streptozotocin-induced Diabetes in Rats on Cardiac Contractile Proteins. Circ.Res. 49:1243 (1981).
3.   J.F. Hoh, P.A. McGrath, P.T. Hale, Electrophoretic Analysis of Multiple Forms of Rat Cardiac Myosin: Effects of Hypophysectomy and Thyroxine Replacement. J.Mol.Cell.Card. 10:1053 (1978).
4.   W.H. Dillmann, S. Berry, N.M. Alexander, A Physiological Dose of Triiodothyronine Normalized Cardiac Myosin Adenosine Triphosphatase Activity and Changes Myosin Isoenzyme Distribution in Semistarved Rats. Endocrinology 112:2081 (1983).
5.   A.M. Lompre, J.J. Mercadier, C. Wisnewsky, P. Bouveret, C. Pantaloni, A. d'Albis, K. Schwartz, Species- and age-dependent Changes in the Relative Amounts of Cardiac Myosin Isoenzymes in Mammals. Developmental Biology 84:286 (1981).
6.   M. Barany, ATPase Activity of Myosin Correlates with Speed of Muscle Shortening. J. Gen.Physiol. 50:197 (1967).
7   C. Delcayre, B. Swynghedauw, A Comparative Study of Heart Myosin ATPase and Light Subunits from Different Species. Pfluegers Arch. 355:39 (1975).
8.   K. Schwartz, Y. Lecarpentier, J.L. Martin, A.M. Lompre, J.J. Mercadier, B. Swynghedauw, Myosin Isoenzymic Distribution Correlates with Speed of Myocard ial Contraction. J. Mol. Cell. Card. 13:1071 (1981).
9.   W.H. Dillmann, A. Barrieux, G.S. Reese, Effect of Diabetes and Hypothyroidism on the Predominance of Cardiac Myosin Heavy Chains Synthesized in vivo or in a Cell-free System. J. Biol. Chem. (In Press).
10. A.M. Sinha, P.K. Umeda, C.J. Kavinsky, C. Rajamanickam, H-J Hsu, S. Jakovcic, M. Rabinowitz, Molecular Cloning of mRNA Sequences for Cardiac α- and β-form Myosin Heavy Chains: Expression in Ventricles of Normal, Hypothyroid and Thyrotoxic Rabbit. Proc. Natl. Acad. Sci. USA 79:5847 (1982).
11. P. Randle, P. Rubbs, The Cardiovascular System 1, the Heart. in: Handbook of Physiology, Sect. 2, R.M. Berne, N. Sperelakis and S.R. Geiser, eds., American Physiological Society, Bethesda, MD. (1974).
12. F.L. Hoch, Metabolic Effects of Thyroid Hormones, in: Handbook of Physiology, Sect. 7: Endocrinology, R.O. Greep, E.B. Astwood, eds., AMerican Physiological Society, Washington, D.C.
13. W.H. Dillmann, Myosin Isoenzyme Distribution and Ca^{++}-activated Myosin ATPase Activity in the Rat Heart is Influenced by Fructose Feeding and Triiodothyronine. Endocrinology (In Press)
14. G. Van den Berghe, Metabolic Effects of Fructose in the Liver. Curr. Top.Cell.Regul.13:97 (1978).
15. W.H. Dillmann, Influence of Thyroid Hormone Administration on Myosin ATPase Activity and Myosin Isoenzyme Distribution in the Heart of Diabetic Rats. Metabolism 31:199 (1982).

16. A.K. Bhan, A. Malhotra, Trypsin Digestion of Canine Cardiac Myosin. Arch.Biochem.Biophys. 174:24 (1976).
17. C.H. Fiske, Y. Subbarow, The Colorimetric Determination of Phosphorus. J.Biol.Chem. 66:375 (1925).
18. E. Laye, Spectrophotometric and Turbidimetric Mettods for Measuring Proteins, in: Methods in Enzymology, S.P. Colowich, N.O. Kaplan, eds. Academic Press, N.Y. (1957).
19. N.M. Alexander, J.F. Jennings, Analyses for Total Serum Thyroxine by Equilibrium Competitive Protein Binding on Small, Reusable Sephadex Columns. Clin.Chem. 20:553 (1974).
20. N.M. Alexander, J.F. Jennings, Radioimmunoassay of Serum Triiodothyronine on Small, Reusable Sepahdex Colums. Clin.Chem. 20:1353 (1974).
21. E. Bernt, U. Bergmeyer, D-fructose, in: Methods in Enzymatic Analysis, H.U. Bergmeyer, ed. Academic Press, N.Y. (1974).
22. F.E. Kaiser, C.N. Mariash, H.L. Schwartz, J.H. Oppenheimer, Inhibition of Malic Enzyme Induction by Triiodothyronine in the Diabetic Rat: Reversal by Fructose Feeding. Metabolism 29:767 (1980).
23. A.E. Farah, A.A. Alousi, The Actions of Insulin on Cardiac Contractility. Life Sciences 29:975 (1981).
24. A.E. Renold, G.W. Thorn, Clinical Usefulness of Fructose. Am.J.Med. 14:163 (1955).
25. G.N. Prager, J.A. Ontko, Direct Effects of Fructose Metabolism on Fatty Acid Oxidation in a Recombined Rat Liver Mitochondria-high Speed Supernatant System. Biochem.Biophys.Acta 424:386 (1976).
26. S.M. Lee, G.F. Tutwiler, R. Bressler, C.H. Kircher, Metabolic Control and Prevention of Nephropathy by 2-tetradecylglycidate in the Diabetic Mouse (db/db). Diabetes 31:12 (1982).
27. F.J. Pearce, J. Forster, J.R. Williamson, G.F. Tutwiler, Inhibition of Fatty Acid Oxidation in Normal and Hypoxic Perfused Hearts by 2-tetradecylglycidic acid. J. Mol. Cell. Card. 11;893 (1979).
28. G.F. Tutwiler, P. Dellevigne. Action of the Oral Hypoglycemic Agent 2-tetradecylglycidic Acid on Hepatic Fatty Acid Oxidation and Gluconeogenesis. J.Biol.Chem. 254:2935 (1979)
29. G.F. Tutwiler, T. Kirsch, R.J. Mohrbacker, W. Ho, Pharmacologic Profile of Methyl 2-tetradecylglycidate (McN-3716) - An Orally Effective Hypoglycemic Agent. Metabolism 27:1539 (1978).
30. G.F. Tutwiler, W. Ho, R.J. Mohrbacker. 2-teradecylglycidic acid. Meth. in Enzymology 72:533 (1981).
31. R.W. Tuman, J. Joseph, C.R. Bowden, H.J. Brentzel, G.F. Tutwiler. Effects of 2-tetradecylglycidic acid (TDGA) on GLucose Metabolism in Skeletal Muscle. Fed. Proc. 41:511 (1982).
32. L.H. Opie, M.J. Tansey, B.M. Kennelly, The Heart in Diabetes Mellitus. Part I. Biochemical Basis for Myocardial Dysfunction. S. Afr. Med. J. 56:207 (1979).

33. G.F. Tutwiler, M.T. Ryzlak, Inhibition of Metochondrial Carnitine Palmitoyl Transferase by 2-tetradecylglycidic acid (McN-3802). Life Sciences 26:393 (1980).
34. T.C. Kiorpes, D. Hoerr, L. Weaner, W. Ho, M. Inman, G.F. Tutwiler, Characterization of 2-tetradecylglycidyl-coenzyme A (TDGA-CoA) as an Irreversible, Active Site-directed Inhibitor of Rat Liver Mitochondrial Carnitine: Palmitoyl Transferase-A (CPT-A). Fed.Proc. 42:2187 (1983).
35. P.B. Garland, P.J. Randle, E.A. Newsholme, Citrate as an Intermediary in the Inhibition of Phosphofructokinase in Rat Heart Muscle by Fatty Acids, Ketone Bodies, Pyruvate, Diabetes and Starvation. Nature 200:169 (1963).
36. P.J. Randle, P.K. Tubbs, Carbohydrate and Fatty Acid Metabolism, in: Handbook of Physiology - The cardiovascular System, Vol.I, American Physiological Society, Bethesda, MD, (1979).
37. J.O. Olubadewo, H.G. Wilcox, M. Heimberg, Effect of Glycerol on Oleate Metabolism by Livers from Triiodothyronine (T3) treated and euthyroid (EU) rats. 65th Annual Meeting The Endocrine Society, San Antonio, Texas (Abstract 484)(1983).

GLYCEROL KINASE DEFICIENCY: COMPARTMENTAL CONSIDERATIONS

REGARDING PATHOGENESIS AND CLINICAL HETEROGENEITY

Edward R.B. McCabe and
William K. Seltzer

Departments of Pediatrics and
Biochemistry, Biophysics and Genetics
University of Colorado School of Medicine
Denver, Colorado

INTRODUCTION

In the past prokaryotic and eukaryotic mutations were used to define the sequence of biochemical pathways. Now we are beginning to use mutations to understand the organization, integration, and regulation of cellular metabolism. Glycerol kinase deficiency (McKusick No. 30703) (1), an inherited disorder involving a compartmented enzyme (2), offers a model for observing the effects that disruption of a reversibly formed microenvironment might have on the functional integrity and energy economy of the cell.

CLINICAL HETEROGENEITY - SAME ENZYME BLOCKED IN PATIENTS WITH DIFFERING PHENOTYPES

Deficient activity of glycerol kinase (ATP:glycerol phosphotransferase, EC 2.7.1.30) was originally reported nearly simultaneously in two very different families (3,4). Two brothers, two and five years of age at the time of diagnosis, evidenced adrenal insufficiency and hypoplasia, psychomotor retardation, nonspecific myopathy, poor somatic growth, and osteoporosis (3,5). Three adult males in another family were noted incidentally because of pseudohypertriglyceridemia in the 70 year old proband, but showed none of the clinical findings of the two children (4). This raised the question initially whether the syndrome described in the children represented only a chance association with this inborn error of metabolism (2). However, as

481

subsequent individuals have been noted with glycerol kinase deficiency, three distinct clinical groupings have been recognized (2,6), known as the infantile, juvenile and adult forms of this enzyme deficiency (Table 1).

To date we are aware of eleven patients (ten male and one female) in six families with the infantile form of glycerol kinase deficiency, all of whom have been noted to be developmentally delayed with adrenal hypoplasia at autopsy or functional evidence of adrenal cortical insufficiency (2,3,5,7-9). Nonspecific myopathy, characterized by Duchenne type changes histologically with markedly elevated serum creatine phosphokinase (CPK) values, has been a prominent feature in many of these patients (2,5,7,8,8a); however, other patients have had normal CPK values and no clinical evidence of myopathy (2,7,8). Osteoporosis and deficient somatic growth are additional features receiving comment in some patients (2,3,5,8,8a), but are frequently not addressed. In general, clinical abnormalities have been noted in the first year of life (2,5,7,8,8a), and in one patient adrenal insufficiency was documented in utero (7).

Two unrelated boys have been described with the juvenile form of glycerol kinase deficiency (2,6,10). Each child presented clinically with his initial episode of vomiting, acidemia and stupor at four years of age. Both have normal adrenal function, normal CPK, and no clinical evidence of myopathy. The one boy with reported developmental test results is well above normal intellectually (6). This child was placed on a low glycerol diet and had no subsequent episodes of coma (6).

Five adult males in three families have been reported with glycerol kinase deficiency and no consistent clinical abnormalities (2,4,11,12). These individuals were identified because of the incidental observation of pseudohypertriglycer-idemia (2,12).

Hyperglycerolemia and glyceroluria are characteristic of affected individuals in all three clinical groups with glycerol kinase deficiency (2). All but one individual with this enzyme deficiency have been male, and pedigrees available for families affected with the infantile and adult forms, as well as biochemical studies of parents of affected individuals, are consistent with X-linked inheritance (2,4,7,12,13).

EVIDENCE FOR COMPARTMENTATION OF GLYCEROL KINASE

Wilson (14) has suggested that the term "ambiquitous" (both places, in analogy with "ubiquitous", all places) should refer to enzymes with rapid and reversible changes in intracellular

482

Table 1. Clinical Subtypes of Glycerol Kinase Deficiency

Clinical Group	Age at Presentation	Clinical Description
Infantile	First year of life	Consistent findings: Adrenal insufficiency and hypoplasia Developmental delay Frequent but not constant observations: Myopathy and elevated serum CPK Variably reported: Osteoporosis Poor somatic growth
Juvenile	4 years old	Vomiting, acidemia, stupor
Adult	21 years and older	Incidental observation of pseudohypertriglyceridemia but no consistent clinical abnormalities

distribution. Enzymes which have been considered in this category include hexokinase (14,15), aldolase (16), and glyceraldehyde 3-phosphate dehydrogenase (16). Recent data from Brdiczka's group as well as ours strongly suggest that glycerol kinase should be considered an ambiquitous enzyme (2,17-19).

Glycerol kinase may be found in either the cytosolic or particulate fraction of the cell with differences in subcellular distribution dependent upon the tissue, developmental stage, and metabolic state at the time of examination (2,17-25). In the particulate fraction glycerol kinase activity is present in both microsomes and mitochondria, though it is the mitochondrial bound activity of this enzyme which varies with the metabolic state of the animal (19). In the mitochondria glycerol kinase is bound to porin, the pore forming protein of the outer mitochondrial membrane (18,19), which is identical to the hexokinase binding protein (18,26,27). Brdiczka (18,19) has suggested a reciprocal

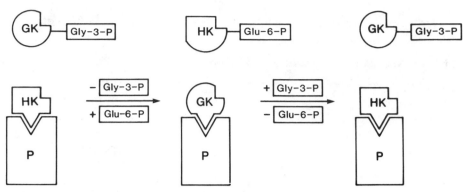

Fig. 1.   Reciprocal regulation in the reversible binding of glycerol kinase and hexokinase to porin. According to this diagram glycerol 3-phosphate leads to solubilization of glycerol kinase and binding of hexokinase to porin; increasing the concentration of glucose 6-phosphate and decreasing the concentration of glycerol 3-phosphate results in debinding of hexokinase and binding of glycerol kinase to porin; diminishing glucose 6-phosphate and increasing glycerol 3-phosphate concentrations reverses the binding and debinding of these two kinases. Certain features which have been incorporated for simplicity in this diagramatic representation should be noted. In this illustration, glycerol 3-phosphate and glucose 6-phosphate have effector affinity sites on their respective kinases, and occupation of an affinity site by the specific effector leads to debinding. However, affinity sites for these effectors may be located on porin or either of the kinase proteins. A single receptor binding site is depicted on porin for these two kinases, but a separate binding site for each kinase is equally possible.

regulation in the reversible binding of glycerol kinase and hexokinase to porin: glucose 6-phosphate leads to debinding of hexokinase and binding of glycerol kinase, and removal of glucose 6-phosphate with addition of glycerol 3-phosphate results in debinding of glycerol kinase and rebinding of hexokinase (Figure 1). Porin is also an important channel for the exchange of adenine nucleotides across the outer mitochondrial membrane (28). This kinase binding pore protein provides a possible molecular explanation of the competition for mitochondrially generated ATP which has been observed between mitochondrial bound hexokinase and added glycerol kinase (2,29,30).

The kinase-porin system is an example of regulated enzyme compartmentation, and, specifically, of a metabolite-mediated, reversibly formed microenvironment not limited or walled off by an organellar membrane (31). As has been pointed out by Welch and DeMoss (32), enzyme organization is valuable to the energy economy of the cell through catalytic facilitation, similar to the catalytic advantage of individual enzyme reactions: enzyme aggregation has potential for significant influence on the free energy of activation of the organized system.

Recent work from our laboratory has focused on the significance of glycerol kinase binding to the function and regulation of this enzyme in bovine adrenal gland (17). This tissue was chosen since the adrenal is consistently affected in the infantile form of glycerol kinase deficiency (Table 1) and the subcellular distribution appears similar for bovine and human adrenals (17,25). Bovine adrenal glycerol kinase was distributed between soluble and particulate fractions in a ratio of approximately 3:1. When glycerol kinase activity was compared between the particulate free 105,000 g supernatant and the mitochondrial fraction, we found that the apparent Kms for both glycerol and ATP were significantly lower for the particulate associated enzyme (Table II).

The subcellular distribution of adrenal glycerol kinase was not static, but could be altered by the presence of specific effectors (17). Although inorganic phosphate (Pi) had no effect on the release of glycerol kinase from the mitochondria, both ATP and glycerol 3-phosphate did modulate debinding in a concentration dependent manner. ATP in the concentration range of 1.0-7.5 mM and in the presence of 5 mM $MgSO_4$ caused release of 20-30% of the total activity which had been initially bound, but had no effect at higher concentrations up to 20 mM. Glycerol 3-phosphate in the presence of 5 mM $MgSO_4$ also produced 20-30% debinding like ATP over this concentration range, but unlike ATP, was just as effective at higher concentrations (10-20 mM). Additionally, the absence of Mg++ promoted debinding of glycerol kinase to a maximum of 44%.

Finally, in the bovine adrenal system we showed that mitochondrial bound glycerol kinase was stimulated by the respiratory substrates ADP and succinate, and was inhibited by 1.25 uM atractyloside either in the presence of respiratory substrates or at low ATP concentration (3 uM) (17). This was interpreted to indicate that the adenine nucleotide carrier was functionally important in the delivery of ATP to the bound glycerol kinase, though the possibility could not be ruled out that carrier bound atractyloside was sterically hindering the binding of ATP to the kinase. Either possibility would indicate a functional intimacy between the outer membrane enzyme and the inner membrane translocase.

Table II. Comparison of Michaelis constants for soluble and bound glycerol kinase from bovine adrenal.

	Soluble	Mitochondrial	
Km Glycerol (uM)	6.3 ± 0.1	4.0 ± 0.3	p=0.01
Km ATP (uM)	12.8 ± 1.5	5.3 ± 1.6	p=0.02

Glycerol kinase activity in the mitochondrial fraction was assayed in the presence of 1.25 uM atractyloside to inhibit ATPase activity and to prevent translocation of ATP into or out of the mitochondria; atractyloside had no effect on soluble glycerol kinase activity. Phosphate was omitted from the soluble and mitochondrial assays to further ensure that mitochondria were not generating ATP. The Km values represent the mean ± SEM from four separate determinations (17).

Brdiczka's group (19) has shown effector mediated, reversible debinding of glycerol kinase from rat liver mitochondria, and has also observed stimulation of bound glycerol kinase activity by succinate and ADP, as well as inhibition by atractyloside, in the rat liver system. Similarly, mitochondrial hexokinase is specifically solubilized by its product, glucose 6-phosphate (15,33), utilizes mitochondrially generated ATP (34-38), and has a Km for ATP which is lower than that for the soluble enzyme (15).

Thus, it would appear that glycerol kinase, like hexokinase, should be considered an "ambiquitous" enzyme (14), demonstrating rapid and reversible changes in intracellular distribution dependent upon cellular energy status and metabolite levels, and showing distinct kinetic properties dependent upon this distribution.

COMPARTMENTAL CONSIDERATIONS IN THE PATHOGENESIS OF GLYCEROL KINASE DEFICIENCY

If we are to understand the pathogenesis and clinical heterogeneity of glycerol kinase deficiency we will be severely limited if we view the system only in terms of possible effects of mutations on the catalytic activity of the enzyme. We must also consider the possible effects of mutations on the mitochondrial binding of glycerol kinase which would alter the dynamic, physiologically modulated compartmentation of this enzyme.

The usual biochemical approaches, focusing on catalytic mutations, have not been revealing. The kinetic properties of the residual glycerol kinase activity have been examined and compared in fibroblasts from individuals with the infantile and adult forms of this disorder (39,40). Cells from both types of individuals showed an increase in the apparent Km for glycerol compared with controls, but the apparent Km for ATP was similar to controls. While the increase in apparent Km for glycerol was slightly higher in fibroblasts from the individual with the infantile form, the variation in the measured values for this parameter (resulting from kinetic measurements of residual activity in cells which have a relatively low activity even in normals) made it impossible to conclude that there was any significant difference between these individuals using this parameter (40). A hybridization panel consisting of fibroblasts from two patients with the infantile form and one individual each with the juvenile and adult forms failed to demonsntrate complementation (39-41).

However, there is evidence that the functional integration of glycerol kinase into cellular metabolism differs in the infantile and juvenile forms of this disorder. Whereas the in vitro glycerol kinase activities from disrupted fibroblasts are quite similar between individuals with the infantile and juvenile forms of this inborn error of metabolism (4-5% of control activity), the in situ incorporation of glycerol into protein by intact fibroblasts is more than 3-fold increased in cells representing the juvenile form compared with in situ activity of intact cells representing the infantile form (9% and 3% of control values, respectively) (6).

The dynamic, porin mediated compartmentation of glycerol kinase should be considered as we attempt to understand the potential impact of different mutations on the functionally intact system. Different mutations might affect binding and/or catalysis (Figure 2). Even more subtle structural variations might be envisaged which would allow porin-kinase binding, but would alter the efficient accessibility of mitochondrial ATP to the affinity site for this substrate on the kinase protein.

SUMMARY AND CONCLUSIONS

Two organs are consistently affected in patients with the infantile form of glycerol kinase deficiency: the brain, with

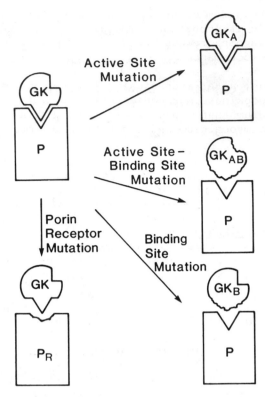

Fig. 2. Possible mutations which might affect the glycerol
kinase-porin system. On the right (from the top) are
depicted mutations affecting glycerol kinase active
site (GK_A), active site and binding site for porin
(GK_{AB}), and binding site for porin (GK_B).
Represented at the lower left is a mutation affecting
the kinase receptor site on porin (P_R).

developmental delay, and the adrenal glands, with functional
insufficiency and structural hypoplasia (Table 1). Both brain and
adrenal evidence significant mitochondrial binding of glycerol
kinase (2,17,25,42-44). The binding of glycerol kinase to outer
mitochondrial membrane porin is regulable and reversible, alters
the kinetic properties of the catalytic activity of the kinase,
and facilitates communication of the kinase with the mitochondrial
matrix. Disruption of the efficient operation of this
microenvironment by mutations affecting catalysis and/or binding
would have particular impact on the normal development and
function of those tissues where binding was significant.

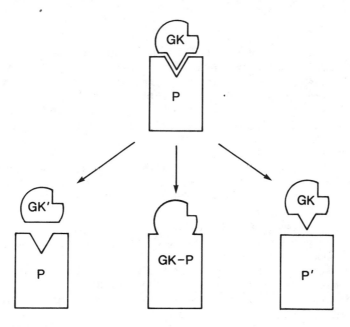

Fig. 3. Examples of engineered proteins which could be
derived from the glycerol kinase-porin system. From
left to right are glycerol kinase without a binding
site for the porin receptor (GK'), a non-dissociable
glycerol kinase-porin complex (GK-P), and porin
lacking the receptor site for glycerol kinase (P').

In our investigation of glycerol kinase deficiency we have
moved from clinical observation to consideration of the
compartmentation of this enzyme at the outer mitochondrial
membrane. Natural mutations allow us to begin the dissection of
this compartmented system. However, modern molecular genetic
approaches will allow us to engineer specific mutations in order
to more clearly understand the structure-function relationships
involved in the organization of this microenvironment (Figure 3).

ACKNOWLEDGEMENTS

This work was supported by an individual research grant from
the National Institute of Arthritis, Metabolic and Digestive
Diseases (RO1 AM26265), a Clinical Research Center Grant from the
Division of Research Resources, (RR-69), a Center Grant (HDMR 5P30
HD0424), a Program Project Grant (5P01 HD08315) and a Training
Grant in Mental Retardation (5T32 HD07096) from the National
Institute of Child Health and Human Development, National Insti-
tutes of Health, and by a Basil O'Connor Starter Research Grant
(No. 5-332) from the March of Dimes Birth Defects Foundation.

REFERENCES

1. V. A. McKusick, "Mendelian Inheritance in Man - Catalogs of Autosomal Dominant, Autosomal Recessive, and X-Linked Phenotypes, Sixth Edition", The Johns Hopkins University Press, Baltimore (1983), p. 1050.
2. E. R. B. McCabe, Human glycerol kinase deficiency: An inborn error of compartmental metabolism, Biochem. Med. 30:215 (1983).
3. E. R. B. McCabe, P. V. Fennessey, M. A. Guggenheim, B. S. Miles, W. W. Bullen, D. J. Sceats, and S. I. Goodman, Human glycerol kinase deficiency with hyperglycerolemia and glyceroluria, Biochem. Biophys. Res. Commun. 78:1327 (1977).
4. C. I. Rose and D. S. M. Haines, Familial hyperglycerolemia, J. Clin. Invest. 61:163 (1978).
5. M. A. Guggenheim, E. R. B. McCabe, M. Roig, S. I. Goodman, G. M. Lum, W. W. Bullen, and S. P. Ringel, Glycerol kinase deficiency with neuromuscular, skeletal and adrenal abnormalities, Ann. Neurol. 7:441 (1980).
6. E. I. Ginns, J. A. Barranger, S. W. McClean, C. Sliva, R. Young, E. Schaefer, S. I. Goodman, and E. R. B. McCabe, A juvenile form of glycerol kinase deficiency with episodic vomiting, acidemia and stupor, J. Peds., in press (1984).
7. J. A. Bartley, D. K. Miller, J. T. Hayford, and E. R. B. McCabe, The concordance of X-linked glycerol kinase deficiency with X-linked adrenal hypoplasia in two families, Lancet (2):733 (1982).
8. J. A. Bartley, J. T. Hayford, J. Perkins, H. I. Firminger, and E. R. B. McCabe, Glycerol kinase deficiency: A X-linked disorder associated with congenital adrenal hypoplasia, myopathy and developmental delay, Proc. Grnwd. Gen. Cen. 2:110 (1983).
8a. W.O. Renier, F.A.E. Nabben, T.W.J. Hustinx, J.H. Veerkamp, B.J. Otten, H.J. Ter Laak, B.G.A. Ter Haar, and F.J.M. Gabreels, Congenital adrenal hypoplasia, progressive muscular dystrophy, and severe mental retardation, in association with glycerol kinase deficiency, in male sibs, Clin. Gen. 24:243 (1983).
9. R. Matalon, L. Librik, J. Wise, and E. R. B. McCabe, unpublished.
10. A. Eriksson, S. Lindstedt, L. Ransnas, and L. von Wendt, Deficiency of glycerol kinase (EC 2.7.1.30), Clin. Chem. 29:718 (1983).
11. D. Pometta, A. Suenram, N. von der Weid, and J. J. Widmann, Liver glycerokinase deficiency in man with hyperglycerolaemia and hypertriglyceridaemia, Europ. J. Clin. Invest. 14:103 (1984)
12. Y. Gousault, E. Turpin, D. Neel, C. Dreux, B. Chanu, R. Bakin, and J. Rouffy, 'Pseudohypertriglyceridemia' caused by hyperglycerolemia due to congenital enzyme deficiency, Clin. Chim. Acta 123:269 (1982).

13. J. Bartley, J. Hayford, and R. Ward, Glycerol kinase activity of fibroblasts from obligate carriers of glycerol kinase deficiency, Amer. J. Hum. Genet. 34:45A (1982).

14. J. E. Wilson, Ambiquitous enzymes: Variation in intracellular distribution as a regulatory mechanism, Trends Biochem. Sci. 3:124 (1978).

15. J. E. Wilson, Brain hexokinase, the prototype ambiquitous enzyme, Curr. Top. Cell Reg. 16:1 (1980).

16. D. J. Winzor, L. D. Ward, and L. W. Nichol, Quantitative considerations of the consequences of an interplay between ligand binding and reversible adsorption of a macromolecular solute, J. Theor. Biol. 98:171 (1982).

17. W. K. Seltzer and E. R. B. McCabe, Subcellular distribution and kinetic properties of soluble and particulate-associated bovine adrenal glycerol kinase, Submitted for publication (1984).

18. C. Fiek, R. Benz, N. Roos, and D. Brdiczka, Evidence for the identity between the hexokinase binding protein and the mitochondrial porin in the outer membrane of rat liver mitochondria, Biochim. Biophys. Acta 688:429 (1982).

19. A.-K. Ostlund, U. Gohring, J. Krause, and D. Brdiczka, The binding of glycerol kinase to the outer membrane of rat liver mitochondria: Its importance in metabolic regulation, Biochem. Med. 30:231 (1983).

20. E. R. B. McCabe, W. K. Seltzer, and W. W. Bullen, Glycerol kinase: Different properties from human liver and fibroblasts, Fed. Proc. 41:879 (1982).

21. W. K. Seltzer, W. W. Bullen, and E. R. B. McCabe, Human glycerol kinase: Comparison of properties from fibroblasts and liver, Life Sci. 32:1721 (1983).

22. E. R. B. McCabe, W. K. Seltzer, R. Hill, and D. Sadava, Glycerol kinase: Developmental biochemistry in man, Pediat. Res. 16:298A (1982).

23. W. K. Seltzer and E. R. B. McCabe, Glycerol kinase activity in human adrenal gland, Pediat. Res. 17:172A (1983).

24. W. K. Seltzer and E. R. B. McCabe, Subcellular distribution and bisubstrate kinetics of rat, bovine and human adrenal glycerol kinase, Fed. Proc. 42:2079 (1983).

25. W. K. Seltzer and E. R. B. McCabe, Human and rat adrenal glycerol kinase: Subcellular distribution and bisubstrate kinetics, Molec. Cell. Biochem., in press (1984).

26. P. L. Felgner, J. L. Messer, and J. E. Wilson, Purification of a hexokinase-binding protein from the outer mitochondrial membrane, J. Biol. Chem. 254:4944 (1979).

27. M. Linden, P. Gellerfors, and B. D. Nelson, Pore protein and the hexokinase-binding protein from the outer membrane of rat liver mitochondria are identical, FEBS Letters 141:189 (1982).

28. N. Roos, R. Benz, and D. Brdiczka, Identification and characterization of the pore forming protein in the outer membrane of rat liver mitochondria, Biochim. Biophys. Acta 686:204 (1982).

29. I. A. Rose and J. V. B. Warms, Mitochondrial hexokinase — release, rebinding and location, J. Biol. Chem. 242:1635 (1967).

30. P. L. Felgner, Studies on the physiological raison d'etre of mitochondrial hexokinase, Fed. Proc. 32:488 (1973).

31. P. A. Srere and R. W. Estabrook, eds., Preface, in: "Microenvironments and Metabolic Compartmentation," Academic Press, New York (1978), p. XIII.

32. G. R. Welch and J. A. DeMoss, Enzyme organization in vivo: Thermodynamic-kinetic considerations, in: "Microenvironments and Metabolic Compartmentation," P. A. Srere and R. W. Estabrook, eds., Academic Press, New York (1978), pp. 323-343.

33. A. S. Chou and J. E. Wilson, Purification and properties of rat brain hexokinase, Arch. Biochem. Biophys. 151:48 (1972).

34. R. E. Gots, F. A. Gorin, and S. P. Bessman, Kinetic enhancement of bound hexokinase activity by mitochondrial respiration, Biochem. Biophys. Res. Commun. 49:1249 (1972).

35. R. E. Gots and S. P. Bessman, The functional compartmentation of mitochondrial hexokinase, Arch. Biochem. Biophys. 163:7 (1974).

36. S. P. Bessman, B. Borreback, P. J. Geiger, and S. Ben-Or, Mitochondrial creatinine kinase and hexokinase — two examples of compartmentation predicted by the hexokinase mitochondrial binding theory of insulin action, in: "Microenvironments and Metabolic Compartmentation," P. A. Srere and R. W. Estabrook, eds., Academic Press, New York (1978), pp. 111-128.

37. M. Inui and S. Ishibashi, Functioning of mitochondria-bound hexokinase in rat brain in accordance with generation of ATP inside the organelle, J. Biochem. 85:1151 (1979).

38. S. P. Bessman and P. J. Geiger, Compartmentation of hexokinase and creatine phosphokinase, cellular regulation, and insulin action, Curr. Top. Cell Reg. 16:55 (1980).

39. E. R. B. McCabe, D. Sadava, W. W. Bullen, H. A. McKelvey, and C. I. Rose, Investigations of fibroblast complementation and enzyme kinetics from clinically distinct individuals with glycerol kinase deficiency, Am. J. Hum. Gen. 32:46A (1980).

40. E. R. B. McCabe, D. Sadava, W. W. Bullen, H. A. McKelvey, W. K. Seltzer, and C. I. Rose, Human glycerol kinase deficiency: Enzyme kinetics and fibroblast hybridization, J. Inher. Metab. Dis. 5:177 (1982).

41. E. R. B. McCabe, unpublished.

42. B. T. Jenkins and A. K. Hajra, Glycerol kinase and dihydroxyacetone kinase in rat brain, J. Neurochem. 26:377 (1976).

43. J. T. Tildon, J. H. Stevenson, and P. T. Ozand, Mitochondrial glycerol kinase activity in rat brain, Biochem. J. 157:513 (1976).

44. J. T. Tildon and L. M. Roeder, Glycerol oxidation in rat brain: Subcellular localization and kinetic characteristics, J. Neurosci. Res. 5:7 (1980).

PHOSPHORYLATED NUCLEOTIDES AND GLYCOLYTIC INTERMEDIATES

IN DIABETIC AND NON-DIABETIC RAT UTERUS IN LATE PREGNANCY

I. Zaidise, P.J. Geiger, D. Boehme, and S.P. Bessman

Department of Pharmacology and Nutrition

University of Southern California, School of Medicine

2025 Zonal Avenue, Los Angeles, California 90033

Insulin is an anabolic hormone known to stimulate any synthetic pathway (Bessman, 1960). Its mechanism of action is still unknown. Bessman (1954, 1970) suggested that the effect of insulin on energy metabolism is accomplished by coupling the hexokinase reaction to the mitochondria, increasing the effectiveness of glucose conversion to glucose-6-phosphate. The ADP created in the reaction produces an acceptor effect on the mitochondria, increasing the rate of oxidative phosphorylation. Since high energy compounds are rate limiting substrates for anabolic reactions, an increase in supply can enhance all of them. The same argument is also valid for insulin's favorable effect on membrane transport, also an energy requiring process.

Several studies found an effect of diabetes and insulin on the mitochondria and energy metabolism. Hall, et al. (1960) showed that mitochondria from diabetic rats were pathological and produced less ATP than normal mitochondria. Ida (1976) perfused guinea pig liver with insulin, then isolated mitochondria and found an increased oxygen consumption. The liver also showed higher levels of ATP and elevated energy charge. Gots and Bessman (1974) found that inhibition of electron transport inhibited the hexokinase reaction even when enough exogenous ATP was supplied. Recently, Mohan (unpublished data) demonstrated an increased oxidation of $2,3-^{14}C$-succinate to CO_2 by insulin and only a trivial effect on oxidation of $1,4-^{14}C$-succinate.

Diabetes during pregnancy is known to be aggravated because of the increase in the demand for insulin, caused by the stress-like effect of the gestational hormones. The effect of the disease on the uterine muscle is unclear. Blood vessels deteriorate in diabetic

495

pregnancy and hypertensive disorders are common. There is no biochemical explanation to this pathology.

In this work we examined the effect of diabetes on the pool
sizes of several high energy nucleotides (ATP, GTP, UTP, CTP, ADP,
CDP) as well as some glycolytic intermediates in rat uterus during
the late stage of pregnancy.

MATERIALS AND METHODS

Female Sprague-Dawley rats 180-200 gr were made diabetic by
streptozotocin (45 mg/kg, injected intravenously). Once diabetes had
been established (non-fasting blood glucose 250-500 mg percent) the
females were mated. A control group was injected with the vehicle
only. The rats were checked daily for vaginal presence of sperm and
a positive finding was considered as day 0 of pregnancy. The rats
received regular diet and water ad libitum. No insulin was administered throughout pregnancy. At days 19 and 21 of gestation the rats
were anesthetized with ether and operated on. A sample of the uterine tissue was quickly excised, frozen in liquid nitrogen, and powdered. The tissue was then extracted with perchloric acid and neutralized with freon and alamine according to the method of Khym
(1975). The neutralized samples were stored at -80°C. All nucleotides and glycolytic intermediates were separated by low pressure
(400-500 psi) liquid chromatography on a 500 x 3 mm glass column and
AGMP-1 resin. Elution was carried out with a gradient mixture of 0.1
ammonium chloride to 0.6 ammonium chloride, each containing 0.5 ammonium borate. The eluent was fractionated, ashed, analyzed and
quantified by the Bessman Automated Phosphate Analyzer (Geiger, 1980).
Internal standards of all nucleotides and glycolytic intermediates
of the highest chemical purity grade purchased from Sigma Chemical Co.
were used for peak identification. External standards of inorganic
phosphate were added at the end of each run for quantitation. Each
uterine sample was run 3-5 times to eliminate machine variations.

RESULTS AND DISCUSSION

No significant differences were noticed in the pool sizes of the
uterine high energy nucleotides and phosphocreatine between the diabetic pregnant rats and the normal ones in both 19 and 21 days of
gestation (Table 1). The level of high energy nucleotides and phosphocreatine increased at day 21 as compared to day 19 in both diabetics and controls, and ranged from 5 to 56%. ATP and PC increased
about 20%. The data concerning glycolytic intermediates are inconsistent (Table 2). This may be due to normal short-term variations
in glycolysis and glycogen synthesis among these animals, or due to
rapid changes in a glycolytic activity during the dissection and
freezing period. Figure 1 is a sample chromatogram of a 19 day

Table 1. High energy nucleotides and phosphocreatine in the uterus of normal and diabetic rats.

Compound	N-19	D-19	N-21	D-21
ATP	3.133 ± 0.433	3.137 ± 0.012	3.745 ± 0.176	3.767 ± 0.148
GTP	0.418 ± 0.053	0.446 ± 0.069	0.500 ± 0.015	0.503 ± 0.072
UTP	0.663 ± 0.148	0.564 ± 0.023	0.702 ± 0.021	0.822 ± 0.154
CTP	0.229 ± 0.047	0.225 ± 0.018	0.312 ± 0.048	0.292 ± 0.041
ADP	0.461 ± 0.027	0.493 ± 0.077	0.621 ± 0.064	0.497 ± 0.080
GDP	0.051 ± 0.004	0.044 ± 0.023	0.068 ± 0.032	0.046 ± 0.006
AMP	0.294 ± 0.010	0.287 ± 0.070	0.276 ± 0.042	0.328 ± 0.002
PC	1.084 ± 0.093	0.906 ± 0.192	1.303 ± 0.220	1.206 ± 0.111
NAD	0.234 ± 0.030	0.219 ± 0.028	0.262 ± 0.001	0.263 ± 0.021
UDPG	0.234 ± 0.033	0.237 ± 0.052	0.274 ± 0.005	0.270 ± 0.011

Uteri of diabetic and control pregnant rat were dissected at days 19 and 21 of pregnancy, frozen in liquid nitrogen and extracted with PCA as described in the materials and methods section. Analysis of phosphorylated compounds was done with the Bessman Automated Phosphate Analyzer. Each sample was chromatographed 3-5 times. Data are presented as micromoles phosphate/g frozen weight. N-19 = Normal 19 days of gestation. D-19 = Diabetic 19 days of gestation. N-21 = Normal 21 days of gestation. D-21 = Diabetic 21 days of gestation.

Table 2. Glycolytic intermediates in the uterus of normal and diabetic pregnant rats.

Compound	N-19	D-19	N-21	D-21
G1P	0.072 ± 0.008	0.090 ± 0.031	0.089 ± 0.020	0.062 ± 0.008
G6P + F6P	0.109 ± 0.008	0.122 ± 0.037	0.100 ± 0.041	0.130 ± 0.001
F-1,6-P	0.044 ± 0.006	0.052 ± 0.021	0.079 ± 0.022	0.046 ± 0.005
2,3-DPG	0.375 ± 0.285	0.366 ± 0.202	0.280 ± 0.082	0.457 ± 0.015

Uteri of diabetic and control pregnant rat were dissected at days 19 and 21 of pregnancy, frozen in liquid nitrogen and extracted with PCA as described in the materials and methods section. Analysis of phosphorylated compounds was done with the Bessman Automated Phosphate Analyzer. Each sample was chromatographed 3-5 times. Data are presented as micromoles phosphate/g frozen weight. N-19 = Normal 19 days of gestation. D-19 = Diabetic 19 days of gestation. N-21 = Normal 21 days of gestation. D-21 = Diabetic 21 days of gestation.

pregnant uterus. The glycolytic intermediate peaks are very small and therefore harder to quantify as compared with the nucleotide ones.

Tissue 2,3-DPG level is negligible. Its presence in the sample related directly to the blood content of the uterus. Calculations, based upon the levels of nucleotides and glycolytic intermediates in rat blood, show insignificant contributions of these compounds to the chromatogram. Uterine blood content was calculated to be 22.3 - 36.4 microliters blood per g frozen weight. The values are comparable to those of Kao (1961).

Data concerning pool sizes of nucleotides and glycolytic intermediates in pregnant uterus are scarce. Values for non-pregnant and early-pregnant rats were reported by Greenstreet and Fotherby (1973a, 1973b). They are twice as high as our data for nucleotides and up to 15 times higher for glycolytic intermediates. The difference in nucleotide pool sizes may have been caused partially by their lack of differentiation between ATP and other tri-nucleotides and by the different metabolic status of our animals (late pregnancy). The higher glycolytic intermediates could have been due to anoxia. ATP levels comparable to ours were reported by Rangachary et al. (1972).

Insulin seems to have no effect on the pool sizes of high energy nucleotides. This lack of effect can be expected assuming that energy is the rate limiting factor of synthetic pathways. Any extra energy (nucleotides) produced is immediately utilized. Therefore, the fluxes of these nucleotides may increase with no change in their pool sizes, as was suggested by Bessman and Pal (1980). Experiments to test this hypothesis are currently underway in our laboratory. [33]P is utilized as a tracer to measure glycolysis and nucleotide fluxes. Another possibility is that insulin affects just a fraction of the mitochondria, or a fraction of the energy produced in each mitochondrion, those involved in synthetic pathways. This hypothesis assumes that energy supply is compartmented and that the major energy expenditure of the cell - maintenance of the sodium potassium pump - is independent of any external hormonal influence. Since the synthetic pathways consume only a few percent of the total energy supply of the cell, insulin effect will not show when the total cell energetics are measured.

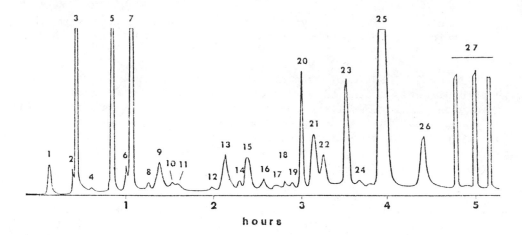

Figure 1. A chromatogram of an acid extract of 19 day old normal pregnant rat uterus.

Uterus of a 19-day old pregnant rat was extracted with PCA and analyzed on the Bessman Automated Phosphate Analyzer as described in the text. Peaks were identified with internal standards as follows:

1 to 4 – phospholipid precursors	18 – fructose 1,6 diphosphate
5 – phosphocreatine	19 – UDP
6 – G1P	20 – 2,3,DPG
7 – Pi	21 – ADP
8 – Unknown	22 – CTP
9 – NAD	23 – UTP
10 – F6P	24 – GDP
11 – G6P	25 – ATP
12 – UMP	26 – GTP
13 – AMP	27 – 20 mmoles Pi
14 – Unknown	
15 – UDPG	
16 – CDP	
17 – PEP	

Internal Standards

REFERENCES

Bessman, S.P., 1954, Fat metabolism, a contribution to the mechanism of diabetes mellitus, in: "Fat Metabolism," V.A. Najjar, ed., The Johns Hopkins Press, Baltimore.

Bessman, S.P., 1960, Diabetes mellitus: observations, theoretical and practical, J. of Pediatrics, 56:191.

Bessman, S.P., Hexokinase acceptor theory of insulin action. new evidence, Isr. J. Med. Sciences, 8:344.

Bessman, S.P., and Pal, N., 1980, Phosphate metabolic control of potassium movement - its effect on osmotic pressure, in: "Advances in Experimental Medicine and Biology," S.G. Massry, E. Ritz, and H. Jahn, eds., Vol. 128, Plenum Press, New York.

Geiger, P.J., Ahn, S., and Bessman, S.P., 1980, Separation and automated analysis of phosphorylated intermediates, in: "Methods in Carbohydrate Chemistry, Vol. III," R. Whistler, ed., Academic Press, New York.

Gots, R.E., Gorin, F.A., and Bessman, S.P., 1972, Kinetic enhancement of bound hexokinase activity by mitochondrial respiration, Biochem. Biophys. Res. Commun., 49:1249

Greenstreet, R.A., and Fotherby, K., 1973a, Carbohydrate metabolism in the rat uterus during early pregnancy, Steroids Lipids Res., 4:84.

Greenstreet, R.A., and Fotherby, K., 1973b, Carbohydrate metabolism in rat uterus during the oestrous cycle, Steroids Lipids Res., 4:341.

Hall, J.C., Sordhal, L.A., and Stefko, P.L., 1960, The effect of insulin on oxidative phosphorylation in normal and diabetic mitochondria, J. Biol. Chem., 235:1536.

Ida, T., Sato, M., Yamaoka, Y., Takeda, H., Kamiama, Y., Kimura, K., Oxawa, K., and Honjo, I., 1976, Effect of insulin on mitochondrial oxidative phosphorylation and energy charge of the perfused guinea pig liver, J. Lab. Clin. Med., 97:925.

Kao, C.Y. and Gams, R.S., 1961, Blood content of uterus and isolated myometrium under estrogen and progesterone domination, Am. J. Physiol., 201:714.

Khym, J.X., 1975, An analytical system for rapid separation of tissue nucleotides at low pressures on conventional ion exchanger, Clin. Chem., 21:1245.

Rangachari, P.K., Paton, D.M., and Daniel, E.C., 1972, Potassium: ATP ratios in smooth muscle, Biochim. Biophys. Acta, 274:462.

EFFECT·OF CALCIUM ANTAGONISTS ON VASOPRESSIN INDUCED CHANGES IN

MYOCARDIAL AND RENAL PYRIDINE NUCLEOTIDES IN THE INTACT RAT

D. DiPette, R. Townsend, J. Guntipalli,
K. Simpson, A. Rogers and E. Bourke

Department of Medicine, Allegheny-Singer Research
Institute, Allegheny General Hospital, Pittsburgh, PA

INTRODUCTION

Recent experimental interest has centered on the role of the calcium antagonists in the preservation of tissue function due to their ability to inhibit intracellular calcium accumulation as well as their potent vasodilatory properties. Most studies to date have centered primarily on myocardial tissue rendered either ischemic or anoxic by coronary artery ligation or manipulation of perfusing solutions. Assessment of myocardial function has included the quantitation of infarct size,[1] ultrastructural histologic changes,[2] or the evaluation of cellular biochemical parameters such as measurement of high energy phosphates,[3] intracellular pH,[4] and pyridine nucleotides.[5]

In contrast to the investigation centering on the myocardium, much less is known concerning the effects of the calcium antagonists on renal tissue, particularly following ischemia. Studies have shown that these agents exert a variety of renal effects, such as inhibition of vasopressin-induced water flow[6] and blockade of vasopressin-induced renal vasoconstriction.[7] However, these agents may differ in their effects on renal blood flow.[8,9] Recent data has shown a key role for the calcium ion in the degree of injury sustained by anoxic tubules.[10] In addition, the calcium antagonist verapamil has been shown to ameliorate the vasoconstriction which follows the injection of radiocontrast media.[11]

The oxidative state of the cell is reflected by the balance between the pyridine nucleotide ratio NAD+–NADH. During ischemic or anoxic conditions, NADH, primarily located in mitochondria,[12] accumulates associated with a decrease in NAD+.[13,14] Our

503

laboratory recently developed an assay, utilizing bioluminescence, capable of determining tissue NAD+ and NADH in picogram quantities. The intense vasoconstrictive properties of vasopressin are well recognized.[15,16,17,18] Elevations in plasma vasopressin have been demonstrated in many clinical settings such as hypotension,[19,20,21] surgery,[19] hypertension,[22,23,24,25] congestive heart failure,[26] hypoxia,[21] and end stage renal disease.[27,28]

This investigation was undertaken to first determine the effect of exogenously administered vasopressin on NAD+—NADH in both myocardial and renal tissue. Second, the effect of pretreatment with two differing calcium antagonists, diltiazem and verapamil, on vasopressin induced changes in NAD+—NADH in each tissue was determined.

METHODS

Twenty-seven male Wistar rats (Charles-River Breeding Laboratories, Wilmington, Massachusetts) weighing between 250-300 grams were used for study. Prior to study, animals were maintained in a temperature and light controlled room and fed standard rat chow (Wayne Lab Blox, Chicago, Illinois) and given tap water ad lib to drink. On the day of study each animal was anesthetized with ether. Under direct vision the right internal iliac artery and right femoral vein were catheterized (PE-50, Clay Adams, Parsippany, New Jersey) allowing hemodynamic monitoring and drug administration respectively. Blood pressure and heart rate were continuously monitored via a Statham (P-23G) transducer and a Hewlett-Packard (7402A) recorder. Following catheter insertion each animal was maintained under light ether anesthesia with blood pressure and heart rate being continuously monitored throughout the experimental period. The study was initiated when heart rate and blood pressure stabilized at the highest possible levels with continued light ether anesthesia (approximately 30-45 minutes). Where indicated, arginine vasopressin (Pitressin, Parke-Davis) was administered via intravenous infusion at a rate of (0.1-0.25 unit/min) for 5-10 minutes. This infusion was titrated in each animal to achieve an approximate mean blood pressure elevation of 30 mmHg. Diltiazem (2.5 mg/kg dissolved in 5% dextrose and administered in a volume of 0.25 ml) was intravenously administered by slow injection over 10 minutes where indicated. Verapamil (1.5 mg/kg diluted with 5% dextrose and administered in a volume of 0.25 ml) was administered via slow i.v. injection over 10 minutes also where indicated.

At the end of study all animals had biopsies obtained of myocardial (left ventricular and renal (cortex) tissue in the following manner. Via a midline abdominal incision, both the right and left kidney were exposed. After decapsulation renal cortical tissue was obtained via a freeze clamp technique with forceps pre-chilled in liquid nitrogen. Immediately following, a sternal incision was made, the heart exposed, and left ventricular tissue obtained in a similar manner. The duration of biopsy never exceeded 10 seconds. Tissue samples were then immediately frozen and stored in liquid nitrogen until later assayed for NAD+ and NADH respectively. Determination of NADH in both myocardial and renal tissue was performed as follows. The snap frozen tissue was rapidly weighed, added to precooled ($-17°C$) alcoholic KOH (0.5M), homogenized (Tissuemizer, Tekmar, Cincinnati, Ohio) and an alkaline extract obtained according to the method of Klingenberg.[29] The supernatant was diluted (1:1) with potassium phosphate buffer (0.1M, pH 6.9) and measured photometrically (Firefly I, Sybron-Brinkman Corp, Westbury, New York) using bioluminescence kit containing purified bacterial oxidoreductase and luciferase (Analytical Luminescence Lab, Inc., San Diego, CA). NAD+ was determined in the following manner. Similarly obtained and weighed tissue was homogenized in perchloric acid (0.6M) and an acid extract obtained and neutralized according to the method of Klingenberg.[29] The supernatant was diluted (1:10) with Tris Buffer (0.2M, pH 8.0) and NAD+ converted to NADH using D-3 hydroxybutyrate (Sigma, St. Louis, Missouri) and 3-hydroxybutyrate (Sigma, St. Louis, Missouri) by the method of Wilkinson.[30] The resultant NADH was measured as above. Both NAD+ and NADH are expressed in pMoles/mg wet weight.

All results are expressed as mean ± SEM. Student's t test for paired and unpaired data and analysis of variance was used where appropriate. A p value of < 0.05 was considered significant.

PROTOCOLS

Four groups of animals were studied as follows. Group A (n=7) - following the stabilization period these animals were maintained under light ether anesthesia for 30 minutes at which time myocardial and renal biopsies were performed. Blood pressure and heart rate were recorded at 10-minute intervals. Thus these animals served as non-infused controls.

Group B (n=7) - similarly prepared and maintained animals as in Group A were infused with vasopressin at such a dose to achieve an increase in mean arterial blood pressure of approximately 10 mmHg.

Group C (n=5) - these animals were prepared and treated as Group B, however, vasopressin infusion was preceded by pretreatment with diltiazem.

Group D (n=8) - these animals were prepared and treated similar to Group C, however, verapamil was administered instead of diltiazem.

Since in Groups C and D the acute administration of both

diltiazem and verapamil decreased mean blood pressure, vasopressin infusion was initiated when mean blood pressure stabilized at approximately 85-90 mmHg post the administration of the respective calcium antagonist.

RESULTS

There was no significant difference in baseline mean blood pressure between any of the four groups of animals studied (A – 96±3; B – 99±3, C – 102±3, D – 108±2 respectively). In the non-infused control animals (Group A) there was no change in mean blood pressure throughout the experimental period. At the time of biopsy, mean blood pressure was 96±3 mmHg. In Group B, the vasopressin infused but not calcium antagonist pretreated animals, vasopressin infusion significantly increased mean blood pressure (baseline – 99±3 to 136±5 mmHg p<0.001). Calcium antagonist administration significantly decreased mean blood pressure in both Group C (diltiazem) and Group D (verapamil). In Group C diltiazem decreased mean blood pressure from a baseline of 102±3 to 84±3 mmHg (p<0.01) while in Group D verapamil decreased mean blood pressure from 108±2 to 78±2 mmHg (p<0.001). In both groups C and D subsequent to calcium administration, vasopressin infusion significantly increased mean blood pressure (Group C – 84±3 to 125±4; Group D – 78±2 to 136±2 mmHg, both p<0.001 respectively).

There was also no significant difference in baseline heart rate between any of the four groups studied (A – 441±16; B – 413±17; C – 405±16; D – 407±8 beats/min respectively). In the non-infused control animals (Group A) there was no change in heart rate throughout the experimental period. At the time of biopsy the heart rate was 432±14 beats/min. In Group B vasopressin infusion significantly decreased heart rate from a baseline of 413±17 to 289±18 beats/min (p<0.01). In Group C following diltiazem infusion there was no change in heart rate (baseline 405±16 to 393±6 beats/min (NS). In Group D following verapamil infusion heart rate significantly decreased (baseline 407±9 to 350±6 beats/min (p<0.001). Vasopressin administration following either calcium antagonist significantly decreased heart rate in both Groups C and D (C – 394±6 to 282±11 (p<0.01) and D – 350±6 to 289±10 beats/min (p<0.001) respectively.

Myocardial (left ventricular) and renal (cortex) NAD+ and NADH determinations are shown in Table 1. Vasopressin infusion alone in Group B decreased both left ventricular and renal cortex NAD+ levels with the left ventricle determinations reaching significance and increased both left ventricle and renal cortex NADH levels with renal cortex determinations reaching significance. Diltiazem pretreatment in Group C significantly prevented the vasopressin induced decrease in NAD+ content in the left ventricle while tending to prevent the decrease in renal cortex. Diltiazem pretreatment also tended to prevent the NADH increase seen following vasopressin infusion in the left ventricle, however, no difference was observed following diltiazem pretreatment in renal cortex. Verapamil pre-treatment (Group D) significantly prevented the vasopressin-induced decrease in renal cortex NAD+ while having little effect on left ventricular NAD+. Verapamil did, however, significantly prevent the vasopressin-induced increase in NADH in both the left ventricle and renal cortex.

TABLE 1

	A(Control)	B(AVP)	C(DZ-AVP)	D(VP-AVP)
NAD+ (pMole/mg)				
Left Ventricle	630±31	512±17**	706±76##	544±24
Renal Cortex	686±77	566±26	635±38	692±36#
NADH (pMole/mg)				
Left Ventricle	297±22	341±43	245±21	172±19##§§
Renal Cortex	127±21	223±37*	211±23§	108±11##

Table 1: NAD+ and NADH determinations for both myocardial (left ventricle) and renal (cortex) in each of the four groups studied. DZ – diltiazem, VP – verapamil.

$$
\begin{array}{lll}
\text{B vs. A} & *p<0.05 & **p<0.001 \\
\text{C or D vs. B} & \#p<0.05 & \#\#p<0.01 \\
\text{C or D vs. A} & \S p<0.05 & \S\S p<0.01
\end{array}
$$

Tissue NAD+ and NADH are expressed as pMole/mg tissue. Results are expressed as mean ± SEM.

The myocardial (left ventricle) NAD+/NADH ratios determined in each of the four groups are shown in Figure 1. Vasopressin infusion (Group B) significantly decreased the NAD+/NADH ratio from that of the control non-infused (Group A) animals. Both calcium antagonists, diltiazem (Group C) and verapamil (Group D) administered prior to vasopressin infusion prevented the decrease in NAD+/NADH ratio following vasopressin infusion. The renal (cortex) tissue NAD+/NADH ratios determined in each of the four groups are shown in Figure 2. Similar to that found in myocardial tissue, vasopressin infusion (Group B) significantly decreased the NAD+/NADH ratio from that of the control (Group A) animals. In contrast to myocardial tissue, diltiazem pretreatment (Group C) did not prevent the vasopressin-induced decrease in the NAD+/NADH ratio while similar to that found in myocardial tissue, verapamil pretreatment did.

507

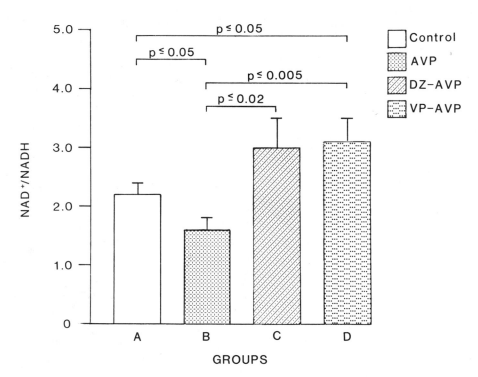

Figure 1: Myocardial (left ventricle) NAD+/NADH ratio determinations in each of the four groups studied. Results expressed as mean ± SEM.

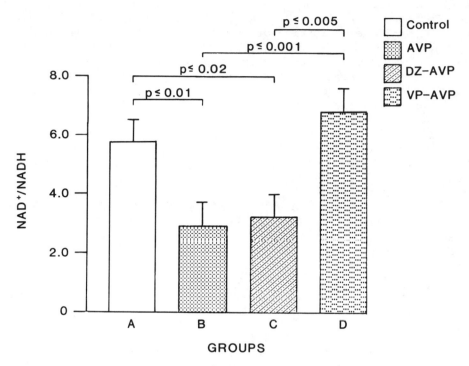

Figure 2: Renal cortex NAD+/NADH ratio determinations in each of the four groups studied. Results expressed as mean ± SEM.

DISCUSSION

The results of this study demonstrate that exogenously administered vasopressin, in a dose sufficient to raise arterial blood pressure, decreased the NAD+/NADH ratio in both myocardial and renal tissue in the intact animal. Since both NAD+ and NADH were determined independently in separate tissue samples, we have shown that NAD+ decreased and NADH increased in both tissues. However, these changes in both individual pyridine nucleotides did not always reach significance as demonstrated by the change in renal NAD+ and myocardial NADH in response to vasopressin administration. Thus the determination of the ratio of the two pyridine nucleotides clearly demonstrated cellular changes better than singular measurement of either NAD+ or NADH alone. Since the NAD+–NADH system reflects the tissue energy demand-supply balance (i.e., oxidative-reductive state), under ischemic conditions NAD+ diminishes and NADH accumulates intracellularly and thus the ratio of the two decreases. The NAD+/NADH ratio reduction in both myocardial and renal tissue in response to administered vasopressin can thus be explained as the response to ischemia induced by intense coronary and renal artery vasoconstriction secondary to vasopressin administration. In support of this, it was noted at the time of biopsy that both organs were intensely cyanotic and mottled. Our study further demonstrated that pretreatment with both the calcium antagonists, diltiazem and verapamil, prevented the reduction in vasopressin-induced NAD+/NADH ratio in myocardial tissue whereas, interestingly, only verapamil prevented the observed decrease secondary to vasopressin in renal tissue.

Our laboratory has recently developed an assay utilizing bioluminescence capable of measuring both NAD+ and NADH in picogram/mg of wet tissue amounts utilizing 25-50 mg of tissue for each determination. Our myocardial levels of both NAD+ and NADH compare favorably with that reported in the literature by others. Swain, et al reported myocardial NAD+ levels of approximately 0.50 umol/gm weight of wet tissues in anesthetized open-chested dogs under control non-intervention conditions.[14] In the same study NAD+ was shown to decrease to approximately 0.40 umol/gm immediately following total coronary artery occlusion.[14] This is in near agreement with both our baseline levels as well as our post vasopressin NAD+ myocardial determinations. Baron, et al reported NADH levels of 285±11 uM/g wet tissue also in anesthetized open-chested dogs under control conditions and an increase to 394±10 uM/g under ischemic conditions induced via total coronary artery occlusion.[31] These levels again compare favorably with our baseline and post-vasopressin NADH determinations. As in myocardium our renal cortex NAD+ determinations are similar to that reported by Burch, et al[32] as well as both NAD+ and NADH being in agreement with that reported by Bourke, et al in the parathyroidectomized volume expanded rat.[33]

The cellular biochemical changes following myocardial ischemia have been previously delineated. These changes include high energy phosphate (i.e. ATP) depletion,[3,34,35] decrease in intracellular pH,[4] and accumulation of intracellular calcium[1,36] particularly in mitochondria.[37,38] Because of their vasodilatory properties but perhaps more importantly their ability to inhibit membrane calcium influx, the calcium antagonists have been investigated as to whether they may preserve ischemic myocardium and/or promote recovery. In this regard, diltiazem and verapamil have been studied. Bush, et al demonstrated that diltiazem decreased infarct size following left circumflex coronary occlusion in the dog.[1] Additionally, intracellular calcium accumulation was attenuated by diltiazem.[1] Ichihara and Abiko showed that diltiazem also attenuates the myocardial intracellular decrease in pH following coronary occlusion in the dog.[4] The effect of diltiazem in rats on reperfusion myocardial creatine kinase release was evaluated by Ashrof, et al.[3] These authors demonstrated that diltiazem decreased the magnitude of creatine kinase release following reperfusion. Additionally, in an ultrastructural histologic study, Fujiwara, et al showed that diltiazem pretreatment consistently decreased myocardial cellular damage following varying durations of ischemia in the pig heart.[2] Verapamil has also been shown to be cytoprotective in myocardium as well. Bolling, et al demonstrated that verapamil administered immediately prior to reperfusion improved left ventricular contractility and compliance in the globally ischemic isolated rabbit heart.[39] During similar global ishemia, verapamil has also been shown by Nayler, et al to decrease intramitochondrial calcium accumulation, thus sparing the decline in ATP generation associated with reperfusion of the ischemic myocardium.[40] Similar results were also demonstrated by Rosenberger, et al.[41] Thus our findings that both dilitiazem and verapamil preserve the NAD+/NADH ratio in myocardium rendered ischemic via vasopressin administration further support a cytoprotective role of these agents in the myocardium. Our study, however, extends these previous reports to include myocardial preservation following vasospasm induced via vasopressin, a known hormone integral in physiologic and perhaps pathophysiologic clinical settings. Further support for our findings is the fact that Kissin and Kilpatrick recently reported that nifedipine, another calcium antagonist with potent vasodilatory properties, decreased the NADH accumulation in myocardium following coronary vasospasm induced via vasopressin administration in the isolated heart.[5] The methodology in this study differed, however, from that of ours in that the isolated heart preparation was utilized and vasopressin was directly perfused to the heart, while we studied the intact animal and administered vasopressin systemically via intravenous infusion. Additionally, Kisin and Kilpatrick determined NADH changes via fluorometry while we directly measure both pyridine nucleotides.[5]

As opposed to the extensive myocardial studies, the effect of the calcium antagonists on renal cytoprotection is less well delineated. In contrast to the homogeneity of myocardial tissue, the kidney is composed of diverse structures including glomeruli, tubules, interstitium and blood vessels. In addition, these structures display differing sensitivity to ischemic and/or anoxic injury thus making a single mechanism operant in renal failure unlikely. Furthermore, the study of ischemic renal failure is encumbered by the difficulty in extrapolating experimental animal models to that which occurs in the clinical situation. Nonetheless, certain features have emerged that deserve consideration. The medullary portion of the nephron segments function in a milieux that is "hypoxic" compared to most other tissues.[42] When this is considered, especially in light of recent data indicating that cytochrome aa_3 is 25-40% oxidized (most tissues contain less than 2%) in kidney tissue, it is apparent that certain portions of the nephron exist on the verge of anoxic conditions.[43] Most animal studies show that following ischemic renal failure the most significant changes occur in the tubules, manifested as loss of villi and mitochondrial swelling, while typically the glomeruli and the vasculature are normal.[44,45]

Similar to myocardium the role of calcium in renal tissue cell death is under investigation. Failure of mitochondria to exclude calcium is felt to be a critical element in irreversible anoxic damage. Wilson, et al have shown that cultured kidney segments survive anoxic stress when calcium is withheld from culture medium immediately following oxygen deprivation.[10] Since calcium plays a role in many cellular processes, attention has focused on the possibility that the calcium antagonists may display renal cytoprotective effects particularly because of the encouraging data from studies on the myocardium. The calcium antagonists have effects upon renal vascular resistance,[46] water handling[6,47] PAH clearance,[48] and renal blood flow.[49,50] Verapamil in particular has been studied. Goldfarb, et al have shown that in rats undergoing contralateral nephrectomy and unilateral ischemia induced by a clamping technique that verapamil afforded an approximate 50% preservation of glomerular filtration rate when administered pre-ishemia.[51] No effect on glomerular filtration rate, however, was demonstrated if verapamil was administered post the ischemic event. Interestingly, Malis, et al were able to show a beneficial effect of pretreatment with verapamil in norepinephrine-induced acute renal failure, while no effect of verapamil was seen with renal failure induced via renal artery clamping.[52] This difference led the authors to conclude that the protective effect of verapamil on post-ischemic renal function was secondary to vasodilation since verapamil antagonized the norepinephrine-induced renal artery vasoconstriction. These authors, however, used a lower dose of verapamil than in that of the study of Goldfarb, et al, nor were contralateral nephrectomys performed in the study of Malis. The different dosing of verapamil, different anesthetic agents administered, different surgical procedures, and different methods of reducing renal blood flow make direct comparisons of these studies difficult. It seems unlikely that vasodilation alone can explain the verapamil protection in the study of Goldfarb, et al since alpha-adrenergic blockade, as performed by Eliahou, et al did not improve renal function after ischemia, despite documented vasodilation.[53] In our study, verapamil preserved the NAD+/NADH ratio when administered prior to vasopressin infusion while diltiazem did not. The kidneys in rats pretreated with verapamil or diltiazem followed by vasopressin infusion were uniformly mottled and cyanosed. Although direct blood flow measurements were not performed in our study, it seems unlikely that vasodilation alone can explain the differing effects on kidney NAD+/NADH ratios seen between verapamil and diltiazem. Diltiazem, if anything, tends to increase renal blood flow while verapamil has been shown to have little effect.[8,9] Thus, this further argues against a vasodilatory explanation of our results. Additionally, as has been shown by Cooper, et al, diltiazem ameliorates the increase in renovascular resistance produced by vasopressin infusion in the isolated perfused rat kidney.[7] Further studies, however, will be necessary to more completely evaluate the mechanism responsible for the differing effects of verapamil and diltiazem in the kidney. Although we can only speculate, it seems clear that any vascular protection afforded by diltiazem is overshadowed by the finding of no difference in the NAD+/NADH ratio in this treatment group from that of the vasopressin infused animals. As opposed to vasodilation, the observed NAD+/NADH difference may be due to a difference in direct cellular effect on kidney tissue between the two agents.

In conclusion, our results demonstrate that exogenously administered vasopressin in blood pressure elevating doses decreases the NAD+/NADH ratio in both myocardial and renal tissue. The calcium antagonists, verapamil and diltiazem, prevented this ratio decrease in myocardium while only verapamil did so in the kidney. The protective mechanism may be related to differences in direct cellular effects between these two agents, however, a vasodilatory mechanism cannot at this time be excluded. Our results support previous studies confirming the utility of both these calcium antagonists in preserving cardiac cellular energy balance following ischemia. The differing renal effects, however, imply that verapamil may potentially be useful in clinical situations producing ischemic renal failure.

REFERENCES

1. Bush LR, Romson JL, Ash JL, Lucchesi BR. Effects of diltiazem on extent of ultimate myocardial injury resulting from temporary coronary artery occlusion in dogs. J. Cardiovas. Pharmacol., 4(2):285-296, 1982.
2. Fujiwara H, Ashra M, Millard RW, Sato S, Schwartz A. Effects of diltiazem, a calcium channel inhibitor, in retarding cellular damage produced during early myocardial ischemia in pigs: a morphometric and ultrastructural analysis. JACC, 3(6): 1427-37, June 1984.
3. Ashraf M, Onda M, Benedict J, Millard R. Prevention of calcium paradox-related myocardial cell injury with diltiazem, a calcium channel blocking agent. Am. J. Cardiol., 49:1675-1681, May 1982.
4. Ishihara K, Abiko Y. Effect of diltiazem, a calcium antagonist, on myocardial pH in ischemic canine heart. J. Pharmacol. Exp. Ther., 222(3):720-725, 1982.
5. Kissin I, Kilpatrick J. Effect of nifedipine on myocardial

energy balance in experimental coronary vasoconstriction and occlusion. J. Cardiovasc. Pharmacol., 4(1):111-115, 1982.

6. Burch R, Halushka P. Verapamil inhibition of vasopressin-stimulated water flow: possible role of intracellular calcium. J. Pharmacol. Exp. Ther., 226(3):701-705, 1983.

7. Cooper C, Malik K. Mechanism of action of vasopressin on prostaglandin synthesis and vascular function in the isolated rat kidney: effect of calcium antagonists and calmodulin inhibitors. J. Pharmacol. Exp. Ther., 229(1): 139-147, 1983.

8. Hof R, Hof A, Neumann P. Effects of PY 108-068, a new calcium channel blocker on general haemodynamics and regional blood flow in anaesthetized cats. A comparison with nifedipine. J. Cardiovasc. Pharmacol., 4:352-362.

9. Hof RP. Calcium antagonist and the peripheral circulation: differences and similarities between PY 108-068, nicardipine, verapamil and diltiazem. Am. J. Pharmacol., 78:375-394, 1983.

10. Wilson PD, Schrier RW. An in vitro model of acute renal failure: calcium restriction protects against ischemic cell death in cultured nephron segments. Clin. Res., 32:460A, 1984.

11. Bakris GL, Larson TS, Burnett JC. The protective role of verapamil against rapid contrast-induced intrarenal vasconstriction. Clin. Res., 32:440A, 1984.

12. Chance B. Pyridine nucleotide as an indicator of the oxygen requirements for energy-linked functions of mitochondria. Circ. Res., 38(1):31-38, 1976.

13. Sugano T, Oshino N, Chance B. Mitochondrial functions under hypoxic conditions: the steady state of cytochrome reduction and of energy metabolism. Biochem. Biophys. Acta., 347:340-358, 1974.

14. Swain JL, Sabina RL, McHale PA, Greenfield JC, Holmes EW. Prolonged myocardial nucleotide depletion after brief ischemia in the open-chest dog. Am. J. Physiol., 242(11):H817-H26, 1982.

15. Altura BM. Comparative cellular and pharmacological actions of neurohypophyseal hormones on smooth muscle. Fed. Proc., 36:1840, 1977.

16. Cowley AW, Switzer S, Guinn M. Evidence and quantification of the vasopressin arterial pressure control system in dogs. Circ. Res., 46:48-67, 1980.

17. Montani JP, Liard JF, Schoun J, Mohring J. Hemodynamic effects of exogenous and endogenous vasopressin at low plasma concentration in conscious dogs. Circ. Res., 47:346-55, 1980.

18. Liard JF, Deriaz O, Schelling P, Thibonnier M. Cardiac output distribution during vasopressin infusion or dehydration in conscious dogs. Am. J. Physio., 243:H663-9, 1982,

19. Cochrane JPS, Forsling ML, Menzies Gow N, Le Quesne LP. Arginine vasopressin release following surgical operations. Br. J. Surg., 68:209-213, 1981.

20. Goldsmith SR, Francis GS, Cowley AW, Cohn JN. Response of vasopressin and norepinephrine to lower body negative pressure in humans. Am. J. Physiol., 243:H970-H973, 1982.

21. Heyes MP, Fraber MO, Manfredi F, Robertshaw D, Weinberger M, Fineberg N, Robertson G. Acute effects of hypoxia on renal and endocrine function in normal humans. Am. J. Physiol. 243:R265-R270, 1982

22. Cowley AW, Cushman WC, Quillen EW, Skelton MM, Langford HG. Vasopressin elevation in essential hypertension and increased responsiveness to sodium intake. Hypertension, 3(1):I93-I100, 1981.

23. Thibonnier M, Aldigier JC, Soto ME, Sassano P, Menard J, Corvol P. Abnormalities and drug-induced alterations of vasopression in human hypertension. Clin. Science, 61:149S-152S, 1981.

24. Thibonnier M, Soto ME, Menard J, Aldiger JC, Corvol P, Milliez P. Reduction of plasma and urinary vasopressin during treatment of severe hypertension by captopril. Eur. J. Clin. Invest., 11:449-453, 1981.

25. Padfield PL. Vasopressin in hypertension. Amer. Heart J., 94:531, 1978.

26. Goldsmith SR, Francis GS, Cowley AW, Levine TB, Cohn JN. Increased plasma arginine vasopressin levels in patients with congestive heart failure. J. Am. Coll. Cardio., 1(6), 1385-90, 1983.

27. Vaziri ND, Skowsky R, Saiki J. Antidiuretic hormone in end-stage renal disease. J. Dialysis., 4(2&3):73-81, 1980.

28. Shimamoto K, Watarai I, Miyahara M. A study of plasma vasopressin in patients undergoing chronic hemodialysis. J. Clin. Endocrinol. Metab., 45:714, 1977.

29. Klingenberg M. Nicotinamide-adenine denucleotides (NAD, NADP, NADH, NADPH); spectrophotometric and fluorimetric methods, H.U. Bergmeyer (ed), Methods of Enzymatic Analysis (2nd edition) New York, Academic Press, Inc., 4:2045-2059, 1974.

30. Wilkenson JH. LDH$_1$, (2-hydroxybutyrate dehydrogenase) UV-assay. In H.U. Bergmeyer (ed), Methods of Enzymatic Analysis (2nd edition), New York, Academic Press, Inc., 2:603-612, 1974.

31. Baron DW, Walls JT, Anderson RE, Harrison CE. Protective effect of lidocaine during regional myocardial ischemia, an altered pathophysiologic response assessed by NADH fluorescence. Mayo Clin. Proc., 57:442-447, 1982.

32. Burch HB, Lowry OH, Von Dippe P. The stability of triphosphopyridine nucleotide and its reduced form in rat liver. J. Biol. Chem., 238(8):2838-2842, 1963.

33. Bourke E, Rogers A, Guntipalli J. Studies on the antiphosphaturic action of insulin (I) independent of parathyroid hormone (PTH). Clin. Research, 31(2), 1983.

34. Jennings RB, Hawkins HK, Lowe JE, Hill ML, Klotman S, Reimer, KA. Relation between high energy phosphate and lethal injury in myocardial ischemia in the dog. Am. J. Pathol., 92:187-214, 1978.

35. Jennings RB, Reimer KA, Hill ML, Mayer SE. Total ischemia in dog hearts, in vitro. 1. Comparison of high energy phosphate

production, utilization and depletion, and of adenine nucleotide catabolism in total ischemia in vitro vs. severe ischemia in vivo. Circ. Res., 49:892–900, 1981.

36. Reimer KA, Jennings RB, Hill ML. Total ischemia in dog hearts, in vitro. 2. High energy phosphate depletion and associated defects in energy metabolism, cell volume regulation, and sarcolemmal integrity. Circ. Res., 49:901–911, 1981.

37. Henry PD, Schuchleib R, Davis J, Weiss ES, Sobel BE. Myocardial contracture and accumulation of mitochondrial calcium in ischemic rabbit heart. Am. J. Physiol., 233(6):H677–H684, 1977.

38. Shen AC, Jennings RB. Kinetics of calcium accumulation in acute myocardial ischemic injury. Am. J. Pathol., 67:441–452, 1972.

39. Bolling SF, Schirmer WJ, Gott VL, Flaherty JT, Bulkley BH, Gardner TJ. Enhanced myocardial protection with verapamil prior to postischemic reflow. Surgery, 283–290, August 1983.

40. Nayler WG, Ferrari R, Williams A. Protective effect of pretreatment with verapamil, nifedipine and propranolol on mitochondrial function in the ischemic and reperfused myocardium. Am. J. Cardiol., 46:242–248, 1980.

41. Rosenberger LB, Jacobs LW, Stanton HC. Evaluation of cardiac anoxia and ischemia models in the rat using calicum antagonists. Life Sci., 34:1379–1387, 1984.

42. Aukland K, Kirg J. Renal oxygen tension. Nature, 188:671, 1960.

43. Epstein FH, Balaban, Ross BD. Redox state of cytochrom aa3 in isolated perfused rat kidney. Am. J. Physiol., 243:F356–F363, 1982.

44. Frega NS, DiBona DR, Guertler B, Leaf A. Ischemic renal injury. Kidney Int., 10:S17–S25, 1976.

45. Venkatachalam MA, Bernard DB, Donohoe JF, Levinsky NG. Ischemic damage and repair in the rat proximal tubule: differences among the S1, S2 and S3 segments. Kidney Int., 14:31–49, 1978.

46. Kanda K, Flaim S. Effects of nifedipine on total cardiac output distribution in conscious rat. J. Pharm. Exp. Ther., 228:711–718, 1984.

47. Humes HD, Simmons CF, Brenner BM. Effect of verapamil on the hydroosmotic response to antidiuretic hormone in toal urinary bladder. Am. J. Physiol., 239:F250–F257, 1980.

48. Dantzler WH, Brokl OH. Verapamil and quinidine effects on PAH transport by isolated perfused renal tubules. Am. J. Physiol., 246:F188–F200, 1984.

49. Hof RP. Selective effects of different calcium antagonists on the peripheral circulation. TIPS, 100–102, 1984.

50. Flaim SF, Zelis R. Effects of diltiazem on total cardiac output distribution in conscious rats. J. Pharm. Exp. Ther., 222:359–366, 1982.

51. Goldfarb D, Iaina A, Serban I, Gavendo S, Kapuler S, Eliahou E. Beneficial effect of verapamil in ischemic acute renal

failure in the rat. Proc. Soc. Exp. Biol. Med., 172:389-392, 1983.

52. Malis CD, Cheung JY, Leaf A, Bonventre HV. Effects of verapamil in models of ischemic acute renal failure in the rat. Am. J. Physiol., 245:F735-742, 1983.

53. Eliahou HE, Brodman RR, Friedman EA. Adrenergic blockers in ischemic acute renal failure in the rat. Proceedings of the Conference on Acute Renal Failure DHEW publication No. (NIH) 74-608, New York, 265-280, 1973.

ACKNOWLEDGEMENTS

The authors thank Karen Klein for secretarial assistance and Debbie Haymaker and Keith Little for illustrations.

Dr. DiPette's research activities partially funded by Allegheny-Singer Research Institute and the Pennsylvania Heart Association.

THE EFFECT OF CREATINE ANALOGUE SUBSTITUTION ON THE POST TETANIC

RESPONSE OF FAST MUSCLE

Graham W. Mainwood and Joanne Totosy de Zepetnek

Department of Physiology
University of Ottawa
Ottawa, Ontario Canada

INTRODUCTION

It is clear that creatine phosphate hydrolysis accounts for most of the heat + work generated during short bursts (1-2 sec) of muscular activity (Curtin and Woledge, 1978). The significance of ATP regeneration by this mechanism in terms of the contractile function of muscle is less clear. The ATP buffer function can be reduced or abolished by either creatine phosphate depletion or creatine kinase inhibitors such as FDNB (Cain & Davies, 1962). Creatine phosphate depletion during ischemia (Gudbjarnason et al., 1970) or fatigue (Spande & Schottelius, 1970) or treatment with FDNB all lead to suppressed contractile force in spite of the fact that a considerable amount of ATP is still present.

These observations however provide little basis for defining a specific role of creatine phosphate in muscle contraction since: a) fatigue and ischemia result in many other parallel intracellular changes, and b) FDNB is a non-specific reagent that reacts with amino groups on many proteins. Creatine depletion by analogue substitution (Fitch et al., 1974) would appear to be a more specific and less ambiguous means of studying the dependence of contraction on the energy buffer system. Sor far, studies of this type have indicated that quite severe depletion of creatine phosphate has little effect on basic contractile parameters (Petrofsky & Fitch, (1980).

In order to examine the effect of the energy buffer system on contraction, we compared the contractile response of rat EDL muscle depleted of creatine phosphate by analogue substitution before and after a brief period of intense activity (1 sec 100 Hz tetanus).

519

METHODS

Sprague-Dawley rats were fed on a diet of Rat Chow containing 1% of β-guanidinopropionate for 4-5 weeks starting from weaning. Control animals were fed the same amount of Rat Chow for the same period of time.

Contraction studies were carried out on exposed, in situ, EDL muscles in rats anaesthetized with sodium pentobarbitol (65 mg/Kg). The distal tendon was attached by a steel wire to a Kulite BG±100 transducer (compliance 1.8×10^{-5}cm.g.$^{-1}$). The muscles were immersed in Tyrode solution at 36°C and stimulated through platinum plate electrodes. Maximal twitch tension was obtained by adjusting muscle length. Muscles were frozen in the rested state between aluminum blocks cooled in liquid nitrogen. Enzymatic assays for ATP and CrP were carried out as described previously (Mainwood & Cechetto, 1980). Creatine was measured by the method of Ennor and Stocken (1948).

RESULTS

Resting EDL muscles from rats fed on a diet containing 1% β-guanidinopropionate for 4-5 weeks contain about 80% less total creatine than normal muscles (Table 1). The CrP:Cr ratio is also reduced so that the muscles of creatine analogue fed rats contain only about 5% of the normal CrP. ATP levels are also considerably reduced.

Table 1. The effect of β-guanidinopropionate feeding on ATP, Cr and CrP in rat EDL.

	ATP	Cr	CrP
Control	5.9 ± .6	26.7 ± 2.7	12.7 ± 2.6
Gp Fed	1.7 ± .3	5.2 ± .6	0.5 ± .2

a) amounts in μmol/g wet wt. (± S.D.)
b) n=8 for both groups

EDL muscles of creatine depleted rats were found to be about 10% smaller than control muscles. When peak twitch tension and tetanic tension are normalized on a weight basis there was no significant difference between the two groups.

When the twitch response after a 1 sec (100 Hz) tetanus is compared with the pre-tetanic twitch the normal muscles show a potentiation of about 80% with a similar increase in the rate of tension development and no significant change in the time to peak tension. Depleted muscles on the other hand show a suppression of about 40% (Fig. 1).

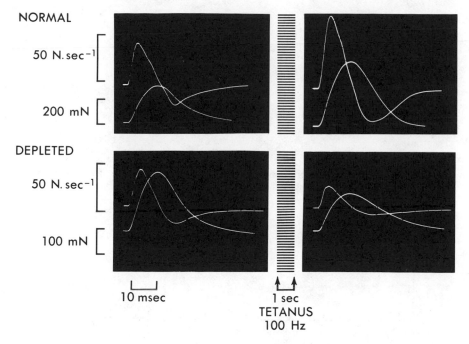

NORMAL

50 N.sec^{-1}

200 mN

DEPLETED

50 N.sec^{-1}

100 mN

10 msec

1 sec
TETANUS
100 Hz

Fig. 1.   The effect of a tetanus on the twitch response of normal
& creatine depleted muscles. Left hand records show
isometric twitch records (lower trace) and first derivative (upper trace) of normal and creatine depleted muscles
before a tetanus. Right hand records show the response of
the same muscles 200 msec after the tetanus.

The suppression is transient and after 1-2 sec it is followed
by a delayed potentiation about 25% of normal. This decays slowly
with a similar time course to normal potentiation decay and
disappears after about 2 min (Fig. 2).

The greatest twitch suppression in depleted muscles is seen
100-200 msec after the tetanus. In order to distinguish between
an effect on the activation mechanism or the contractile element
the muscle was stimulated with trains of pulses instead of a single
stimulus after the conditioning tetanus.

When normal muscles were stimulated without a conditioning
tetanus the maximum rate of rise was given when the interval between
pulses was 2-3 msec. Peak tension was reached with 20 pulses at
2.5 msec intervals. When this stimulus train was applied before
and after a tetanus the peak developed tension showed a similar
small decline in both normal and depleted muscles (Fig. 3). This

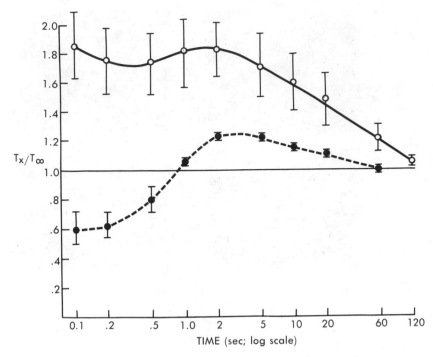

Fig. 2. Peak twitch tension after a 1 sec (100 Hz) tetanus as a function of time (log scale). Ordinate: twitch tension at a time x (T_x) as a fraction of rested state tension (T_0). Upper curve (o) shows the response of a normal EDL (mean ± SE, n=6) and the lower curve (●) of a creatine depleted muscle (n=6).

clearly showed that the twitch was not suppressed because of the limited ability of the muscle to develop tension. However the maximum rate of rise of tension was about 30% less in the depleted muscles after the tetanus whereas in the normal muscles it was about 5% greater. The rate of relaxation was about 50% slower following a tetanus in the depleted muscle and only slightly slower in normal muscles.

At normal intracellular pH (7.0) the hydrolysis of CrP is accompanied by an uptake of protons while ATP hydrolysis generates protons (Alberty, 1969). In order to test the hypothesis that post tetanic suppression results from a fall in pH around the myofilaments the intracellular pH was reduced to 6.5. At this pH there is no net proton production (Alberty, 1969). Intracellular pH was lowered by 30% CO_2 (Clancy and Brown, 1966).

Under these conditions, post tetanic suppression was slightly

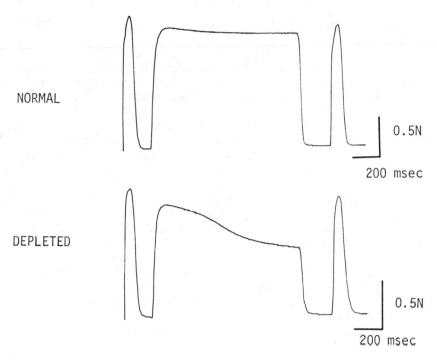

NORMAL

0.5N

200 msec

DEPLETED

0.5N

200 msec

Fig. 3.   The response of normal and depleted muscles to a train of
stimuli causing maximal activation before and after a
tetanus.   Initial contraction shows response to a train
of 20 pulses at 2.5 msec intervals.   The muscle is then
stimulated at 100 Hz for 1 sec.   200 msec later the initial
train is repeated.   Note: the mean 'sag' of tension in a
1 sec (100Hz) tetanus was about -24% in depleted muscles
and -8% in normal muscles.

decreased but a large component of the suppression remained.   Normal
muscles under the same conditions showed an enhancement of the
potentiation from 80% to about 110%.

DISCUSSION

It has been proposed that post tetanic twitch potentiation in
mammalian fast muscles is due to the increased effectiveness of the
activation process (Close and Hoh, 1968). Our observations support
this since the ability of the contraction mechanism to develop
force during maximal activation is not increased but slightly decreased.   This suggests that in the post tetanic state there is
either an increased calcium release or an increased sensitivity of
the contractile system to calcium.   The latter would seem more
likely in view of the fact that calcium transients, at least in frog

muscle are decreased following a tetanus (Blinks et al., 1978).

Creatine depletion appears to reverse the effect of a tetanus on the activation process. The transient suppression appears to be superimposed on a small potentiation which becomes evident 2 sec after the tetanus when the transient suppression is over.

While a small component of this transient suppression could be due to a pH fall associated with net ATP hydrolysis, the CO_2 experiment seems to rule this out as the major cause of the suppression. It seems likely that the suppression results from an increase in ADP or a fall in ΔG_{ATP}. A reasonable interpretation of the relationship between lowered ΔG_{ATP} and suppressed activation is provided by the proposal of Hasselbach and Oetliker (1983). They show that the free Ca^{2+} level within the SR is critically dependent on the free energy of hydrolysis of ATP.

The free Ca^{2+} level within the SR presumably provides the driving force for Ca^{2+} release during the activation process. Ca^{2+} release would therefore be reduced following a reduction of ΔG_{ATP}. At the same time the rate of Ca^{2+} removal from the cytosol would be slowed. This mechanism would thus account for both the reduced twitch activation and the slowed relaxation seen in creatine depleted muscles after a tetanus.

These experiments then suggest that creatine phosphate is important in the maintenance and potentiation of the activation process during brief bursts of activity in skeletal muscle. Depletion of the energy buffer system results in suppression of activation.

While the proposal is speculative, it is attractive since it provides a useful protective feedback mechanism. Diminished energy levels would suppress activation and so reduce the energy demand. Under unfavourable conditions such as ischemia or during prolonged activity when a steady state can not be maintained this could protect the cell by preventing ATP from falling below a critical level.

ACKNOWLEDGEMENTS

This work was supported by the Medical Research Council of Canada.

REFERENCES

Alberty, R.A., 1969, Standard Gibbs free energy, enthalpy, and entropy changes as a function of pH and pMg for several reactions involving adenosine phosphates. J. Biol. Chem. 244:3290-3302.

Blinks, J.R., Rudel, R. and Taylor, S.R., 1978, Calcium transients in isolated amphibian skeletal muscle fibres: detection with aequorin. J. Physiol. 277:291-323.

Cain, D.F. and Davies, R.E., 1962, Breakdown of ATP during a single contraction of working muscle. Biochem. Biophys. Res. Comm. 8:361-366.

Clancy, R.L. and Brown, E.B., 1966, In vivo CO_2 buffer curves of skeletal and cardiac muscle. Am. J. Physiol. 211: 1309-1312.

Close, R. and Hoh, J.F.Y., 1968, The after effects of repetitive stimulation on the isometric twitch contraction of the rat fast skeletal muscle. J. Physiol. 197:461-477.

Curtin, N.A. and Woledge, R.C., 1978, Energy changes and muscular contraction. Physiol. Rev. 58:690-761.

Ennor, A.M. and Stocken, L.A., 1948, The estimation of creatine. Biochem. J. 42:557-563.

Fitch, C.D., Jellinek, M. and Mueller, E.J., 1974, Experimental depletion of creatine and phosphocreatine from skeletal muscle. J. Biol. Chem. 249:1060-1063.

Gudbjarnason, S., Mathes, P. and Ravens, K.G., 1970, Functional compartmentation of ATP and CrP in heart muscle. J. Mol. Cell Cardiol. 1:325-339.

Hasselbach, W. and Oetliker, M., 1983, Energetics and electrogenicity of the sarcoplasmic reticulum calcium pump. Ann. Rev. Physiol. 45:325-339.

Mainwood, G.W. and Cechetto, D., 1980, The effect of bicarbonate concentration on fatigue and recovery in isolated rat diaphragm. Can. J. Physiol. Pharmacol. 58:624-632.

Petrofsky, J.S. and Fitch, C.D., 1980, Contractile characteristics of skeletal muscles depleted of phosphocreatine. Pflugers Arch. 384:123-129.

Spande, J.I. and Schottelius, B.A., 1970, Chemical basis of fatigue in isolated mouse solcus muscle. Am. J. Physiol. 219:1490-1495.

CALCIUM COMPARTMENTATION IN

MAMMALIAN MYOCARDIUM

G.A. Langer

Departments of Medicine and Physiology
Cardiovascular Research Laboratory
UCLA School of Medicine
Center for the Health Sciences
Los Angeles, California

INTRODUCTION

Since I have written recently published (Langer et al., 1982) or soon to be published (Langer, 1984) reviews on various aspects of calcium (Ca) compartmentation this report will serve as a brief summary of my present concepts of compartmentation with a focus on recent work from the Cardiovascular Research Laboratory at UCLA. These studies support the concept that Ca is distributed on and within the cell very differently dependent upon conditions of perfusion and functional demands.

CALCIUM AT THE SARCOLEMMA

A simple modification of Ringer's experiments on frog ventricle indicates the importance of rapidly exchangeable Ca in the support of contractile force in mammalian ventricle (Philipson and Langer, 1979). Removal of Ca from the arterial perfusate caused contractile force to fall with a $t\frac{1}{2} \sim 50$ seconds. Replacement of Ca after force had declined to near-zero level produced force redevelopment with a $t\frac{1}{2} \sim 10$ seconds or approximately 5 times the rate of loss upon Ca removal. Moreover, addition of lanthanum (La, 0.2 mM), a competitor for Ca at binding sites, uncoupled excitation from contraction with a $t\frac{1}{2} < 10$ seconds. The asymmetry of the rates of loss and regain of force and the rapidity of the response to La which binds to the sarcolemma and does not penetrate intracellularly strongly suggested that sarcolemmal-bound Ca plays a crucial role in the support of contractile force.

527

This concept was directly supported by the demonstration that Ca bound to highly purified sarcolemmal vesicles was in direct proportion to the level of contractile force of intact ventricle as $[Ca]_o$ was varied from 0.05 to 10 mM (Bers et al., 1981). In addition modification of sarcolemmal binding by alteration of perfusate sodium ($[Na]_o$) concentration (Philipson et al., 1980b) or by addition of various competitive cations (Bers and Langer, 1979) produced closely proportional changes in contractile force.

The specific molecular locus of bound Ca at the cellular surface was originally proposed to be within the glycocalyx - possibly the sialic acid in this structure (Langer et al., 1976). Though this remains a possibility, quantitatively the phospholipids (PL) of the sarcolemmal bilayer appear to be more likely candidates (Philipson et al., 1980a). The PL account for 80-85% of the binding sites at physiological $[Ca]_o$.

Though sialic acid within the glycocalyx seems to be of importance in the maintenance of selective permeability of the cell to Ca (Langer et al., 1981) recent studies add support to the concept that PL may be the sites related to contractile control on the basis of their ability to bind Ca:
1). Polymyxin B (PXB) is an amphiphilic peptidolipid with a positively charged head-group (diaminobutyric acids) and lipophilic tail. There is strong evidence that the tail inserts into the sarcolemmal lipid bilayer while the positively charged head group interacts specifically with negatively charged phospholipid. PXB is a potent displacer of Ca from isolated sarcolemmal membrane (Burt and Langer, 1983) and from cultured cardiac cells (Burt et al., 1983). We also have preliminary evidence that PXB acts to uncouple excitation from contraction.
2). Treatment of sarcolemmal membrane with phospholipase D (PLD) specifically cleaves the nitrogenous base from the phospholipids, producing phosphatidic acid, and thereby increases the net anionic charge on the membrane. Such treatment significantly increases (by 60%) the amount of Ca bound (Langer and Nudd, 1983). Philipson and Nishimoto (1984) have shown that PLD treatment of purified sarcolemmal vesicles from dog heart stimulates Na-Ca exchange by 300-400%. Finally work in progress demonstrates that PLD treatment of isolated rabbit papillary muscle is strongly positively inotropic.

Therefore, specific modification of the sarcolemmal PL results in predictable changes in Ca binding with the expected inotropic consequences. Our current hypothesis visualizes the PL as surface "storage" sites for Ca in rapid equilibrium with extracellular Ca. These sites would provide Ca to the Na-Ca exchanger and, probably, to the Ca channels - the two routes through which Ca influx occurs. The mechanism by which Ca could be released to the exchanger and channel upon excitation can only be speculated upon.

Perhaps the affinity of the PL is regulated by the level of the membrane potential as proposed by Lüllman and Peters (1977). The dipole moment (μ) of polarized membrane constituents is related to the electric field (E, determined by membrane potential and membrane thickness) and the polarizability of the charged sites (β) according to $\mu = \beta E$. With membrane potential high, as in the polarized state, the dipole will be high and proton binding increased within the membrane. This relatively high intramembranous pH will facilitate binding of Ca ions to the acidic phospholipids. As membrane depolarization proceeds, the magnitude of the dipole decreases, protons are released, pH falls and Ca would be released - possibly to the channel or to the exchanger or both.

CALCIUM AT THE MITOCHONDRIA

Experiments utilizing the tissue culture model have enabled us to either exclude or include mitochondrial Ca exchange dependent upon the exclusion or inclusion, respectively, of a proton donor in the perfusate. In HEPES-buffered perfusate which contains chloride as the only inorganic anion all of the exchangeable Ca is rapidly exchangeable ($t\frac{1}{2} < 1$ minute) and approximately 80% La-displaceable. Addition of phosphate at relatively low pH ($<$ 7.2) adds a slow component of exchange ($t\frac{1}{2} \sim 40$ min) which is not La-displaceable (Langer and Nudd, 1980). According to the scheme proposed and demonstrated in vitro by Lehninger (1974) phosphate serves as a proton donor as it enters the mitochondrial matrix. The reaction is equivalent to entry of H_3PO_4 with loss of a proton which is then removed via electron transport in respiring mitochondria. The resulting excess anion provides the milieu for Ca accumulation as the phosphate salt. In the presence of 1.0 mM Ca addition of 10 mM phosphate to the perfusate adds a mitochondrial compartment which exchanges Ca at a rate of approximately 2.5 x 10^{-5} mol/kg dry wt/min. This slow rate is compatible with the low rate of mitochondrial exchange found in vivo by Robertson et al. (1982).

The fact that either Warfarin or Antimycin-A, specific inhibitors of mitochondrial respiration, completely eliminate the phosphate-induced slow component in the cultured cells (Langer and Nudd, 1980) essentially proves its mitochondrial locus. In addition caffeine has no effect on this slow component of exchange as would be expected for mitochondrial Ca exchange.

The cultured cells beat well and synchronously in HEPES-buffered medium in which all exchangeable Ca is rapidly exchangeable with no evidence of mitochondrial participation. Therefore it seems Ca can cycle between sarcolemmal sites and myofilaments without, in effect, exchanging with the mitochondria. The role of the sarcoplasmic reticulum (SR) was then investigated.

CALCIUM AT THE SR

The Ca uptake pattern in HEPES perfused (all rapidly exhange-
able) and phosphate (pH < 7.2) perfused (addition of mitochondrial
component) is unaffected by 10 mM caffeine (Langer et al., 1983).
Since caffeine is believed to promote release and prevent uptake
of Ca by the SR the lack of effect, in both culture and rabbit
ventricle, of caffeine under the specific perfusion conditions suggested that the SR was not participating in cellular Ca exchange.
If, however, the rate of cellular Ca uptake was increased above
the level present under the designated perfusion conditions, caffeine then had a marked effect on Ca uptake pattern.

In the presence of phosphate, elevation of pH to 7.35-7.50
causes a marked increase in Ca uptake rate (Ponce-Hornos et al.,
1982). This additional uptake is not affected by inhibitors of
mitochondrial respiration and is believed due to product inhibition by phosphate (PO_4^{3-}), of the Na-K pump of the cell
(Ponce-Hornos and Langer, 1982) with subsequent stimulation of
Na-Ca exchange. The latter is proposed to be the basis for the
augmented Ca uptake. In the presence of this augmented Ca uptake
rate, caffeine now causes a further increase in uptake indicative
of Ca retention within the cell. The effect of phosphate at pH
7.35-7.50 and its production of caffeine sensitivity is demonstr-
able both in cultured cells and rabbit ventricle (Langer et al.,
1983).

Further results in rabbit ventricle (Langer et al., 1983)
provide additional evidence that SR participation in cellular Ca
exchange is dependent upon the level of cellular Ca uptake or
"load." As indicated above, 10 mM caffeine added to the perfusion
of rabbit interventricular septa under conditions of "low level"
Ca uptake (HEPES perfusate) induces no progressive contracture nor
change in rate of ^{45}Ca uptake. If, however, ouabain is added in
order to stimulate Ca uptake, caffeine now causes a marked increase in ^{45}Ca uptake rate and progressive contracture.

Finally, it was demonstrated (Langer et al., 1983) that low
dose sodium orthovanadate (1-3 μM) added to the HEPES-perfusate
consistently induced caffeine sensitivity in the rabbit ventricle.
At this low dosage vanadate inhibits neither the Na-K pump nor SR
Ca uptake but does inhibit the sarcolemmal Ca-Mg ATPase significantly. This enzyme regulates the sarcolemmal Ca pump (Caroni and
Carafoli, 1981). Vanadate, prior to caffeine administration, had
no effect on force development nor on rate of Ca uptake. Addition
of caffeine in the presence of vanadate, however, induced progressive contracture and marked increase in the rate of Ca uptake.

The above results are interpreted as follows: Without ouabain or vanadate the level of cellular Ca is not sufficient to

530

stimulate Ca uptake by the SR. If little or no SR uptake is taking place the action of an inhibitor, caffeine, is not manifest either functionally (production of contracture) or on Ca uptake pattern (increased retention of Ca). Ouabain induces augmented transsarcolemmal uptake, raises cellular Ca to a level which stimulates SR uptake so that caffeine inhibition results in contracture and Ca retention. Vanadate, on the other hand, inhibits the sarcolemmal Ca pump which increases cellular Ca level which, in turn, stimulates the formerly inactive SR Ca pump. Again, caffeine inhibition of the SR now is manifest. The series of experiments, both in cultured cells and adult mammalian ventricle, suggest that Ca may move through the cell during the contraction-relaxation cycle without SR exchange under conditions of relatively low Ca "load."

CONCLUSION

Presently available results indicate that Ca bound to sarcolemmal sites in rapid equilibrium with extracellular Ca is of critical importance in the control of contractile force. Evidence favors the concept that these sarcolemmal sites are phospholipid molecules which, at $[Ca]_o$ of 1.0-1.5 mM, can bind 500-700 µmoles Ca/kg wet tissue. Under conditions of relatively low Ca uptake or "load" the bound fraction cycles from sarcolemma to myofilaments and returns to the sarcolemma without distribution to more slowly exchangeable cellular sites. As Ca uptake or cellular Ca "load" is increased the SR is activated to exchange Ca and, according to Fabiato (1983), to serve as an amplifier of cellular Ca levels by the process of calcium-induced calcium release. The level of Ca at which the SR is activated probably varies greatly dependent upon species (Fabiato and Fabiato, 1978) and experimental conditions (e.g., catecholamine level, drug administration). The mitochondria will participate at a low rate of Ca exchange if a proton donor (e.g., phosphate, bicarbonate) is provided to the cell.

REFERENCES

Bers, D.M., and Langer, G.A., 1979, Uncoupling cation effects on cardiac contractility and sarcolemmal Ca^{2+} binding. Am. J. Physiol. 237:H332-H341

Bers, D.M., Philipson, K.D, and Langer, G.A., 1981, Cardiac contractility and sarcolemmal calcium binding in several cardiac muscle preparations. Am. J. Physiol. 240:H576-H583

Burt, J.M., and Langer, G.A., 1983, Ca^{2+} displacement by Polymyxin B from sarcolemma isolated by "gas dissection" from cultured neonatal rat myocardial cells. Biochim. Biophys. Acta 729:44-52

Burt, J.M., Duenas, C.J., and Langer, G.A., 1983, Influence of Polymyxin B, a probe for anionic phospholipids, on calcium binding and calcium and potassium fluxes of cultured cardiac cells. Circ. Res. 53:679-687

Caroni, P., and Carafoli, E., 1981, The Ca^{2+}-pumping ATPase of heart sarcolemma. Characterization, calmodulin dependence, and partial purification. J. Biol. Chem. 256:3263-3270

Fabiato, A., 1983, Calcium-induced release of calcium from the cardiac sarcoplasmic reticulum. Am. J. Physiol. 245:C1-C14

Fabiato, A., and Fabiato, F., 1978, Calcium-induced release of calcium from the sarcoplasmic reticulum of skinned cells from adult human, dog, cat, rabbit, rat and frog hearts and from fetal and new-born rat ventricles. Am. J. Physiol. 307:491-522

Langer, G.A., Frank, J.S., Nudd, L.M., and Seraydarian, K., 1976, Sialic acid: Effect of removal on calcium exchangeability of cultured heart cells. Science 193:1013-1015

Langer, G.A., and Nudd, L.M., 1980, Addition and kinetic characterization of mitochondrial calcium in myocardial tissue culture. Am. J. Physiol. 239:H769-H774

Langer, G.A., Frank, J.S., and Philipson, K.D., 1981, Correlation of alterations in cation exchange and sarcolemmal ultrastructure produced by neuraminidase and phospholipases in cardiac cell culture. Circ. Res. 49:1289-1299

Langer, G.A., Frank, J.S., and Philipson, K.D., 1982, Ultrastructure and calcium exchange of the sarcolemma, sarcoplasmic reticulum and mitochondria of the myocardium. Pharmac. Therap. 16:331-376

Langer, G.A., and Nudd, L.M., 1983, Effects of cations, phospholipases and neuraminidase on calcium binding to "gas dissected" membranes from cultured cardiac cells. Circ. Res. 53:482-490

Langer, G.A., Rich, T.L., and Nudd, L.M., 1983, Calcium compartmentalization in cultured and adult myocardium: Activation of a caffeine-sensitive component. J. Mol. Cell. Cardiol. 15:459-473

Langer, G.A., 1984, Calcium at the sarcolemma. J. Mol. Cell. Cardiol. 16: In press

Lehninger, A.L., 1974, Role of phosphate and other proton-donating anions in respiration-coupled transport of Ca^{2+} by mitochondria. Proc. Natl. Acad. Sci. 71:1520-1524

Lüllman, H., and Peters, T., 1977, Plasmalemmal calcium in cardiac excitation-contraction coupling. Clin. Exp. Pharmacol. Physiol. 4:49-57

Philipson, K.D., and Langer, G.A., 1979, Sarcolemmal bound calcium and contractility in the mammalian myocardium. J. Mol. Cell. Cardiol. 11:857-875

Philipson, K.D., Bers, D.M., and Nishimoto, A.Y., 1980a, The role of phospholipids in the Ca^{2+} binding of isolated cardiac sarcolemma. J. Mol. Cell. Cardiol. 12:1159-1173

Philipson, K.D., Bers, D.M., Nishimoto, A.Y., and Langer, G.A., 1980b, Binding of Ca^{2+} and Na^+ to sarcolemmal membranes: relation to control of myocardial contractility. Am. J. Physiol. 238:H373–H378

Philipson, K.D., and Nishimoto, A.Y., 1984, Stimulation of Na^+-Ca^{2+} exchange in cardiac sarcolemmal vesicles by phospholipase D. J. Biol. Chem. In press

Ponce-Hornos, J.E., and Langer, G.A., 1982, Effects of inorganic phosphate on ion exchange, energy state, and contraction in mammalian heart. Am. J. Physiol. 242:H79–H88

Ponce-Hornos, J.E., Langer, G.A., and Nudd, L.M., 1982, Inorganic phosphate: its effects on Ca exchange and compartmentalization in cultured heart cells. J. Mol. Cell. Cardiol. 14:41–51

Robertson, S.P., Potter, J.D., and Rouslin, W., 1982, The Ca^{2+} and Mg^{2+} dependence of Ca^{2+} uptake and respiratory function of porcine heart mitochondria. J. Biol. Chem. 257:1743–1748

CALCIUM CHANNEL BLOCKERS, BETA BLOCKERS

AND THE MAINTENANCE OF CALCIUM HOMEOSTASIS

Winifred G. Nayler and W.J. Sturrock

Department of Medicine
University of Melbourne
Austin Hospital
Heidelberg, Victoria
Australia

INTRODUCTION

A properly functioning myocardium is well equipped to maintain ionic homeostasis. Each myocyte is surrounded by a selectively permeable membrane into which are inserted the various ionic pumps, the ion-selective, voltage-activated and receptor operated channels, and the ion transporters, including the Na^+-Ca^{2+} exchanger (Figure 1). In addition the cells contain an abundant capacity to synthesize energy-rich phosphates, provided that the supply of precursors, cofactors, substrate and oxygen does not become rate limiting. These energy-rich phosphates are needed not only as substrate for the myosin ATPase enzyme; they also provide the substrate for the various ionic pumps that are involved in maintaining intracellular ionic homeostasis. These pumps include the Na^+-K^+ ATPase, the plasmalemmal Ca^{2+} ATPase (Figure 1) and the Ca^{2+} ATPases of the mitochondria and the sarcoplasmic reticulum (S.R).

This paper is concerned with the events that occur when cardiac muscle cells lose their capacity to maintain ionic homeostasis with respect to calcium. Two conditions will be considered - the calcium paradox and post-ischaemic reperfusion. These conditions have been selected because in both instances they result in a loss of ionic homeostasis with respect to Ca^{2+}, a condition which then triggers a cascade of events that ultimately ends in cell death and tissue necrosis.

535

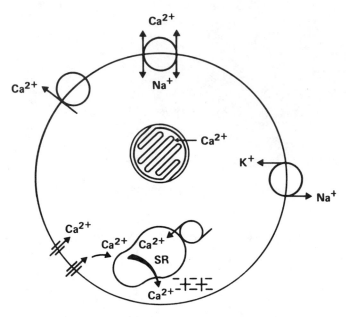

Fig. 1. Schematic representation of the various ionic pumps, ion-selective channels, ionic exchangers and subcellular organelles involved in maintaining ionic homeostasis with respect to Ca^{2+}.

The Calcium Paradox

The paradoxical response of hearts to calcium repletion after a short period of calcium-free perfusion was first described by Zimmerman and Hulsmann, in 1966. This phenomenon, now known as "the calcium paradox", is characterized by extensive ultrastructural damage (Muir, 1968; Yates and Dhalla, 1975; Frank et al., 1977; Ruigrok et al., 1980), a rapid and massive release of intracellular constituents (Zimmerman and Hulsmann, 1966; Hearse et al., 1978;1980), depletion of the energy rich phosphate reserves (Boink et al., 1978), a loss of K^+ (Crevey et al., 1978) and a gain in Na^+ and Ca^{2+} (Alto and Dhalla, 1978; Nayler and Grinwald, 1981). Although the gain in Ca^{2+} that occurs under these conditions is of critical importance its route of entry has not yet been established (Grinwald and Nayler, 1981). The known normal routes of Ca^{2+} entry include a small component due to passive inward diffusion, entry in exchange for Na^+ (Reuter, 1974) and entry through ion-selective, voltage-activated channels (Reuter and Scholz, 1977). However, in the case of the calcium-paradox it seems probable that more than one route of Ca^{2+} entry is involved. Because of the rapidity with which ionic homeostasis with respect to Ca^{2+} is lost during the paradox it has been difficult to establish the temporal sequence of events that ultimately results in massive Ca^{2+}-overloading and cell death.

Table 1. Effect of Ca^{2+}-free Perfusion on Intracellular Ca^{2+} and Na^+

Minutes of Ca^{2+}-free perfusion	Control		Na^+-loaded	
	Ca^{2+}_i	Na^+_i	Ca^{2+}_i	Na^+_i
0	3.46 ± 0.3	56.5 ± 2.6	2.72 ± 0.57	129.5 ± 10.2
1.0	3.34 ± 0.45	76.8 ± 6.3	2.69 ± 0.41	125.3 ± 13.3
1.5	3.11 ± 0.54	100.3 ± 7.4	2.42 ± 0.26	149.1 ± 14.1
10.0	1.64 ± 0.33	73.8 ± 13.4	1.73 ± 0.28	156.2 ± 11.4

Table 1. Each result is mean±SE of 5-6 experiments. Ca^{2+}_i and Na^+_i are expressed as µmoles/g dry wt. The hearts, obtained from adult Sprague Dawley rats, were equilibrated with normal or 'Na$^+$-loading' Krebs buffer for 20 minutes before they were Ca^{2+}-depleted by removing Ca^{2+} from and adding 0.1 mM EDTA to the perfusion buffer. Perfusions were retrograde, at 37 °C and at a perfusion pressure of 60-80 mM Hg pressure.

Routes of Ca^{2+} Entry in the Calcium Paradox

Plasmalemmal vesicles that are harvested from Ca^{2+}-depleted hearts are not freely permeable to Ca^{2+} (Nayler et al., 1984). Hence, unless a Ca^{2+}-free induced membrane defect that renders the membrane freely permeable to Ca^{2+} is lost or concealed when the vesicles are isolated it is difficult to account for the Ca^{2+}-paradox-induced gain in Ca^{2+} simply in terms of an enhanced passive inward movement of Ca^{2+} along its concentration gradient, which is about 1000:1. It is equally difficult to account for this gain in Ca^{2+} solely in terms of an enhanced entry of Ca^{2+} in exchange for Na^+, because although the Na^+-Ca^{2+} exchange mechanism survives the paradox (Nayler et al., 1984) and although intracellular Na^+ rises during Ca^{2+}-depletion (Goshima et al., 1980; Nayler et al., 1984) we have already shown that the gain in Ca^{2+} that occurs after 10 minute's of Ca^{2+}-free perfusion correlates poorly with the intracellular Na^+ at the start of repletion. However there is evidence that some of the Ca^{2+} that enters early upon Ca^{2+}-repletion does enter in exchange for Na^+. This evidence comes from experiments in which the time-course for the gain in Ca^{2+} has been followed in isolated rat hearts the ionic milieu of which has been manipulated so that the cells contain either normal (56.5 ± 2.6 μmoles/ gm dry wt) or raised (129.5 ± 10.2 μmoles/gm dry wt) levels of Na^+ at the time of Ca^{2+} repletion. Na^+-loading was achieved as described by Glitsch et al. (1970), by replacing some of the K^+ in the perfusion buffer with mannitol and lowering the Ca^{2+} from the control level of 1.3 to 0.15 mmoles/l during the period of equilibration. The hearts were divided into several groups: in one group the Na^+-loaded hearts were Ca^{2+}-depleted for 10 minutes whilst in the other group the period of Ca^{2+}-free perfusion was reduced to 1.0 or 1.5 minutes. Table 1 shows that immediately prior to Ca^{2+} repletion the Na^+-loaded hearts contained significantly more Na^+ ($p < 0.001$) than their respective controls, which had been perfused for the same period of time but with normal followed by Ca^{2+}-free Krebs perfusion buffer.

The results of these experiments are summarized in Figure 2A and B and Figure 3. Figure 2 (A and B) shows that neither the initial rate (Fig 2A) nor the total gain (Fig 2B) in intracellular Ca^{2+} caused by 10 minute's repletion after 10 minutes of Ca^{2+}-free perfusion was affected by Na^+-loading, even although the Na^+-loaded hearts contained 156.2 ± 11.4 μmoles Na^+/gm dry weight immediately before repletion (Table 1) whereas the control hearts had contained only 73.8 ± 13.4 μmoles Na^+/gm dry wt (Table 1). However it is premature to conclude that a raised intracellular Na^+ does not affect the amount of Ca^{2+} that is gained under these conditions because a slightly different picture emerges when the duration of the Ca^{2+}-free perfusion is

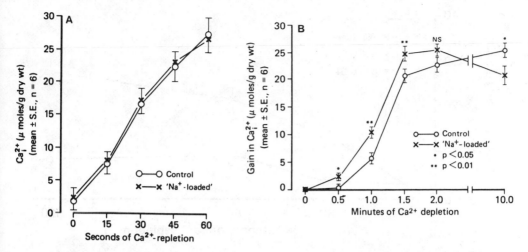

Fig. 2.A: The time course of the gain in intracellular Ca^{2+} during the first 60 seconds of Ca^{2+} repletion in control and "Na^+-loaded" hearts after 10 min Ca^{2+}-depletion. B: Effect of "Na^+-loading" on gain in intracellular Ca^{2+} during 10 min repletion after the indicated times of Ca^{2+}-depletion. N.S, not significant, p=0.05

reduced. Hence, as the data in Figure 2B shows Ca^{2+}-repletion of Na^+-loaded hearts which had been perfused with Ca^{2+}-free buffers for relatively short periods of time (0.5, 1 or 1.5 minutes) gained excess Ca^{2+} during 10 minute's repletion relative to the hearts which had not been Na^+-loaded. After 10 minute's repletion, however, such an effect had totally disappeared.

These results indicate the possibility that some of the early gain in Ca^{2+} that occurs upon repletion involves an entry of Ca^{2+} in exchange for Na^+. Further data that is relevant to this possibility was provided by experiments in which conditions of a "mild paradox" were used. This was achieved by reducing the period of Ca^{2+}-free perfusion to one minute (Figure 3), and following the rate of repletion at 30 second intervals, instead of measuring it only after 10 minute's of Ca^{2+} repletion. Under these conditions (Figure 3) we find unequivocal evidence of the fact that upon Ca^{2+} repletion the Na^+-loaded hearts gain Ca^{2+} at a faster rate (p<0.01) than the Ca^{2+}-depleted controls. Since intracellular Na^+ is known to rise during perfusion with Ca^{2+}-

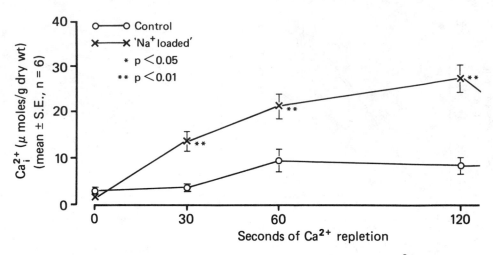

Fig. 3. Time course of the gain in intracellular Ca^{2+} during Ca^{2+}-repletion after 1 minute of Ca^{2+}-depletion in control and "Na^+-loaded" hearts.

free buffers (Alto and Dhalla, 1979) and since the $Na^+:Ca^{2+}$ exchanger survives Ca^{2+} depletion and repletion, we can conclude that at least some of the Ca^{2+} that is taken up by the myocytes when Ca^{2+}-containing buffers are re-introduced after a period of Ca^{2+}-free perfusion involves the entry of Ca^{2+} in exchange for Na^+. However this cannot be the only route of entry, because if this had been the case then the discrepancy between the intra-cellular Na^+ content at the start of repletion and the amount of Ca^{2+} that was gained should have persisted throughout the 10 minute's of repletion. Since this did not happen other routes of Ca^{2+} entry must be involved.

Another possible route of Ca^{2+} entry involves entry through the slow channels. Measurements of Ca^{2+} gain that relate to tissue levels of Ca^{2+} found in hearts that have been Ca^{2+} repleted for 10 minutes after 10 minute's Ca^{2+}-free perfusion have consistently shown (Ruigrok et al., 1980; Nayler and Grinwald, 1981; Nayler et al., 1984) that the slow channel

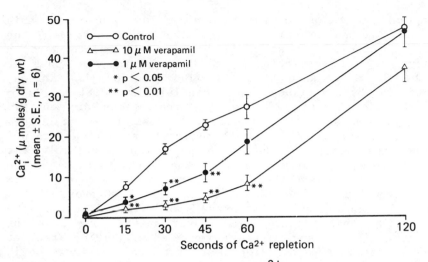

Fig. 4.Changes in intracellular Ca^{2+} during the first 2 minute's Ca^{2+}-repletion. When verapamil was present it was added before, during and after Ca^{2+}-depletion.

blocker verapamil (1 and 10 μ g/1) fails to prevent the repletion-induced gain in Ca^{2+}. However (Figure 4) by looking at the time-course of the gain in Ca^{2+} a transitory inhibitory effect of verapamil can be detected.

In general, therefore, it seems possible that the <u>early</u> gain in Ca^{2+} that occurs when Ca^{2+}-containing buffers are re-admitted to hearts which have been perfused with Ca^{2+}-free buffers could involve the entry of Ca^{2+} through normal physiological pathways. Thus during the first few seconds of Ca^{2+} repletion some Ca^{2+} probably enters in exchange for some of the Na^+ that has accumulated during the phase of Ca^{2+}-depletion. In addition some Ca^{2+} enters through the slow channels. However (Fig 2,3 and 4) other routes of entry that are slow channel blocker - and Na^+-insensitive must also be involved and become predominant after the first few minutes of repletion. Enzyme and myoglobin release profiles (Hearse et al., 1978,1980; Nayler and Grinwald, 1981) indicate that massive cellular damage is not co-incidental with repletion. Instead there appears to be one or two minute's delay. Of course this delay could be an artifact due to the time course of the washout. It could just as easily reflect the existence of a secondary stage in repletion that is triggered, in part at least, by the early gain in Ca^{2+}. The question that arises, therefore, is why the tissue cannot handle this additional Ca^{2+}-load. Certainly it is not because the hearts are energy-deficient at the start of repletion, because as Boink et al. (1976) have shown, the ATP and CP reserves are well maintained throughout the period of Ca^{2+}-free perfusion. Probably the answer to this conundrum lies in the fact that Ca^{2+}-free perfusion alters the architecture of the sarcolemma and inter-calated discs (Muir, 1968; Frank et al., 1977; Crevey, 1978). It is well known that Ca^{2+}-free perfusion distorts the glycocalyx, so that its outermost layer splits away from the inner-layer. It has been argued (Crevey et al., 1978; Frank et al., 1977) that this deformation leads to a massive increase in permeability with respect to Ca^{2+}. It is equally possible that it weakens the sarcolemmal complex, thereby rendering the underlying plasmalemma more susceptible to deformation and distortion. This brings us to another facet of the Ca^{2+}-paradox that is beginning to attract attention (Ganote et al., 1980) - that is, the changed appearance of the intercalated discs, which separate from one another at the fascia adherens and macula adherens junctions during Ca^{2+}-free perfusion. This separation, which was first described by Muir (1968), must drastically influence the distribution of forces between adjacent cells. Hence, at the time of Ca^{2+}-repletion we have cells with high ATP and CP reserves, but with ultrastructural abnormalities involving the intercalated discs and the sarcolemma. These cells, it seems, are almost primed for destruction, and the "trigger" must be associated with the readmission of Ca^{2+} to the perfusion buffer. The sequence of events could be as shown in Fig 5.

Protection
_____

Under these circumstances the slow channel blockers will not prevent (Grinwald and Nayler, 1981) although they may reduce (Hearse et al., 1980) the severity and slow the progression of the paradox. Nor can the β-blockers be expected to provide protection, because the failure of the cells to maintain homeostasis with respect to Ca^{2+} is not due to energy-depletion. In all probability it is due to a weakening effect Ca^{2+}-depletion exerts on the integrity of the fascia adherens and macula adherens junctions of the intercalated discs, and the cohesiveness of the glycocalyx. The early influx of Ca^{2+}, therefore, need only trigger a rapid contraction to disrupt the intercalated discs and the sarcolemma. Such an explanation is quite compatible with the observation that ATP-depleted hearts

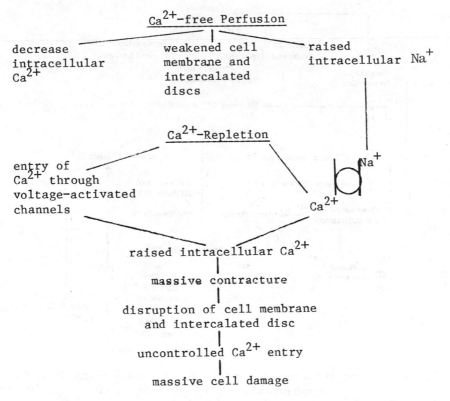

Fig. 5. Schematic representation of the cascade of events involved in the loss of Ca^{2+} homeostasis during the Ca^{2+} paradox.

are protected against the Ca^{2+}-paradox (Ruigrok et al., 1978). It is also compatible with the fact that foetal hearts are protected (Chizzonite and Zak, 1981; Frank and Rich, 1983) because these hearts have simplified intercalated discs. The fact that hypothermia protects (Holland and Olsen, 1975; Baker et al., 1983; Rich and Langer, 1982; Boink et al., 1980) could be anticipated, because hypothermia slows the $Na^+:Ca^{2+}$ exchanger. In addition, it will affect the "fluidity" of the membranes, including those of the intercalated discs and the plasmalemma.

Post-ischaemic reperfusion

The mammalian myocardium is an aerobic organ with comparatively little capacity for anaerobic metabolism. Moreover its

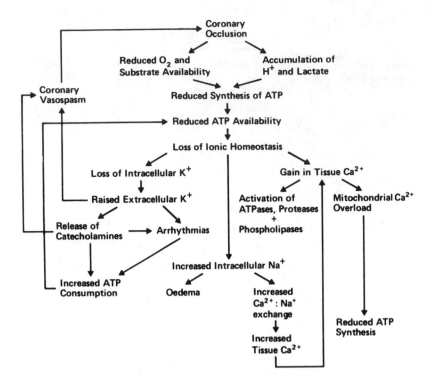

Fig. 6. Schematic representation of the events involved in loss of Ca^{2+} homeostasis during post-ischaemic reperfusion.

storage capacity for ATP and CP is relatively low, whilst its rate of ATP and CP usage is high. These three factors ensure that should the blood supply to the myocardium be interrupted even momentarily, there is a rapid depletion of the energy-rich phosphate reserves. The consequences of this are widespread and include (Figure 6) a loss of homeostasis with respect to Ca^{2+}. Catecholamines are also released, K^+ leaks out of the cells to accumulate in the extracellular space (Hirche et al., 1980), intracellular H^+ concentration rises (Cobb and Poole-Wilson, 1980) and the cells become electrically unstable.

Reperfusion causes a massive exacerbation of the damage caused by the pre-existing period of ischaemia (Figure 6) largely because the cells are now being presented with an almost unlimited supply of Ca^{2+} at a time when their stores of ATP and CP are either reduced or depleted, depending upon the duration of the ischaemic episode. Under these conditions intracellular Ca^{2+} rises rapidly (Figure 7), to trigger cell death and tissue necrosis. Some of the increase in cytosolic Ca^{2+} that occurs under these conditions can probably be attributed to Ca^{2+}

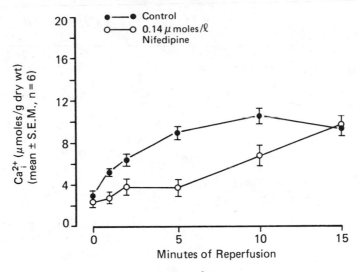

Fig. 7. Gain in intracellular Ca^{2+}, and the effect of 0.14 μmoles/1 nifedipine on that gain during reperfusion after 60 minute's low coronary flow (0.1 ml/minute) ischaemia in isolated rat hearts.

leaking out from its internal storage areas - including from within the sarcoplasmic reticulum. In addition, a large amount of Ca^{2+} floods in across the cell membrane (Figure 7). Hence the reperfused ischaemic heart resembles the Ca^{2+}-paradox heart in that it ultimately accumulates an excess of Ca^{2+}. However, whereas the gain in Ca^{2+} that is exhibited by the reperfused ischaemic hearts is preceded by a depletion of the energy rich phosphate reserves the reverse holds true for the calcium-paradox hearts, which maintain their full compliment of ATP and CP until Ca^{2+} repletion is instigated (Ruigrok et al., 1978).

Routes of Ca^{2+} entry during post-ischaemic reperfusion

Theoretically the gain in Ca^{2+} that occurs during the reperfusion of an ischaemic heart involves any one of the routes of entry discussed for the paradox. Figure 7 shows quite clearly that this gain in Ca^{2+} can be slowed, but not completely blocked by the Ca^{2+}-channel blocker, nifedipine. This

Table 2. Effect of Na^+-Depletion on Ca^{2+} Gain During Post-Ischaemic Reperfusion

	CONTROL		Na^+-DEPLETED	
After 30 min equilibration				
	Na^+	Ca^{2+}	Na^+	Ca^{2+}
	51.5 ± 10.6	4.53 ± 0.12	8.58 ± 0.38	4.01 ± 0.76
After 45 min ischaemia plus 15 min reperfusion				
		12.2 ± 0.9	4.67 ± 1.40	13.31 ± 1.31
After 60 min ischaemia plus 15 min reperfusion				
		18.6 ± 1.2	4.95 ± 0.94	16.32 ± 2.83

Table 2. Each result is mean ± SE of 5-6 expts. Results are presented as μ moles/gm dry wt and refer to intracellular Ca^{2+} and Na^+. Na^+-depleted hearts were reperfused with Na^+-free buffer, and controls with Tyrode.

protective effect of nifedipine is not a peculiar property of the dihydropyridines, since pretreatment with verapamil (Nayler et al., 1980) has also been shown to reduce Ca^{2+} overload during post-ischaemic reperfusion.

Because of their proven ability to slow the reperfusion-induced gain in Ca^{2+} some investigators have argued that the additional Ca^{2+} is entering through the slow channels. Whilst this may be true there is another explanation for these results – namely, that these drugs are protective because of their "energy-sparing" activity (Nayler et al., 1980), a property which ensures that more ATP will be around to act as substrate for the ATP-supported ionic pumps. One such pump is the Ca^{2+} ATPase of the sarcolemma (Nayler et al., 1980).

Another route of Ca^{2+} entry which theoretically may be involved in the inward movement of Ca^{2+} during post-ischaemic reperfusion is the $Na^+:Ca^{2+}$ exchanger (Figure 1). The data listed in Table 2 shows, however, that hearts in which the intracellular Na^+ content was reduced from the normal levels of 51.5 ± 10.6 to 8.58 ± 0.38 μmoles/gm dry weight before they were subjected to 60 minute's ischaemia and then reperfused with Na^+-free Tyrode's solution gained the same amount as Ca^{2+} as the controls, which were not Na^+ depleted and were reperfused with normal Tyrode's solution. Had the $Na^+:Ca^{2+}$ exchanger played a predominant role we would have expected a reduced Ca^{2+} gain in the Na^+-depleted hearts. Nevertheless, because intracellular Na^+ rises early during reperfusion (Shen and Jennings, 1972), presumably because the ischaemic-induced depletion of the

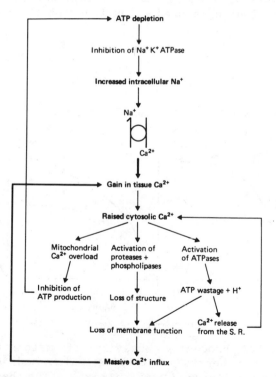

Fig. 8. Schematic representation of the possible involvement of Na^+-Ca^{2+} exchange during the loss of Ca^{2+} homeostasis caused by post-ischaemic reperfusion.

endogenous stores of ATP results in substrate-depletion induced inhibition of the Na^+ K^+ ATPase (Figure 8), some of the Ca^{2+} that enters upon reperfusion would enter in exchange for Na^+. Certainly the $Na^+:Ca^{2+}$ exchanger survives periods of ischaemia and reperfusion. In all probability, therefore, Ca^{2+} enters by a variety of routes upon reperfusion. Early during reperfusion the routes of entry may be physiological but, because of the ATP-depleted state of the myocardium, cytosolic Ca^{2+} rises in an uncontrolled manner. This in turn would lead to activation of the various phospholipases and proteases, with the consequent loss of membrane structure and function. At this stage large holes or rents may appear, allowing the free entry of Ca^{2+}. Hence in post-ischaemic reperfusion the end result mimics that of the paradox, with the loss of Ca^{2+} homeostasis being the vital event.

Protection against the loss of Ca^{2+} homeostasis due to post-ischaemic reperfusion

If the massive loss of function that persists despite post-ischaemic reperfusion is used as an index of the severity of the

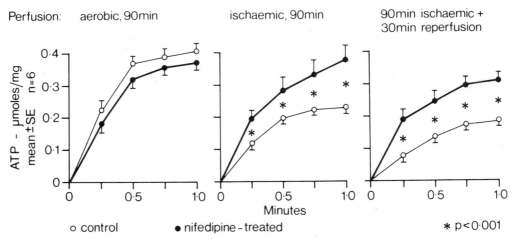

Fig. 9. The ATP producing activity of mitochondria isolated from the hearts of rabbits which had been pretreated with nifedipine (1 mg/kg/day). The hearts were perfused aerobically, made globally ischaemic or made ischaemic at 37°C as indicated before the mitochondria were harvested.

548

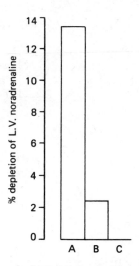

A 15 min ischaemia, 15 min reperfusion

B 15 min ischaemia, 15 min reperfusion
with 10 μg/ℓ nifedipine *added at reperfusion*

C 15 min ischaemia, 15 min reperfusion,
10 μg/ℓ nifedipine throughout

Fig. 10. Effect of 10 μg/1 nifedipine on the loss of cardiac noradrenaline caused by 15 minute's global ischaemia and reperfusion. Each bar is the mean of 6 experiments on rat hearts.

loss of Ca^{2+} homeostasis then it is possible to evaluate whether various "protective" regimes that have been proposed are, in fact, protective.

Slow channel blockers. Although it is often argued that the prophylactic use of slow channel blockers provides effective protection because they have a direct effect on the additional entry of Ca^{2+} that occurs upon reperfusion this argument may be erroneous. This is because it is based on the assumption that the slow channels are the major route of Ca^{2+} entry for the additional Ca^{2+} that is accumulated. An alternative, and we believe a more satisfactory argument, is to assume that these agents are protective because they indirectly preserve mitochondrial function, so that when the supply of oxygen and

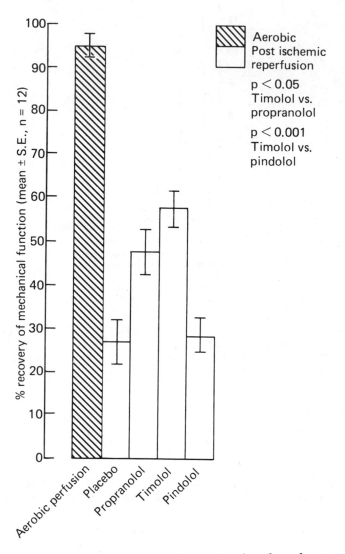

Fig. 11. Percentage recovery of peak developed tension in isolated rabbit hearts reperfused after 60 min global ischaemia at 37°C. The hearts in the experimental group were pretreated with 12.6 µg/1 timolol, 25.9 µg/1 propranolol or 12.4 µg/1 pindolol.

metabolic substrates is restored the mitochondria can regenerate the energy-rich phosphates needed as substrate for the ionic pump. Evidence of the ability of the slow channel blocker nifedipine, to preserve mitochondrial function in hearts which have been made ischaemic for sixty minutes and then reperfused is shown in Figure 9. These particular experiments were carried out with rabbit hearts, and the rabbits were pretreated with nifedipine for three days before the hearts were isolated, made ischaemic and then reperfused (Nayler et al., 1980). The data illustrates two important points; firstly, oxidative-phosphorylating activity of cardiac mitochondria is severely impaired during ischaemia and reperfusion. Secondly, pretreatment with a calcium channel blocker can attenuate the damaging effect of ischaemia and reperfusion (Bourdillon and Poole-Wilson, 1982; Bersohn and Shine, 1983). Under these conditions, therefore we could expect a greater regeneration of ATP upon the restoration of flow and substrate supply. It is of interest to note that under these same conditions the ischaemia and reperfusion-induced exacerbation of noradrenaline release is attenuated (Figure 10).

Beta-adrenoceptor blockade

The widespread use of β-adrenoceptor antagonists in the management of ischaemic heart disease provides ample proof of their efficacy. Animal studies have provided similar proof. For example when hearts from rabbits which have been pretreated with a variety of beta blockers are made ischaemic and then reperfused they all recover a greater percentage of the mechanical function, relative to the controls (Figure 11). Obviously some of these beta antagonists are more effective than others (Figure 11). A possible reason for this difference between the efficacy of the various blockers can be gleaned from the data shown in Figure 12. This shows that the various beta blockers protected the mitochondria from becoming overloaded with Ca^{2+}, a condition which is known to impair their oxidative phosphorylating capacity. This protective effect must be an indirect consequence of beta adrenoceptor blockade, because when added directly to the mitochondria these agents fail to alter mitochondrial function. Once again, however, it can be argued that because of their energy sparing activity these agents slow the rate of ischaemic induced depletion of the energy-rich phosphate reserves so that upon reperfusion the tissue has sufficient energy in the form of ATP to ensure maintenance of ionic homeostasis.

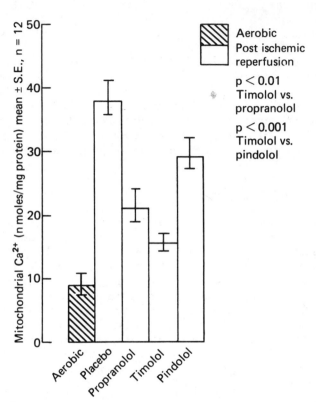

Fig. 12 Ca^{2+} content of mitochondria isolated from aerobically perfused rabbit hearts, after 60 minute's ischaemia and 20 minute's reperfusion with either timolol (12.6 µg/1), propranolol (25.9 µg/1), or pindolol (12.4 µg/1). When the drugs were present they were added before as well as after the ischaemic episode.

Conclusion

Because Ca^{2+}-repletion and post-ischaemic reperfusion injury is characterized by a massive cellular uptake of Ca^{2+} it has been natural to look for holes or rents in the sarcolemma to account for the breakdown of the sarcolemmal barrier to Ca^{2+}. Severe disruption of the sarcolemma becomes obvious after prolonged periods of Ca^{2+}-free perfusion and during reperfusion after prolonged periods of ischaemia. In the former case this disruption may contribute to the uncontrolled entry of Ca^{2+} that occurs upon repletion. However it is equally feasable that the Ca^{2+}-free perfusion sensitizes the plasmalemma and the intercalated discs so that when Ca^{2+} enters through a normal pathway and triggers a rapid contraction, the cells pull apart and distort, causing gross disruption of the sarcolemma and discs. The Ca^{2+} channel blockers can only delay and not prevent this phenomenon.

During post-ischaemic reperfusion an entirely different set of conditions prevail, because of the decline in the tissue levels of ATP and CP caused by the ischaemic insult. This ischaemic-induced decline in tissue ATP and CP ensures that homeostasis with respect to Ca^{2+} is lost prior to reperfusion. However the expression of that loss of homeostasis depends upon the unlimited supply of Ca^{2+} that accompanies reperfusion. It is not surprising therefore, that agents which slow the rate of depletion of the tissue stores of ATP and CP will slow the loss of Ca^{2+} homeostasis during the ischaemic episode, so that upon reperfusion, some enhanced recovery of function will be assured.

ACKNOWLEDGEMENTS

These experiments were undertaken during the tenure of a grant from the National Health and Medical Research Council of Australia.

REFERENCES

Alto, L.E., and Dhalla, N.S., 1979, Myocardial cation contents during induction of calcium paradox, Am. J. Physiol., 237:H713-H719.

Baker, J.E., Bullock, G.R., and Hearse, D.J., 1983, The temperature dependence of the calcium paradox: Enzymatic, functional and morphological correlates of cellular injury, J. Mol. Cell. Cardiol., 15:393-411.

Baker, J.E., and Hearse, D.J., 1983, Slow calcium channel blockers and the calcium paradox: comparative studies in the rat with seven drugs, J. Mol. Cell. Cardiol., 15:475-485.

Bersohn, M.M., and Shine, K.I., 1983, Verapamil protection of ischemic isolated rabbit heart: dependence on pretreatment, J. Mol. Cell Cardiol., 15:659-671.

Boink, A.B.T.J., Ruigrok, T.J.C., Maas, A.H.J., and Zimmerman, A.N.E., 1976, Changes in high-energy phosphate compounds of isolated rat hearts during Ca^{2+}-free perfusion and reperfusion with Ca^{2+}, J. Mol. Cell. Cardiol., 8:973-979.

Boink, A.B.T.J., Ruigrok, T.J.C., de Moes, D., Maas, A.H.J., and Zimmerman, A.N.E., 1980, The effect of hypothermia on the occurrence of the calcium paradox, Pfluegers Arch., 385:105-109.

Bourdillon, P.D., and Poole-Wilson, P.A., 1982, The effects of verapamil, quiescence and cardioplegia on calcium exchange and mechanical function in ischemic rabbit myocardium, Circ. Res., 50:360-369.

Chizzonite, R.A., and Zak, R., 1981, Calcium-induced cell death: susceptibility of cardiac myocytes is age-dependent, Science., 213:1508-1510.

Cobbe, S.M., and Poole-Wilson, P.A., 1980, The time of onset and severity of acidosis in myocardial ischaemia, J. Mol. Cell. Cardiol., 12:745-760.

Crevey, B.J., Langer, G.A., and Frank, J.S., 1978, Role of Ca^{2+} in the maintenance of rabbit myocardial cell membrane structural and function integrity, J. Mol. Cell. Cardiol., 10:1081-1100.

Frank, J.S., Langer, G.A., Nudd, L.M., and Seraydarian, K., 1977, The myocardial cell surface; its histochemistry and the effect of sialic acid and calcium removal on its structure and cellular ionic exchange, Circ. Res., 41:702-714.

Frank, J.S., and Rich, T.L., 1983, Ca depletion and repletion in rat heart: age-dependent changes in the sarcolemma, Am. J. Physiol., 245:H343-H353.

Ganote, C.E., Liv, S.Y., Safavi, S., and Kaltenbach, J.P., 1980, Hypoxia, calcium and contracture as mediators of myocardial enzyme release, J. Mol. Cell. Cardiol., 12:47.

Glitsch, H.G., Reuter, H., and Scholz, H., 1970, The effect of the internal sodium concentration on calcium fluxes in isolated guinea-pig auricles, J. Physiol., 209:25-43.

Goshima, K., Wakabayashi, S., and Masuda, A., 1980, Ionic mechanisms of morphological changes of cultured myocardial cells on successive incubation in media without and with Ca^{2+}, J. Mol. Cell. Cardiol., 12:1135-1157.

Grinwald, P.M., and Nayler, W.G., 1981, Calcium entry in the calcium paradox, J. Mol. Cell. Cardiol., 13:867-880.

Hearse, D.J., Baker, J.E., and Humphrey, S.M., 1980, Verapamil and the calcium paradox, J. Mol. Cell. Cardiol., 12:733–740.

Hearse, D.J., Humphrey, S.M., and Bullock, G.R., 1978, The oxygen paradox and calcium paradox: two facets of the same problem, J. Mol. Cell. Cardiol., 10:641–688.

Hirche, H.J., Franz, C.H.R., Bos, L., Bissig, R., Lang, R., and Schramm, M.,1980, Myocardial extracellular K^+ and H^+ increase and noradrenaline release as possible cause of early arrhythmias following acute coronary artery occlusion in pigs, J. Mol. Cell. Cardiol., 12:579–593.

Holland, C.E., and Olsen, R.E., 1975, Prevention by hypothermia of paradoxical necrosis in cardiac muscle, J. Mol. Cell. Cardiol., 7:917–928.

Muir, A.R., 1968, A calcium-induced contracture of cardiac muscle cells, J. Anat., 102:148–149.

Nayler, W.G., Elz, J.S., Perry, S.E., and Daly, M.J., 1984, The biochemistry of uncontrolled calcium entry, Eur. Heart J., (In press).

Nayler, W.G., Ferrari, R., and Williams, A., 1980, Protective effect of pretreatment with verapamil, nifedipine and propranolol on mitochondrial function in the ischemic and reperfused myocardium, Am. J. Cardiol., 46:242–8.

Nayler, W.G., and Grinwald, P.M., 1981, The effect of verapamil on calcium accumulation during the calcium paradox, J. Mol. Cell. Cardiol., 13:435–441.

Reuter, H., 1974, Exchange of calcium ions in the mammalian myocardium, Circulation., 34:599–605.

Reuter, H., and Scholz, H., 1977, A study of the ion selectivity and kinetic properties of the calcium-dependent slow inward current in mammalian cardiac muscle, J. Physiol., 264:17–47.

Rich, T.L., and Langer, G.A., 1982, Calcium depletion in rabbit myocardium: calcium paradox protection by hypothermia and cation substitution, Circ. Res., 51:131–141.

Ruigrok, T.J.C., Boink, A.B., Slade, A., Zimmerman, A.N.E., Meijler, F.L., and Nayler, W.G., 1980, The effect of verapamil on the calcium paradox, Am. J. Pathol., 98:769–782.

Ruigrok, T.J.C., Boink, A.B.T., Spies, F., Blok, J., Maas, A.H.J., and Zimmerman, A.N.E., 1978, Energy dependence of the calcium paradox, J. Mol. Cell. Cardiol., 10:991–1002.

Shen, A.C., and Jennings, R.B., 1972, Myocardial calcium and magnesium in acute ischemic injury, Am. J. Pathol., 71:417–40.

Yates, J.C., and Dhalla, N.S., 1975, Structural and functional changes associated with failure and recovery of hearts after perfusion with Ca^{2+}-free medium, J. Mol. Cell. Cardiol., 7:91–104.

Zimmerman, A.N.E., and Hulsmann, W.G., 1966, Paradoxical influence of calcium ions on the permeability of the cell pembranes of the isolated rat heart, <u>Nature.</u>, 211:646-647.

SODIUM-CALCIUM EXCHANGE: CALCIUM REGULATION AT THE SARCOLEMMA

Kenneth D. Philipson and Malcolm M. Bersohn

Departments of Medicine and Physiology
Cardiovascular Research Laboratories
UCLA School of Medicine
Center for the Health Sciences
Los Angeles, California

INTRODUCTION

Regulation of intracellular Ca is of paramount importance in maintaining the contractile, electrophysiological, and metabolic integrity of the myocardium. Myocardial cells regulate cytoplasmic Ca by multiple transport pathways in the sarcolemma and intracellular organelles. The sarcolemma can transport Ca by Na-Ca exchange, an ATP-dependent Ca pump, and a voltage-sensitive Ca channel. In addition, the sarcoplasmic reticulum and the mitochondria both possess Ca uptake and release mechanisms. Because of this complexity, it is often difficult to unequivocably assign to a specific transport pathway a Na or Ca flux or a current measured in intact tissue. In myocardial tissue, Na-Ca exchange is usually studied by introducing large interventions such as altering the external Na or Ca concentration. One must assume that these interventions have no effect on other Na or Ca transport mechanisms. In addition, as internal Na and Ca concentrations adjust in response to the change in the extracellular milieu, cellular metabolic and electrophysiologic properties may change. Thus there is often uncertainty in identifying and quantitating Na-Ca exchange in myocardial tissue.

Recently, reliable techniques have been developed for measuring Na-Ca exchange in isolated cardiac sarcolemmal vesicles (Reeves and Sutko, 1979). Briefly, Na-loaded vesicles are rapidly diluted into a Na-free, isosmotic medium containing ^{45}Ca. Under these conditions, a rapid exchange of internal Na for external Ca occurs. The uptake of Ca is strictly dependent on internal Na and occurs only with intact sarcolemmal vesicles. Initial rates of Na_i-dependent Ca uptake can be as high as 20-30 nmol Ca/mg protein/s. This is comparable with the highest rates of Ca transport reported for cardiac sarcoplasmic reticulum. The exchange process is reversible; Ca efflux can be readily stimulated by elevating the extravesicular Na concentration. Techniques for the measurement of vesicular Na-Ca exchange are detailed by Philipson (1984).

Some of the recent results from our laboratory on the Na-Ca exchange of cardiac sarcolemmal vesicles have physiologic and pathophysiologic significance. These particular findings will be briefly reviewed here. Effects of membrane potential, pH, ischemia, and membrane environment on Na-Ca exchange will be discussed. A more general review on the properties of Na-Ca exchange in plasma membrane vesicles is available (Philipson, 1985). Langer (1982) and Reuter (1982) have written reviews on myocardial Na-Ca exchange which emphasize experiments performed with intact myocardium.

ELECTROGENICITY

One area which has been addressed very successfully using sarcolemmal vesicles is the electrogenicity of Na-Ca exchange. If Na-Ca exchange is the countertransport of 3 or more Na ions for each Ca ion, then each transport cycle involves the net movement of charge. Specifically, vesicular Na_i-dependent Ca uptake will be accompanied by a net outward movement of positive charge. An inside negative membrane potential will develop, which will inhibit further outward charge movement, and Na-Ca exchange will be inhibited. That this is indeed the case is clearly demonstrated by experiments which relieve inhibition through the use of valinomycin-generated, K-diffusion potentials (Philipson and Nishimoto, 1980). By varying the [K] in the presence of valinomycin the voltage can be "clamped" at positive values, and Na_i-dependent Ca uptake can be stimulated by 50-100%. The enhanced Ca uptake is due to stimulation of voltage-sensitive Na-Ca exchange and is not secondary to effects of membrane potential on other sarcolemmal transport activities. The electrogenicity of sarcolemmal Na-Ca exchange has also been demonstrated in other laboratories with different techniques (Reeves and Sutko, 1980; Caroni et al., 1980). An electrogenic Na-Ca exchange has obvious physiological significance (Mullins, 1979). During the depolarization phase of the cardiac action potential, calcium influx via Na-Ca exchange will be accelerated. This Ca could contribute to the Ca-activated contractile response. With repolarization, the Na-Ca exchange mechanism will favor Ca efflux and muscle relaxation will occur. The exact role of Na-Ca exchange in the excitation-contraction process will depend on intra- and extracellular ion activities, change vis-a-vis other cellular Ca transport pathways.

pH SENSITIVITY

The Na-Ca exchange of cardiac sarcolemmal vesicles is very dependent on pH (Philipson et al., 1982). The dependence of the initial rate of Na_i-dependent Ca uptake on pH is sigmoidal. At pH 6.7, Na-Ca exchange is markedly inhibited, and at pH 8.0, exchange is significantly enhanced compared to pH 7.4. The protons apparently compete with Ca for binding sites on the exchange protein. That is, the effects of pH on Na-Ca exchange are much more noticeable at low Ca levels than at high Ca levels. This is demonstrated in Table 1.

Table 1. Effect of pH on Na_i-dependent Ca-Uptake in Cardiac Sarcolemmal Vesicles

[Ca] (mM)	pH	Na-Ca Exchange (nmol/mg/s)	Inhibition
0.005	7.4	4.4 ± 0.7	
	6.7	1.7 ± 0.3	61%
1.0	7.4	25.9 ± 1.8	
	6.7	25.3 ± 3.1	2%

Thus, in the intact myocardium, a change in extracellular pH would have little effect on Na-Ca exchange due to the high external Ca concentration. In contrast, a fall in intracellular pH could drastically inhibit Na-Ca exchange due to the effective competition of increased proton activity with the low intracellular Ca activity. Since it is a fall in intracellular pH which appears to account for the negative inotropic response to acidosis, the results are consistent with a role for Na-Ca exchange in this response. Changes in pH, of course, have multiple cellular effects. Nevertheless, Na-Ca exchange should be considered in the interpretation of the effects of pH on myocardial Ca transport.

ISCHEMIA

Many of the detrimental effects of myocardial ischemia may be secondary to altered Ca metabolism. We therefore examined what effects ischemia had on sarcolemmal Na-Ca exchange (Bersohn et al., 1982). Sarcolemmal vesicles were isolated from control rabbit hearts and from rabbit hearts subjected to 1 hr global ischemia. Na-Ca exchange is inhibited by 50% after the ischemic insult due to a decrease in V_{max} while K_m for Ca ($\sim$ 35 μM) remains unchanged. The inhibition is not due to differential purification of sarcolemma after ischemia, nor is it due to an increased Ca permeability.

The ischemia-induced inhibition of Na-Ca exchange could possibly be due to the activation of proteinases during ischemia. However, we find that if vesicles are treated with a variety of different proteinases, Na-Ca exchange is actually markedly stimulated (up to 200% above control levels) (Philipson and Nishimoto, 1982). Harsh proteolysis is necessary before inhibition of sarcolemmal Na-Ca exchange occurs. The mechanism whereby proteinase treatment stimulates Na-Ca exchange is unknown. We tentatively conclude that proteolysis is not responsible for the inhibition of Na-Ca exchange which occurs during ischemia.

Another possibility to account for the altered ion transport during ischemia is the accumulation of lysophosphatidylcholine (LPC) and other amphiphiles (Corr et al., 1982). We find that 30 μM LPC, added exogenously to the sarcolemmal vesicles, inhibits Na-Ca exchange by 50% (Bersohn and Philipson, 1983). However, LPC also causes a substantial increase in the passive permeability of the vesicles to Ca, i.e. the vesicles become leaky. This contrasts strikingly with ischemia which caused no detectable increase in the passive permeability of the isolated sarcolemmal vesicles. Thus, although build up of lysophospholipids may be important in the pathology of ischemia, LPC does not mimic the effects of ischemia on sarcolemma isolated from ischemic tissues. This implies that other still unknown factors are important in the response to ischemia.

As discussed in the previous section, intracellular pH declines during ischemia. This factor by itself will decrease Na-Ca exchange activity. Functionally, the declining pH will exacerbate the ischemia-induced inhibition of Na-Ca exchange activity. Thus, during ischemia, Na-Ca exchange will be inhibited by the changing environment (declining pH) and by alterations which remain detectable after sarcolemmal isolation. This combination of inhibiting factors may have drastic consequences in vivo.

INTERACTION WITH PHOSPHOLIPIDS

Based on experiments with phospholipases (Philipson et al., 1983; Philipson and Nishimoto, 1984), we have advanced the hypothesis that Na-Ca exchange could be stimulated by negatively charged phospholipids. The most direct evidence to support this

560

hypothesis comes from experiments using phospholipase D. When phospholipase D has converted about 10% of sarcolemmal phospholipids to phosphatidic acid, Na-Ca exchange is stimulated by about 300%. Langer and Nudd (1983) observe an increase in sarcolemmal-bound Ca after phospholipase D treatment. Possibly, the increase in sarcolemmal-bound Ca is related to the stimulation of Na-Ca exchange.

The stimulation of Na-Ca exchange by phosphatidic acid may be important in the "phosphatidylinositol response." In this phenomenon, increased turnover of plasma membrane phosphatidylinositol has been associated with a large number of stimulus-response coupling mechanisms in a wide variety of tissues (Berridge, 1981). A prevalent model has been that the phosphatidylinositol is metabolized to phosphatidic acid. The phosphatidic acid then acts as a Ca ionophore, Ca influx occurs, and the appropriate response is elicited. This model has not been verified. The striking stimulation of Na-Ca exchange after phospholipase D treatment provides direct evidence for an effect of phosphatidic acid on a well defined Ca transport pathway. This effect may be an important part of the "phosphatidylinositol response."

CONCLUSION

In vitro studies have contributed greatly to an understanding of the various myocardial Ca transport mechanisms. What is now needed are experiments which differentiate the relative physiologic roles of the different Ca pathways. It is probable that Na-Ca exchange is prominent in myocardial Ca regulation, but an exact role needs to be resolved.

ACKNOWLEDGMENT

This research was supported by the USPHS (R01-HL27821), the AHA, Greater Los Angeles Affiliate, and the Castera Foundation. KDP is an Established Investigator of the American Heart Association.

REFERENCES

Berridge, M.J., 1981, Phosphatidylinositol hydrolysis: a multifunctional transducing mechanism, Mol. Cell. Endocrinol., 24:115.
Bersohn, M.M., and Philipson, K.D., 1983, Lysophosphoglycerides and sodium-calcium exchange in cardiac sarcolemma, Circulation (Suppl. II), 68:III-167 (Abstract).

Bersohn, M.M., Philipson, K.D., and Fukushima, J.Y., 1982, Sodium-calcium exchange and sarcolemmal enzymes in ischemic rabbit hearts, Am. J. Physiol., 242:C288.

Caroni, P., Reinlib, L., and Carafoli, E., 1980, Charge movements during the Na^+-Ca^{2+} exchange in heart sarcolemmal vesicles, Proc. Natl. Acad. Sci. USA. 77:6354.

Corr, P.B., Gross, R.W., and Sobel, B.E., 1982, Arrhythmogenic amphiphilic lipids and the myocardial cell membrane, J. Molec. Cell. Cardiol., 14:619.

Langer, G.A., 1982, Sodium-calcium exchange in the heart, Ann. Rev. Physiol., 44:435.

Langer, G.A., and Nudd, L.M., 1983, Effects of cations, phospholipases, and neuraminidase on calcium binding to "gas-dissected" membranes from cultured cardiac cells, Circ. Res., 53:482.

Mullins, L.J., 1979, The generation of electric currents in cardiac fibers by Na/Ca exchange, Am. J. Physiol., 236:C103.

Philipson, K.D., 1984, Methods for measuring sodium-calcium exchange in cardiac sarcolemmal vesicles, in: "Methods in Studying Cardiac Membranes, Vol. 1," N. Dhalla, ed., CRC, Boca Raton, FL.

Philipson, K.D., 1985, Sodium-calcium exchange in plasma membrane vesicles, Ann. Rev. Physiol., in press.

Philipson, K.D., Bersohn, M.M., and Nishimoto, A.Y., 1982, Effects of pH on Na^+-Ca^{2+} exchange in canine cardiac sarcolemmal vesicles, Circ. Res., 50:287.

Philipson, K.D., Frank, J.S., and Nishimoto, A.Y., 1983, Effects of phospholipase C on the Na^+-Ca^{2+} and Ca^{2+} permeability of cardiac sarcolemmal vesicles, J. Biol. Chem., 258:5905.

Philipson, K.D., and Nishimoto, A.Y., 1980, Na^+-Ca^{2+} exchange as affected by membrane potential in cardiac sarcolemmal vesicles, J. Biol. Chem., 255:6880.

Philipson, K.D., and Nishimoto, A.Y., 1982, Stimulation of Na^+-Ca^{2+} exchange in cardiac sarcolemmal vesicles by proteinase treatment, Am. J. Physiol., 243:C191.

Philipson, K.D., and Nishimoto, A.Y., 1984, Stimulation of Na^+-Ca^{2+} exchange in cardiac sarcolemmal vesicles by phospholipase D, J. Biol. Chem., 259:16.

Reeves, J.P., and Sutko, J.L., 1979, Sodium-calcium ion exchange in cardiac membrane vesicles, Proc. Natl. Acad. Sci. USA, 76:590.

Reeves, J.P., and Sutko, J.L., 1980, Sodium-calcium exchange activity generates a current in cardiac membrane vesicles, Science, 208:1461.

Reuter, H., 1982, Na-Ca countertransport in cardiac muscle, in: "Membranes and Transport, Vol. 1," A.N. Martonosi, ed., Plenum, New York.

THE CALCIUM PUMPING ATPase

OF HEART PLASMA MEMBRANE

Ernesto Carafoli and
Pico Caroni

Lab. of Biochemistry
Swiss Federal Institute
of Technology (ETH)
8092 Zurich, Switz.

INTRODUCTION

At each beat, Ca^{2+} penetrates into heart cells through a gated channel. According to the prevailing theory, this promotes the release of a much larger amount of Ca^{2+} from sarcoplasmic reticulum to activate contraction. It is immediately evident that the trigger Ca^{2+} that has entered the cell must be reexported to prevent cellular Ca^{2+} overload. Since Ca^{2+} in the cytosol of heart cells is μM or less, whereas in the extracellular spaces it is mM, re-export evidently requires active transport. Two systems are responsible for it, a Na^{+}/Ca^{2+} exchanger and a specific ATPase: they work in parallel, but have different kinetic properties, which qualify them for different roles. The ATPase has high Ca^{2+} affinity but low pumping rate, and can thus be considered as the fine tuner of cell Ca^{2+}, which functions in heart in the same way as in all other cells where it has been demonstrated. The Na^{+}/Ca^{2+} exchanger has lower Ca^{2+} affinity but high transport rate, and may thus be assumed to function at peak activation, when large amounts of Ca^{2+} must be ejected, but high affinity is not necessarily required due to the presumably increased concentration of Ca^{2+} at the inner side of the sarcolemma.

The Ca^{2+} pumping ATPase of heart sarcolemma has been documented conclusively only recently (Caroni and Carafoli, 1980) but has already been the subject of a number of studies that have considerably advanced knowledge on its structure and function. In this article, a survey of the properties of the ATPase will be presented, with special attention to the enzyme in the purified state.

GENERAL PROPERTIES OF THE CALCIUM PUMPING ATPase IN HEART SARCOLEMMA

An experiment published by Caroni and Carafoli in 1980 demonstrated conclusively the existence of an ATP-dependent Ca^{2+} pump in heart sarcolemma. The point is of importance, since until recently it was assumed that excitable cells like heart ejected Ca^{2+} through the well known Na^{+}/Ca^{2+} exchanger only, and not through a specific ATPase. The latter was considered typical of non-excitable cells, of which erythrocytes were the classical example. Caroni and Carafoli (1980) (Figure 1) documented the existence of an ATP-dependent Ca^{2+} pumping system in a preparation of dog heart sarcolemma. Per se, the observation was not striking, since it can be expected that heart sarcolemmal preparations are contaminated by sarcoplasmic reticulum vesicles, which are known to contain a Ca^{2+}-pumping ATPase.

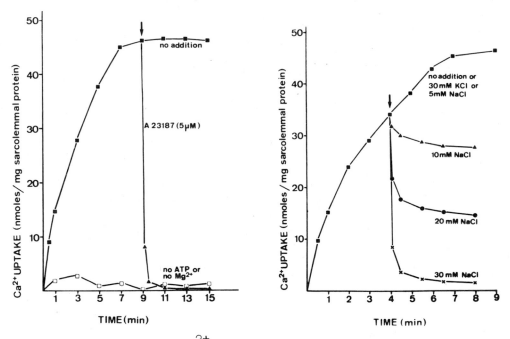

Fig. 1.   ATP-dependent Ca^{2+} accumulation in dog heart sarcolemmal vesicles, and discharge of the accumulated Ca^{2+} by Na^{+}. The Figure is taken from Caroni and Carafoli (1980), where a detailed description of the experiment is given. Sarcolemma vesicles were exposed to 75 μM $^{45}Ca^{2+}$ and 1 mM ATP. Ca^{2+} was accumulated in the vesicular space, since it was discharged by the specific Ca^{2+} ionophore A23187 (left panel). Addition of increasing amounts of Na^{+} during the Ca^{2+} uptake process reversed it partially or completely depending on the amount of Na^{+}. Ca^{2+} uptake was measured by Millipore filtration.

The novelty of the observation was in the fact that the accumulated Ca^{2+} could be specifically discharged by the addition of Na^+, implying that the ATP-dependent system had pumped Ca^{2+} into vesicles which also contained Na^+/Ca^{2+} exchange activity: i.e., into sarcolemmal vesicles.

The properties of the ATP-dependent pump were then investigated in detail (Caroni and Carafoli, 1981a), and it became soon clear that the enzyme was a classical ATPase of the E_1E_2 type, inhibitable by low concentrations of vanadate and having high affinity for Ca^{2+} (K_m, < 1 µM). However, the matter of the affinity for Ca^{2+} turned out to be a complex matter, since it could be shown that the ATPase, in agreement with studies carried out at about the same time on the Ca^{2+}-ATPase of erythrocytes, was sensitive to calmodulin (Figure 2)

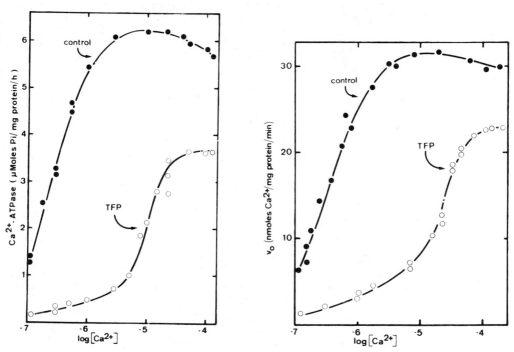

Fig. 2. Effect of trifluoperazine on the Ca^{2+}-ATPase and ATP-dependent Ca^{2+} transport in dog heart sarcolemmal vesicles. A detailed description of the experiment is given in Caroni and Carafoli (1981a), from which the Figure has been modified. The free Ca^{2+} concentrations shown on the abscissa were obtained by EGTA buffering. The ATPase activity (left panel) was measured with a coupled enzyme assay, the uptake of Ca^{2+} (right panel) isotopically, using $^{45}Ca^{2+}$ and a millipore filtration system. The initial velocity of the uptake process was determined from a series of samplings made at 15 sec intervals. ATP concentration, 1 mM, trifluoperazine (TFP) concentration 30 µM.

The latter shifted the enzyme from a state of low Ca^{2+} affinity (K_m, about 20 μM) to a state of high Ca^{2+} affinity (K_m, about 0.5 μM). At variance with erythrocytes, where a simple wash with EDTA-containing solutions suffices to remove the calmodulin bound to the ATPase, in the case of heart sarcolemma harsher extraction procedures had to be used before effects of added calmodulin on the Ca^{2+}-ATPase (and on the associated Ca^{2+} transport) could be observed. Therefore, it was found convenient to use anticalmodulin drugs, rather than calmodulin extraction procedures, to demonstrate the calmodulin sensitivity of the process. The demonstration of the existence of a high affinity Ca^{2+} pumping system in heart sarcolemma was of particular interest in view of the finding that the Na^+/Ca^{2+} exchanger has a very low Ca^{2+} affinity (Reeves and Sutko, 1979), and cannot thus be expected to operate under "resting" conditions, when cytosolic Ca^{2+} presumably falls below 1 μM. The presumed respective roles of the 2 Ca^{2+} transporting systems have been discussed in the Introduction section.

REGULATION OF THE CALCIUM PUMPING ATPase of HEART SARCOLEMMA BY PHOSPHORYLATION/DEPHOSPHORYLATION

Caroni and Carafoli (1981b) found that the ATP-dependent Ca^{2+}-pumping system of dog heart sarcolemma was influenced by phosphorylation. Since normally prepared heart sarcolemma vesicles are phosphorylated to a high degree, the demonstration of the effect of phosphorylation on the ATP-dependent Ca^{2+} pumping required previous dephosphorylation of the vesicles by an exogenous phosphatase (Figure 3). The incorporation of hydrohylamine-resistant ^{32}P-phosphate from γ ^{32}P-ATP was inhibited by an inhibitor of cAMP dependent protein kinase, and so was the stimulation of the Ca^{2+} pumping by pretreatment of dephosphorylated vesicles with ATP (not shown in the Figure). However, the inhibition was not complete, suggesting that another kinase, not depending on cAMP, was also involved in the reactivation process. That this second kinase might be of the Ca^{2+}-calmodulin type was indicated by the observation (Caroni and Carafoli, 1981b) that the addition of EGTA during the preincubation with ATP prevented the full reactivation of the Ca^{2+}-pumping reaction. It was demonstrated conclusively by Vetter et al. (1982), who found that the preincubation of sarcolemmal vesicles with calmodulin and the catalytic subunit of the protein kinase cAMP-dependent produced additive stimulations of the ATP-dependent Ca^{2+} uptake. The vesicles used by Vetter et al. (1982) contained relatively little endogenous cAMP-dependent kinase, and higher amounts of the calmodulin-dependent kinase. One problem, here, is the nature of the immediate target of the 2 phosphorylation systems, which work by Caroni et al. (1983) has shown not to be the Ca^{2+}-pumping ATPase proper. Lamers et al. (1981) have obtained evidence that it might be a protein of 9 KDa, which originates from the dissociation (induced by boiling) of a 24 KDa component. The situation appears to be similar to that of heart sarcoplasmic reticulum, where 2 protein

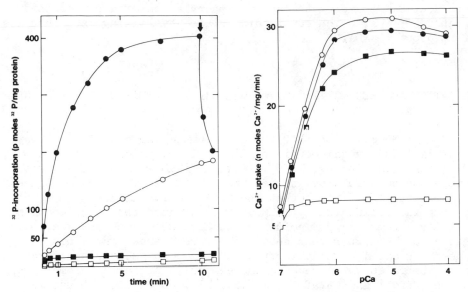

Fig. 3. Phosphorylation-dephosphorylation of heart sarcolemmal vesicles; effects on the ATP-dependent uptake of Ca^{2+}. Experimental conditions are described in detail in Caroni and
Carafoli (1981b), from which the Figure has been modified.
Left panel, incorporation of hydroxylamine-resistant ^{32}P -
phosphate from ATP into sarcolemmal vesicles. γ ^{32}P- ATP
was 40 µM, free Ca^{2+} 5 µM (buffered with EGTA), cAMP 5 µM,
$MgCl_2$ 20 µM, phosphorylase phosphatase, 2 µg, protein kinase
inhibitor, cAMP-dependent 20 µg. Reaction volume 150 µl.
The vesicles were incubated 5 min with the above reagents
as indicated in the Figure, 10 additional min with 0.6 M
hydroxylamine in Na OH, and then filtered through Millipore
filters for radioactivity counting ■ = controls. □, protein
kinase inhibitor. ● vesicles treated with phosphorylase phosphatase and Mg^{2+}. The same reagents added at the arrow.
○, phosphatase-treated vesicles plus protein kinase inhibitor. Right panel, ATP-dependent Ca^{2+} uptake. Vesicles
preincubated 10 min in a medium to which 1 mM ATP and 1 mM
$MgCl_2$ were added at the times indicated in the Figure. After
the preincubation, ^{45}Ca-EGTA were added to obtain the free
Ca^{2+} concentrations indicated. Aliquots were removed and
filtered at 10 sec intervals to obtain the initial rate of
uptake. ●,■ , ATP-Mg^{2+} added 10 min before Ca^{2+}. ○,□ , ATP-
Mg^{2+} added 5 sec before Ca^{2+}. ●,○, control vesicles. ■ □,
dephosphorylated vesicles (vesicles treated with phosphorylase phosphatase, washed and resuspended.

kinases, one cAMP, one calmodulin-dependent also stimulate the ATP-dependent Ca^{2+} pumping through phosphorylation of a proteolipid of M_r about 25 KDa, which can be dissociated by boiling into subunits of M_r about 11 KDa.

ISOLATION AND RECONSTITUTION OF THE CALCIUM PUMPING ATPase OF HEART SARCOLEMMA

The demonstration that the Ca^{2+} pumping ATPase of erythrocytes was stimulated by calmodulin by direct interaction (Niggli et al., 1979; Lynch and Cheung, 1979) provided Niggli et al. (1979) with a simple and powerful tool to isolate the ATPase from the membrane environment. The finding that the Ca^{2+} pumping ATPase of heart sarcolemma was stimulated by calmodulin indicated that a calmodulin affinity chromatography column might have been successful also in this case. The experiment shown in Figure 4 shows that this was indeed the case. Calmodulin-free, detergent dissolved heart sarcolemma membranes were loaded on a calmodulin affinity-chromatography column (Caroni and Carafoli, 1981a). Elution of the unbound material with Ca^{2+} liberated from the column more than 99% of the applied protein, and a very considerable amount of ATPase activity (top panel of the Figure). The latter, however, was not Ca^{2+}-dependent. Elution with EGTA following the Ca^{2+} wash produced a very small amount of protein, having very high Ca^{2+}-dependent ATPase activity. SDS-polyacrylamide gel electrophoresis of the EGTA-eluted peak showed an essentially homogeneous protein having M_r of about 140 KDa (middle and lower panel of Figure 4), which formed an acyl-phosphate intermediate upon incubation with Ca^{2+} and ATP. These properties are very similar to those of the Ca^{2+}-pumping ATPase isolated from erythrocytes (Niggli et al., 1979), with which, indeed, the isolated heart enzyme was found to cross-react immunologically (Caroni et al., 1983). By contrast, immunological cross-reactivity experiments have ruled out similarities with the Ca^{2+}-pumping ATPase of heart sarcoplasmic reticulum. The isolated heart sarcolemma enzyme was found to be shifted to the high Ca^{2+} affinity state by calmodulin (Figure 5, bottom panel) as in the case of the erythrocyte enzyme. Also in agreement with findings made on the erythrocyte ATPase (Niggli et al., 1981) transition to the high Ca^{2+}-affinity state could be induced in the absence of calmodulin by acidic phospholipids and by a limited proteolytic treatment with trypsin (Figure 5, a and b). The pattern of trypsin proteolysis was essentially similar to that of the purified erythrocyte enzyme, which has now been studied in considerable detail (Zurini et al., 1984). It has also been possible to reconstitute the Ca^{2+}-pumping activity in liposomal vesicles, and to observe that the reconstituted heart sarcolemmal ATPase transported Ca^{2+} with a stoichiometry of 1 with respect to the hydrolyzed ATP (Caroni et al., 1983).

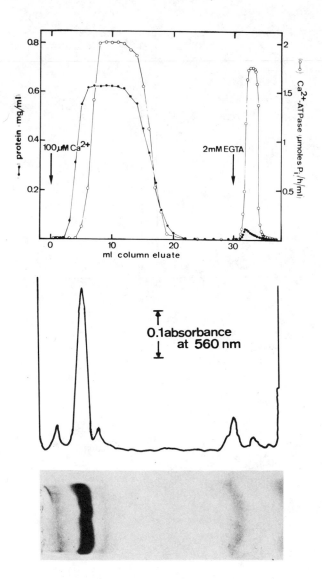

Fig. 4. Purification of the Ca^{2+}-pumping ATPase of heart sarcolemma on a calmodulin affinity chromatography column. Full
details are given in Caroni and Carafoli (1981a), from
which the Figure has been modified. Top panel, elution
profile of the sarcolemmal components from the calmodulin
affinity chromatography column (the membranes were dissolved with Triton X-100, and the column was equilibrated with
Triton X-100 and phosphatidyl-serine). The ATPase activity
was measured with a coupled enzyme assay. Mid panel, a
densitrometric trace of the SDS polyacrylamide gel electrophoresis of the EGTA-eluted protein (bottom panel).

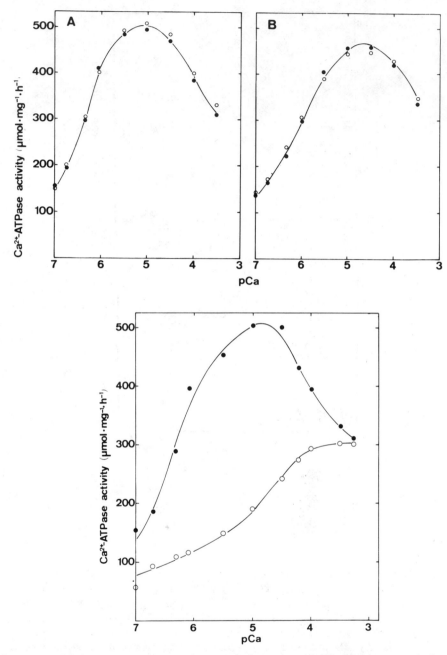

Fig. 5. Effect of calmodulin, acidic phospholipids, and limited proteolysis on the affinity of the purified heart sarcolemmal Ca^{2+}-ATPase for Ca^{2+}. Complete experimental details are given in Caroni et al. (1983), from which the Figure has been modified. The Triton X-100 enzyme was prepared

in the presence of phosphatidylcholine. The free Ca^{2+} concentrations shown on the abscissae have been obtained by EGTA buffering. The ATPase activity was measured with a coupled enzyme assay. A, ● control (2.5 μg calmodulin per 0.7 μg ATPase),o, no calmodulin, 50 μg phosphatidyl-serine per 0.7 μg ATPase. B,●= calmodulin-ATPase as in A. o, 0.8 μg ATPase trypsinized for 5 min at 0°. Lower panel, ● , 2 μg calmodulin, 0.7 μg enzyme per ml.o , no calmodu-lin.

CONCLUSIONS

The presence of a Ca^{2+} pumping ATPase in heart sarcolemma, different from the Ca^{2+} pump of sarcoplasmic reticulum, is now conclusively documented. The ATPase is similar (or identical) to the Ca^{2+} pump of erythrocytes, and will probably be shown in the future to share properties with Ca^{2+} pumping ATPases of other plas-ma membranes. It interacts with Ca^{2+} with very high affinity, but pumps it at a relatively low rate: these properties qualify the enzyme for functioning continuously during the heart activity cycle. It most likely is the only system active in extruding Ca^{2+} during the diastolic period, whereas immediately after peak activation it will be powerfully supplemented by the higher capacity Na^+/Ca^{2+} exchanger.

REFERENCES

Caroni, P., and Carafoli, E., 1980, An ATP-dependent calcium pumping system in dog heart sarcolemma, Nature, 283:765.

Caroni, P., and Carafoli, E., 1981a, The Ca^{2+}-pumping ATPase of heart sarcolemma, J. Biol. Chem., 256:3263.

Caroni, P., and Carafoli, E., 1981b, Regulation of Ca^{2+}-pumping ATPase of heart sarcolemma by a phosphorylation-dephosphorylation process, J. Biol. Chem., 256:9371

Caroni,P., Zurini, M., Clark, A., and Carafoli, E., 1983, Further characterization and reconstitution of the purified Ca^{2+}-pumping ATPase of heart sarcolemma, J. Biol. Chem.,258:7305.

Lamers, J.M.J., and Stinis, J.T., 1983, Inhibition of Ca^{2+}-dependent protein kinase and Ca^{2+}/Mg^{2+}-ATPase in cardiac sarcolemma by the anti-calmodulin drug calmidazolium, Cell Calcium, 4:281.

Lynch, Th.J., and Cheung, W.J., 1979, Human erythrocyte Ca^{2+}-Mg^{2+}-ATPase: mechanism of stimulation by Ca^{2+}, Arch. Biochem. Biophys.,194:165.

Niggli, V., Penniston, J.T., and Carafoli, E., 1979, Purification of the $(Ca^{2+} + Mg^{2+})$-ATPase from human erythrocyte membrane using a calmodulin affinity column, J. Biol. Chem., 254:9955.

Niggli, V., Adunyah, E.S., and Carafoli, E., 1981, Acidic phospholipids, unsaturated fatty acids, and limited proteolysis mimic the effect of calmodulin on the purified erythrocyte Ca^{2+}-ATPase, J. Biol. Chem., 256:8588.

Reeves, J.P., and Sutko, J.L., 1979, Sodium-calcium exchange in cardiac membrane vesicles, Proc. Nat. Acad. Sci., USA, 76:590.

Vetter, R., Haase, H., and Will, H., 1982, Potentiating effect of calmodulin and catalytic subunit of cyclic AMP-dependent protein kinase on ATP-dependent Ca^{2+} transport by cardiac sarcolemma, FEBS Letters, 148:326.

Zurini, M., Krebs, J., Penniston, J.T., and Carafoli, E., 1984, Controlled proteolysis of the purified Ca^{2+}-ATPase of the erythrocyte membrane. A correlation between the structure and the function of the enzyme. J. Biol. Chem., 259:618.

CALCIUM COMPARTMENTATION AND REGULATION IN MYOCYTES

John R. Williamson, Andrew P. Thomas, Rebecca J. Williams,
Janette Alexander, and Mary A. Selak

University of Pennsylvania
Dept. of Biochemistry and Biophysics
Philadelphia, Pennsylvania 19104 USA

SUMMARY

The cytosolic free Ca^{2+} concentration of isolated rat myocytes
that were resistant to addition of external Ca^{2+} (Ca^{2+}-tolerant) has
been measured by two independent methods, the null point titration
technique and by use of Quin 2 as an intracellular Ca^{2+} probe.
Values obtained for quiescent cells were in the range of 170 to
270 nM. Using Quin 2-Ca^{2+} fluorescence to monitor changes of cytosolic free Ca^{2+} ($[Ca^{2+}]_i$) in the presence of 0.65 mM external Ca^{2+},
separate additions of the Ca^{2+} ionophore ionomycin, the mitochondrial
uncoupling agent 1799 or the respiratory inhibitor KCN each caused
an increase of $[Ca^{2+}]_i$ of about 3-fold. The Quin 2 loaded myocytes
responded to electrical stimulation by a transient increase of
$[Ca^{2+}]_i$, which peaked about 75% above the resting level. The rise
of $[Ca^{2+}]_i$ was complete within 50 ms and declined gradually to the
resting level. The β-agonist isoproterenol caused up to a 100%
increase in the amplitude of the Quin 2-Ca^{2+} fluorescence change,
with a half maximal effect at 130 nM. The stimulation-induced
$[Ca^{2+}]_i$ transient was abolished by addition of 100 μM propanolol
after 10 μM isoproterenol.

The distribution of calcium within the myocyte was measured by
addition of the mitochondrial uncoupling agent FCCP to release mitochondrial calcium followed by the Ca^{2+} ionophore A23187 to release
calcium from other vesicular pools, using arsenazo III as an extracellular Ca^{2+} indicator. Over the range of total releasable cell
calcium from 0.5 to 4.5 nmol/mg cell dry weight, the ratio of the
distribution of mitochondrial to sarcoplasmic reticulum was approximately constant at 1:2. The role of mitochondria in regulating and

573

buffering cytosolic free Ca^{2+} and possible regulation of mitochondrial Ca^{2+}-dependent dehydrogenases by the intramitochondrial free Ca^{2+} during the cardiac contraction cycle is discussed.

INTRODUCTION

A number of different techniques are in principle available for measurement of cytosolic free Ca^{2+} concentrations (for reviews see 1, 2). These fall into the following categories: bioluminescent indicators, of which aequorin has been most widely used; metallochromic indicators such as arsenazo III and antipyrylazo III; fluorescent indicators, notably Quin 2, and Ca^{2+}-selective microelectrodes. Each has advantages and disadvantages for specific applications and have different systematic errors and problems. With all of them, calibration of the signal in terms of the absolute free Ca^{2+} concentration in the cytosol is difficult, but relative changes of the intracellular free Ca^{2+} can be measured more reliably. The techniques most amenable to calibration are Quin 2, Ca^{2+}-selective microelectrodes, and arsenazo III when used for null point tirations after permeabilizing the cell with digitonin or saponin. However, the latter two techniques are unsuitable for following rapid changes of the cytosolic free Ca^{2+} because of the relatively slow response time of Ca^{2+} electrodes at submicromolar Ca^{2+} concentrations, while the null point titration is essentially a static technique. Aequorin has been used extensively to follow Ca^{2+} transients in excitable cells such as muscle and nerve (1). Its use with isolated cardiac muscle preparations such as papillary muscle, Purkinje fibers or atrial trabeculae requires micro-injection into multiple superficial cells and averaging of up to several hundred successive signals during repetitive stimulation for acceptable signal to noise ratios. Aequorin responds to increases or decreases of Ca^{2+} with a response time in the order of 10 ms, but suffers from the nonlinearity of the light emissions with Ca^{2+} concentration, which increases in proportion to the power of Ca^{2+} up to factors of 2.5. This means that if differences of free Ca^{2+} distribution exist within the cell, the aequorin signal will be dominated by contributions from those regions with highest free Ca^{2+} so that a given amount of Ca^{2+} in the cell will give a brighter signal when its distribution is uneven than when it is uniformly distributed. However, it still remains to be established whether extreme intracellular free Ca^{2+} heterogeneities really do occur, even during the rapid Ca^{2+} transients associated with excitation-contraction coupling. A further problem with aequorin is that since the Ca^{2+} concentration-light emission curve flattens out at Ca^{2+} concentrations in the region of 0.2 μM, it is a very insensitive indicator at resting cytosolic free Ca^{2+} concentrations.

On the other hand, Quin 2 (3, 4) is an excellent Ca^{2+} indicator in the region of 0.1 to 0.5 μM free Ca^{2+} since its Ca^{2+} dissociation constant (in the presence of 1 mM Mg^{2+}, pH 7.05, 37°C) is 115 nM (5).

It has a very low affinity for Mg^{2+} and H^+, a relatively high fluor-escence quantum yield of the Ca^{2+}-bound complex and little or no detectable binding to membranes. Quin 2 is a quinoline derivative with four free carboxyl groups that are involved in Ca^{2+} binding, with a 1:1 stoichiometry between Ca^{2+} and the molecule. A major advantage of the compound is that it can be made permeable to cells by converting the free carboxyl groups to acetoxymethyl esters (Quin 2/AM), which are subsequently hydrolysed by intracellular esterases present in most cells thereby producing the essential impermeable Quin 2 in the cell. It appears to be a true indicator of cytosolic free Ca^{2+} since it is apparently excluded from intracellular organelles (5). The rate constants for binding and unbinding of Ca^{2+} to Quin 2 have not yet been accurately measured, but they appear to be at least as fast as those for aequorin. Potential disadvantages with the use of Quin 2 as an indicator for rapid changes of the cytosolic free Ca^{2+} are its buffering effect, the nonlinearity of the Ca^{2+} concentration dependency above its K_d, and interference from changes of pyridine nucleotide fluorescence due to a large degree of overlap in their excitation and emission spectra. This latter problem can be partially overcome by a judicious selection of transmission wavelengths for the excitation and emission filters. In fact, simultaneous measurement of fluorescence changes attributable primarily to the Quin 2-Ca complex or to pyridine nucleotides, as in the fluorometer used in our studies (6), offers advantages for interpretation of changes of cell metabolism in relation to alterations of calcium homeostasis. However, an acceptable discrimination between Quin 2-Ca fluorescence and pyridine nucleotide fluorescence in the Quin 2 channel with a reasonable signal to noise ratio requires intracellular Quin 2 loadings of about 0.5 mM. The presence of Quin 2 in the cell at this concentration does buffer the intracellular calcium, as indicated by a net gain of cellular calcium equal to about half the Quin 2-loading (5, 7)[1] when the loading is performed in the presence of extracellular Ca^{2+}. Under these conditions, the basal level of cytosolic free Ca^{2+} in lymphocytes has been shown to be independent of the Quin 2 content up to 5 mM, also with no evidence of cellular toxicity (5). In contrast, when cells are loaded with Quin 2 in the absence of external Ca^{2+}, the cytosolic free Ca^{2+} falls to about 20 nM (5)[1]. The extent to which Ca^{2+} transients are blunted in Quin 2-loaded cells has not been fully evaluated, but from the results presented in this paper with electrically stimulated Quin 2-loaded myocytes, this effect does not appear to be as severe as has been conjectured (1). Nevertheless, the nonlinearity of the Quin 2-Ca fluorescence response due to saturation of the indicator with Ca^{2+} makes Quin 2 a very insensitive indicator of free Ca^{2+} changes above about 0.6 μM.

The purpose of the present paper is to report our preliminary

---

[1] J. R. Williamson, S. K. Joseph and K. E. Coll, unpublished observations.

studies on the use of Quin 2 to measure cytosolic free Ca^{2+} in isolated myocytes and the intracellular Ca^{2+} transients induced by electrical stimulation of the cells. In addition, we review data on the intracellular distribution of calcium in myocyte and reassess the role of mitochondrial Ca^{2+} cycling both as a buffering system for the cytosolic free Ca^{2+} and in the regulation of mitochondrial Ca^{2+}-dependent enzymes during normal cardiac contractions and after stimulation by inotropic interventions.

EXPERIMENTAL METHODS

Calcium tolerant heart cells, prepared as previously described (8), were incubated at 37°C in Hank's medium containing 0.65 mM Ca^{2+} and were equilibrated with 100% O_2. The cells (5-10 nmol/mg cell dry weight/ml) were loaded with Quin 2 by a 45 min incubation with Quin 2/AM (5-10 nmol/mg cell dry weight of the tetraacetoxymethyl ester) and subsequently washed twice with fresh Hank's medium to remove excess Quin 2 ester and free Quin 2. The intracellular concentration of Quin 2 was in the range of 0.5 to 1 mM, as determined by the use of [$G-^3H$] Quin 2-tetraacetoxymethyl ester. For measurements of the Quin 2 fluorescence, aliquots of the myocytes suspension were incubated at 37°C in a quartz cuvette at a concentration of 1 to 2 mg dry weight/ml (final vol. of 1.5 ml) in a modified Johnson Research Foundation Electronics Shop fluorometer. The cuvette was fitted with two platinum electrodes for field stimulation, one immediately above the stirrer but below the light path and one just above the light path, with the leads attached to a Grass Stimulator. Excitation light from a mercury source passed through a primary 335 nm interference filter, while fluorescent light passed to two photomultipliers each at 90° to the incident light. During experiments, the gain of the two photomultipliers was adjusted to be the same. Quin 2 fluorescence was selected by secondary filters with a band pass of 490-570 nm and pyridine nucleotide fluorescence was measured using 420-450 nm secondary filters (6). Currently, no electronic corrections are applied to the Quin 2 signal to account for the relatively small pyridine nucleotide spillover. Calibration of the Quin 2-Ca signal in terms of the cytosolic free Ca^{2+} concentration was made at the end of each run as follows (see Ref. 5). Addition of EGTA in tris base (pH 8.3) decreased the extracellular free Ca^{2+} to below 1 nM and records the extracellular Quin 2-Ca fluorescence due to leakage of Quin 2 from the cells. Subsequent addition of a detergent such as Triton X-100 releases Quin 2 from the cells where it is accessible to external Ca^{2+} calibration, but also causes an artifactual large fluorescence decrease due to a variety of factors including light scattering changes, dilution of NAD(P)H and different quenching of Quin 2-Ca^{2+} fluorescence between the intracellular and extracellular environments. Finally, excess Ca^{2+} was added to the detergent-treated cells to obtain F_{max} for the sum of the Quin 2-Ca fluorescence attributable to

Quin 2 that was extra cellular plus that released from the cells. This deflection was corrected by subtracting the deflection obtained after the initial EGTA addition. However, there is some ambiguity for calibration of the Quin 2–Ca^{2+} fluorescence changes in terms of absolute intracellular free Ca^{2+} concentrations due to the difficulty of determining the correct F_{min} after Triton addition. This deflection was biphasic, and the endpoint was taken as the point of inflexion. This method yielded values for the cytosolic free Ca^{2+} for control cells in the region from 150–200 nM.

Other methods are the same as those reported previously (8).

RESULTS

Cytosolic Free Ca^{2+} and Calcium Distribution in Quiescent Myocytes

Fig. 1 shows a null point titration (9) of cytosolic free Ca^{2+} concentration in heart cells obtained by plotting the net changes of medium Ca^{2+} upon addition of 10 µg of digitonin/mg of cell dry weight against the initial extracellular free Ca^{2+} concentration as measured with arsenazo III. The cytosolic free Ca^{2+} concentration is obtained by extrapolation to determine the extracellular free Ca^{2+} concentration at which no net Ca^{2+} flux occurs when the plasma membrane permeability barrier is removed. The particular experiments shown in Fig. 1 gave a value of 0.26 µM for the cytosolic free Ca^{2+} concentration. The mean ± SEM for determinations on 8 separate myocyte preparations was 0.27 ± 0.03 µM.

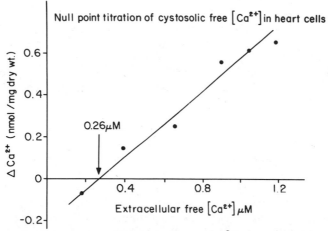

Fig. 1. Measurement of cytosolic free Ca^{2+} concentration in rat myocytes. Myocytes (1 mg dry weight/ml) were incubated at 37°C in modified Hank's medium, pH 7.4, containing 50 µM arsenazo III and 1 µM ruthenium red. The amount of calcium taken up or released from the cells upon addition of 10 µg of digitonin/mg of cell dry weight is plotted against the initial extracellular free Ca^{2+} concentration.

577

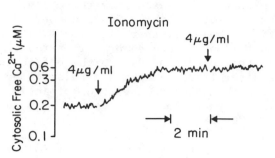

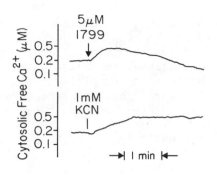

Fig. 2. Effect of ionomycin on the cytosolic free Ca^{2+} concentration of non-stimulated isolated myocytes incubated at 37°C in Hank's medium containing 0.65 mM Ca^{2+}.

Fig. 3. Effects of uncoupler (1799) and KCN on the cytosolic free Ca^{2+} concentration of non-stimulated isolated myocytes loaded with Quin 2.

Quin 2 is a much more convenient intracellular Ca^{2+} indicator, and Fig. 2 illustrates the effect of the Ca^{2+} ionophore ionomycin on Quin 2-Ca fluorescence changes of quiescent myocytes incubated in Hank's medium containing 0.65 mM Ca^{2+}. The ionophore caused a release of calcium from both the mitochondria and the sarcoplasmic reticulum, which resulted in an increase of the cytosolic free Ca^{2+} from 0.2 to 0.6 μM within 2 min. A second addition of ionophore produced no further deflection of the Quin 2-Ca trace, suggesting either that the intracellular Quin 2 was saturated with Ca^{2+} or that ionomycin was not affecting Ca^{2+} influx at the plasma membrane. Further experiments showed that the latter possibility was correct, since a further increase of the Quin 2-Ca fluorescence could be obtained if the extracellular Ca^{2+} concentration was increased to 30 mM.

Fig. 3 (top trace) shows the effect of the nonfluorescent mitochondrial uncoupling agent 1799 on the Quin 2-Ca fluorescence. In this case the increase of the cytosolic free Ca^{2+} to 0.5 μM was transient. Further studies are required to evaluate the meaning of this response. The lower trace of Fig. 3 shows that inhibition of the mitochondrial respiratory activity with KCN caused a stable increase of the cytosolic free Ca^{2+}, presumably as a consequence of collapse of the mitochondrial membrane potential and release of calcium from the mitochondrial pool.

When myocytes are incubated in Ca^{2+}-free medium in the presence of an extracellular Ca^{2+} indicator such as arsenazo III, the total amount of calcium released after addition of uncoupling agents or

Ca^{2+} ionophores can be quantitated. Fig. 4 shows a representative trace of the Ca-arsenazo absorbance changes following successive additions of the uncoupling agent FCCP and the Ca^{2+} ionophore A23187. Ruthenium red (RR) was added to the suspension of heart cells to inhibit further uptake of calcium into mitochondria of cells with leaky plasma membranes. This normally induced only a small Ca^{2+} release due to the activity of the mitochondrial Ca^{2+}/Na^{+} exchange carrier. Addition of FCCP caused a release of about 2 nmol of calcium, which can be attributed to the mitochondrial calcium pool (8, 10). Subsequent addition of A23187 caused a larger release of calcium from the remaining vesicular calcium pools, notably the sarcoplasmic reticulum.

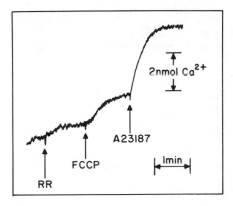

Fig. 4. Quantitation of FCCP-releasable and A23187-releasable calcium from suspensions of isolated rat myocytes. The cells (1 mg dry weight/ml) were incubated at 37°C in modified Hank's medium, pH 7.4, containing 50 μM arsenazo III. The concentrations of additions were: ruthenium red (RR), 1 μM; FCCP, 2 μM; A23187, 2 μM.

Fig. 5 shows the effect of varying the total content of calcium in the myocytes on the distribution of calcium within the cell. The cell calcium content was varied either by preincubating the cells in the absence of Ca^{2+} or with 1 mM Ca^{2+} for varying times up to 30 min. In all cases, ruthenium red was added prior to additions of FCCP and A23187, as in Fig. 4. Over the range of releasable calcium contents up to 4.5 nmol/mg of cell dry weight, the amount of calcium released was directly proportional to the cell calcium content, with the slope of the A23187-releasable calcium linear regression line being about twice that for the FCCP-releasable calcium. Unlike previous studies with hepatocytes (10), no evidence was obtained for saturation of the A23187-releasable calcium pool. At higher initial cell calcium contents, the myocytes readily lost accumulated calcium when incubated in Ca^{2+}-free medium, and stable Ca-arsenazo absorbance baselines could not be obtained. Consequently, on the assumption that sequential additions of FCCP and A23187 provide a valid monitor for the mitochondrial and sarcoplasmic reticular calcium pools, respectively, it may be concluded that mitochondria account for about one third of the total cell calcium. At physiological levels of total myocardial cell calcium (8), this corresponds to about 1.2 nmol/mg of cell dry weight. If a slightly higher estimate of 330 mg mitochondrial protein/g of heart, dry weight for the mitochondrial content of heart is used[2], compared with the previous estimate of 250 mg mitochondrial protein/g of heart, dry weight (8), the mitochondria in the intact heart cell are calculated to contain 3.6 nmol of calcium/mg protein. Using the value of 1.36 nmol/mg.μM for the ratio of total/free Ca^{2+} in heart mitochondria (11), the mitochondrial matrix free Ca^{2+} concentration is estimated to be in the region of 2.6 μM.

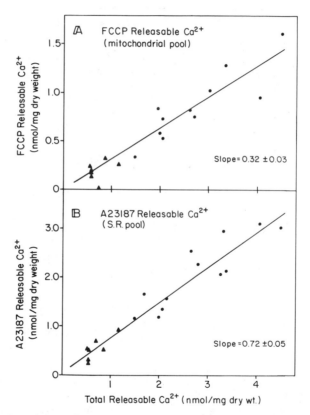

Fig. 5. Relationship of the FCCP-releasable and subsequent A23187-releasable Ca^{2+} to the total releasable Ca^{2+} of rat myocytes. The cells were preincubated either in the absence of Ca^{2+} (▲) or for various times up to 30 min in the presence of 1 mM Ca^{2+} (●). Subsequently the cells were washed with Ca^{2+}-free Hank's medium and the calcium pool sizes were determined as in Fig. 4.

---

[2] Personal communication, Ruth Altschuld

Cytosolic Free Ca^{2+} Transients in Electrically Stimulated Myocytes

Suspensions of isolated myocytes contract synchronously, independently of their orientation, when subjected to field stimulation via platinum electrodes. A supramaximum stimulating voltage of 70 volt and a duration of 1.5 ms was used routinely for the present experiments. The mechanical contraction, however, was attenuated in Quin 2-loaded cells. Fig. 6 shows that the Quin 2-Ca signal responded to electrical stimulation of the myocytes with a Ca^{2+} transient, showing a rapid upstroke and a slower downstroke in synchrony with the imposed stimulation. On the basis of the calibration method used, the cytosolic free Ca^{2+} increased from a resting level of 178 nM to a peak of 243 nM. Addition of a maximum concentration of the β-agonist isoproterenol (10 μM) caused an increase in the amplitude of the Quin 2-Ca signal to a maximum value within 6 beats, corresponding to a peak cytosolic free Ca^{2+} concentration of about 500 nM. Fig. 6B is a continuation of the trace in Fig. 6A and shows that the Quin 2-Ca transient kept pace with an increase of the beat frequency from 10 to 37 beats/min but with a decrease of maximum amplitude. Finally, addition of excess of the β-antagonist propanolol abolished the Quin 2-Ca transients despite continued stimulation. These data show, therefore, that the Quin 2-Ca transient is dependent on electrical stimulation and is responsive to both the stimulation frequency and to inotropic interventions.

The average amplitude of the Quin 2-Ca transient reached a constant value after the first few contractions with isoproterenol, and a dose-response curve for the increase of the amplitude of the Quin 2-Ca signal with isoproterenol is shown in Fig. 7. A half maximal effect was obtained with 130 nM isoproterenol, which is within the range observed with this agonist for half maximal increases of contractile activity and phosphorylase activity in various isolated heart preparations (12–15).

The random noise in the traces shown in Fig. 6 was considerably reduced by connecting the fluorometer output to a storage oscilloscope or a Gould Brush 260 recorder. Representative traces of the Quin 2-Ca fluorescence and pyridine nucleotide fluorescence using the Brush recorder are shown in Fig. 8, using a stimulation frequency of 1 per sec and an overall time constant of about 10 msec. Addition of 0.1 μM isoproterenol increased the peak cytosolic free Ca^{2+} by 43% (*c.f.* Fig. 6). The rate of the increase of the Ca^{2+} transient appeared to remain constant (approximately 35 ms), but the rate of fall of the cytosolic free Ca^{2+} from its peak value was clearly increased by isoproterenol. The reproducibility of the contraction-induced Ca^{2+} transient is shown at the right hand side of the figure by changing to a slower chart speed to record more transients. The changes of pyridine nucleotide fluorescence recorded at the same sensitivity as the Quin 2-Ca fluorescence during the contractions of the cells are also shown in Fig. 8. These were small relative to the

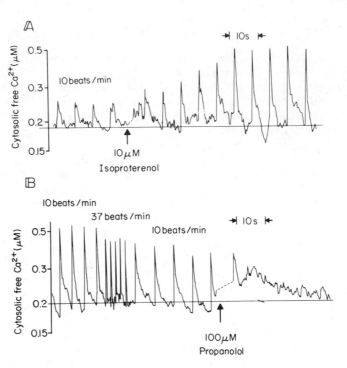

Fig. 6.   Effects of isoproterenol and propanolol on cytosolic free
Ca^{2+} transients of contracting isolated myocytes.   The myocytes were
loaded with Quin 2 and incubated with stirring at 37°C in Hank's
medium containing 0.65 mM Ca^{2+} at a concentration of 2 mg dry weight/
ml.   Contractions were induced by stimulation pulses of 70 volts and
1.5 msec duration.

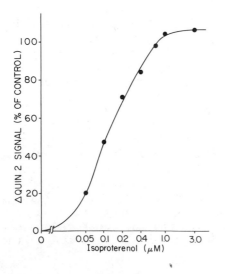

Fig. 7.   Dependency of the amplitude of the Quin 2-Ca fluorescence
change in contracting heart cells
on isoproterenol concentration.
The data were obtained from experiments similar to that shown in
Fig. 6.

Quin 2 signal, indicating relatively little spillover of the pyridine nucleotide fluorescence into the Quin 2-Ca fluorescence. According to Fig. 8, contraction of the myocytes was associated with a rapid pyridine nucleotide reduction followed by a slower reoxidation, with the peak reduction occurring shortly after the peak of the Quin 2-Ca signal.

These preliminary studies clearly show, in contrast to earlier predictions (1), that Ca^{2+} transients in stimulated, isolated myocytes can be recorded with the fluorescent Ca^{2+} indicator Quin 2. Questions remain, however, concerning the absolute accuracy of the calibration and the degree to which the presence of Quin 2 damps the Ca^{2+} transients. Quin 2 itself is unable to measure intracellular free Ca^{2+} concentrations above 0.8 μM since it becomes saturated with calcium in this range. Hopefully other similar compounds will soon become available that remedy some of the present deficiencies of Quin 2, namely fluorescent indicators with a higher K_d, a higher quantum yield and/or a shift of fluorescence emission to higher wavelengths (2). In any case, the usefulness and limitations of Quin 2 in measuring the Ca^{2+} transient in stimulated, isolated myocytes can be further evaluated by varying the amount of Quin 2 in loaded cells so that the degree of its Ca^{2+} buffering effect can be quantitatively assessed. Presently we have not ascertained the lower limit for Quin 2 loading compatible with acceptable signal to noise ratio of the fluorescence change.

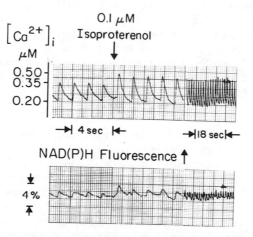

Fig. 8. Comparison of Ca^{2+} transients measured with Quin 2 and pyridine nucleotide fluorescence changes in stimulated, isolated myocytes. The cells were incubated as in Fig. 1 and stimulated at the rate of 1 beat/sec by 70 volt pulses of 1.5 msec duration. The fluorescence signals were recorded on a Gould Brush 260 recorder with an overall time constant of about 10 msec.

DISCUSSION

The present measurements of intracellular free Ca^{2+} transients obtained using Quin 2 can be compared with light emission signals recorded from muscles injected with aequorin (16-22). This latter system has the advantage that contraction of the muscle can be measured simultaneously with the aequorin light emission. In mammalian myocardium, the aequorin signal rises much more rapidly than tension, and declines to near basal levels by the time that peak tension is achieved. In the studies of Morgan and Blinks (18) using cat papillary muscle with a stimulus interval of 4 s, norepinephrine increased the peak of light emission, increased tension, shortened the time to peak light and at submaximal concentrations abbreviated the decline of light intensity. The cytosolic free Ca^{2+} transient measured with aequorin is thus very similar to the Quin 2-Ca transient, and illustrates the dual effect of catecholamines in augmenting the cytosolic free Ca^{2+} and stimulating its rate of sequestration by the sarcoplasmic reticulum through a cyclic AMP-dependent mechanism (22). In addition, Kurihara and Allen (19) have shown that in rat ventricular muscle strips (unlike cat muscle) an increase of the stimulation frequency from 30 to 120 beats/min caused a decrease of both tension development and the peak of the light transient, which is similar to the decrease of the Quin 2-Ca signal seen in Fig. 6 with an increased stimulation frequency. Notable differences between the aequorin light transient and the Quin 2-Ca fluorescence transient are that the latter signal appears to be considerably more prolonged and shows a smaller peak increase. These differences presumably reflect the buffering action of Quin 2 and the different linearity of response between the two Ca^{2+} indicators, with Quin 2 more accurately measuring the lower cytosolic free Ca^{2+} concentrations but less accurately measuring the peak Ca^{2+} due to saturation of the dye at Ca^{2+} concentrations in the region of 0.8 μM. Thus, use of Quin 2-loaded myocytes would seem to offer a useful alternative to aequorin-injected muscle preparations for studies of excitation-contraction coupling and intracellular Ca^{2+} homeostasis in cardiac muscle.

Over the last few years there has been renewed interest and speculation concerning the relationship between the cytosolic free Ca^{2+} concentration in cardiac tissue and the mitochondrial calcium content. Denton and McCormack (24-30) have pioneered the concept that several Ca^{2+}-dependent enzymes in the mitochondrial matrix are regulated *in vivo* through changes of the matrix free Ca^{2+} concentration in response to alterations of the cytosolic free Ca^{2+}. This suggestion arose from observations that the activities of three exclusively mitochondrial enzymes are increased several fold by an increase of free Ca^{2+}, all with half maximal activation constants of about 1 μM. These are pyruvate dehydrogenase phosphatase, which when activated by Ca^{2+} increases the effective V_{max} of pyruvate dehydrogenase by decreasing the proportion of the enzyme in the inactive phosphorylated form (31), the α-ketoglutarate dehydrogenase complex (27) and NAD^+-linked isocitrate dehydrogenase (25). The effect of Ca^{2+} on the latter two enzymes is to decrease their apparent K_m values for α-ketoglutarate and isocitrate, respectively, with no effect on the enzyme activities at saturating substrate concentrations. Since these mitochondrial Ca^{2+}-dependent enzymes are involved in the regulation both of the rate of production of acetyl-CoA and its rate of oxidation in the citric acid cycle, the proposition is most attractive that the increase of the time averaged cytosolic free Ca^{2+} induced by positive inotropic agents in heart muscle is the common factor causing, a) an augmentation of glycogenolysis by Ca^{2+} activation of phosphorylase kinase, b) an increased contractile state and myofibrillar ATPase activity by increased Ca^{2+} binding to troponin C and c) an increased rate of ATP synthesis by increasing the mitochondrial free Ca^{2+} concentration (29, 32).

In order to prove that Ca^{2+} is acting in a concerted manner to regulate energy metabolism according to the above suggestion, a number of criteria have to be met. Essentially, the free Ca^{2+} concentration of the mitochondrial matrix should be shown to be increased, together with an increase of flux of the Ca^{2+}-dependent enzymes over their Ca^{2+}-sensitive range, when the cytosolic free Ca^{2+} concentration of contracting heart muscle is increased on a beat-to-beat basis or time averaged basis after intervention of positive inotropic agents. Since this is presently impossible using direct experimental techniques, a number of indirect approaches have been used. In the first instance, it is particularly important to define the content of calcium in mitochondria in the intact cell and determine whether changes of the calcium content in this pool can account for changes in the activity of the mitochondrial Ca^{2+}-dependent enzymes. Crompton et al (32) approached this problem by isolating mitochondria from rat hearts perfused under control conditions and with the $α_1$-agonist methoxamine or with β-adrenergic agents. The relationships between the endogenous Ca^{2+} content of the mitochondria and the time period that elapsed between homogenization and sedimentation of the mitochondria was measured, and it was ascertained that between 10 and 35 min the relationships were linear for each condition. Extrapolation to time zero provided a value of 1.75 nmol/mg protein for the mitochondrial calcium content of control hearts, with increases of 48%, 100%, and 140% for 10 μM methoxamine, 1 μM isoproterenol and 1 μM epinephrine-treated hearts, respectively. This estimate for the mitochondrial calcium content of control (Ca^{2+} perfused) hearts is half our estimate of the mitochondrial calcium content of Ca^{2+}-tolerant myocytes, and is also considerably lower than that reported by Kessar and Crompton (33) using a rapid cell disruption technique with isolated myocytes. No data are currently available concerning the effect of α or β-agonists on the mitochondrial calcium content of isolated myocytes, although such studies are in progress in the author's laboratory. Nevertheless, despite problems inherent in extrapolating data from isolated mitochondria to the intact tissue, the apparent increase of the mitochondrial calcium content after stimulation of hearts with positive inotropic agents is consistent with the time averaged increase of cytosolic free Ca^{2+} and with an increase in the amount of active pyruvate dehydrogenase in hearts under these conditions (29, 34). Furthermore, the increase of active pyruvate dehydrogenase induced by positive inotropic agents or external Ca^{2+} in perfused rat hearts could be prevented by addition of ruthenium red, which presumably entered the cell and caused inhibition of the mitochondrial Ca^{2+} uniporter (35).

The interconversion between the active (nonphosphorylated) and inactive (phosphorylated) forms of pyruvate dehydrogenase is also influenced by several metabolites, notably pyruvate, acetyl-CoA and NADH, which affect pyruvate dehydrogenase kinase, as well as by Mg^{2+}, which is required for pyruvate dehydrogenase phosphatase activity (36, 37). Consequently, it is difficult to rule out the possibility that an effector other than calcium is also changing when measurements of pyruvate dehydrogenase activity are made using intact heart preparations. In fact, it is well known that an increase of the contractile state, induced by β-adrenergic agents, Ca^{2+} or increased pre- or afterload, will cause a fall of the mitochondrial $NADH/NAD^+$ ratio as a consequence of an increased flux through the electron transport chain due to an enhanced requirement of the tissue for ATP synthesis (38). Ample proof has been provided in studies with both perfused hearts and isolated cardiac mitochondria to show that a delicately balanced coordination of control at pyruvate dehydrogenase, NAD-linked isocitrate dehydrogenase and α-ketoglutarate dehydrogenase is exerted by the $NADH/NAD^+$ ratio in response to changes of phosphate acceptor availability (for reviews see Refs. 36, 38-40). Hence, a demonstration of the regulation of the dehydrogenase activities by Ca^{2+} requires that the other effectors of enzyme activity, particularly NADH, should not change simultaneously. This problem has been addressed in part (24, 27, 34), but is difficult to resolve conclusively because of compartmentation of the effector molecules within the cell and between free and bound forms, and the inherent difficulty of knowing the mitochondrial free Mg^{2+} concentration. Use of α-ketoglutarate dehydrogenase as the Ca^{2+}-dependent monitoring system offers some advantages over measurements of pyruvate dehydrogenase activity in studies with isolated mitochondria since the enzyme activity is subject to fewer regulators. Measurements of α-ketoglutarate dehydrogenase activity in rat heart mitochondria at subsaturating α-ketoglutarate concentrations have shown that half maximum activation by Ca^{2+} is achieved at mitochondrial calcium contents of 0.5 - 1 nmol/mg of protein, with maximal activation at 2-3 nmol of Ca^{2+}/mg of protein (11, 41, 42). These values for the Ca^{2+} requirements for half maximum and maximum activation of α-ketoglutarate dehydrogenase are somewhat lower (by a factor of about 2) than the estimates of the mitochondrial calcium content of control and hormone-stimulated cardiac muscle, respectively, but are sufficiently close to support the suggestion that the mitochondrial dehydrogenases are regulated by physiological relevant changes of mitochondrial calcium rather than always being saturated with Ca^{2+} as we have previously suggested (8, 36). In fact, the data in Fig. 8 indicate that the mitochondrial dehydrogenases may sense the change of cytosolic free Ca^{2+} on a beat-to-beat basis since electrical stimulation of the myocytes caused a stimulus-dependent reduction of the pyridine nucleotides. Isolated myocytes contract against a zero load resistance, so that the extra energy requirements for contraction are very small. Under these circumstances it may be envisioned that a Ca^{2+}-dependent activation of the dehydrogenases is revealed by a reduction of the pyridine nucleotides, rather than the pyridine nucleotide redox state being dominated by activation of the electron transport chain.

A number of factors that are present in the intact cell but absent or altered under conditions of the experiments with isolated mitochondria may be responsible for changing the sensitivity of the mitochondrial Ca^{2+} uniporter or the intramitochondrial dehydrogenases to Ca^{2+}. Differences in the Mg^{2+} content or the intramitochondrial ATP/ADP (GTP/GDP) ratio between isolated mitochondria and mitochondria in the intact cell might account for a 2-3-fold decrease in the sensitivity of the dehydrogenases to Ca^{2+}. The possibility that heart mitochondria respond to beat-dependent cytosolic Ca^{2+} transients with an increased rate of Ca^{2+} uptake and release has generally been discounted because of the very high apparent K_m for Ca^{2+} uptake in the presence of Mg^{2+} relative to the fluctuations of the cytosolic free Ca^{2+} concentration (43, 44). However, recent work from this laboratory (45), has shown that the polyamines, spermine, and spermidine at physiological concentrations will lower the apparent K_m values for Ca^{2+} of both the Ca^{2+} uniporter and the mitochondrial Ca^{2+} efflux carriers of isolated liver and heart mitochondria and saponin-permeabilized cells incubated in the presence of Mg^{2+}, thereby allowing the mitochondria to cycle Ca^{2+} down to physiological extramitochondrial free Ca^{2+} concentrations of 0.2 μM. Consequently, the relative roles of the mitochondria and sarcoplasmic reticulum in buffering and regulating the cytosolic free Ca^{2+} in relation to the mitochondrial Ca^{2+} content (46), may require reevaluation.

REFERENCES

1. J. R. Blinks, W. G. Wier, P. Hess, and F. G. Prendergast, Measurement of Ca^{2+} concentrations in living cells, Progr. Biophys. Molec. Biol. 40: 1-114 (1982).
2. R. Y. Tsien, Intracellular measurements of ion activation, Ann. Rev. Biophys. Bioeng. 12: 91-116 (1983).
3. R. Y. Tsien, New calcium indicators and buffers with high selectivity against magnesium and protons: design, synthesis and properties of prototype structures, Biochemistry 19: 2396-2404 (1980).

4. R. Y. Tsien, A non-disruptive technique for loading calcium buffers and indicators into cells, Nature 290: 527-528 (1981).

5. R. Y. Tsien, T. Pozzan, and R. J. Rink, Calcium homeostasis in intact lymphocytes: cytoplasmic free calcium monitored with a new intracellularly trapped fluorescent indicator, J. Cell. Biol. 94: 325-334 (1982).

6. A. P. Thomas, Alexander, J. and J. R. Williamson, Relationship between inositol polyphosphate production and the increase of cytosolic free Ca^{2+} induced by vasopressin in isolated hepatocytes, J. Biol. Chem., in press.

7. R. Charest, P. F. Blackmore, B. Berthon, and J. H. Exton, Changes in free cytosolic Ca^{2+} in hepatocytes following α-adrenergic stimulation. Studies on Quin 2-loaded hepatocytes, J. Biol. Chem. 258: 8769-8773 (1983).

8. J. R. Williamson, R. J. Williams, K. E. Coll, and A. P. Thomas, Cytosolic free Ca^{2+} concentration and intracellular calcium distribution of Ca^{2+}-tolerant isolated heart cells, J. Biol. Chem. 258: 13411-13414 (1983).

9. E. Murphy, K. E. Coll, T. L. Rich, and J. R. Williamson, Hormonal effects on calcium homeostasis in isolated hepatocytes. J. Biol. Chem. 255: 6600-6608 (1980).

10. S. K. Joseph, K. E. Coll, R. H. Cooper, J. S. Marks, and J. R. Williamson, Mechanisms underlying calcium homeostasis in isolated hepatocytes, J. Biol. Chem. 258: 731-741 (1983).

11. K. E. Coll, S. K. Joseph, B. E. Corkey, and J. R. Williamson, Determination of the matrix free Ca^{2+} concentration and kinetics of Ca^{2+} in liver and heart mitochondria, J. Biol. Chem. 257: 8696-8704 (1982).

12. W. R. Kukovetz, M. E. Hess, J. Shanfeld, and N. Haugaard, The action of sympathomimetic amines on isometric contraction and phosphorylase activity of the isolated rat heart, J. Pharmacol. Exp. Therap. 127: 122-127 (1959).

13. W. R. Ingebretsen, W. F. Friedman, and S. E. Mayer, Isoproterenol-induced restoration of contraction in K^+-depolarized hearts: relationship to cAMP, Am. J. Physiol. 241: H187-H193 (1981).

14. K. Hermsmeyer, R. Mason, S. H. Griffen, and P. Becker, Rat cardiac muscle single cell automaticity responses to α and β-adrenergic agonists and antagonists, Circ. Res. 51: 532-537.

15. J. E. Holl, Selective additive effect of phenylephrine to the inotropic action of isoproterenol on rabbit left atria, Naunyn-Schmiedeberg's Arch. Pharmacol. 318: 336-339 (1982).

16. D. G. Allen and J. R. Blinks, Calcium transients in aequorin injected frog cardiac muscle, Nature 273: 509-513 (1978).

17. W. G. Wier, Calcium transients during excitation-contraction coupling in mammalian heart: aequorin signals of canine purkinje fibers, Science 207: 1085-1087.

18. J. P. Morgan and J. R. Blinks, Intracellular Ca^{2+} transients in the cat papillary muscle, Can. J. Physiol. Pharmacol. 60: 524-528 (1982).

588

19. S. Kurihara and D. G. Allen, Intracellular Ca^{2+} transients and relaxation in mammalian cardiac muscle, Japn. Circ. J. 46: 39-43.

20. D. G. Allen and S. Kurihara, The effects of muscle length on intracellular calcium transients in mammalian cardiac muscle, J. Physiol. 327: 79-94 (1982).

21. W. G. Wier and G. Isenberg, Intracellular $[Ca^{2+}]$ transients in voltage clamped cardiac purkinje fibers, Pflügers Arch. 392: 284-290 (1982).

22. Eisner, D. A., C. H. Orchard, and D. G. Allen, Control of intracellular ionized calcium concentration by sarcolemmal and intracellular mechanisms, J. Mol. Cell. Cardiol. 16: 137-146 (1984).

23. R. W. Tsien, Cyclic AMP and contractive activity in the heart, Adv. Cyclic Nucleotide Res. 8: 363-420 (1977).

24. R. M. Denton and J. G. McCormack, On the role of calcium transport cycle in heart and other mammalian mitochondria, FEBS. Lett. 119: 1-8.

25. R. M. Denton, D. A. Richards and J. G. Chin, Calcium ions and the regulation of NAD$^+$ linked isocitrate dehydrogenase from the mitochondria of rat heart and other tissues, Biochem. J. 176: 899-906.

26. R. M. Denton, J. G. McCormack, and N. J. Edgell, Role of calcium ions in the regulation of intramitochondrial metabolism, Biochem. J. 190: 107-117.

27. J. G. McCormack and R. M. Denton, The effects of calcium ions and adenine nucleotides on the activity of pig heart 2-oxoglutarate dehydrogenase complex, Biochem. J. 180: 533-544 (1979).

28. J. G. McCormack and R. M. Denton, Role of calcium ions in the regulation of intramitochondrial metabolism, Biochem. J. 190: 95-105 (1980).

29. J. G. McCormack and R. M. Denton, The activation of pyruvate dehydrogenase in the perfused rat heart by adrenaline and other inotropic agents, Biochem. J. 194: 639-643 (1981).

30. J. G. McCormack and R. M. Denton, Role of Ca^{2+} ions in the regulation of intramitochondrial metabolism in rat heart, Biochem. J. 218: 235-247 (1984).

31. R. M. Denton, P. J. Randle, and B. R. Martin, Stimulation by calcium ions of pyruvate dehydrogenase phosphate phosphatase, Biochem. J. 128: 161-163 (1972).

32. M. Crompton, P. Kessar and I. Al-Nasser, The α-adrenergic-mediated activation of the cardiac mitochondrial Ca^{2+} uniporter and its role in the control of intramitochondrial Ca^{2+} in vivo, Biochem. J. 216: 333-342 (1983).

33. P. Kessar and M. Crompton, The sequestration of Ca^{2+} by mitochondria in rat heart cells, Cell Calcium 4: 295-305 (1983).

34. T. Hiraoka, M. Debuysere, and M. S. Olson, Studies of the effects of β-adrenergic agonists on the regulation of pyruvate dehydrogenase in the perfused rat heart, J. Biol. Chem. 255: 7604-7609 (1980).

35. J. G. McCormack and P. J. England, Ruthenium red inhibits the activation of pyruvate dehydrogenase caused by positive inotropic agents in the perfused rat heart, Biochem. J. 214: 581-585 (1983).

36. J. R. Williamson and R. H. Cooper, Regulation of the citric acid cycle in mammalian systems, FEBS Lett. 117: K73-K92 (1980).

37. P. J. Randle, Phosphorylation-dephosphorylation cycles and the regulation of fuel selection in mammals, Curr. Topics Cell. Regul. 18: 108-129 (1981).

38. J. R. Williamson, Mitochondrial function in the heart, Ann. Rev. Physiol. 41: 485-506 (1979).

39. R. G. Hansford, Control of mitochondrial substrate oxidation, Curr. Topics Bioenerg. 10: 217-278 (1980).

40. P. J. Randle and P. K. Tubbs, Carbohydrate and fatty acid metabolism, in: "Handbook of Physiology", Section 2, The Cardiovascular System, R. M. Berne, ed., Am. Physiol. Soc., Bethesda (1979).

41. R. G. Hansford and F. Castro, Effects of micromolar concentrations of free calcium ions in the reduction of heart mitochondrial NAD(P) by 2-oxoglutarate, Biochem. J. 198: 522-533 (1981).

42. R. G. Hansford and F. Castro, Intramitochondrial and extramitochondrial free calcium ion concentrations with very low plausibly physiological, contents of total calcium, J. Bioenerg. Biomembr. 14: 361-376 (1982).

43. T. Kitazawa, Physiological significance of Ca uptake by mitochondria in the heart in comparison with that by cardiac sarcoplasmic reticulum, J. Biochem. (Tokyo) 80: 1129-1147 (1976).

44. S. P. Robertson, J. P. Potter and W. Rouslin, The Ca^{2+} and Mg^{2+} dependence of Ca^{2+} uptake and respiratory function of porcine heart mitochondria, J. Biol. Chem. 257: 1743-1748 (1982).

45. C. V. Nicchitta and J. R. Williamson, Spermine: A regulator of mitochondrial calcium cycling, J. Biol. Chem., in press.

46. D. G. Nicholls and K. Åkerman, Mitochondrial calcium transport, Biochim. Biophys. Acta 683: 57-88 (1982).

ACKNOWLEDGMENTS

This work was supported by NIH grant HL-14461.

Ca^{++}-DEPENDENT AND Ca^{++}-INDEPENDENT EFFECTS OF Mg^{++} ON CANINE RIGHT ATRIA

W.T. Woods, Jr.

Department of Physiology and Biophysics
University of Alabama in Birmingham
University Station
Birmingham, AL   35294

INTRODUCTION

Mg^{++} and Ca^{++}, the divalent cations that exist in highest concentrations in biological fluids, interact with cardiac cell membranes by binding to them or by crossing them through carriers or channels. Binding and transmembrane movement of Ca^{++} directly affect electrogenesis and contractility in cardiac cells. Mg^{++} has been thought to act less directly on electromechanical function by facilitating active transport or competing with Ca^{++} and other cations for membrane binding sites.

Competition between Mg^{++} and Ca^{++} at the cell membrane comes about because of similarities between them (extracellular concentrations, ionic diameters, valencies, etc.). Physiologic consequences of this competition depend on whether Mg^{++} can activate the same event or play the same role as Ca^{++} when it contacts a Ca^{++}-sensitive site on the membrane. Mg^{++} can substitute for Ca^{++} in preventing the so-called Ca^{++} paradox (Rich and Langer, 1982), in binding to sarcolemmal vesicles (Bers and Langer, 1979), and in promoting development of tension in papillary muscles (Bers and Langer, 1979). However, Mg^{++} is considered to be a competitive antagonist of Ca^{++} in cardiac electrical and mechanical events that occur at physiologic concentrations (Pappano and Sperelakis, 1969; Pappano, 1970; Bers and Langer, 1979; Rich and Langer, 1982.

Since Mg^{++} is present in body fluids in relatively high concentrations (0.85 mmol./l. in canine blood), it is important to know whether its physiologic effect is the result of competition

591

with Ca^{++} or simply the direct effect of Mg^{++}. Therefore, the present studies were carried out to elucidate the mechanism by which Mg^{++} alters pacemaker firing rate and tension in the canine atrial cells. They suggest that not all of the effects of Mg^{++} on atrial electromechanical function can be explained by competition with Ca^{++}.

METHODS

Right atria were excised from 5 mongrel dogs less than 6 months old. They were pinned with the endocardial surface down in a 25 ml. wax-bottomed dish, and a solution containing (in mmol./l.) Na^+, 145; K^+, 4.20; Ca^{2+}, 1.27; Mg^{2+}, 1.00; Cl^-, 124; SO_4^{2-}, 1.00; $H_2CO_3^-$, 25.0; dextrose, 5.60 (pH 7.4 and temperature $36\pm1°C$) was perfused through the sinus node artery as described previously (Woods et al., 1976). The perfusate was removed after one pass through the sinus node artery by a suction tube at the bath surface; it was kept at a volume of 25 ml. and was not recirculated. Flow was 5 ± 1 ml./min. $[Mg^{++}]$ and $[Ca^{++}]$ were changed as described in Results and perfused for 10.0 min. into the sinus node pacemaker regions. The 10 min. period during which new suffusates were tested was not long enough to lower or raise all cells' extracellular $[Mg^{++}]$'s and $[Ca^{++}]$'s to the levels contained in the suffusate. Therefore, the responses observed reflected early decreases or increases in extracellular concentrations, not stable responses to long term perfusion with a particular concentration of Mg^{++} or Ca^{++}. Bipolar silver surface electrodes (1 mm. interpolar distance) were placed on the epicardial surface in the sulcus terminalis. These provided a bipolar surface electrogram which served as the trigger for a tachogram providing a continuous monitor of atrial rate.

To monitor changes in atrial contraction amplitude the outer edge of the atrial preparation (posterior right atrial surface) was tied with thread to a strain gauge lever arm; compliance was 0.25 mm./g. (f.). The strain gauge output was linearly proportional to the atrial displacement. A 1.0 g. (f.) atrial contraction produced a 25.0 mm. pen displacement on the recorder chart.

Atropine (5 mg./l.) and propranolol (10 mg./l.) were perfused into the sinus node artery after they dissolved in the perfusing solution. 10 min. exposure to these drugs produced complete adrenergic and cholinergic blockade in the sinus node and atrium. The full perfusion procedure and the effects of atropine and propranolol on sinus rate in the isolated perfused canine right atrium have been described in detail (Woods et al., 1978).

Data were analyzed for statistical significance with Student's t test. Paired differences were used when appropriate and are so designated. Differences are reported as significant when the P value is less than 0.05. When mean values are reported, one standard deviation is included (mean ± S.D.).

RESULTS

Effect of $[Mg^{++}]$ on Sinus Rate

Mg^{++} at concentrations of 2.50, 1.25, and 0.05 mmol./l. was added to the solution perfusing the pacemaker regions (sinus nodes) of the right atria in the presence of a constant $[Ca_{++}]$ (2.50, 1.25, or 0.05 mmol./l.). Figure 1 shows that when $[Mg^{++}]$ was lowered, sinus rate increased (P<0.05) at each of the 3 different $[Ca^{++}]$'s. When $[Ca^{++}]$ was decreased, sinus rate fell slightly as reported previously (Woods et al., 1979).

Effect of $[Mg^{++}]$ on Atrial Resting Tension

During exposure to the arterial perfusates containing 2.50, 1.25, and 0.05 mmol./l. Mg^{++}, resting tension was measured as the minimum tension recorded between contractions. Table 1 shows that lowering $[Mg^{++}]$ was consistently without significant effect (P<0.05) on resting tension except when $[Ca^{++}]$ was 2.5 mmol./l. in which case 0.05 mmol./l. Mg^{++} caused a substantial increase (P<0.05) in resting tension. When $[Ca^{++}]$ was 0.05 mmol./l., resting tension always increased, but the $[Mg^{++}]$ had no effect (P<0.05) on the amount of increase.

Table 1. Atrial Resting Tensions Observed When $[Mg^{++}]_o$ and $[Ca^{++}]_o$ Were Changed

$[Mg^{++}]_o$ (mmol./l.)	2.50	$[Ca^{++}]_o$ (mmol./l.) 1.25		0.05
2.50	0 ±0	0 ±0	*	192 ±48
1.25	36 ±72 *	0 ±0	*	188 ±60
0.05	120 ±76	76 ±100	*	160 ±104

*between 2 entries denotes significant difference (p<0.05) between them.

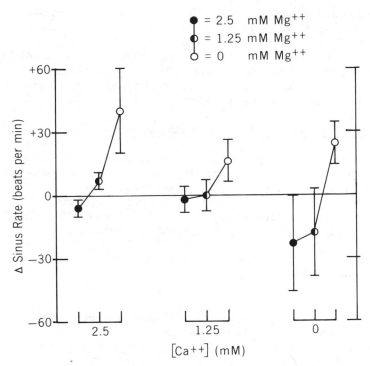

Figure 1. This graph shows the changes in sinus rate associated with 10 min perfusion of solutions containing different $[Mg^{++}]$ and $[Ca^{++}]$. For any one $[Ca^{++}]$, response to lowering $[Mg^{++}]$ can be read from left to right. Points are means + 1 S.D.

Effect of $[Mg^{++}]$ on Atrial Developed Tension

During exposure to the arterial perfusates containing 2.50, 1.25, and 0.05 mmol./l. Mg^{++}, developed tension was measured as the difference between the total tension recorded minus the preceding resting tension. Figure 2 shows that lowering $[Mg^{++}]$ was consistently without significant effect (P>0.05) on developed tension except when $[Ca^{++}]$ was 2.50 mmol./l. in which case omission of Mg^{++} (0.05 mmol./l.) caused a substantial <u>decrease</u> (P<0.05) in developed tension. Conversely, in all other combinations of Mg^{++} and Ca^{++}, higher $[Ca^{++}]$'s were always associated with higher developed tensions.

Rate–Dependency of Mg^{++}/Ca^{++} Effects

The rise in resting tension and concomitant fall in developed tension observed at $[Ca^{++}]$=2.50 mmol./l., $[Mg^{++}]$=0.05 mmol./l. was accompanied by an increase in firing rate of 40±20 beats/min. (the largest increase in rate observed in this study). Therefore, 5 atria were exposed to 2.5 mmol./l. Ca^{++}, 1.2 mmol./l. Mg^{++} and paced by electrode at 40 beats/min. higher than the observed firing rate. In 3 of these atria developed tension increased slightly; in 2 it did not change; in none did it decrease.

DISCUSSION

The relationship between muscle tension and extracellular $[Ca^{++}]$ has been studied extensively. In this study the question of how $[Mg^{++}]$ alters this relationship was explored. With respect to resting atrial tension, these observations confirmed that it is directly related to extracellular $[Ca^{++}]$. Extracellular $[Mg^{++}]$ had no significant effect on resting tension except in one special case. When $[Ca^{++}]$ was raised to 2.50 mmol./l. while $[Mg^{++}]$ was 0.05 mmol./l., resting tension became substantially higher. Since resting tension is a function of the amount of intracellular $[Ca^{++}]$ available to contractile elements at rest, this raises the possibility that lowering extracellular $[Mg^{++}]$ raises intracellular $[Ca^{++}]$. Further experimentation will be necessary to determine whether this could result from higher membrane permeability to Ca^{++} or lower affinity binding of intracellular Ca^{++}.

Data from this study relating to active tension support the hypothesized relationship between extracellular $[Mg^{++}]$ and intracellular $[Ca^{++}]$. Extracellular $[Mg^{++}]$ was without effect on the development of tension during atrial contraction except when $[Ca^{++}]$ was 2.50 mmol./l. and $[Mg^{++}]$ was 0.05 mmol./l. Under these conditions active tension fell substantially, and combined with the concomitant rise in resting tension, the atrium appeared to be

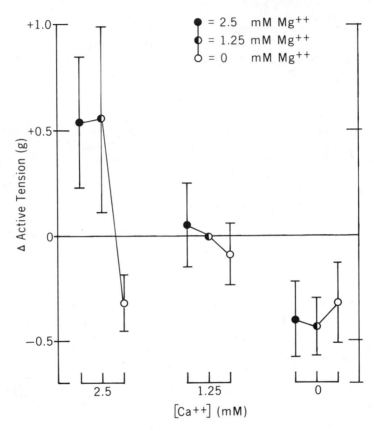

Figure 2. This graph shows the changes in atrial active (developed) tension associated with perfusion of solutions containing different [Mg^{++}] and [Ca^{++}]. For any one [Ca^{++}], response to lowering [Mg^{++}] can be read from left to right. Points are means ± 1 S.D.

in an early stage of contracture. In separate studies, continued perfusion with a solution of this Mg^{++} and Ca^{++} composition caused irreversible contracture within 30 min. (data not shown). Since contracture is associated with increased intracellular $[Ca^{++}]$ and contracture was never observed when $[Mg^{++}]$ was 1.25 or 2.50 mmol./l., these observations support the hypothesis that extracellular $[Mg^{++}]$ promotes lower intracellular $[Ca^{++}]$. This could explain why in the presence of very low extracellular $[Mg^{++}]$, contracture that was characteristic of "Ca^{++} overload" could occur in atrial cells.

Previous studies (Chesnais et al., 1971, 1975) led to the hypothesis that in the cardiac action potential extracellular $[Mg^{++}]$ impedes movement of Na^+ more than it does movement of Ca^{++}. One study suggested that the decreased rate of firing of sinus node pacemaker cells observed when extracellular $[Mg^{++}]$ becomes elevated, is associated with depressed Na^+ influx rather than depressed Ca^{++} influx (Woods et al., 1979). The present observations are consistent with that hypothesis since, for example, sinus rate always fell when $[Mg^{++}]$ was lowered, but extracellular $[Ca^{++}]$ had no effect on the amount of fall. In fact, sinus rate always fell by the same amount regardless of $[Ca^{++}]$.

The periods (10 min.) of suffusion with the altered cation concentrations tested in this study were intentionally too brief to allow complete equilibration with the extracellular fluid of the tissue. The intent was to establish the direction and magnitude of early responses so that change in extracellular rather than intracellular concentrations could be evaluated (Page and Polimeni, 1974).

The results suggest that extracellular $[Mg^{++}]$ in physiologic concentration can be an important regulator of atrial electromechanical activity. While it may impede or compete with transmembrane Ca^{++} movement, other effects, such as interference with transmembrane movement of Na^+ may be of equivalent physiologic importance.

REFERENCES

Bers, D. M., and Langer, G. A., 1979, Uncoupling cation effects on cardiac contractility and sarcolemmal Ca^{2+} binding, Amer. J. of Physiol. 237(3):H332-H341.

Chesnais, J. M., Coraboeuf, E., Sauviat, M. P., and Vassas, J. M., 1971, Inhibition par les ions magnesium de la conductance sodique lente apparaissant sous l'effet de depolarisations membranaires au niveau des fibres atriales de Grenouille, C. R. Acad. Sc. Paris, 273:1594-1597.

Chesnais, J. M, Coraboeuf, E., Sauviat, M. P., and Vassas, J. M., 1975, Sensitivity to H, Li and Mg ions of the slow inward sodium current in frog atrial fibres, J. Molec. Cell. Cardiol., 7:627-642.

Polimeni, P. I., and Page, E., 1974, Further observations on magnesium transport in rat ventricular muscle, Recent Advances in Studies on Cardiac Structure and Metabolism, 4(Myocardial Biology):217-232.

Pappano, A. J., 1970, Calcium-dependent action potentials produced by catecholamines in guinea pig atrial muscle fibers depolarized by potassium, Circ. Res., 27:379-390.

Pappano, A. J., and Sperelakis, N., 1969, Spike electrogenesis in cultured heart cells, Amer. J. of Physiol., 217:615-624.

Rich, T. L., and Langer, G. A., 1982, Calcium depletion in rabbit myocardium, Circ. Res., 51:131-141.

Woods, W. T., Katholi, R. E., Urthaler, F., and James, T. N., 1979, Electrophysiological effects of magnesium on cells in the canine sinus node and false tendon, Circ. Res., 44:182-188.

Woods, W. T., Urthaler, F., and James, T. N., 1976, Spontaneous action potentials of cells in the canine sinus node, Circ. Res., 39:76-82.

Woods, W. T., Urthaler, F., and James, T. N., 1978, Progressive postnatal changes in sinus node response to atropine and propranolol, Amer. J. of Physiol., 234:H412-H415.

CHRONOTROPIC AND INOTROPIC EFFECTS OF $[Mg^{++}]_o$ NOT DEPENDENT UPON $[Ca^{++}]_o$

W.T. Woods, Jr.

Department of Physiology & Biophysics, University of

Alabama School of Medicine, Birmingham, Alabama

Within its physiologic range of concentrations, Mg^{++}_o (extra-cellular Mg^{++}) can depress both cardiac rate and mechanical activity. Mechanisms by which Mg^{++}_o concentration ($[Mg^{++}]_o$) alters the firing rate of cardiac pacemaker cells and the mechanical tension (resting and developed) of cardiac working muscle tissue have not been identified. Influx of Ca^{++} occurs during pacemaking and tension generation. Therefore, this study was designed to determine whether certain chronotropic and inotropic effects of Mg^{++}_o share similar Ca^{++}-dependent mechanisms.

Studies were performed in 30 isolated right atria that had been excised from pentobarbital-anesthetized (30 mg/kg) dogs (6 ± 2 kg), and that were perfused through their sinus node arteries. $[Ca^{++}]$'s and $[Mg^{++}]$'s were altered in the physiologic perfusion solutions (containing normal canine blood electrolytes) such that a concentration of 2.50 mmoles/l, 1.25 mmoles/l, or 0 (less than 50 micromoles/l) of each divalent cation was tested in the presence of each different concentration of the other.

- Sinus Rate: Whenever $[Mg^{++}]_o$ was lowered, sinus rate increased. The maximum amount of increase (36 ± 10 beats per minute) and percentage (30 ± 5%) change were always the same regardless of $[Ca^{++}]_o$.
- Resting Tension: Lowering $[Mg^{++}]_o$ was without effect on resting tension except when $[Ca^{++}]_o$ was 2.50 mmole/l. At this higher $[Ca^{++}]_o$ only, omission of Mg^{++} from the perfusate caused an increase of 0.120 ± 0.760 g in resting tension.
- Developed Tension (total tension minus resting tension): Lowering $[Mg^{++}]_o$ was without effect on developed tension

except when $[Ca^{++}]_o$ was 2.50 mmole/l. At this higher $[Ca^{++}]_o$ only, omission of Mg^{++} from the perfusate caused a substantial decrease in developed tension (0.52 ± 0.50 to -0.35 ± 0.1 g). For each experiment in which a change in tension was accompanied by a change in rate of firing, the atrium was paced at a constant rate while the experiment was repeated. This procedure demonstrated that changes in rate per se could not account for the observed changes in tension.

Conclusion: Within a physiologic range of concentrations, Mg^{++}-induced changes in the pacemaker cell firing rate and atrial tension are not dependent upon $[Ca^{++}]_o$. However, lowering $[Mg^{++}]_o$ while $[Ca^{++}]_o$ is elevated promotes contracture of atrial muscle.

SODIUM MODULATION OF RESTING FORCE, CONTRACTILE PROPERTIES, AND
METABOLISM WITH PARTICULAR EMPHASIS ON ITS ROLE IN THE DEVELOPMENT
OF CALCIUM OVERLOAD STATES

Dale G. Renlund, Edward G. Lakatta and Gary Gerstenblith

Cardiology Division, Department of Medicine, The Johns
Hopkins University School of Medicine, and the
Cardiovascular Section, Gerontology Research Center
National Institute on Aging, NIH, Baltimore, Maryland

This work was supported in part by National Heart, Lung
and Blood Institute Specialized Center of Research Grant
#P-50-HL17655-08, Bethesda, Maryland and Coronary Heart
Disease Research, a program of the American Health
Assistance Foundation

The crucial role of extracellular calcium in modulating
cardiac muscle function has been recognized for over 100 years
(1). The manner in which changes in extracellular calcium result
in altered cellular calcium and therefore changes in resting and
active force development, however, is still being explored. A
study of factors influencing cellular calcium is relevant not only
because cellular calcium controls cardiac force development but
also because calcium overload is now recognized to be an
accompaniment and perhaps contributor to the functional and
metabolic derangements which occur during certain pathologic
states (2).

Increases in extracellular calcium may increase cellular
calcium via a voltage dependent channel, a nonspecific "leak" down
the eletrochemical trans-sarcolemmal calcium gradient or via
coupled exchange with cellular sodium (3,4). This exchange occurs
via a carrier, and its magnitude and direction is dependent on the
trans-sarcolemmal calcium gradient, the transmembrane voltage, pH,
temperature and, most importantly for the purposes of this
discussion, the trans-sarcolemmal sodium gradient. For any given
extracellular sodium, the gradient is determined by the
intracellular sodium level and therefore variations in cellular

601

sodium would be expected to directly influence cellular calcium content. For the past several years, we have explored the importance of modifications of cellular sodium on cellular calcium in cardiac muscle and on properties dependent on the cellular calcium content (5-7).

Several interventions are known to affect intracellular sodium activity. Reduction of extracellular sodium via substitution with substances such as lithium has been shown to cause a rapid decrease in intracellular sodium (8). Removal of perfusate potassium and the addition of cardiac glycosides are known to raise intracellular sodium by inhibiting the Na-K-ATPase pump (9,10). Thus one can devise interventions which raise or lower intracellular sodium and assess the effect of these interventions on the relationship between extracellular calcium and calcium activity as evidenced by changes in resting force, calcium dependent light scattering properties and mechanical, metabolic and ionic parameters. The effect of interventions which would vary cellular sodium was studied in three conditions. The first was during step increases in extracellular calcium concentration from 1 to 4 mM (5). The second was during a period of ischemia prior to reperfusion (6) and the third was at the time of reintroduction of calcium following a period of calcium free perfusion (7).

In the first set of experiments (5) right ventricular papillary muscles from male Wistar rats were used. The muscles were mounted horizontally between lucite clamps and perfused with HEPES buffered solution at 29 $^\circ$ C containing, in mM NaCl = 140, KCl = 4.2, $CaCl_2$ = 1.0, $MgCl_2$ = 1.2, Dextrose = 10, and HEPES = 4 which was bubbled with 100% oxygen. The muscles were paced at 24 beats per minute and were at the peak of their length tension curve. Following equilibration, pacing was discontinued and the change in resting force monitored while perfusate calcium was changed from 1 to 4 mM under conditions of varying external sodium concentration, in the presence and absence of ouabain, and under normal and absent extracellular potassium.

Sodium was lowered in unstimulated, nonbeating preparations by equilibrating muscles in perfusate in which lithium was substituted for sodium with LiCl equal to 75%, 50%, 25%, or 0% of the initial value of 140mM NaCl. After allowing 20 minutes for equilibration at each level of lithium substitution, extracellular calcium was increased from 1 to 4 mM and the peak change in resting force was measured. In some experiments, light scattering properties were also measured. Intensity fluctuations in coherent light are due to calcium dependent microscopic cellular motion (11). Changes in intensity fluctuations in many experimental conditions reflect changes in calcium load and coupled with changes in calcium dependent resting force are believed to provide

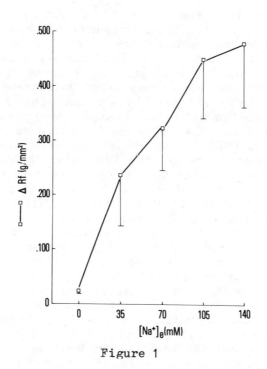

Figure 1

The effect of an increase in extracellular calcium from 1 to 4 mM on the change in resting force (delta RF) as a function of the perfusate sodium in which the calcium step was made. Baseline resting force = 0.749 ± 0.25 g/mm^2; developed force = 2.48 ± 0.54 g/mm^2 before discontinuing stimulation. Redrawn from Walford et al (5).

an indirect monitor of changes in cellular calcium. Extracellular calcium was then returned to 1 mM, the sodium back to 140 mM and the muscle paced until steady state was reached. Pacing was then discontinued again and another level of extracellular sodium was introduced followed by the same calcium step. In other experiments, the calcium step was performed in the presence of increased cellular sodium by perfusing with 1 mM ouabain or with potassium free solution.

Figure 1 depicts the increase in resting force when the calcium step was performed after the muscles had been equilibrated in the presence of varying concentrations of extracellular sodium. As can be seen, the change in resting force a parameter reflecting cellular calcium gain, is less when the calcium step from 1 to 4 mM is made in muscles while have been equilibrated in perfusate containing lowered extracellular and presumably lowered intracellular sodium. Similar changes are present in light scattering properties. The influence of sodium was exaggerated in the presence of caffeine indicating that sarcoplasmic reticulum likely buffers some of the calcium that enter the cell during step calcium increases and that the sodium effect in the absence of caffeine is not due to an effect on the amount of calcium released by the SR rather than an effect on calcium influx. The change in resting force accompanying the calcium step, as shown in Figure 2, was exaggerated in the presence of ouabain and zero potassium, two interventions which would raise cellular sodium, in the presence of constant external sodium concentration. These results indicate that calcium influx resulting from a step increase in external calcium vary with conditions that alter intracellular sodium prior to the calcium step, i.e. the greater the cellular sodium loading, the greater the calcium influx. This sodium dependence would not be expected on the basis of calcium influx via a passive leak since the trans-sarcolemmal calcium gradient would not be altered in a manner so as to increase calcium gain nor as a competition between sodium and calcium at the cell surface since if such were the case, a step increase in external calcium in the presence of **reduced** external sodium would be expected to result in an exaggerated calcium influx. These results could also not be explained on the basis of a change in resting membrane potential since calcium steps per se and the ranges of external sodium employed would not be expected to vary the steady state membrane potential. The most reasonable interpretation of these results is that, in unstimulated rat cardiac muscle, increases in extracellular calcium result in increased cellular calcium levels via a coupled exchange with intracellular sodium and that the greater the cellular sodium at the time of the step increase in extracellular calcium, the greater will be the resultant calcium influx.

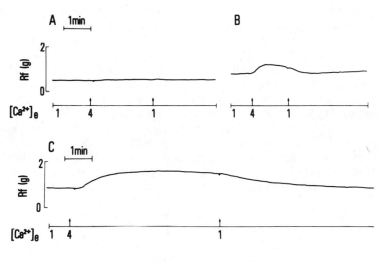

Figure 2

An example of the effect of potassium free perfusate and ouabain
on the change in resting force in response to an increase in
perfusate calcium from 1 to 4 mM. In Panel A, perfusate
potassium = 4.2 mM and ouabain is absent. Note that the change
in perfusate calcium from 1 to 4 mM does not appear to cause an
appreciable change in resting force because the sensitivity of
the recording apparatus is too low. In contrast to this note
that in panel B, after the muscle had been equilibrated in
potassium free perfusate and in panel C, when 1 mM ouabain had
been added prior to the increase in perfusate calcium, the change
in resting force is of substantially greater magnitude when the
calcium step is made. Redrawn from Walford et al (5).

The second area which will be discussed is the role of interventions which alter cellular sodium on myocardial recovery during reperfusion following an ischemic period (6). These experiments were prompted by several prior reports. Jennings and his co-workers were probably the first to report massive calcium gain following reperfusion of ischemic myocardium (12). Calcium overload of cells and mitochondria is a process which requires respiratory energy but which can also impair mitochondrial production of ATP (13). As early as 1962 it was reported that isolated kidney mitochondria could actively accumulate substantial amounts of calcium in a respiratory dependent process (14). Massive calcium loading required respiratory energy, ATP, magnesium, and inorganic phosphate. On the basis of similarities noted between the processes of oxidative phosphorylation and calcium transport, competition between the two has been investigated (15). It was shown that upon the simultaneous pulsed addition of ADP and calcium, calcium transport preceeded ADP phosphorylation and that it was only after calcium accumulation occurred that ADP phosphorylation began. This apparent domination of calcium translocation over oxidative phosphorylation has been reported for mitochondria isolated from numerous tissues (16).

The mechanism for the massive calcium loading which occurs during reperfusion is not fully understood. There is considerable evidence to suggest that the calcium gain does not occur via non-specific entry through sarcolemmal damage. This is supported by studies demonstrating an unimpaired ability to exclude barium at the same time the calcium gain is occurring (17). In addition, the inability of quiescence (18) or the calcium channel blockers verapamil (18) or nifedipine (19) to prevent calcium gain or improve functional recovery during reperfusion argues against calcium influx via the time and voltage dependent so called "slow" channel.

Another major source of calcium influx is via the above described sodium-calcium exchange mechanism (3,4). Under conditions of depleted cellular ATP, including ischemia, cellular sodium rises (20). This is likely due to increased membrane leakiness in the presence of a large electrochemical gradient favoring sodium entry and decreased activity of the ATP dependent Na-K-ATPase pump. Although cellular sodium rises, there are several factors during ischemia which would tend to inhibit sodium dependent calcium entry and mitochondrial calcium uptake. Two of the most important are the intracellular acidosis, which inhibits sodium-calcium exchange (21), and the lack of energy, which is required for mitohondrial calcium uptake (13). In addition free myoplasmic calcium levels might be elevated by mitochondrial calcium loss induced by increased extra-mitochondrial sodium and hydrogen ions and the lessened attachment of calcium to myofibrils associated with intracellular acidosis (22-24). Upon reperfusion, these conditions are reversed and in particular oxygen is restored enabling the production of ATP and pH is returned to normal. Under these conditions, the intracellular sodium might be expected to prompt a calcium gain coupled with sodium loss. If such occurred, the cellular and mitochondrial calcium gain would be expected to impair metabolic recovery and cause contracture. This might result in sarcolemmal disruption and increased cellular calcium entry because of movement down its electro-chemical gradient.

If sodium gain during ischemia mediates in part calcium gain during reperfusion which in turn impaired functional and metabolic recovery, interventions which would be expected to modify the sodium gain would also alter recovery during reperfusion. The next series of experiments examined this hypothesis (6). Hearts were removed from anesthetized, heparinized New Zealand white rabbits and mounted as shown in Figure 3 in an isovolumic

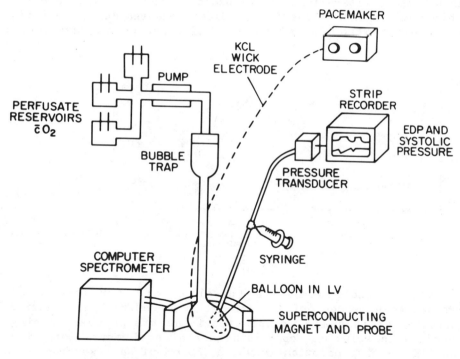

Figure 3

Experimental preparation which allows the simultaneous and continuous measurement of isovolumic left ventricular pressure and high energy phosphates via 31-phosphorous nuclear magnetic resonance.

preparation. This preparation allows simultaneous and continuous monitoring of left ventricular pressure and high energy phosphates, the latter via 31- phosphorous NMR (25). During the pre-ischemic control period, as well as during 60 minutes of reperfusion, all hearts were perfused at 28 ml/minute with oxygenated modified HEPES buffer at pH 7.4 and 37°C containing in mM: Na = 142, Ca = 2.0, Mg = 1.2, Cl = 149.4, K = 3.0, PO_4 = 2.0, and glucose = 5.0. During 60 minutes of ischemia, the flow was reduced to 0.1 ml/minute in all hearts. In Group 1 hearts (n = 9) no change was made in perfusate composition. Group 2 hearts (n = 9) were exposed during ischemia only to perfusate in which 120 mM of sodium had been replaced with lithium and a third group of hearts (n = 9) were exposed to perfusate containing no potassium.

Control values for mean developed pressure, end diastolic pressure and planimeterd areas of ATP and PCr did not differ among the three groups. The changes in high energy phosphates during the 60 minutes of ischemia are shown in Figure 4 and did not differ among the three groups. In addition, the fall in systolic pressure and rise in end diastolic pressure also did not differ. Although these alterations in perfusate composition had no effect on biochemical and mechanical indices measured during ischemia, they significantly altered recovery of these parameters during

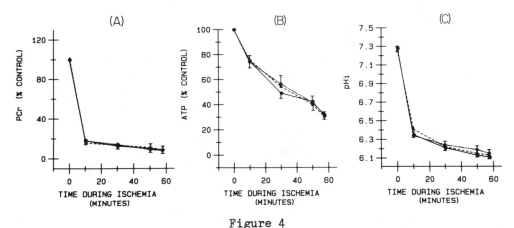

Figure 4

The fall in phosphocreatine (panel A) and ATP (panel B), expressed as a percent of the pre-ischemic control value during 60 minutes of ischemia are plotted in hearts perfused during ischemia with solution containing normal sodium and potassium (Group 1■——■), solution in which 120 mM of NaCl was replaced by 120 mM of LiCl (Group 2▲— — —▲), and solution containing no potassium (Group 3◆-- --◆). There is no statistically significant difference among any of the groups for each of the measured indices. Redrawn from Renlund et al (6).

608

reperfusion as is shown in Figure 5. Hearts perfused during
ischemia with solution in which 120 mM of sodium was replaced by
lithium (Group 2) exhibited the best recovery of PCr, ATP, and
developed pressure, and the lowest end diastolic pressure. Those
perfused with normal sodium and potassium during ischemia showed
intermediate recovery values and those perfused with zero
potassium during ischemia showed the poorest recovery of high

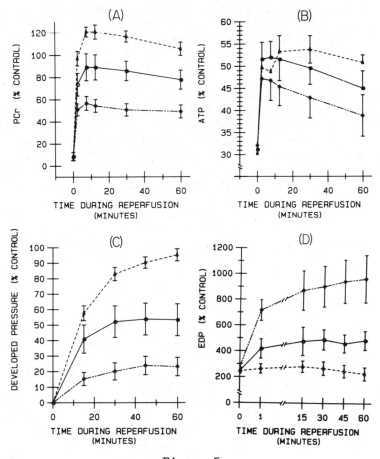

Figure 5

Effect of perfusate solution during ischemia on phosphocreatine
(panal A), ATP (panel B), developed pressure (panel C) and end
diastolic pressure (panel D) during 60 minutes of reperfusion
plotted as a percent of control. The symbols for each group
correspond to those depicted in Figure 4. The overall test of
difference among the groups for developed pressure,
phosphocreatine and end diastolic pressure is significant at the
p < .04 level. Redrawn from Renlund et al (6).

energy phosphates and developed pressure and the highest end diastolic pressure. It is likely that these interventions exerted their effect by altering the trans-sarcolemmal sodium gradient at the end of the ischemic period so as to lessen or reverse a sodium dependent calcium influx. This may have been accomplished by lowering cell sodium during ischemia and then exposing the cells to a higher extracellular sodium at the item of reperfusion.

The influence of altered sodium gradients on calcium loading was investigated more directly in another example of massive calcium overload, the calcium paradox model. This occurs when perfusion with calcium containing solution following a transient exposure to calcium-free perfusate results in massive calcium loading and cell death (26). Sodium gain occurs during calcium free perfusate in cardiac muscle (27,28) and disaggregated cardiac cells (29). Sodium-calcium exchange cannot occur, however, since extracellular calcium is not present. At the time of reintroduction of calcium, however, sodium-calcium exchange could be responsible for bringing in large amounts of cellular calcium which could result in mitochondrial calcium overload and contracture with sarcolemmal disruption. Unlike the ischemic model, it is possible to measure cellular sodium and calcium under control conditions, at the time of hypothesized sodium gain, i.e. at the end of the period of calcium free perfusion, and following the reintroduction of calcium. We therefore conducted experiments during which sodium gain during the calcium free period was varied by lithium substitution and the use of ouabain and measured the effect of these interventions on ionic contents before and after the re-introduction of calcium (7).

In these experiments the rabbit interventricular septal preparation was used. The septa were cannulated and then perfused with HEPES buffer at 30 $^{\circ}$C containing in mM NaCl = 140, KCl = 4.4, $MgCl_2$ = 1.2, $CaCl_2$ = 1.0, KCoEDTA = 1.0, and glucose = 10. The septa were paced at a rate of 60 beats per minute. Following equilibration, they were perfused with calcium free solution for 30 minutes and then calcium was re-introduced for a period of 30 minutes. In control septa, no modification of the perfusate was made, other than the removal of calcium during calcium free perfusion. In a second group of septa, ouabain was added at a concentration of 5×10^{-5} M 10 minutes after the onset of the calcium free period and remained present for the duration of the experiment. In the third group, perfusate sodium was lowered to 46.7 mM via lithium substitution at the onset of the calcium free period and restored to normal at the time of the reintroduction of calcium. In each of these groups, certain septa were removed and analyzed for ionic content via atomic absorption, at different periods in the protocol. Using cobalt as a marker for the extracellular space (30), cellular ionic contents could be calculated.

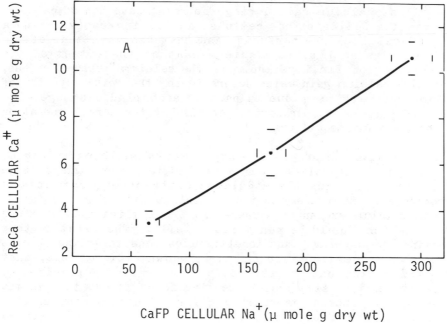

CaFP CELLULAR Na$^+$(μ mole g dry wt)

Figure 6

Cell calcium contents following calcium re-introduction (ReCa) expressed as a function of cell sodium at the end of the calcium free period (CaFP). Redrawn from Ruano-Arroyo et al (7).

Cellular sodium and calcium contents in the three groups are presented in Figure 6. Mean cell sodium rose 124% during calcium free perfusate with normal sodium. Note that the intended gradation was achieved. In the group perfused with low sodium, mean cellular sodium was only 47% of control but in the ouabain group rose to 214% of control values.Calcium gain following the reintroduction of calcium varied with the cellular sodium content at that time. Calcium gain was highest in the group which had been exposed to ouabain, 10.6 ± 0.7 u mol/g dry weight, intermediate in the group exposed to normal sodium, 6.5 ± 1.0 u mol/g dry weight, and lowest in the group perfused with low sodium containing solution, 3.4 ±0.5 u mol/g dry weight. Thus in the high sodium group, a 152% gain in cellular calcium above control was found, in the regular sodium group a 55% increase in calcium above control occurred while in the low sodium group, there was no calcium gain. Similar gradations were found in the extent of contractile recovery with the best recovery occurring in the group perfused with low sodium during the calcium free period which had the smallest calcium gain during the reintroduction of calcium. These results indicate that cellular sodium increases during a period of calcium free perfusion and that the magnitude of the sodium gain is an important determinant of the extent of the constellation of findings known as the calcium "paradox." Thus, the massive calcium gain which occurs during the reintroduction of calcium is likely to be due in part to a coupled exchange with sodium and thus not be paradoxical at all but the normal operation of a thermodynamic equilibrium.

In summary, although these experiments employed different species, models, techniques, and methodologies, they all indicate that sodium significantly modulates contractile properties and metabolic parameters in a fashion consistent with the function of a sodium calcium exchanger. There are two implications of these findings which should be mentioned briefly. The first is that these findings may have functional implications regarding species differences in cardiac muscle. It is known, for example, that higher concentrations of extracellular calcium are required to produce a change in steady state resting force in cat than in rat cardiac muscle. Indeed, there is a gradation across many species (31) despite the fact that force-calcium curves of skinned preparations are similar among species (32). Some species variation therefore, may be due to a variation in cellular calcium content due to species variations in cellular sodium or sodium-calcium exchange. The second implication of these findings is that they may provide a further mechanism of ischemic damage. To date, most interventions to reduce ischemic damage have focused on preserving high energy phosphates and intracellular pH during the ischemic period itself (33). These results suggest that another accompaniment of ischemia, i.e. the rise in cellular sodium, may also contribute to impaired recovery during reperfusion and suggest that interventions to reduce the sodium gain during ischemia, or the calcium gain at the time of reperfusion, may also improve functional and metabolic recovery following an ischemic period. Although ion selective electrodes would allow the measurement of sodium activity, direct measurements of cellular sodium and calcium during ischemia using the methods described above are not feasible since they are dependent on an equilibration between the perfusate and the extracellular space. It may be possible to further test these hypotheses in the hypoxia-reoxygenation model.

ACKNOWLEDGEMENT

The authors would like to acknowledge Elsie Beard for excellent statistical assistance.

REFERENCES

1. Ringer, S: A further contribution regarding the influence of
    the different constituents of the blood on the contractililty
    of the heart.   J Physiol (London) 4:29-42, 1882.

2. Katz AM, Reuter H: Cellular calcium and cardiac cell death.
    Am J Cardiol 44:188-190, 1979.

3. Langer GA: Sodium-calcium exchange in the heart.   Ann Rev
    Physiol 44:435-449, 1982.

4. Mullins LJ: The generation of electric currents in cardiac
    fibers by Na/Ca exchange.   Am J Physiol 236:C103-110, 1979.

5. Walford GD, Gerstenblith G, Lakatta EG: Na$^+$ modulation of
    Ca^{2+}-dependent resting force of isolated rat cardiac muscle
    (In Press).

6. Renlund DG, Gerstenblith G, Lakatta EG, Jacobus WE, Kallman
    CH, Weisfeldt ML: Perfusate sodium during ischemia modifies
    post ischemic functional and metabolic recovery in the rabbit
    heart.   J Mol Cel Cardiol (In Press).

7. Ruano-Arroyo G, Gerstenblith G, Lakatta EG: "Calcium
    Paradox" in the heart is modulated by cellular Na during the
    Ca-free period.   J Mol Cel Cardiol (In press).

8. Ellis D: The effeects of external cations and ouabain on the
    intracellular sodium activity of sheep heart Purkinje fibers.
    J Physiol (London) 273:214-240, 1977.

9. Eisner DA, Lederer WJ, Vaughn-Jones RD: The dependence of
    sodium pumping and tension on the intracellular sodium
    activity in voltage-clamped sheep Purkinje fibers.   J Physiol
    (London) 317:163-187, 1981.

10. Ellis D and Deitmer JW: The relationship between the intra
    and extracellular sodium activity of sheep heart Purkinje
    fibers during inhibition of the Na-K pump.   Pfluegers Arch
    377:209-215, 1978.

11. Stern MD, Kort AA, Bhatnagar GM, Lakatta EG: Scattered-light
    intensity fluctuations in diastolic rat cardiac muscle caused
    by spontaneous Ca^{++}- dependent cellular mechanical
    oscillations.   J Gen Physiol 82:119-153, 1983.

12. Shen AC and Jennings RB: Kinetics of calcium accumulation in acute myocardial ischemic injury. Am J Pathol 67:441-452, 1972.

13. Chance B: The energy-linked reaction of calcium with mitochondria. J Biol Chem 240:2729-2748, 1965.

14. Vasington FD and Murphy JV: Ca^{++} uptake by rat kidney mitochondria and its dependence on respiration and phosphorylation. J Biol Chem 237:2670-2677, 1962.

15. Rossi CS and Lehninger AL: Stoichiometry of respiratory stimulation, accumulation of Ca^{++} and phosphate, and oxidative phosphorylation in rat liver mitochondria. J Biol Chem 239:3971-3980, 1964.

16. Carafoli E and Lehninger AL: A survey of the interaction of calcium ions with mitochondria from different tissues and species. Biochem J 122:681-690, 1971.

17. Shine KI, Douglas AM, Ricchiuti NV: Calcium, strontium and barium movements during ischemia and reperfusion in right ventricle: Impllications for myocardial preservation. Circ Res 43:712-720, 1978.

18. Bourdillon PDV and Poole-Wilson PA: The effects of verapamil, quiescence, and cardioplegia on calcium exchange and mechanical function in ischemic rabbit myocardium. Circ Res 50:360-368, 1982.

19. Henry PD, Shuchleib R, Davis J, Weiss SE, Sobel BE: Myocardial contracture and accumulation of mitochondrial calcium in ischemic rabbit heart. Am J Physiol 233:H677-H684, 1977.

20. Regan TJ, Broisman L, Haider B, Eaddy C, Oldewurtel HA: Dissociation of myocardial sodium and potassium alterations in mild versus severe ischemia. Am J Physiol 238:H575-580, 1980.

21. Philipson KD, Bersohn MM, Nishimoto AY: Effects of pH on Na^+-Ca^{2+} exchange in canine cardiac sarcolemmal vesicles. Circ Res 50:287, 1982.

22. Fishkum G and Lehninger AL: The mechanisms and regulation of mitochondrial calcium transport. Fed Proc 39:2432-2436, 1980.

23. Crompton M and Heid I: The cycling of calcium, sodium, and protons across the inner membrne of cardiac mitochondria. Eur J biochem 91:599-608, 1978.

24. Fabiato A and Fabiato F: Effects of pH on the myofilaments and the sarcoplasmic reticulum of skinned cells from cardiac and skeletal muscles. J Physiol (London) 276:233-255, 1978.

25. Flaherty JT, Weisfeldt ML, Bulkley BH, Gardner TJ, Gott VL, Jacobus WE: Mechanisms of ischemic myocardial cell damage assessed by phosphorous-31 nuclear magnetic resonance. Circulation 65:561-571, 1982.

26. Zimmerman ANE: Morphological changes of heart muscle caused by successive perfusion with calcium-free and calcium-containing solutions (calcium paradox). Cardiovasc Res 1:201-209, 1967.

27. Deitmer JS and Ellis D: Changes in the intracellular sodium activity of sheep heart purkinje fibres produced by calcium and other divalent cations. J Physiol (London) 277:437-453 (1978).

28. Tritthart H, MacLeod DP, Stierle HE, Krause H: Effects of Ca-free and EDTA-containing tyrode solution on transmembrane electrical activity and contraction in guinea pig papillary muscle. Pfluegers Arch 338:361-376, 1973.

29. Goshima K, Wakabayashi S, Masuda A: Ionic mechanisms of morphological changes of cultured myocardial cells on successive incubation in media without and with Ca^{2+}. J Mol Cell Cardiol 12:1125-1157, 1980.

30. Bridge JHB, Bersohn MM, Gonzales F, Bassingthwaighte JB: Synthesis and use of radio cobaltic EDTA as an extracellular marker in rabbit heart. Am J Physiol 242:H671-676, 1982.

31. Kort AA and Lakatta EG: Light scattering identifies diastolic myoplasmic Ca^{2+} oscillations in diverse mammalian cardiac tissues (Abstract). Circulation 64(4):IV-162, 1981.

32. Fabiato A and Fabiato F: Calcium-induced release of calcium from adult human, dog, cat, rabbit, and frog hearts and from fetal and new born rat ventricles. NY Acad Sci 307:491-522, 1978.

33. Maroko PR, Kjekshus JK, Sobel BE, Wantabe T, Covell JW, Ross J Jr, Braunwald E: Factors influencing infarct size following experimental coronary artery occlusions. Circulation 43:67-82, 1971.

THE EFFECT OF SHORT CHAIN FATTY ACID ADMINISTRATION ON HEPATIC

GLUCOSE, PHOSPHATE, MAGNESIUM AND CALCIUM METABOLISM

Richard L. Veech[1], William L. Gitomer[1], Michael T. King[1], Robert S. Balaban[2], Jonathan L. Costa[3], and E. David Eanes[4]

1. Laboratory of Metabolism, NIAAA, Rockville, MD, 20852
2. Laboratory of Kidney and Electrolyte Metabolism NHLBI, Bethesda, MD, 20205
3. Clinical Neuropharmacology Branch, NIMH, Bethesda, MD 20205
4. Mineralized Tissue Research Branch, NIDR, Bethesda MD, 20205

ABSTRACT

Intra peritoneal administration of the short chain fatty acids, acetate, propionate and butyrate, in amounts calculated to reach 20 mM in total body water were given to fed and 48 hour starved male Wistar rats. One half hour after administration, the livers were freeze-clamped and the hepatic contents of various intermediary metabolites were measured. The liver content of total glycolytic intermediates was elevated by short chain fatty acids. In fed animals, the portion of glycolysis from fructose 1,6-bisphosphate (FBP) to PEP was elevated 2 to 4 fold. In 48 hour starved animals, where gluconeogenesis is active, the portion of the gluconeogenetic pathway from FBP to glucose was elevated 1.5 to 3.5 fold with the exception of the butyrate treated animals where blood glucose was not elevated. The metabolites of the hexose-monophosphate pathway that were measured, namely 6-phosphogluconate, ribulose 5-phosphate and xylulose 5-phosphate were increased in both fed and starved animals. The free cytoplasmic $[NAD^+] / [NADH]$, $[NADP^+] / [NADPH]$, and $[\Sigma ATP] / [\Sigma ADP] \times [\Sigma Pi]$ ratios were all decreased in both fed and starved animals after short chain fatty acid administration. The liver content of calcium increased 1.2 to 2 fold in fed animals and 2 to 3 fold in starved animals while total liver magnesium was either unchanged or increased only 1.2 times. The liver pyrophosphate (PPi) content increased a minimum of 10 fold in fed animals and over 100 fold in starved animals. In all cases no PPi

617

could be detected in vivo by ^{31}P NMR even though in the starved rats the PPi levels approached those of ATP. The liver content of inorganic Pi increased 1.3 to 1.5 fold in fed animals and 1.5 to 2 fold in starved animals. The total "rapidly metabolizing" Pi pool, that includes adenine and guanine nucleotides, glycolytic and shunt intermediates, Pi and PPi increased 1.3 times in fed animals (from 13.8 umole/g fresh weight) and 1.5 to 1.7 fold in starved animals (from 15.7 umol/g fresh weight). The total phosphate taken up from blood and entering the rapidly turning over pool of liver phosphate ranged between 4 and 12 umols/g of liver. It is concluded that the administration of short chain fatty acids whose activation produces inorganic PPi in the cytoplasm and/or the mitochondria have a profound effect on cellular metabolism by: (a) changing the distribution of energy between the various nucleotide pools such as the free cytoplasmic [NADP+] / [NADPH] , [NAD+] / [NADH] , and [ΣATP] / [ΣADP] x [ΣPi] ratios, (b) elevating the steady state hepatic content of the metabolites of the hexosemonophosphate pathway and the glycolytic pathway, (c) altering the free cytoplasmic PPi and thus changing blood glucose concentrations according to the relation,

$$K_g = \frac{[glucose\text{-}6\text{-}P] \, [Pi]}{[glucose] \quad [PPi]} = 45.9, \text{ and}$$

(d) increasing Pi, Ca and Mg transport into the liver.

INTRODUCTION

Biochemists in the 1960s and 1970s observing the ubiquitous and highly active inorganic pyrophosphatases present in nearly all tissue homogenates concluded that inorganic pyrophosphate (PPi) simply did not exist in living cells (1, 2). More recently it has been shown that PPi will act as a phosphoryl donor in place of ATP in a number of biosynthetic reactions (3, 4). Nonetheless, there remains an indifference to the potential importance of PPi. This is particularly so among those biochemists engaged in studying the reactions involved with the synthesis of DNA and RNA where inorganic PPi is at least theoretically capable of reversing the process of nucleotide polymerization (5, 6).

In this paper we show that administration of common short chain fatty acids to the rat at a final concentration of about 20 mM resulted in the accumulation of as much as 2.5 umoles PPi/g wet weight of liver. Concomittant with this large accumulation of PPi was a large increase in the hepatic content of calcium and a small increase in the content of magnesium. It is likely that other divalent and transition metals that bind PPi strongly also increased in concentration (7, 8, 9).

This large increase in calcium is reminiscent of the effect parathyroid hormone has on liver. It has been shown that parathyroid hormone increases the bidirectional transport of calcium in rat liver (10) and into rat liver mitochondria (11, 12). In addition to its effect on calcium, parathyroid hormone has been shown to stimulate the liver to increase glucose (13) and urea (14) production. Since formation of PPi within the liver mimics the calcium and glucose effects, it raises the possibility that the effect of parathormone may be exerted by PPi itself and not simply by c-AMP. Likewise the ability of the pyrophosphate analogue ethane-1-hydroxy-1-diphosphonate to block calcitonin induced lowering of plasma inorganic Pi (15) raises another possibility that PPi plays a role in the action of this hormone since influx of Pi into the liver far in excess of that required to form PPi is one of the most striking and puzzling aspects of this study. Work by Lehninger and his collegues has established that mitochondria, in the presence of acetate or phosphate, undergo massive calcium loading (16, 17) using energy from the electron transport chain. Whether this in vitro mechanism found in isolated mitochondria accounts for these in vivo findings is currently under investigation.

A role for inorganic PPi in glucose metabolism in rat liver has previously been proposed (18) as has a role for PPi in nucleotide metabolism in the avian liver (19). In this paper we show that PPi is linked to the reduction of the free cytoplasmic [NADP+]/[NADPH] found after administration of short chain fatty acids. This effect is similar to that seen after the administration of glucagon or prolonged treatment with thyroxine (20) both treatments which are known to cause a concomittant increase in hepatic c-AMP.

Finally the effects of short chain fatty acids in raising intracellular PPi and Ca may give an explanation for the diverse effects butyrate has on gene expression and cell morphology in certain cell lines (21, 22). While it is true that butyrate inhibits the acetylation of nuclear histones, acetylation fails to adequately explain all the effects observed after butyrate treatment (23). Clearly changes in PPi and Ca might be expected to effect not only nucleotide metabolism, but also the intracellular proteins that alter cell shape during "detransformation".

MATERIALS AND METHODS

Male Wistar rats (220-290 g body wt) were purchased from Charles River Labs (Wilmington, MA) and received food (NIH stock diet) and water ad lib. For starved animals, food was removed 48 h before sacrifice.

Butyric acid was purchased from Sigma Chemical Co. (St. Louis, MO). Acetic acid was purchased from J. T. Baker Chemical Co. (Phillipsburg, N.J.). Commercially available enzymes were obtained from Boehringer-Mannheim (Indianapolis, IN). All other materials were reagent grade or better and obtained from commercial sources.

Rats were injected intraperitoneally with 1.0 ml/100 g body wt sodium acetate (2.0 M, pH 7.4), sodium propionate (2.0 M, pH 7.4), sodium butyrate (2.0 M, pH 7.4) or physiological saline. The rats were sacrificed 30 min after injection by cervical dislocation and the livers were removed and rapidly frozen by clamping between aluminum discs pre-cooled in liquid nitrogen (24). The frozen tissue was ground under liquid nitrogen and stored at $-90^{o}C$ until use. Perchloric acid extracts were prepared as in (25).

The measurement of adenine and guanine nucleotides and the determination of IMP was done using a Waters High Performance Liquid Chromatograph (HPLC) (26). The values of total ADP are somewhat lower with the HPLC method since the enzymatic method also measures GDP. All other metabolites were measured using standard enzymatic assays as described previously (25) with the exception of inorganic PPi which was also measured enzymatically (27).

The near-equilibrium reactions used to calculate the redox states, phosphorylation potential and various free metabolite concentrations are given in Table I.

All NMR spectra were collected using a Nicolet 360WB spectrometer detecting ^{31}P at 146 MHz. The spectra of the neutralized PCA extracts of the liver were collected using 12 mm NMR tubes in a standard Nicolet NMR probe. The in vivo experiments were performed by placing an anesthetized animal, phenobarbital 50mg/kg, in a custom designed animal cradle and placing a surface coil (28) (two turn coil 1.25 cm in diameter) over the liver after it had been surgically exposed as described earlier (29). After injecting the starved rats with butyrate the animals fell into a deep "sleep". Thus, in several experiments we took advantage of this condition to collect spectra on non-anesthetized rats to avoid the effects of anesthesia on the generation of pyrophosphate. The ^{31}P NMR spectra of the liver were obtained without surgery by increasing the pulse width on the surface coil placed on the skin over the liver to in excess of 70 usec. As described earlier (30) this resulted in the saturation of the muscle and skin layer resulting in most of the signal originating from the liver, indicated by a large decrease in creatine phosphate. Due to the geometry and size of the liver the added focusing by topical magnetic resonance required for studies on the kidney (30) were not required in these studies.

Table 1. Near-Equilibrium Reactions Used to Calculate Redox-States, Phosphorylation States and Free Metabolite Levels in Various Tissue Compartments.

Values are for $T = 38°$, $I = 0.25$ and free $[Mg^{2+}]$ as specified.

Calculation of Free Nucleotide Ratios   Reference

(1) Cytoplasmic free $[NAD^+] / [NADH]$

$$K_{LDH} = \frac{[pyruvate][NADH][H^+]}{[lactate][NAD^+]} = 1.11 \times 10^{-11}M \qquad (32)$$

(2) Mitochondrial free $[NAD^+]/[NADH]$

$$K_{HBDH} = \frac{[acetoacetate][NADH][H^+]}{[\beta\text{-hydroxybutyrate}][NAD^+]} = 4.93 \times 10^{-9}M \qquad (32)$$

(3) Cytoplasmic $[NADP^+] / [NADPH]$

$$K_{ICDH} = \frac{[\alpha\text{-ketoglutarate}^{-2}][CO_2][NADPH]}{[isocitrate^{-3}][NADP^+]} = 1.17M \qquad (33)$$

(4)

$$K_{6PGDH} = \frac{[ribulose\ 5\text{-}P^{-2}][CO_2][NADPH]}{[6\text{-phosphogluconate}^{-3}][NADP^+]} = 1.72 \times 10^{-1}M \qquad (33)$$

(5) Cytoplasmic free $\dfrac{[\Sigma ATP]}{[\Sigma ADP][Pi]}$

$$\frac{K_{G+G}}{K_{LDH}} = \frac{[3PG][\Sigma ATP][lactate]}{([DHAP]/22)[\Sigma ADP][Pi][pyruvate]} = 1.65 \times 10^7\ M^{-1} \qquad (25)$$

free $[Mg^{2+}]$ = 1mM

Calculation of free cytoplasmic metabolite concentrations

(6) Free cytoplasmic $[GAP]$

$$[GAP] = \frac{[measured\ DHAP]}{K_{TPI}} \qquad (34)$$

where $K_{TP1} = \dfrac{[DHAP]}{[GAP]} = 22$

Table 1 (Continued)

(7) Free cytoplasmic [Fl,6BP]

$$[Fl,6BP] = \frac{[\text{measured DHAP}]^2}{0.99 \times 10^{-4}M \times 22} \qquad (34)$$

(8) Free cytoplasmic [PPi]

$$[PPi] = \frac{1}{K_{UDPG-PP_iase}} \quad \frac{[\text{measured UTP}][\text{measured G1P}]}{[\text{measured UDPG}]} \qquad (18)$$

where $K_{UDPG-PPiase}$ = 4.5

The determination of Ca_2PPi and Mg_2PPi solubility products was performed in closed polypropylene vessels at 37 $\pm$ 0.1°C. Precipitations were initiated by adding rapidly, with stirring, 30 ml solutions containing twice the cation concentrations required to equal volumes of solutions containing twice the required phosphate concentrations as well as 50 mM $NaHCO_3$. The ionic strength of all solutions was adjusted to 0.25 M with NaCl and KCl (Na/K = 0.77) prior to addition. Precipitation commenced immediately following mixing of the reactants. The suspensions were stirred continuously under 5% CO_2/95% air, and the pH was maintained at 7.40 $\pm$ 0.01 with 0.07 N HCl by means of a pH-stat. The solution concentrations were chosen in order that analytically measurable levels of all reactants remained in solution after precipitation. The data reported herein are from experiments which were terminated at 30 minutes. This reaction time was chosen to facilitate comparison with the in vivo results obtained in this paper. With the exception of the precipitations which contain Mg^{2+} as the only divalent cation, solid/solution equilibration was apparently reached by this time, since extending the reaction to 90 minutes did not change solution reactant levels. In addition, these levels were rapidly restored in 30 minute old Ca_2 PPi suspensions diluted 1:2 or 1:5 with NaCl/KCl solutions (u = 0.25 M). Incongruent dissolution of the solids made it impractical, however, to assess solution stability in the other precipitation reactions by this dilution/reequilibration method. At the completion of each reaction, portions of the suspension were filtered rapidly through 0.22 um cellulose membrane filters. Residues were washed briefly with ammoniated water (pH 10) and lyophilized. Both filtrates and solids were analyzed for Ca, Mg, Pi and PPi. Solids were also analyzed for Na and K. Pi and PPi were analyzed colorimetrically by the method of Putnins and Yamata (31). Ca, Mg, Na, and K were determined using a Perkin Elmer atomic absorption spectrometer model 603.

RESULTS AND DISCUSSION

Activation of Short Chain Fatty Acids

The pathways of the activation of the three free fatty acids given are shown in figure 1. On the basis of in vitro studies of the subcellular localization of acetyl CoA synthetase (EC 6.3.1.1), it was predicted that 80-90% of the acetate would be activated in the cytoplasm with only 10-20% activated within the mitochondria. With propionate 40% would be predicted to be activated in the cytoplasm and 60% in the mitochondria (36). Butyryl-CoA synthetase (EC 6.2.1.2) acts on C-4 to C-11 chain length fatty acids and is localized entirely within the mitochondrial matrix (37). Except for the small fraction of butyrate activated by acetyl CoA synthetase, due to the lack of absolute substrate specificity of this enzyme, it would be expected that all the butyrate would be activated in the mitochondrial matrix and thus all of the PPi formed during butyrate activation would also be formed in the mitochondrial matrix.

While the scheme presented in figure 1 would appear reasonable, analysis of the short chain acyl CoA's in liver under these conditions suggests that such a proposal may not be entirely correct since succinyl CoA, a metabolite localized exclusively in the mitochondria, decreases in propionate and butyrate treated fed animals but does not change in the starved animals given butyrate (Table 2). Furthermore, the free CoA fails to decrease with butyrate treatment. It, therefore, would seem that the activation scheme proposed should be viewed as tentative pending further work.

The Intermediates of Glycolysis and Gluconeogenesis

Table 3 gives the results of the enzymatic analysis of the hepatic metabolites after short chain fatty acid administration to ad lib fed rats. The summary of results is presented in the proportionate change diagram given in figure 2a. It can be seen that short chain fatty acids have very small effects on the amount of glycolytic intermediates after dihydroxyacetone phosphate (DHAP). In the glycolytic pathway prior to DHAP there is essentially a two fold elevation of all metabolites from fructose-1,6-bisphosphate (FBP) to glucose. It should, however, be remembered that the measured FBP is a relatively meaningless number since the bulk of the FBP measured is bound.

Table 4 gives the results of the enzymatic analysis of hepatic metabolites after short chain fatty acid administration to 48 h starved rats. It should be noted that malate, citrate, and glucose are elevated only in the propionate and acetate treated group where presumably inorganic PPi is being generated in both the cytoplasm and the mitochondria. The complete set of gluconeogenic metabolites

PATHWAYS OF ACETATE, PROPIONATE AND BUTYRATE METABOLISM

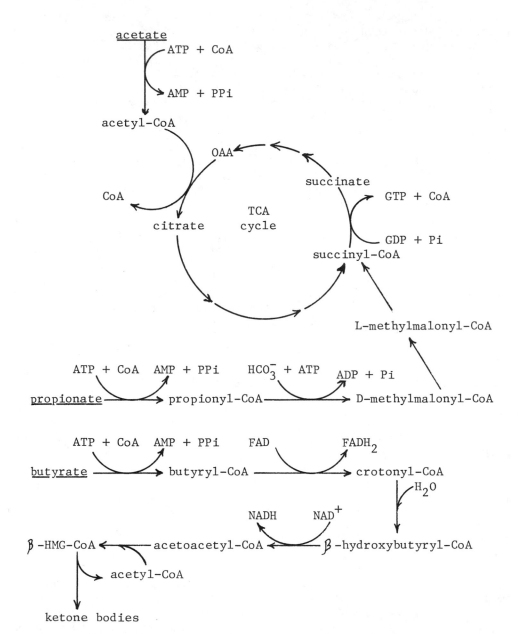

Figure 1. The pathways of short chain fatty acid metabolism in rat liver. The transport of the cytosolically formed acetyl-CoA and propionyl-CoA into the mitochondria via the acetyl-carnitine transferase carrier is omitted for clarity.

Table 2. Effect of Short Chain Fatty Acid Administration of the
Level of Soluble Acyl-CoAs.

Values are given as means $\pm$ S.E.M. in nmol/gm wet weight.

Ad lib FED	Saline (n=6)	Acetate (n=6)	Propionate (n=4)	Butyrate (n=4)
Malonyl	10.92 $\pm$ 2.09	23.58 $\pm$ 4.18	14.43 $\pm$ 0.81	---
Free	50.02 $\pm$ 3.40	60.77 $\pm$ 5.43	19.23 $\pm$ 1.81	54.4 $\pm$ 4.06
Me Malonyl	9.59 $\pm$ 0.88	9.90 $\pm$ 1.57	102 $\pm$ 4	---
Succinyl	32.75 $\pm$ 1.79	20.27 $\pm$ 1.38	4.61 $\pm$ 1.31	5.35 $\pm$ 0.97
HMG	4.07 $\pm$ 0.48	4.50 $\pm$ 0.44	1.94 $\pm$ 0.20	1.79 $\pm$ 0.19
Acetyl	26.92 $\pm$ 1.68	30.80 $\pm$ 1.57	10.45 $\pm$ 1.00	26.87 $\pm$ 1.92
Propionyl	---	---	75.00 $\pm$ 7.47	1.70 $\pm$ 0.13
Crotonyl	---	---	---	1.56 $\pm$ 0.17
Butyryl	---	---	---	18.57 $\pm$ 1.39

48 Hour Starved	(n=5)	(n=5)	(n=4)	(n=5)
Malonyl	13.98 $\pm$ 1.66	20.08 $\pm$ 1.53	20.05 $\pm$ 1.86	22.72 $\pm$ 3.32
Free	75.72 $\pm$ 8.98	98.84 $\pm$ 6.03	38.58 $\pm$ 2.78	82.14 $\pm$ 4.61
Me Malonyl	9.8 $\pm$ 2.0	13.4 $\pm$ 1.6	89.80 $\pm$ 11.92	12.4 $\pm$ 1.7
Succinyl	25.92 $\pm$ 3.80	28.36 $\pm$ 3.02	13.68 $\pm$ 1.40	28.80 $\pm$ 3.68
HMG	2.70 $\pm$ 0.06	2.57	1.2 $\pm$ 0.3	2.19 $\pm$ 0.14
Acetyl	56.46 $\pm$ 4.34	70.34 $\pm$ 6.41	26.70 $\pm$ 0.60	78.08 $\pm$ 4.42
Propionyl	---	---	136 $\pm$ 11	---
Crotonyl	---	---	---	17.46 $\pm$ 0.86
Butyryl	---	---	---	48.06 $\pm$ 8.19

Table 3. Measured Metabolites of Freeze-Clamped Liver from Ad Lib
Fed Rats.

Values are given as mean $\pm$ S.E.M. in nmol/gm wet weight. A *
indicates a significant difference from saline value at $P < 0.02$ as
judged by the Students T-test.

	Saline	Acetate	Propionate	Butyrate
n	5	6	8	6
10^{-3} x glucose	8.40$\pm$.27	13.77*$\pm$.70	17.86*$\pm$.67	14.10*$\pm$.63
glucose-6-P	149$\pm$12	386*$\pm$27	527*$\pm$38	442*$\pm$29
glucose-1-P	12$\pm$1	26*$\pm$2	34*$\pm$3	26*$\pm$2
fructose-6-P	51$\pm$4	106*$\pm$7	144*$\pm$11	112*$\pm$9
fructose-1,6-bis-P	5.5$\pm$.7	12.3$\pm$3.2	10.9*$\pm$.8	11.5*$\pm$1.1
DHAP	46$\pm$3	53$\pm$5	51$\pm$3	51$\pm$5
3-phospho-glycerate	294$\pm$15	405$\pm$27	474*$\pm$19	315$\pm$21
PEP	135$\pm$7	181$\pm$15	222*$\pm$6	140$\pm$12
pyruvate	158$\pm$13	98*$\pm$9	170$\pm$15	61*$\pm$3
L-lactate	727$\pm$36	743$\pm$70	1287*$\pm$125	767$\pm$72
L-malate	252$\pm$21	961*$\pm$41	421*$\pm$25	830*$\pm$90
α-keto-glutarate	269$\pm$14	305$\pm$39	173*$\pm$24	242$\pm$8
isocitrate	26$\pm$2	81*$\pm$1	30$\pm$2	82*$\pm$3
citrate	300$\pm$17	1573*$\pm$44	397*$\pm$27	1625*$\pm$103
acetoacetate	100$\pm$19	117$\pm$8	261*$\pm$9	1578*$\pm$102
β-hydroxy-butyrate	117$\pm$20	151*$\pm$12	223*$\pm$15	1429*$\pm$72
UDP-glucose	768$\pm$58	616$\pm$19	599$\pm$33	614$\pm$46
UTP	543$\pm$82	364$\pm$34	379$\pm$30	392$\pm$41

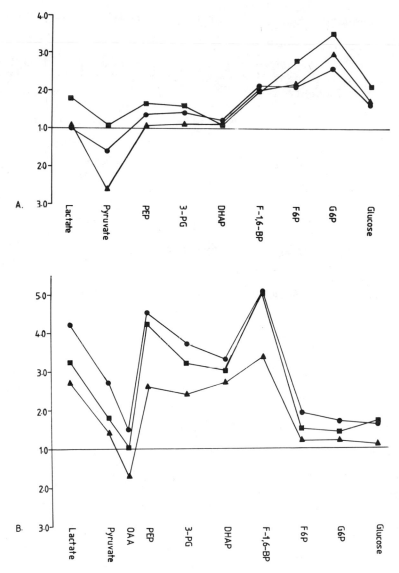

Figure 2.   Relative change diagram of A. glycolytic metabolites from
ad lib fed rats and B. gluconeogenic metabolites from 48
hour starved rats.   Both fed and starved rats were
treated with ● acetate, ■ propionate or ▲ butyrate.

is presented in the proportionate change diagram given in figure 2b.
There it can be seen that in starved rats given acetate or
propionate the end portion of gluconeogenesis from fructose-6-

Table 4. Measured Metabolites of Freeze-Clamped Liver From 48 Hour
Starved Rats.

Values are given as mean $\pm$ S.E.M. in   nmol/gm wet weight.   A *
indicates a significant difference from saline value at $P < 0.05$ as
judged by the Students T-test.

n	Saline 13	Acetate 10	Propionate 10	Butyrate 10
10^{-3} x glucose	4.81+.21	7.94*+.42	8.30*+.43	5.45+.33
glucose-6-P	59+2	99*+10	84*+9	70*+7
glucose-1-P	7+1	11*+1	9*+1	8+1
fructose-6-P	17+1	32*+3	25+4	20+2
fructose-1,6-bis-P	4.6+.4	23*+6	23*+3	20+4
DHAP	11+1	36*+4	33*+1	30*+3
3-phospho-glycerate	156+14	581*+62	497*+36	372*+32
PEP	73+5	330*+40	305*+29	190*+19
pyruvate	10+1	27*+6	18*+2	14+2
L-lactate	171+17	721+208	554*+35	456*+71
L-malate	268+28	592*+84	532*+44	274+21
α-keto-glutarate	118+13	86+17	49*+5	79+10
isocitrate	17+2	41*+3	23+2	21+2
citrate	308+42	944*+85	458*+33	385+27
acetoacetate	638+33	643+66	704+55	2631*+201
β-hydroxy-butyrate	1643+75	983*+83	945*+44	2098*+152
UDP-glucose	350+15	367+25	431*+19	365+22
UTP	205+9	186+8	181+11	187+14

phosphate (F6P) to glucose is elevated. Butyrate however did not elevate F6P, glucose-6-phosphate (G6P), glucose 1-phosphate or glucose to nearly as great an extent as did acetate or propionate. In the initial portion of gluconeogenesis, the metabolites from phosphoendpyruvate (PEP) to FBP are elevated in all groups treated with short chain fatty acids. This pattern of elevation of this portion of glycolysis is the classic pattern seen with glucagon or other hormones that stimulate c-AMP formation (20). Butyrate, however, differs from acetate, propionate or glucagon by not elevating glucose in the starved animal.

Currently, it is widely held that the elevation of PEP following glucagon treatment of the starved animal is a result of the "slowing" of the "futile cycling" of PEP and pyruvate (38, 39). Such evidence based on isotopic data, fails to consider the possibility of the existence of pyrophosphate phosphotransferase reactions that might indeed cause cycling of isotopic label, but that would not be futile in the sense of being energy wasteful. This is so since the PPi would be conserved during cycling between OAA and PEP. Since a PPi dependent PEP carboxykinase (PEPCK) (EC 4.1.1.38) is known to exist in lower organisms, the elevation of PEP under the conditions of increased PPi reported here make such an enzyme, or more likely a variant of such an enzyme, an intriguing possibility. The other possibility is that short chain fatty acid "activates" the enzyme PEPCK (EC 4.1.1.32). In data not shown, there is no evidence for a change in the GTP/GDP x Pi ratio to account for this. No activators of the GTP dependent PEPCK are known although recent workers have expressed doubt that the acute regulation of PEPCK activity is fully understood (40).

The changes in the steady state levels of metabolites between PEP and FBP reflect changes in the cytoplasmic $[NAD^+]/[NADH]$ and cytoplasmic $[\Sigma ATP]/[\Sigma ADP] \times [\Sigma Pi]$ ratios as well as each other (25). As figure 2b and Table 5 show, once the PEP level is elevated in starved animals given short chain fatty acids, the steady state levels of 3-phosphoglycerate (3-PG), DHAP and FBP must also increase since there is no net change in $[NADH]/[NAD^+] \times [\Sigma ATP]/[\Sigma ADP] \times [\Sigma Pi]$. Thus the primary change in the gluconeogenic state must occur in the step converting oxaloacetate to PEP.

The values of the free phosphorylation and redox states of fed and starved animals are given in Table 5. In fed animals, short chain fatty acids cause a decrease in the free cytoplasmic $[NAD^+]/[NADH]$ ratio since the redox state of the fatty acids being metabolized in the treated group is more reduced than the carbohydrate the fed control animal is metabolizing. In the starved animal that is already metabolizing free fatty acid and making glucose, the decrease in free cytoplasmic $[NAD^+]/[NADH]$ ratio is not as great or as consistent since the control animals liver is already

Table 5.   Free Nucleotide Ratios in Freeze-Clamped Liver From Ad Lib Fed and 48 Hour Starved Rats.

Values are given as mean $\pm$ S.E.M.   A * indicates a significant difference from control value at P < 0.02 as judged by Students T-test.

FED (n)	Saline (5)	Acetate (6)	Propionate (8)	Butyrate (6)
cytoplasmic				
$\dfrac{[NAD^+]}{[NADH]}$	1944$\pm$94	1209*$\pm$88	1235*$\pm$125	745*$\pm$67
$10^3 \times \dfrac{[NADP^+]}{[NADPH]}$	10.7$\pm$.7	3.7*$\pm$.5	5.7*$\pm$.7	2.9*$\pm$.1
$\dfrac{[\Sigma ATP]}{[\Sigma ADP][\Sigma Pi]}$ M-1	25800$\pm$3200	13700*$\pm$2600	11200*$\pm$1300	10400*$\pm$1900
mitochondrial				
$\dfrac{[NAD^+]}{[NADH]}$	18.2$\pm$2.3	17.4$\pm$2.6	24.7$\pm$23	22.6$\pm$1.6
STARVED (n)	(13)	(10)	(8)	(10)
cytoplasmic				
$\dfrac{[NAD^+]}{[NADH]}$	587$\pm$86	391$\pm$35	294*$\pm$28	321*$\pm$49
$10^3 \times \dfrac{[NADP^+]}{[NADPH]}$	7.3$\pm$.7	2.1*$\pm$.3	2.2*$\pm$.3	3.7*$\pm$.3
$\dfrac{[\Sigma ATP]}{[\Sigma ADP][\Sigma Pi]}$ M-1	3710$\pm$580	2090$\pm$280	1650*$\pm$180	2360$\pm$440
mitochondrial				
$\dfrac{[NAD^+]}{[NADH]}$	8.1$\pm$.7	13.8*$\pm$1.4	15.2*$\pm$1.1	26.4*$\pm$2.4

metabolizing fatty acids and amino acids. Associated with the decreases in free cytoplasmic [NAD+]/[NADH] ratio is a decrease in the free cytoplasmic [ΣATP]/ΣADP] x [ΣPi] as would be expected from eqn 5 in Table 1.   This equation shows the link between the ATP and NAD+ systems that occurs because of the stoiciometry of the glyceraldehyde-3-phosphate (EC 1.1.1.29) and 3-phosphoglycerate kinase (EC 2.7.2.3) reactions.

Table 6. The Apparent K_{eq} In Vivo of the Metabolites of a Glucose
PPi Phosphotransferase Reaction.

Values are given in umoles/g fresh wet liver $\pm$ S.E.M.

FED

	Saline	Acetate	Propionate	Butyrate
n	5	6	8	6
Glucose	8.40 $\pm$ .27	13.77* $\pm$ .70	17.86* $\pm$ .67	14.10* $\pm$ .63
Glucose 6 P	0.149 $\pm$ .012	0.386 $\pm$ .027	0.527 $\pm$ .038	0.442 $\pm$ .029
Pi	3.19 $\pm$ .16	4.67* $\pm$ .26	5.51* $\pm$ .21	4.32* $\pm$ .23
Calculated free PPi	0.0018 $\pm$ .0002	0.0034 $\pm$ .0004	0.0048 $\pm$ .0005	0.0037 $\pm$ .0004
$\dfrac{[G\ 6\ P][Pi]}{[Glucose][free\ PPi]} = 45.9$	31	39	34	37

STARVED

n	13	10	10	10
Glucose	4.84 $\pm$.21	7.94* $\pm$.42	8.30* $\pm$.43	5.45 $\pm$.33
Glucose 6 P	0.059 $\pm$.002	0.099 $\pm$.010	0.084 $\pm$.009	0.069 $\pm$.004
Pi	4.22 $\pm$.12	7.95* $\pm$.80	9.61* $\pm$.42	8.86* $\pm$.68
Calculated free PPi	0.0009 $\pm$.0001	0.0013 $\pm$.0001	0.0009 $\pm$.0001	0.0009 $\pm$.0001
$\dfrac{[G\ 6\ P][Pi]}{[Glucose][free\ PPi]} = 45.9$	59	83	114	123

It has previously been proposed that the steady state level of glucose is in near-equilibrium with a liver glucose-PPi phosphosphotransferase reaction (18). The value expected at equilibrium for this reaction is 45.9. The values obtained in this study are given in Table 6. They agree quite well with the predicted value.

The Relationship of the Hexose-Monophosphate Pathway to Glycolysis

Tables 2, 3, and 7 show that elevation of either F6P or DHAP causes elevation of shunt intermediates. This is to be expected since the final products of the shunt are F6P and GAP and thus changes in either should affect the steady state level of shunt intermediates.

The equilibrium constant for the reaction catalysed by 6-phosphogluconate dehydrogenase is 0.17 M (Table 1). Whether this reaction is near-equilibrium _in vivo_ was tested using the $[NADP^+]/[NADPH]$ ratio calculated from the isocitrate dehydrogenase reaction (Table 1, eqn 3) and the levels of measured metabolites of the reaction. The values determined range from 0.11 M to 0.36 M. It may, therefore, be concluded that the $[isocitrate]/[\alpha\text{-ketoglutarate}]$ and $[6\text{-phosphogluconate}]/[ribulose\ 5\text{-P}]\times[CO_2]$ ratios both fairly well approximate the free $[NADP^+]/[NADPH]$ ratio in cytoplasm as originally proposed (33).

The non-oxidative portion of the hexose-monophosphate pathway has been recognized for some time to be a near-equilibrium system of rather complex isomerases (40) that in brain achieve near-equilibrium (41). The realization that the 6-phosphogluconate dehydrogenase reaction is usually in near-equilibrium with the cytoplasmic $[NADP^+]/[NADPH]$ ratio as calculated from the isocitrate dehydrogenase catalysed reaction (33) means that changes in CO_2 pressure and thus $[NADP^+]/[NADPH]$ will effect metabolite levels in the shunt. The steady state level of the metabolites of the hexose-monophosphate pathway are also linked to the glycolytic pathway via F6P and glyceraldehyde-3-phosphate (GAP).

The formal relationship relating the steady state levels of the first portion of glycolysis to the shunt and the $NADP^+$ redox and pyrophosphorylation state of the cell is given by:

$$K_{S-G} = 0.027M = \frac{[glucose]^{2/3}\,([DHAP]/22)^{1/3}[CO_2]}{[6P\text{-Gluconate}]} \times \frac{[PPi]^{2/3}}{[Pi]^{2/3}} \times \frac{[NADPH]}{[NADP^+]} \quad (I)$$

The values of this _in vivo_ constant agree fairly well, except in the fed butyrate and starved acetate samples (Table 8). This suggests that just as changes in the steady state levels of metabolites of the later half of glycolysis may reflect changes in the cytoplasmic $[NAD^+]/[NADH]$ and $[\Sigma ATP]/[\Sigma ADP]\times[\Sigma Pi]$ (25) changes in the first half ofglycolysis including the blood and liver glucose may reflect changes in free cytoplasmic $[NADP^+]/[NADPH]$ and the cytoplasmic pyrophosphorylation state, i.e. $[\Sigma PPi]/[\Sigma Pi]$.

Table 7. Effect of Short Chain Fatty Acids on Liver Metabolites.

Values reported as mean + SEM. All values with units are umol/gm wet weight tissue. A * represents a p<0.05 compared to the saline control as determined by student's T-test.

	Ad Lib Fed				48 h Starved			
n	saline (5)	acetate (6)	propionate (6)	butyrate (6)	saline (5)	acetate (6)	propionate (5)	butyrate (6)
glucose	8.40 ± .27	13.77* ± .70	17.86 ± .67	14.10* ± .63	4.84 ± .21	7.94* ± .42	8.30* ± .43	5.45 ± .33
6-phospho-gluconate	0.011 ± .001	0.024* ± .002	0.029* ± .002	0.025* ± .003	0.0034 ± .0007	0.0090* ± .0009	0.0072 ± .0007	0.0066 ± .0007
ribulose 5-phosphate	0.0074 ± .0013	0.0099 ± .0008	0.0118 ± .0003	0.0108 ± .0009	0.0026 ± .0003	0.0042* ± .0005	0.0035 ± .0005	0.0040* ± .0003
xylulose 5-phosphate	0.013 ± .003	0.018 ± .001	0.020* ± .001	0.019 ± .002	0.0037 ± .0006	0.0063* ± .0003	0.0063* ± .0004	0.0068* ± .0003
dihydroxy-acetone phosphate	0.023 ± .001	0.025 ± .002	0.033* ± .002	0.023 ± .002	0.011 ± .001	0.036* ± .004	0.033* ± .001	0.030* ± .003
cytosolic a $\dfrac{NADPH}{NADP+}$	97 ± 8	270* ± 36	189 ± 25	345 ± 12	137 ± 13	476 ± 68	455 ± 62	270 ± 22
cytosolic b $\dfrac{PPi}{Pi}$ X 10^{-4}	5.29 ± 0.84	6.80 ± 0.74	8.26* ± 0.61	8.06 ± 1.17	2.02 ± 0.10	1.41* ± 0.18	0.84* ± 0.07	0.93* ± 0.10

a. Calculated from isocitrate dehydrogenase reaction as described in methods.
b. Calculated form UDP-glucose pyrophosphorylase reaction as described in methods.

Table 8. The Effect of Short Chain Fatty Acids on some Near-Equilibrium Relationships of the Hexose Monophosphate Shunt.

FED

	saline	acetate	prop	but
6-phosphogluconate dehydrogenase $\dfrac{[Ru5P]}{[6PG]}$ $[CO_2]$ X $\dfrac{[NADPH]}{[NADP^+]}$ = 0.17 $\underline{M}$	.11	.18	.12	.24
Ribulose-phosphate 3-epimerase $\dfrac{[X5P]}{[Ru5P]}$ = 2	1.6	1.9	1.7	1.7
K_{S-G} = .027$\underline{M}$	.039	.085	.073	.115

STARVED

	saline	acetate	prop	but
6-phosphogluconate dehydrogenase $\dfrac{[Ru5P]}{[6PG]}$ $[CO_2]$ X $\dfrac{[NADPH]}{[NADP^+]}$ = 0.17 $\underline{M}$	.17	.36	.35	.26
Ribulose-phosphate 3-epimerase $\dfrac{[X5P]}{[Ru5P]}$ = 2	1.3	1.5	1.8	1.7
K_{S-G} = .027$\underline{M}$	.051	.110	.092	.047

where:

$$K_{S-G}= \frac{[glucose]^{2/3}([DHAP]/22)^{1/3}[CO_2]}{[6\text{-}P\ Gluconate]} \ X \ \frac{[PPi]^{2/3}}{[Pi]^{2/3}} \ X \ \frac{[NADPH]}{[NADP^+]}$$

In mongrel dogs maintained on a respirator, it has been shown that hyperventilation in the presence of elevated blood sugar (18.6 mM) led to a decrease in serum inorganic Pi to 1/2 normal values while the phosphorylated intermediates in muscle increased. Thus in muscle G6P increased 3 fold, ATP increased 1.5 fold, creatine phosphate increased 1.5 fold and muscle inorganic Pi increased 1.7 fold (44). Hyperventilation has long been known to cause a decrease in serum phosphorus (45). These findings coupled with a doubling of blood lactate concentration in animals hyperventilated to lower arterial pCO_2 lead investigators to postulate that glycolysis in muscle was increased due to a decrease in intracellular hydrogen ion concentration.   The explanation of these events was attributed to the fact that a decrease of hydrogen ion concentration activated the enzyme phosphofructokinase (EC 2.7.1.11) (46).   Rather illogically the increase in G6P was also attributed to the fact that the rate of glycolysis was increased, although one would have imagined that if PFK were stimulated, the G6P concentration should have decreased since G6P is in equilibrium with F6P which is a substrate for PFK.

It had earlier been shown that elevation of arterial pCO_2 induced by breathing 10 to 30% CO_2 gas mixtures lead in brain to a 50% decrease in the rate of glycolysis accompanied by 2 fold rise in G6P, a 1.5 fold rise in Pi, a 3 fold elevation of brain hydrogen ion concentration and a decrease in creatine phosphate (42).   In this set of experiments the rise in G6P and fall in DHAP coupled with a decrease in overall glycolytic rate was again attributed to the fact that, in vitro, phosphofructokinase is more sensitive to inhibition by ATP and citrate in the presence of an elevation of intracellular hydrogen ion concentration (47).   However, changes in hydrogen ion concentration in a living animal are paradoxically accompanied by decreases in pCO_2 in spite of the equilibrium relationship between hydrogen ion, bicarbonate and pCO_2 as defined by Henderson and Hasselbach (48), namely:

$$pH = pK_a' + log \frac{[HCO_3^-]}{[CO_2]} \text{, where } pK_a' = 6.1.$$

Therefore, an increase in hydrogen ion concentration usually causes a decrease in CO_2 concentration due to the minute to minute control of pCO_2 by the mid-brain respiratory center.   Thus, an increase in CO_2 concentration could subsequently then cause a change in the concentration of the other components of the 6-phosphogluconate dehydrogenase catalysed reaction.   These changes would then be reflected in changes in the concentration of all the metabolites of the non-oxidative portion of the shunt including its products F6P and GAP.   As a consequence of the near-equilibrium relationship of the metabolites of the non-oxidative portion of the shunt, changes in the concentration of one shunt metabolite usually are reflected in changes of the concentration of the other metabolites.   And since the shunt and glycolysis share the common metabolites, F6P and GAP, these two metabolic pathways are interdependent.   Hence, just as CO_2 may affect the steady state level of glycolytic intermediates through the $[NADP^+]$ / $[NADPH]$ linked metabolites of the hexosemonophosphate pathway, so may the administration of short chain fatty acids effect the metabolite levels of the shunt through changes in the metabolite levels of glycolysis.

Changes in the levels of hexose-monophosphate pathway metabolites are now being reported by NMR measurements in newborn human infants (43) as well as in certain forms of malignancy. It is unlikely that these are isolated elevations of ribose 5-phosphate as suggested, but rather, they are likely an accumulation of many shunt intermediates.

The administration of short chain fatty acids, could represent an acid burden to the cell since it is assumed that the acids enter the cell in the neutral protonated form and would subsequently dissociate since their pK's are less than 5. One might think therefore that changes in phosphate and the phosphorylated metabolites are a direct consequence of this lowering of intracellular pH. This possibility is currently under investigation.

Effects of Short Chain Fatty Acids on Total Liver Content of Ca, Mg, Pi and Adenine Nucleostides

In Table 9 are given the net changes in total liver content of Ca, Mg, Pi and adenine nucleotides induced by the administration of short chain fatty acids. As stated previously, total PPi content rose 100 fold or more in starved animals which is the largest proportional change, but by no means the largest absolute change. The total Ca plus Mg increased in the starved animals between 4 to 6 umoles per g wet weight while the total inorganic Pi increased 3.7 to 5.4 umoles/gm wet weight. It therefore appears possible that in some instances the transfer of Ca^{2+} plus Mg^{2+} into the liver from circulating blood was accompanied by HPO_4^{2-}. In the fed animals, the increase in total liver Ca plus Mg ranged from about 2 to .1 umoles/g wet weight while Pi increased 2 to 1.3 umoles/g. The phosphate increase in the fed animals given butyrate was far in excess of the increase in Ca and Mg. This suggests that short chain fatty acids may increase liver phosphate independent of Ca movement, perhaps in exchange for intracellular OH^- or its equivilent.

The primary change after the administration of short chain fatty acids is the generation of PPi, either in mitochondria and/or cytoplasm. Even though the rate of PPi generation did not markedly differ between fed and starved animals, the elevation of PPi in fed animals was usually 10 fold less. The reasons why fed animals accumulate less PPi than starved animals is presently being investigated.

The marked increase in Ca over Mg strongly suggests that the reason total PPi is so elevated is due to the formation of an insoluble Ca_2PPi or CaMgPPi complex. Since there is no great difference between the solubility products of Ca_2PPi and Mg_2PPi, there is no thermodynamic reason for the preferential uptake of Ca over Mg (Table 10). It follows that the excessive Ca uptake in the presence of excess PPi is due to complex formation between Ca and

Table 9. Change in Mg Ca and Phosphate Compounds in Liver Following Short Chain Fatty Acid Aministration.

Values are in umoles/g wet weight.

| | FED | | | | STARVED | | | | |
	Fed Control 16	Acetate 16 Δ	Prop 8 Δ	But 1 Δ	Starved Control 13	Ace 10 Δ	Prop 10 Δ	But 10 Δ	Fed Fructose[a] (4)
n									
Ca	1.06	+0.70	+1.06	+0.23	1.33	+2.89	+4.16	+2.92	---
Mg	11.76	+1.18	+1.22	+0.14	10.1	+1.8	+2.0	+1.1	---
PPi	0.018	+0.18	+0.62	+0.22	0.024	+2.00	+2.91	+2.44	---
Pi	3.19	+1.36	+1.96	+1.23	4.22	+3.73	+5.39	+4.64	1.67
Σ Adenine Nucleotide Pi	7.95	+1.48	+0.65	+1.78	9.32	+0.07	-0.16	-0.3	3.05
Σ Guanine Nucleotide Pi	1.56	+0.41	+0.18	+0.27	1.76	+0.19	+0.14	+0.02	---
Σ Glycolytic Pi	0.65	+0.6	+0.91	+0.46	0.36	+0.86	+0.69	+0.4	9.16
Σ Pi Increase from All measured metabolites	13.75	+4.22	+4.94	+4.17	15.71	+8.85	+11.89	+9.65	13.88

a. Taken from Woods, H. F., Eggleston, L. V. and Krebs, H. A. (1970) Biochem. J. 119:501-510.

637

Table 10. Initial and Final Solution Concentrations of Precipitation Incubations used to Determine Solubility Product of PPi with Ca and Mg.

All incubations were performed at 37°C, pH 7.4, I = 0.25. The ionic strength was adjusted with NaCl and KCl (Na/K = 0.77).

Solution Concentration (mM)
30 Min After Initiation of Preparation

Ca	Mg	Pi	PPi	Solubility Product, M^3
.76 ± .01	-	-	.12 ± .01	6.9×10^{-11}
-	1.10 ± .05*	-	.30 ± .03*	3.6×10^{-10}*
.69 ± .01	0.32 ± .01	-	.26 ± .01	---
3.06 ± .03	---	1.92 ± .01	.45 ± .02	---
---	7.96 ± .01	4.63 ± .02	1.70 ± .02	---
2.60 ± .04	1.13 ± .02	2.19 ± .02	.52 ± .01	---

Solubility product = $M^2 \times PPi$, where M = Ca or Mg.

*Solution Mg and PPi concentrations and the calculated solubility product at 90 min were 0.62 and 0.14 m$\underline{M}$ and 5.4×10^{-11} M^3, respectively.

PPi in a cellular compartment where Ca is present at higher concentrations than Mg. While the free Mg^{2+} in the cytoplasm of liver is estimated by the measured citrate/isocitrate ratio to be about 0.7 mM (35) the free cytoplasmic Ca^{2+} is about 0.2 uM. Precipitation of Ca PPi in cytoplasm is therefore not possible. The highest estimate for free Ca^{2+} in rat liver mitochondrial matrix is about 10 uM (50). Given a solubility product of Ca or Mg_2PPi to be about 5×10^{-11} M^3 and assuming all the measured PPi were in the mitochondrial matrix at 25 mM concentration, it would require about 45 uM free mitochondrial Ca^{2+} to precipitate Ca_2PPi. Since it is not likely that all the measured PPi is present and free in mitochondrial matrix at 25 mM concentrations, it suggests that in the intact liver, the free mitochondrial matrix Ca^{2+} in vivo may be very much higher than estimated on the basis of experiments in isolated mitochondria. To achieve precipitation the free mitochondrial Ca^{2+} would have to approach 1 mM.

Studies of in vivo rat liver with ^{31}P NMR show that the 2.5 mM PPi present in these animals is not detectable (figure 3), therefore, the conclusion that the vast majority of the PPi exists as a complex with Ca is compatible with this NMR silence. Alternately the PPi could be present in a compartment where the concentration of a paramagnetic ion is in high enough concentration so that the PPi signal is broadened to invisability. The fact that the ATP lines are not broadened, makes it seem certain that the PPi is not in the same compartment as the NMR visible ATP, namely cytoplasm (25). The concentration of PPi present is sufficient to be easily detected by ^{31}P NMR as can be seen in the spectra of a liver extract of a butyrate treated rat (figure 4b).

At present, therefore, it must be concluded that based on the fact that butyrate forms PPi almost exclusively in the mitochondrial matrix, the excessive Ca and PPi that accumulates is probably localized there. Direct evidence to substantiate this point is, however, lacking given the inadequate level of our current methodology.

Table 9 also shows that treatment of rats with short chain fatty acids causes an increase in the total rapidly turning over cellular Pi by 30% in the fed and by over 50% in the starved animals. In fed animals, short chain fatty acids even increased the total adenine nucleotide pool, (ATP + ADP + AMP) by 0.65 to 1.80 umole/g. The pool of phosphorylated glycolytic intermediates either doubled or tripled. This finding was completely unexpected. The implications of the increase in the total phosphate burden of the cell are now under study.

It is of interest to compare the changes in cellular Pi and nucleotides after short chain fatty acid administration to that occuring after fructose administration (52). In that case, internal liver Pi is entirely taken up with the formation of 8 mM fructose-1-phosphate (F1P), total liver Pi drops to 1.67 umoles/g and the total adenine nucleotide pool is cut in half while the free cytoplasmic $[\Sigma ATP]/[\Sigma ADP] \times [\Sigma Pi]$ increases to an incredible value of 73,000 M^{-1}. Pi is literally taken from adenine nucleotides to form F1P. Even though later Pi in the cell increases somewhat, there does not appear to be the large Pi uptake into the liver which characterizes the administration of short chain fatty acids.

Parathyroid hormone has long been known to stimulate Ca uptake into HeLa or Ehrlich ascites cells (53, 54). The fact that parathyroid hormone is also reported to stimulate glucose and urea production in isolated liver cells due to stimulation of liver adenyl cyclase (14) is particularly interesting since glucagon does not characteristically elevate fed rat liver phosphate from its normal value of 3.94 umol/g wet weight. The differences in various

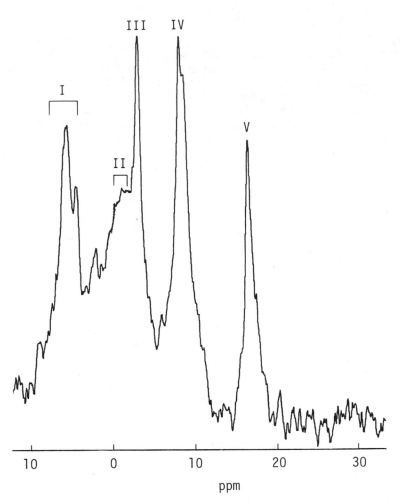

Figure 3. NMR spectrum of the in vivo rat liver collected over a 20 minute period after the injection of Na-butyrate. This spectrum was collected using a 75 usec pulse duration with a 10 sec delay between each pulse. 100 scans were averaged for this spectrum and 25 Hz linebroadening was applied. The sweep width was 10,000 Hz. The coil, a 1.25 cm surface coil, was placed over the liver just below the sternum of the rat. The 75 usec pulse was sufficient to remove any significant contribution by the skin as indicated by the small creatine phosphate peak. Peak assignments I) monophosphate esters, II) creatine phosphate, III) gamma phosphate of ATP, IV) alpha phosphate of ATP, and V) beta phosphate of ATP.

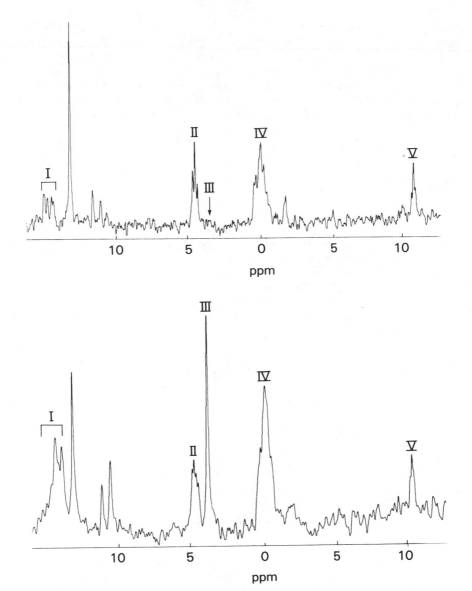

Figure 4. ^{31}P NMR spectra of rat liver extracts. All spectra were collected using magnetization flips of 90° with 10 sec delay between each flip. 300 scans were averaged per spectrum and 10 Hz line broadening was applied. Sweep width was 12,050 Hz. The peak assignments are I) monoester phosphates, II) gamma phosphate of ATP and Beta phosphate of ADP, III) Pyrophosphate, and VI) alpha phosphates of ATP and ADP. A) saline control extract. B) Na-Butyrate treatment extract.

hormone effects may be related to difference in Pi and PPi effects not simply c-AMP. The reports that calcitonin increases the Pi content of bone cells in culture (55) likewise may not be an isolated phenomena but may also apply to liver cells since the changes in nucleotide metabolism found in bone cells are also present in liver cells when PPi and Pi content is changed. The study of PPi metabolism is therefore likely in the future to effect not only glucose metabolism, but nucleotide metabolism and Ca, Pi and Mg homeostatis and provide understanding of metabolic processes that previously were obscure.

REFERENCES

1. Shatton, J. B., Shah, H., Williams, A., Morris, H. P., and Weinhouse, S. (1981) Activities and properties of inorganic pyrophosphatase in normal tissues and hepatic tumors of the rat. Cancer Research 41, 1866-1872.

2. Nordlie, R. C. and Arion, W. J. (1964) Evidence for the common identity of glucose 6-phosphatase, inorganic pyrophosphatase and pyrophosphate-glucose phosphotransferase. J. Biol. Chem. 239, 1680-1685.

3. Reeves, R. E. (1976) How useful is the energy in inorganic pyrophosphate? Trends in Biochem. Sci. 1, 53-55.

4. Wood, H. G. (1977) Some reactions in which inorganic pyrophosphate replaces ATP and serves as a source of energy. Fed. Proc. 36, 2197-2205.

5. Bessman, M. J., Lehman, I. R., Simons, E. S., and Kornberg, A. (1958) An enzymatic synthesis of desoxyribonucleic acid. J. Biol. Chem. 233, 171-177.

6. Kornberg, A. (1981) in DNA Replication pp 55-56, W. H. Freeman, San Francisco.

7. Merryfield, M. L. and Lardy, H. A. (1982) Ca^{2+} mediated activation of phosphoenolpyruvate carboxykinase occurs via release of Fe^{2+} from rat liver mitochondria. J. Biol. Chem. 257, 3628-3655.

8. Konopka, K. and Romslo, I. (1981) Studies on the mechanism of pyrophosphate mediated uptake of iron from transferrin by isolated rat-liver mitochondria. Eur. J. Biochem 117, 239-244.

9. Simkiss, K. (1981) Calcium, pyrophosphate and cellular pollution. Trends in Biochem. Sci. 6, 3-5.

10. Chausmer, A. B., Sherman, B. S., and Wallack, S. (1972) The effect of parathyroid hormone on hepatic cell transport of calcium. Endo. 90, 663-672.

11. Rasmussen, H., Nagata, N., Feinblatt, J., and Fast, D. (1968) in "Parathyroid Hormone and Thyrocalcitonin" (P.V. Talmage and L. F. Belanger, eds.) p 299, Exerptor Medica Foundation, Amsterdam.

12. Deluca, H. F. and Sallis, J. D. (1965) in "The Parathyroid Gland" (Gailhard, P. J., Talmage, R. V. and Budy, A. M., eds.) p 181, University of Chicago Press, Chicago.

13. Hems, D. A., Harmon, C. S., and Whitton, P. D. (1975) Inhibition by parathyroid hormone of glycogen synthesis in the perfused rat liver. FEBS Lett. 58, 167-169.

14. Moxley, M. A., Bell, N. H., Nagle, S. R., Allen, D. O., and Ashmore, J. (1974) Am. J. Physiol 227, 1058-1061.

15. Talmage, R. V., Weil, C. J. V., and Matthews, J. L. (1981) Calcitonin and Phosphate. Mol. and Cell. Endo. 24, 235-251.

16. Lohninger, A. L., Carafoli, E. and Rossi, C. S. (1967) Energy-linked ion movements in mitochondria Adv. Enzymol. 29, 259.

17. Lenhinger, A. L., Brand, M. D. and Reynafarje, B. (1975) Pathways and stoiciometry of H+ and Ca+ transport coupled to mitochondrial electron transport, in Electron Transfer Chains and Oxidative Phosphorylation (E. Quagliariello, S. Papa F. Palmieri, E. C. Slater, and N. Siliprandi, eds) pp 329-334, North Holland, Amsterdam.

18. Lawson, J. W. R., Guynn, R. W., Cornell, N. W., and Veech, R. L. (1976) in "Gluconeogenesis" (Hanson, R. W. and Mehlman, M. A., eds.) pp. 481-512, John Wiley, New York.

19. Krebs, H. A. and Mapes, J. P. (1978) Rate-limiting factors in urate synthesis and gluconeogenesis in avian liver. Biochem J. 172, 193.

20. Veech, R. L., Nielsen, R., and Harris, R. L. (1975) in "Frontiers of Pineal Physiology" (Altschule, M. D., ed) pp 177-196, MIT Press, Cambridge, Mass.

21. Ginsburg, E., Solomon, D., Sreeralsan, T., and Freese, E. (1973) Growth inhibition and morphological changes caused by lipophilic acids in mammalian cells. Proc. Natl. Acad. Sci., USA 70, 2457-2461.

22. Wright, J. A. (1973) Morphology and growth rate changes in Chinese hamster cells cultured in presence of sodium butyrate Exp. Cell. Res. 78, 456-460.

23. Boffa, L. C., Gruss, R. J., and Allfrey, V. G. (1981) Manifold effects of sodium butyrate on nuclear functions. J. Biol. Chem. 256, 9612-9621.

24. Wollenberger, A., Ristan, O., and Schoffa, G. (1960) Pflugers Archiv. Gesante Menschien Tiere 270, 399-412.

25. Veech, R. L., Lawson, J. W. R., Cornell, N. W., and Krebs, H. A. (1979) Cytosolic Phosphorylation Potential. J. Biol. Chem. 254, 6538-6547.

26. Reiss, P., Zuurendonk, P., and Veech, R. L. Anal. Biochem. (in press).

27. Cook, G. A., O'Brien, W. E., Wood, H. G., King, M. T., and Veech, R. L. (1978) A rapid enzymatic assay for the measurement of inorganic pyrophosphate. Analytical Biochem. 91, 557-565.

28. Ackerman, J. J. H., Grove, T. H., Wong, G. G., Gadian, D. G., and Radda, G. K. (1980) Nature 283, 167-170.

29. Griffiths, J. R., Stevens, A. N., Gadian, D. G., Iles, R. A., and Porteous, R. (1980) Biochem. Soc. Trans. 8, 641.

30. Balaban, R. S., Gadian, D. G., and Radda, G. K. (1980) Kid. Int. 20, 575-579.

31. Putnins, R. F. and Yamada, E. W. (1975) Anal. Biochem. 68, 185-195.

32. Williamson, D. H., Lund, P., and Krebs, H. A. (1967) The redox state of the free nicotinamide-adenine dinucleotide in the cytoplasm and mitochondria of rat liver. Biochem J. 103, 514-517.

33. Veech, R. L., Eggleston, L. V., and Krebs, H. A. (1969) The redox state of free nicotinamide-adenine dinucleotide phosphate in the cytoplasm of rat liver. Biochem. J. 115, 609-619.

34. Veech, R. L., Raijman, L., Dalziel, K., and Krebs, H. A. (1969) Disequilibrium in the triose phosphate isomerase system in rat liver. Biochem. J. 115, 837-842.

35. Veloso, D., Guynn, R. W., Oskarsson, M., and Veech, R. L. (1973) The concentration of free and bound magnesium in rat tissues. J. Biol. Chem. 248, 4811-4819.

36. Aas, M. and Bremer, J. (1968) Biochem. Biophys. Acta 164, 157-166.

37. Barth, C., Sladek, M., and Decker, K. (1971) Biochim. Biophys. Acta 248, 24-33.

38. Clark, D. G., Rognstad, R., and Katz, J. (1973) Isotopic evidence for futile cycles in liver cells. Biochem. Biophys. Res. Comm. 54, 1141-1148.

39. Rognstad, R. and Katz, J. (1972) J. Biol. Chem. 247, 6047.

40. Ray, P. D. (1983) in Biochemistry of Metabolic Processes (Lennon, D., Stratman, W., and Zahlten, R. M., eds.) pp 111-124.

41. Kauffman, F. C., Brown, J. G., Passonneau, J. V., and Lowry, O. H. (1969) Effects of change in brain metabolism on levels of pentose phosphate pathway intermediates. J. Biol. Chem. 244, 3647-3653.

42. Miller, A. L., Hawkins, R. A., and Veech, R. L. (1975) Decreased rate of glucose utilization by rat brain in vivo after exposure to atmospheres containing high concentrations of CO_2. J. Neurochem. 25, 553-558.

43. Cady, E. B., Dawson, M. J., Hope, P. L., Tofts, P. S., Costello, A. M., Delpy, D. T., Reynolds, E. O. R., and Wilkie, D. R. (1983) Non-invasive investigation of cerebral metabolism in newborn infants by phosphorus nuclear magnetic resonance spectroscopy. Lancet 1059-1060.

44. Brautbar, N., Leibovici, H., and Massry, S. (1983) On the mechanism of hypophosphatemia during acute hyperventilation: evidence for increased muscle glycolysis. Mineral Electrolyte Metab. 9, 45-50.

45. Haldane, J. B. S., Wigglesworth, V. B., and Woodrow, C. E. (1924) The effect of reaction changes in human inorganic metabolism. Proc. R. Soc. B. 96, 1-12.

46. Mansour, T. E. (1963) Studies on heart phosphofructokinase. J. Biol. Chem. 238, 2285-2292.

47. Uyeda, K. and Racker, E. (1965) J. Biol. Chem. 240, 4682-4688.

48. Henderson, L. J. (1928) *Silliman Lectures*, Yale University Press.

49. Bessman, S. P. and Geiger, P. J. (1979) Compartmentation, Cellular regulation and insulin action, in *Curr*. *Topics in Cell Reg*. (Horecker, B. L. and Stadtman, E. L., eds) Acedemic Press, New York.

50. Coll, K. E., Joseph, S. K., Corkey, B. E., and Williamson, J. R. (1982) Determination of matrix free Ca^{2+} concentration and kinetics of Ca^{2+} efflux in liver and heart mitochondria. *J*. *Biol*. *Chem*. 257. 8696-8704.

51. Zuurendonk, P. F. and Tager, J. M. (1974) *Biochem*. *Biophys*. *Acta* 333, 393-399.

52. Woods, H. F., Eggleston, L. V., and Krebs, H. A. (1970) The cause of hepatic accumulation of fructose 1-phosphate on fructose loading. *Biochem*. *J*. 119, 501-510.

53. Tenenhouse, A., Meier, R., and Rasmussen, H. (1966) *J*. *Biol*. *Chem*. 241, 1314.

54. Bork, A. B. and Neuman, W. F. (1965) *J*. *Cell*. *Biol*. 36, 567.

55. Carnes, D. L. and Campbell, J. W. (1979) *Int*. *J*. *Biochem*. 27, 239-246.

LESSONS FOR MUSCLE ENERGETICS FROM ^{31}P NMR SPECTROSCOPY

Martin J. Kushmerick
Division of Nuclear Magnetic Resonance
Department of Radiology
Harvard Medical School
Boston, Massachusetts 02115

INTRODUCTION

The basic paradigm of muscle energetics has two aspects: (1) there is a net decrease in chemical potential energy content during muscular activity, the net reaction being the splitting of PCr; and (2) there is a recovery period after mechanical relaxation in which oxidative metabolism uses substrate to regenerate the initial pre-contraction steady-state levels of high-energy phosphate compounds, and so restores the initial chemical potential. At least under certain experimental conditions, it is possible to separate completely the processes occurring in the contraction phase (e.g., PCr splitting) from those occurring in the recovery phase (e.g., oxygen consumption above the basal rate).

What distinguishes muscle cells from most other cells is that the dynamic range of metabolic activity is so large. For example, the steady state of ATP production in unstimulated frog sartorius muscle is approximately 1 nmole ATP/g muscle/s. During a maximal tetanic stimulation, the rate of energy utilization can be a thousand times higher. In mammalian skeletal muscle, this range is approximately ten times lower, because the unstimulated so-called resting rate is higher than in amphibians, and because the rate of actomyosin ATP utilization, especially in mammalian slow-twitch and cardiac muscles, is lower than in frog muscle.

The basic energetic paradigm is schematically illustrated in Fig. 1. The phase of contraction is diagrammed on the left as a rise of isometric force. During the recovery period there is no mechanical activity. In panel B of the figure, the ATPase rate is plotted as the measure of energy utilization. Before stimulation

647

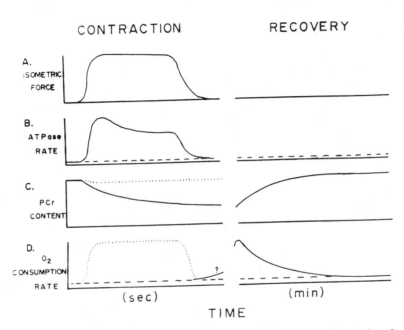

CONTRACTION   RECOVERY

A.
ISOMETRIC
FORCE

B.
ATPase
RATE

C.
PCr
CONTENT

D.
O_2
CONSUMPTION
RATE

(sec)   (min)

TIME

Fig. 1. An idealized representation of chemical and mechanical changes during muscle contraction is shown as a function of time (on the left). The restoration of these changes to the initial steady state of unstimulated muscles occurs during the recovery period (on the right).

648

there is a small ATPase rate equivalent to the basal rate of metabolism. Stimulation induces a rapid rise in the rate, which is initially somewhat higher than afterwards. The main point is that the isometric rate is many times larger than the basal rate. As a consequence of the increased rate of ATP utilization and of the near-equilibrium status of the creatine kinase reaction, there is not a decrease in ATP, but rather a decrease in PCr levels in the cell, as shown in panel C. The oxygen consumption increases little if at all during a very brief tetanus, though of course it does either in a long tetanus or after contractile activity. Following contractile activity mitochondrial respiration is stimulated so that oxygen consumption rapidly increases, and later declines as an apparent first order process during the recovery period, provided there is no further stimulation. Thus in the recovery phase oxidative phosphorylation generates ATP and gives rise to increasing PCr levels (by reversal of the creatine kinase reaction), thereby asymptotically reaching the pre-contraction level. Simultaneously, the rate of oxygen consumption declines as a pseudo-first order process to its initial basal rate. These events are illustrated on the right set of panels.

Another pattern of cellular energetics is illustrated. Consider the possibility that the rate of ATP utilization can be matched by the rate of oxidative ATP synthesis. Thus during contractile activity in this type of cell, PCr levels would decline little; possibly the decrease is undetectable. In this case there would be an increase of ATPase above the basal level associated with contractile processes, but net decrease in PCr would be minimal because increased respiration is in this model proportional to the ATPase rate; this case is diagrammed by the dotted lines. Obviously in this case there is no distinction between a contraction and recovery phase.

PATTERN OF ENERGY UTILIZATION IN MAMMALIAN MUSCLES

The energetic pattern in mammalian muscles appears to be basically similar to what is observed in amphibians (for reviews, see Curtin & Woledge, 1978; Homsher & Keane, 1978; Kushmerick, 1983), and is consistent with the basic paradigm of energetics described. Recently, a detailed study of the energetics of a predominantly fast-twitch muscle, the mouse extensor digitorum longus (EDL), and of a predominantly slow-twitch muscle, the mouse soleus, was completed (Crow & Kushmerick, 1982a). Some important qualitative and quantitative differences were found. First, as the data in Fig. 2 show, the energy cost normalized to the isometric force per cross-sectional area was independent of the chemical potential of the high-energy phosphate pool; the latter decreased whereas force and isometric energy cost was constant. The longest of these contractions (15 s) was sufficient to deplete most of the high-energy phosphate pool. In the EDL, there was a decrease in the energy cost for force maintenance after approximately 9 s of tetanus. It is no longer clear that the mechanism for

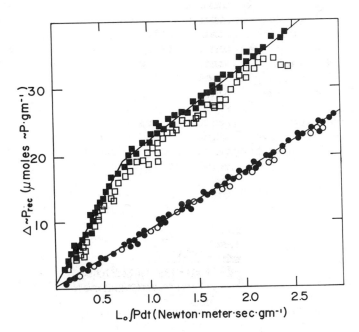

Fig. 2.   The relationships between total high-energy phosphate utilization ($\Delta\tilde{}P_{rec}$) and the tension-time integral for isometric
tetani of mouse EDL (squares) and soleus (circles) at 20°C.
$\Delta\tilde{}P_{rec}$ is expressed in µmole $\tilde{}P/g$, and is the amount of high-
energy phosphate resynthesized as calculated from recovery
oxygen consumption alone (open symbols) or from recovery
oxygen consumption plus recovery lactate production (closed
symbols). The lines drawn through the data are linear functions fitted by least squares. Figure from Crow & Kushmerick
(1982a), which should be consulted for details.

this decrease in rate of energy utilization is phosphorylation of
the so-called regulatory light chain of myosin (18,000 dalton light,
or LC-2f) (compare Crow & Kushmerick, 1982b; Butler et al., 1983).
Because there is definitely a decrease in the rate of cross-bridge
turnover as judged from the maximal velocity of shortening (Crow &
Kushmerick, 1983), it appears that in mouse EDL as well as in very
long contractions of the soleus (Edwards & Jones, 1975), other fac-
tor(s) must be involved in the change in rate of energy utilization;
possible mechanisms include regulation by intracellular acidosis, Pi
accumulation, or lowered ATP/ADP ratios. Unfortunately, the mechanism for this important aspect of muscle energetics and mechanics
remains unknown. For brief tetani, the energy cost in the fast-twitch
EDL was 2.9 times that of the slow-twitch soleus. This was expected
from the greater actomyosin-ATPase activity from EDL versus soleus
muscle. After some 10 s of tetanus, however, the force-normalized
energy cost in the EDL was reduced, so that it was only 1.5 times
that of the soleus. Because the mouse soleus contains a significant
fraction of fast-twitch fibers, this three-fold dynamic range in ATP
utilization rates represents an underestimate of the true range in
mammalian muscle cells. These findings were based on recovery metabolism, measured as the total oxygen consumption above the baseline
induced by contractile activity.

In mouse soleus, a further observation was made. It was clear
that in a fully aerobic soleus muscle, a steady state was possible
during a tetanus in which the rate of ATP synthesis matched the rate
of ATP splitting. That is, in a continuous tetanic stimulation, the
oxygenated muscle could be in a steady state wherein there was no
further measurable extent of reaction involving inorganic phosphate
(Pi), PCr, or ATP. This fact is illustrated by the data in Fig. 3,
open symbols. If the soleus were anaerobic, the measured extent of
high-energy phosphate splitting increased continuously during the
maintained tetanus, i.e., chemical changes were not confounded by
aerobic resynthesis. This observation illustrates the wide dynamic
range of aerobic capacity in the mouse soleus, and implies that the
mitochondrial density and diffusion of oxygen and substrates were
sufficient to maintain PCr and ATP levels even during an isometric
tetanus. This large aerobic capacity was not found in the fast-
twitch EDL muscle, which also has a three-fold higher ATPase rate.
These two muscles of the mouse illustrate nicely the extreme of
energetic patterns in striated muscle (Kushmerick, 1983). The faster
EDL can be described as a "twitch now, pay later" type of cellular
oxidative pattern. The slower soleus, which also has a greater
mitochondrial density, follows more of a "pay as you go" strategy of
cellular respiration found also in smooth and cardiac muscles. The
"twitch now, pay later" strategy corresponds to the first energetic
model described above, whereas the "pay as you go" strategy typifies
the second paradigm.

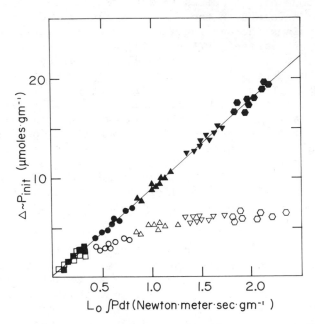

Fig. 3. The relationship between directly-measured initial chemical
breakdown and tension-time integral in the soleus. Units
are the same as in Fig. 2. Each data point represents the
initial chemical breakdown ($\Delta\sim P_{init}$) in a single muscle compared with its control from observed changes in content of
ATP, PCr, and Pi. The open symbols represent the initial
chemical change assessed under aerobic conditions, whereas
the closed symbols represent the initial chemical change
assessed under anaerobic conditions. The solid line is the
linear regression function fitting the anaerobic data: the
different symbols represent muscles stimulated for different
tetanus durations. The symbols used are (□, ■), 1 s; (○,
●), 3 s; (△, ▲), 6 s; (▽, ▼), 9 s; (⬡, ⬢), 12 and 15 s.
From Crow & Kushmerick, 1982a.

The ability of modern nuclear magnetic resonance spectrometers to measure the tissue content of phosphate compounds relevant to cellular energetics has been well established (Gadian, 1982). Sufficiently large magnets exist to monitor these intracellular metabolites in intact human limbs (Ross et al., 1981).

The first observation based on NMR results which is relevant to our purposes here is that the inorganic phosphate content of muscles in normal human limbs, in rat muscles, and in well-perfused fast-twitch muscles (Meyer et al., 1982) is substantially lower (i.e., approximately 1 μmole/g) than is usually reported from analyses of extracts of rapidly frozen tissues (i.e., 5-7 μmole/g). It is likely that most of the discrepancy, if not all, is due to artefactual breakdown of phosphorylcreatine, a much more labile compound than ATP, during the extraction and/or freezing procedures. Since Pi levels increase in proportion to the amount of PCr split (except for the increase in hexose phosphates), and because the PCr levels are on the order of 20-30 mM, the range of Pi concentrations during normal activity ranges from about 1-30 mM. Pi therefore may be an important metabolic regulatory signal.

The second NMR observation I wish to call to your attention is that there are important qualitative differences in the intracellular pH in response to contractile activity. It is well established that the intracellular pH can be measured from the chemical shift or spectral position of the inorganic phosphate peak (Moon & Richards, 1973). During stimulation and subsequent recovery, the intracellular pH changes are characteristically different in the fast-twitch and slow-twitch muscle. For example, during a 15-min period of steady-state twitches, the purely slow-twitch soleus of the cat undergoes a marked intracellular alkalinization from a control value of pH 7.1 to about pH 7.4 (Fig. 4A). In these experiments, the extracellular pH was maintained with bicarbonate/CO_2 buffer at pH 7. The mechanism for the alkalinization is proton uptake during net PCr breakdown. In the recovery period of the cat soleus, there was a moderate acidification to about pH 6.9. By way of contrast, in the fast-twitch biceps muscle little alkalinization was detected, even though the PCr breakdown was more rapid and proceeded to a greater molar extent per unit volume muscle. The lack of alkalinization with an acidification instead (Fig. 4B) is due to a greater intracellular buffer capacity in the fast-twitch muscle than in the slow-twitch, and to a concomitant glycolytic lactate production. During the recovery period, the acidification became quite marked, reaching values as low as pH 6.2. The biceps is a mixed muscle, with approximately equal proportions of fast oxidative-glycolytic (FOG) and fast glycolytic (FG) fibers. Interestingly, the shape of the Pi peak broadened considerably during the recovery period in the biceps, but not in the soleus. This observation indicates a heterogeneity in fiber-to-fiber intracellular

CHEMICAL SHIFT OF Pi DURING STIMULATION-RECOVERY

soleus
60 twitches/min
2 min scans

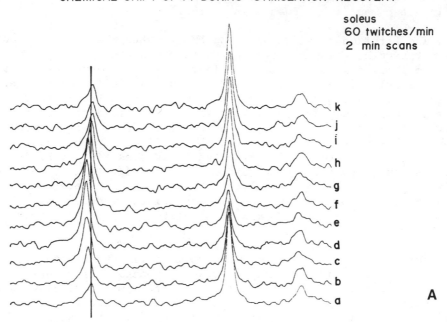

A

Fig. 4.   Portions of ^{31}P-NMR spectra which show the chemical shift of
the inorganic phosphate peak as a measure of intracellular
pH during a stimulation-recovery cycle. Panel A: cat soleus
was perfused with an erythrocyte containing physiological
saline (Meyer et al., 1982) at 25°C and mounted in a Bruker
HX-270 spectrometer. The spectra were acquired in the
Fourier transform mode using 90° pulses at intervals of 15 s
at a frequency of 109.3 MHz. The three peaks shown are,
left to right, Pi, PCr, and ATP (phosphorus). Each set of
spectra is aligned vertically at the frequency of PCr which
is independent of pH under the conditions of this experiment.
The vertical line through the Pi region indicates an intracellular pH of 7.1. A shift to the left indicates an alkalinization, and a shift to the right indicates an intracellular
acidification. Sequential spectra taken every 2 min, 8 scans
averaged. a, unstimulated control; b-f, sequential spectra
during a 10-min period of maximal isometric twitches at 60/
min, showing an increase of intracellular pH to 7.4; g-h,
sequential spectra during the next 10-min period of recovery.

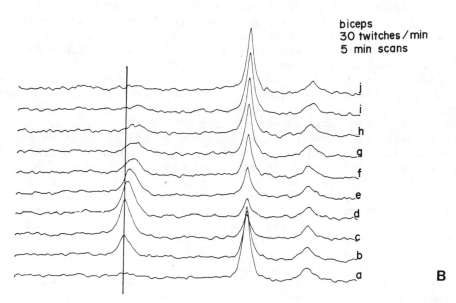

Fig. 4 (cont.). Panel B: a similar experiment in the fast-twitch
   biceps, showing a decrease in pH of about 0.3 units. Each
   spectrum at 5-min intervals, 20 scans averaged. a, unstimulated; b-d, stimulated at 30 switches/min; e-j, recovery.
   Figures taken from Kushmerick et al., 1983.

pH not present in the homogeneous soleus muscle, but clearly demonstrated in the biceps. Thus there are detectable differences in the
kinetics of metabolic responses in FOG and FG fibers, which comprise
the heterogeneous cat biceps, whereas there are only slow-twitch
fibers in the soleus, and it behaves homogeneously

The third and most important set of ^{31}P NMR observations that
bear on our topic is that twitch stimulations at various frequencies
produce steady-state graded levels of intracellular PCr and Pi. That
is, provided that the maximal aerobic capacity of the muscle is not
exceeded, the graded decreased levels of PCr and increased levels of
Pi are accompanied by graded levels of oxygen consumption. The data
which demonstrate these conclusions were derived from studies of
isolated cat biceps and soleus muscles perfused through their arterial
tree by a suspension of red cells in Krebs Henseleit buffer (Meyer
et al., 1984). The range of oxygen consumption rates at 30°C in both
types of in vitro perfused cat muscles are shown in Fig. 5. Contractile activity was induced by applying supra-maximal twitches for 15
min to obtain the steady-state rate of oxygen consumption measured by
arterio-venous differences in the total oxygen content of the perfusate delivered at constant flow. Whereas the biceps reached a maximal oxygen consumption rate of about 60 μmole oxygen/min/100 g muscle.
at 40 twitches/min, it was not established what the maximal rate of
oxygen consumption of the soleus was--it probably was more than
double that of the biceps. Figure 5B shows that the levels of PCr
and of Pi attained in the steady state are functions of the oxygen
consumption; all of these data were obtained under conditions in which
we were certain there was no limitation of oxygen supply, as the data
in panel A indicate. Graded levels of intracellular metabolites in
steady-state twitch contractions were also observed in the gastrocnemius muscles of anesthetized rats studied by ^{31}P surface coils, in
which the twitches (2-10 Hz) were delivered to the muscles via the
sciatic nerve; an example is given in Fig. 6 (Kushmerick & Meyer,
1984.

THE ROLE OF PHOSPHORYLCREATINE AND CREATINE KINASE

The rapid equilibration between phosphorylcreatine and ATP is
considered to be important in muscle function as a rapidly-available
source of energy. While not analyzing this and other possible
aspects of the physiological significance of creatine kinase function
in the detail possible (Meyer et al., 1984; Jacobus & Ingwall, 1980),
I would like to discuss what may be the most basic metabolic function
of this reaction and the basis for understanding other secondary
functions: that creatine kinase serves to buffer the ADP levels in
the μM range is probably more important than its buffering of cellular
ATP levels. This is a point we have emphasized (Meyer et al., 1984)
in some detail. Creatine kinase reaction not only buffers cellular
ATP/ADP ratio, but simultaneously generates inorganic phosphate

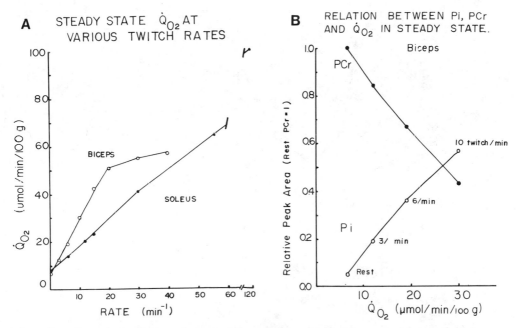

Fig. 5. Panel A shows the steady-state oxygen consumption of cat
biceps and soleus muscles isolated and arterially perfused
with an erythrocyte suspension at various frequencies of
isometric twitch stimulation. Panel B shows the relationship
between PCr and Pi levels measured by ^{31}P-NMR (in arbitrary
units) during steady state of oxygen consumption given in
Panel A. Data taken from Meyer et al., 1984, in press.

657

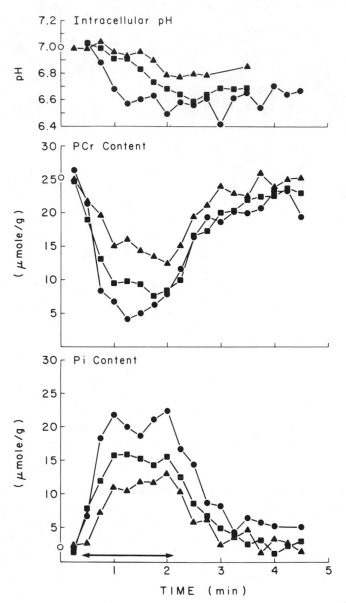

Fig. 6. Chemical changes in a rat lower limb musculature before, during and after 1.8-min stimulation of sciatic nerve at 2 Hz (▲), 4 Hz (■), and 10 Hz (●), obtained from ^{31}P surface coil NMR spectra. Top panel, intracellular pH; middle panel, PCr; bottom panel, Pi. Open symbols at origin represent average of control values for this animal obtained from resting muscle before stimulation and at least 15 min after each stimulation period. Figure from Kushmerick & Meyer, 1984, in press.

levels in the 1-30 mM range, as pointed out above. The cytosolic ADP level is well known to be an important metabolic regulator, including that of mitochondrial respiration (Lawson & Veech, 1979; Moredeth & Jacobus, 1982), and Pi may well prove to be important in the regulation of glycolysis and the modification of actomyosin kinetics.

These aspects of creatine kinase function are easily appreciated by consideration of two sets of reactions. The first is:

$$ATP \leftrightarrow ADP + Pi + \alpha \; H^+ \qquad\qquad \text{[Equation 1]}$$

where α is a function of pH; near pH 7, $\alpha = 0.5$. This reaction is written reversibly, but of course different enzyme systems catalyze each direction. Actomyosin ATPase and other ATP hydrolases catalyze the reaction to the right. Mitochondrial respiration catalyzes the reactions to the left. Substrate level phosphorylation is also a mechanism for ATP generation, but is quantitatively irrelevant for our purposes because the net extent of reaction is quantitatively small in the fully aerobic state.

The second reaction to consider is the truly reversible reaction catalyzed by creatine kinase:

$$PCr + ADP + H^+ \leftrightarrow ATP + Cr \qquad\qquad \text{[Equation 2]}$$

The evidence for this reaction being reversible and near equilibrium in muscle cytosol and probably other cells containing creatine kinase has been well discussed elsewhere (e.g., Meyer et al., 1984). The net reaction, which has been demonstrated to occur in a great variety of muscles during contractile activity and discussed so far in this paper, is the following:

$$PCr + (1 - \alpha) \; H^+ \leftrightarrow Cr + Pi \qquad\qquad \text{[Equation 3]}$$

Because the forward and reverse fluxes of Equation 2 are faster than the total cellular ATPase activity and ATP synthesis rate (i.e., the fluxes of Equation 1), then Equation 2 can be considered near or at equilibrium. By writing the apparent equilibrium constant for Equation 2 for any particular pH, and rearranging, we obtain:

$$\frac{PCr}{Cr} = \frac{1}{Kck} \frac{ATP}{ADP} \qquad\qquad \text{[Equation 4]}$$

It is easily seen that the PCr:Cr ratio is directly proportional to the ATP:ADP ratio. At pH 7 and 1 mM Mg^{2+}, the value of the apparent equilibrium constant (Kck) is on the order of 100. The cellular concentration of PCr, Cr and ATP are in the mM range, typically 25, 6, and 7 mM for unstimulated fast-twitch muscles, respectively. However, ADP concentration is in the range of 10 μM. Thus for a tenfold change in the ratio of PCr:Cr, a ten-fold change in the ratio of

ATP:ADP is easily accomplished with no measurable decrement in ATP, and with an increase in cytosolic ADP, perhaps to 100 µM, a concentration which is above the apparent K_m for the nucleotide translocase, but below the limits of detectability in typical ^{31}P NMR experiments. Of course, a small decrease in ATP of about 0.1 mM must occur when ADP increases.

There is also evidence that the more thermodynamically appropriate quantity that regulates mitochondrial respiration in the cell is the phosphorylation potential (Erecinska et al., 1978), which is defined as:

$$PP = \frac{ATP}{ADP \ Pi}$$

It should be emphasized that this quantity ignores the large and differential changes in specific fiber types in intracellular pH that are known to occur during and after contractile activity, as I have emphasized in the preceding sections. Thus on thermodynamic as well as factual grounds, the phosphorylation potential has its limitations for mechanistic interpretation. Nonetheless, there are expected and observed correlations between the magnitude of the phosphorylation potential and the PCr, Cr and Pi levels and metabolic regulation, i.e., between any metabolic function coupled to the phosphorylation potential and Equation 3.

Combining Equation 1 with Equation 3, we get:

$$\frac{PCr}{Cr} \cdot \frac{1}{Pi} = \frac{PP}{Kck}$$

The point of all these quantitative aspects is the view that PCr:Cr ratio bears a predictable relationship to the ATP:ADP ratio in the cell. Thus the observed simple relationship between the steady-state levels of PCr and Pi and oxygen consumption described in our particular examples in Figs. 5 and 6 are easily understood.

POORLY-METABOLIZABLE SUBSTRATES FOR THE CREATINE KINASE REACTION

For some years, several laboratories (e.g., Fitch et al., 1975; Mahanna et al., 1980; Woznicki & Walker, 1980) have studied the effect of analogues of creatine on muscle function and energetics. The most common of these is β-guanidopropionate, which can be phosphorylated by the reversal of Equation 2, but very slowly, since the K_m for βGPA is higher, and the V_{max} is substantially lower than that of creatine under comparable conditions. When the analogue is fed to animals over the course of 6-12 weeks, the analogue is incorporated into the muscles, hearts, and brains of the animals, displaces much of the creatine phosphate and creatine normally present, and is itself phosphorylated. In prolonged contractile activity, it can be shown that the phosphorylated βGPA can be split very slowly, but in bursts of brief contractile activity this does not occur. One might argue that the mere fact that these treated animals live and function without serious limitation to their daily activity demonstrates that the creatine kinase reaction plays no role in normal muscle function.

On the basis of the previous discussion, I propose that it is relatively easy to understand the energy metabolism of these animals, as well as in normals, and to see the important role of the creatine kinase reaction. Whether or not other metabolic adaptations have occurred (and this has not been tested systematically), in the analogue-treated animals contractile activity should induce large changes in the ATP:ADP ratio even with relatively mild contractile efforts because of the absence or near-absence of Equation 2. In these analogue-fed animals, one would expect the oxygen consumption not to show the graded response obtained in normals, but be turned on to the muscles' maximal capacity, and more rapidly in time following the onset of contractile activity precisely because of the absence of the creatine kinase reaction (Equation 2). That is, in the absence of the creatine kinase reaction, the ATP:ADP ratio is not well buffered. We have shown in preliminary experiments that analogue-fed animals in which the phosphorylated form of βGPA accumulates in rat skeletal muscle and heart, and in which the creatine phosphate levels are no more than 5% of normal values, can be induced to run on a treadmill and have nearly the same maximal oxygen consumption as control animals. So there is no obvious limit to the approximately normal maximal oxygen consumption in the presence of the analogue. To date, there is no evidence regarding the kinetics of oxygen consumption following exercise, either in these animals or in their isolated muscles, to my knowledge. The prediction is straightforward, and the experiment is relatively easy to do.

ACKNOWLEDGEMENTS

The experimental work reported here was done in collaboration with T.R. Brown, M.T. Crow, R.A. Meyer and H.L. Sweeney, and was supported primarily by grants from NIH (AM 14485) and from the Muscular Dystrophy Association of America. S.A. Byers edited and prepared the typescript.

REFERENCES

Butler, T.M., Siegman, M.J., Mooers, S.U., and Barsotti, R.J., 1983, Myosin light chain phosphorylation does not modulate cross-bridge cycling rate in mouse skeletal muscle, Science, 220:1167.

Crow, M.T., and Kushmerick, M.J., 1982a, Chemical energetics of slow- and fast-twitch muscles of the mouse, J. Gen. Physiol., 79:147.

Crow, M.T., and Kushmerick, M.J., 1982b, Phosphorylation of myosin light chains in mouse fast-twitch muscle associated with reduced actomyosin turnover rate, Science, 217:835.

Crow, M.T., and Kushmerick, M.J., 1983, Correlated reduction of velocity of shortening and the rate of energy utilization in mouse fast-twitch muscle during a continuous tetanus, J. Gen. Physiol., 82:703.

Curtin, N.A., and Woledge, R.C., 1978, Energy changes and muscular contraction, Physiol. Rev., 58:690.

Edwards, R.H.T., Hill, D.K., and Jones, D.A., 1975, Metabolic changes associated with the slowing of relaxation in fatigued mouse muscle, J. Physiol. (London), 251:287.

Erecinska, M., Wilson, D.F., and Nishiki, K., 1978, Homeostatic regulation of cellular energy metabolism: experimental characterization in vivo and fit to a model, Am. J. Physiol., 234 (Cell Physiol. 3):C82.

Fitch, C.D., Jellinek, M., Fitts, R.H., Baldwin, K.M., and Holloszy, J.O., 1975, Phosphorylated β-guanidopropionate as a substitute for phosphocreatine in rat muscle, Am. J. Physiol., 228:1123.

Gadian, D.G., 1982, "Nuclear Magnetic Resonance and its Application to Living Systems," Clarendon, Oxford.

Homsher, E., and Kean, C.J., 1978, Skeletal muscle energetics and metabolism, Ann. Rev. Physiol., 40:93.

Jacobus, W.E., and Ingwall, J.S., eds., 1980, "Heart Creatine Kinase," Williams and Wilkins, Baltimore.

Kushmerick, M.J., 1983, Energetics of muscle contraction, in: "Handbook of Physiology," L. Peachey, R. Adrian, and S.R. Geiger, eds., American Physiological Society, Bethesda.

Kushmerick, M.J., and Meyer, R.A., 1984, Chemical changes in rat leg muscle by ^{31}P NMR, Am. J. Physiol. (Cell Physiol.), in press.

Kushmerick, M.J., Meyer, R.A., and Brown, T.R., 1983, Phosphorus NMR spectroscopy of cat biceps and soleus muscles, in: "Oxygen Transport to Tissue," vol. 4, H.I. Bicher and D.F. Bruley, eds., Plenum, New York.

Lawson, J.W.R., and Veech, R.L., 1979, Effects of pH and free Mg^{2+} on the K_{eq} of the creatine kinase reaction and other phosphate hydrolyses and phosphate transfer reactions, J. Biol. Chem., 254:6528.

Mahanna, D.A., Fitch, C.D., and Fischer, V.W., 1980, Effects of β-guanidopropionic acid on murine skeletal muscle, Exp. Neurol., 68:114.

Meyer, R.A., Brown, T.R., and Kushmerick, M.J., 1984, Phosphorus 31 NMR of fast- and slow-twitch muscle, Am. J. Physiol. (Cell Physiol.), in press.

Meyer, R.A., Kushmerick, M.J., and Brown, T.R., 1982, Application of ^{31}P-NMR spectroscopy ot the study of striated muscle metabolism, Am. J. Physiol., 242 (Cell Physiol. 11):C1.

Moon, R.B., and Richards, J.H., 1973, Determination of intracellular pH by ^{31}P magnetic resonance, J. Biol. Chem., 248:7276.

Moreadith, R.W., and Jacobus, W.E., 1982, Creatine kinase of heart mitochondria. Functional coupling of ADP transfer to the adenine nucleotide translocase, J. Biol. Chem., 257:899.

Ross, B.D., Radda, G.K., Gadian, D.G., Rocker, G., Esiri, M., and Falconer-Smith, J., 1981, Examination of a case of suspected McArdle's syndrome by ^{31}P nuclear magnetic resonance, N. Eng. J. Med., 304:1338.

Woznicki, D.T., and Walker, J.B., 1980, Utilization of cyclocreatine phosphate, an analogue of creatine phosphate, by mouse brain during ischemia and its sparing action on brain energy reserves, J. Neurochem., 34:1247.

METABOLIC DEPLETION PRECEDING CYTOLYSIS INDUCED BY ANTIBODY AND

COMPLEMENT AS REVEALED BY ^{31}P-NMR SPECTROSCOPY

Reuven Tirosh, *Hadassa Degani and Gideon Berke

Departments of Cell Biology and *Isotope Research
The Weizmann Institute of Science
Rehovot 76100, Israel

SUMMARY

The mechanism whereby fixation of the membrane attack complex of complement (C') induces irreversible membrane damage ultimately leading to cell death may not be an exclusive membrane event. We investigated possible involvement of cellular metabolism in the lysis of nucleated cells induced by antibody (Ab) against cell surface antigens and C'. Using ^{31}P-NMR spectroscopy we observed a marked reduction of creatine phosphate and relatively unaltered ATP levels shortly after the application of C', but prior to the onset of lysis. These metabolic changes preceded uptake of vital stains (e.g., eosine), or release of isotopically ($Na_2^{51}CrO_4$)-labeled cytoplasmic components. Monitoring the course of natural cell death over a 6-hr period revealed a comparable depletion of creatine phosphate prior to cell death. We would like to propose that membrane fixation of the C' attack complex induce metabolic depletion of high energy components which in turn cause irreversible cell swelling and membrane damage leading to cytolysis.

The vast biochemical and structural knowledge of the complement (C') cascade and its membrane fixation (1-4) is not matched by a clear understanding of how irreversible damage to the target finally occurs. It is well accepted today that the plasmalema is the primary site of the attack. Evidence has been presented that membrane-bound C' components [C5b-C9]n form (trans)membrane 'channels' (the 'doughnut' model; 5, 6) and/or 'leaky patches (3, 7), suggesting that these perturb ion conductance of the membrane allowing net influx of water and 'colloid-osmotic' lysis. A detergent-like effect of C' action, possibly irrelevant to a

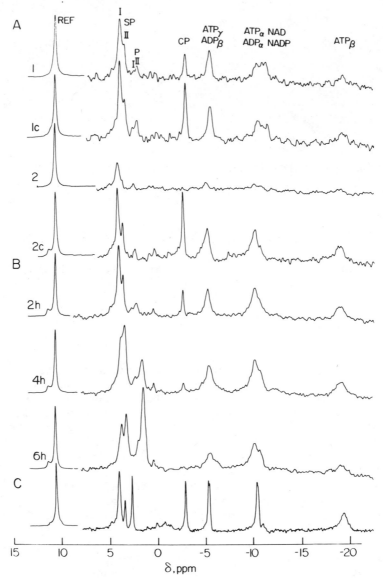

FIGURE 1. ^{31}P proton coupled NMR spectra at 121.5 MHz of leukemia EL4 cells exposed to antibody and complement.

Cells were obtained from the peritoneal cavities of C57BL/6 mice, 4-7 days after intraperitoneal inoculation, by washing with phosphate-buffered saline supplemented with newborn calf serum (10%). Preliminary measurements indicated that a 30-min preincubation of the tumor cells at 37°C was required to raise creatine

666

(FIGURE 1, continued)

phosphate (CP) levels found otherwise to be low immediately after cell preparation. Cells (20×10^6/ml) were exposed to BALB/c (H-2^d) anti-EL4 (H-2^b) hyperimmune serum (Ab) 1/100, for 30 min at 4°C, with constant shaking. Complement (C'), guinea pig serum, was added and the cell suspension was reincubated at 37°C with constant shaking. For NMR measurements, 4×10^8 treated cells were washed twice with ice-cold phosphate-free Krebs–Ringer buffer solution that contained 140 mM NaCl, 5.6 mM KCl, 3.0 mM CaCl$_2$, 1.4 mM MgSO$_4$, 1 mg/ml glucose and 20 mM HEPES buffer, pH 7.4 (at room temperature). Cell pellets were resuspended in 1 ml of a 30% (v/v) ^{2}H$_2$O in Krebs–Ringer HEPES buffer. The total volume of about 1.5 ml was kept on ice and then transferred to A 10 mm NMR glass tube. In the tube an additional coaxial capillary was held containing 10 ml of reference solution composed of 1 M H$_3$PO$_4$, 1 M HCl and 115 mM PrCl$_3$. Spectra were recorded with a Bruker CXP-300 spectrometer, at 4°C, without sample spinning. 400 pulses were applied with an interval of 0.69 sec between transients. The external reference signal (REF) in all spectra was recorded with a 10 times lower gain. 0 ppm refers to 85% H$_3$PO$_4$. Line broadening and the number of scans of the records in (A) and (B) were 15 Hz and 1300 to 3000 and in (C), 5 Hz and 10,000, respectively.
    A. ^{31}P-NMR spectra of Ab+C' treated cells. 1, 2: C' diluted 1/15 for 10 min and 30 min, respectively, at 37°C. 1c, 2c: Controls treated and untreated with antibody, respectively, both without C'. Cells treated with complement alone gave a spectrum comparable to the controls (not shown). B. 2h-6h: Spectra of the control A2C sample maintained at 4°C in the spectrometer and monitored 2, 4 and 6 hrs later. C. Spectrum of perchloric acid extract of EL4 cells preincubated at 37°C, as above. For extraction, 4×10^8 cells in 1.5 ml Krebs–Ringer-HEPES ^{2}H$_2$O (20%) were treated with 0.15 ml HCLO$_4$ 70% (Fluka) for 20 min on ice. After neutralizing with KHCO$_3$ powder and centrifuging to remove KCLO$_4$ and cellular debris the clear supernatant was examined. REF, reference solution; SP, sugar phosphate; P, inorganic phosphate; CP, creatine phosphate,ATP, adenosine triphosphate; ADP, adenosine diphosphate; NAD NADP, nicotinamide adenine dinucleotides. By integrating the various peaks, approximate values can be obtained for intracellular concentrations of various phosphate compounds, as follows: C = (RI x PR) / (NC x CV), where RI, ratio of integrals of a specific over the reference peaks; PR, phosphate reference, 10 umole; NC, number of cells in the NMR tube (4×10^8 cells); CV, average cellular volume of EL4 (1800 u^3). For example, from A1c [SP] = 4.2 mM; [CP] = 1.6 mM; [ATP] = 0.7 mM; [ADP] = 0.9 mM; [NAD+NADP] = 1.0 mM.

physiological settings, has been considered in certain liposomal
and viral systems ('noncolloid-osmotic'; 2, 3). At the present
time, however, it is not entirely clear whether insertion of the
membrane attack complex of C' alone is both required and sufficient to bring about cytolysis. For example, recent studies on

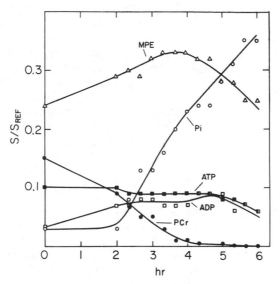

FIGURE 2. Changes in phosphate compounds in control EL4 cells
incubated under limited oxygen supply at $4^{\circ}C$.

The cells employed are those in Fig. 1B. Successive NMR spectra
were automatically collected at 20 min intervals, beginning 2 hrs
after that in Fig. 1A2C. The integrated area of each peak (S) is
normalized to that of the reference (S_{REF}). MPE, monophosphoes-
ters (equivalent to SP above).

C'-dependent bacteriolysis suggest metabolic involvement (8). In
addition, evidence has been presented that C' attack on nucleated
cells can be influenced by drugs which affect cellular metabolism,
including cAMP levels (9, 10) and by the cell cycle (11).
Furthermore, electrical and isotopic measurements of cells undergoing Ab+C' attack have revealed membrane depolarization and
changes in ion conductance, including channel-flickering prior to
uptake of vital stains (12, 13). Under limited C' attack, insufficient for inducing uptake of vital strains, these changes have

668

been fully reversible. These findings are difficult to reconcile
with formation of terminally lethal 'holes' by C' as an exclusive
lytic mechanism. As an alternative, we suggest that persistent
membrane depolarization induced by C' fixation can affect cellular
metabolism ultimately resulting in cell death. Membrane depolarization induced by C' is probably followed by voltage-dependent
gating of Ca^{2+} (14, 15), a well-known trigger of cellular activi-
ty.Here we present data suggesting C'-induced depletion of high
energy metabolites to be a major pre-lytic event. Such a depletion can cause loss of membrane permeability barriers culminating
in colloid-osmotic lysis.

Using ^{31}P-NMR spectroscopy (16, 17), we monitored high energy
metabolites of leukemia EL4 cells of C57BL/6 mice subjected to
BALB/c anti-EL4 hyperimmune serum (Ab) and guinea pig serum (C'),
and of control cells treated with either Ab or C', as well as of
untreated cells undergoing spontaneous death. Under mild attack
of Ab+C', causing only 4% lysis (10%/6% control) as determined by
eosine dye exclusion or by release of radioactivity from
$Na_2^{51}CrO_4$-labeled EL4 cells, we detected considerable depletion of
intracellular creatine phosphate (CP) but only small changes in
other phosphate containing compounds (Fig. 1A1, A1c). Total
depletion of CP was detected (Fig. 1A2, A2c) under C' attack where
37% of cells were stained by eosine. In the latter case, taking
the sugar phosphate (SP) peak in Fig. 1A2 as an indicator for the
number of metabolite-possessing cells, there appeared some ATP
depletion per remaining cell as compared to controls (Fig. 1A2C).
Comparable control spectra were obtained for cells incubated with
either Ab or C' (not shown). Taken together, these results
indicate that under Ab+C' attack, cells undergo depletion of CP
prior to lysis. A 6-hr long process of 'natural death' was then
followed in the NMR tube at $4^{\circ}C$ in the absence of an external
oxygen supply (Fig. 1B; Fig. 2). The depletion of CP as well as
the unaltered levels of cellular nucleotides appeared similar to
those detected in cells undergoing Ab+C' attack. The increasing
second peak of inorganic phosphate (Pi_{II}) and its chemical shift
to increasing magnetic field, could indicate accumulation of
external Pi and acidification due to glycolysis. The more
alkaline peak of internal inorganic phosphate (Pi_I) showed a
smaller acidic shift relative to that of Pi_{II}. This homeostatic
control of internal pH and Pi concentration suggested integrity of
the cell membrane. ATP levels remained constant as long as CP was
detectable; it was only after 5 hr at $4^{\circ}C$ that the ATP signal
began to decrease. In Fig. 1C, a high resolution spectrum was
obtained for perchloric acid extract of control EL4 cells like
those shown in Fig. 1A2C. The marked variations in the CP and Pi
peaks (compared to Fig. 1A2C) were probably due to perchloric acid
effects on these and other compounds. The single Pi signal clearly suggested that the increasing peak in Fig.1B represented external accumulation of Pi and concomitant acidification.

Most of our understanding of C'-mediated lysis comes from studies on RBC, their ghosts, and synthetic liposome model systems. Insertion of terminal C' components into the membrane and membrane spanning has been demonstrated by several groups (18-22). The common view that terminal C' components (C5b-C9) exert their lytic effect(s) by creating hydrophilic pores through the lipid membrane of the target is supported by some but not all observations (4). While Bhakdi et al. (23) reported water-filled membrane structures from freeze-etching studies, Sims and Lauf (24) and Sims (25) observed distinct variations between estimated and calculated dimensions of 'leaky' pores induced by C' (3). Undoubtedly, distinct C'-dependent membrane structures and pores are observed in membranes during and following C' attack (26). But whether the mere formation of these structures is required and sufficient for inducing lysis is not entirely clear.

Briefly stated, the alternative model suggests that irreversible damage to the membrane leading to cytolysis is the end result of intracellular events, initiated by C' fixation to the membrane. The need for an alternative model of C'-induced lysis comes primarily from studies on lysis of nucleated cells exhibiting a number of characteristics which suggest a more complex series of events following C' attack. A large body of evidence shows triggering of non-lethal cellular events prior to the onset of C'-mediated killing. For example, Stephens and Henkart (12) have demonstrated nonlethal and reversible membrane depolarization and changes in ion conductance in glioma-neuroblastoma cells under Ab+C' attack. The finding of early membrane depolarization is compatible with nonlethal increase in the flux of ^{86}Rb following C' attack (27) prior to lysis. The important observation of full recovery from Ab+C' attack of (depolarized) cells whose ion conductance was initially changed (12) shows that C'-induced membrane depolarization alone cannot be responsible for C'-dependent lethal effects. It suggests that membrane depolarization triggers an additional step(s) ultimately leading to lysis. In a more recent related study, Jackson et al. (13), using an extracellular patch electrode, reported single channel currents during antibody and C' attack. Interestingly, channels appeared to flicker between ion conducting and non-conducting states. Channel flickering and the recovery from membrane depolarization appear incompatible with lethal membrane lesion induced by C'. We have suggested that membrane depolarization induced by C' binding triggers Ca^{2+} gating, which can lead to activation of a multitude of metabolic and cellular processes. Direct measurement of the increase in intracellular concentration of free calcium ions in response to the action of complement was reported (28). Indirect evidence indicating prelytic Ca^{2+} influx during C' attack on nucleated (mast) cells has been presented (29). Earlier studies have shown a role for divalent ions in the lethal fixation of Ab+C' to target cells (10, 14). It is noteworthy that uncontrolled influx of Ca^{2+}

by and of itself may be cell damaging. Thus, toxicity of the Ca^{2+} ionophore A23817 is markedly enhanced in the presence of Ca^{2+} (29). C' may function in an analogous way, inducing influx of Ca^{2+} and thereby causing metabolic activation and exhaustive depletion of high energy metabolites. Additional evidence implicating altered metabolic process(es) during C' attack stem from experiments showing that the susceptibility of nucleated cells to Ab+C' attack can be altered (enhanced or depressed) by a wide range of drugs (10). Influence of the cell-cycle phase excluding antigen density has also been presented (11). Furthermore, the strong temperature dependence of C'-mediated lysis of nucleated cells (30), showing great resemblance to CTL-mediated lysis (31), is highly compatible with metabolic involvement.

The fixation of the C' complex in cell membrane may capitalize on Ca^{2+} regulation of cellular activities. Persistent cellular activation can lead to exhaustive ATP and CP consumption, as is the case in the ischemic heart. Osmotic balance across the cell membrane is maintained by the ATP-fuelled Na^+-pumping.. Hence, depletion of ATP could interfere with normal osmotic functions, finally resulting in colloid-osmotic swelling and lysis. This can explain the observation that osmotic protection against swelling not only prevents Ab+C' induced lysis but can rescue affected cells (30), possibly by allowing metabolic recovery. A similar CP-depletion and recovery prior to cell death has been observed in the ischemic myocardium (32); Ca^{2+}-channel blockers induced recovery (33), possibly by slowing down metabolic activities, thus allowing replenishment of CP and ATP. The higher susceptibility of RBC to Ab+C' showing, in addition, less recovery than nucleated cells, may be related to the lower metabolic capacity of RBC.

Finally we would like to draw an analogy between the response of cells to Ab+C' and to a wide range of stimulators, including growth and chemotactic factors (34, 35). This analogy is promoted by a common early depolarization, followed by Ca^{2+} influx and metabolic stimulation. The size and structure of (C5b-C9) and its sustained membrane fixation, unlike hormones and growth factors which undergo rapid clustering and endo- or exocytosis, may be a key factor in determining the lethal sequence of events initiated by its binding to the membrane. In experiments under way, we are exploiting the above approach to test whether lymphocyte mediated cytolysis, like the effects of Ab+C', involves metabolic depletion of the target prior to lysis.

REFERENCES

1. H. Müller-Eberhard, Complement. Ann. Rev. Biochem. 44:697 (1975).

671

2. M.M. Mayer, D.W. Michaels, L.E. Ramm, M.B. Whitlow, J.B. Willoughby, and M.L. Shin, Membrane damage by complement, Crit. Rev. Immunol. 2:133 (1981).
3. A.F. Esser, Interactions between complement proteins and biological and model membranes, in: "Biological Membranes," D. Chapman, ed., Academic Press, New York (1972), p. 277.
4. P.J. Lachmann, Complement, in: "The Antigens," M. Sela, ed., Academic Press, New York (1979), p. 283.
5. M.M. Mayer, Membrane attack by complement (with comments on cell-mediated cytotoxicity), In: "Mechanisms of Cell-Mediated Cytotoxicity," W.R. Clark and P. Golstein, eds., Plenum Press, New York, (1981), p. 193.
6. L.E. Ramm and M.M. Mayer, Life-span and size of the transmembrane channel formed by large doses of complement. J. Immunol. 124:2281 (1980).
7. E.R. Podack, G. Biesecker, and H.J. Müller-Eberhard, Membrane attack complex of complement: Generation of high affinity phospholipid plasma proteins, Proc. Natl. Acad. Sci. USA 76:897 (1979).
8. B.W. Taylor, H.P. Knoll, and S. Bhakdi, Killing of Escherichia coli LP1092 by human serum, Immunobiology 164:304 (1983).
9. M. Kaliner and K.F. Austen, Adenosine 3',5'-monophosphate: Inhibition of complement-mediated cell lysis, Science 183:659 (1974).
10. S.H. Ohanian, S.I. Schlager, and T. Borsos, Molecular interactions of cells with antibody and complement: Influence of metabolic and physical properties of the target on the outcome of humoral immune attack, Contemp. Top. Mol. Immunol. 7:153 (1978).
11. W.U. Shipley, Immune cytolysis in relation to the growth cycle of Chinese hamster cells, Cancer Res. 31:1925 (1971).
12. C.L. Stephens and P.A. Henkart, Electrical measurements of complement-mediated membrane damage in cultured nerve and muscle cells, J. Immunol. 122:3455 (1979).
13. M.B. Jackson, C.L. Stephens, and N. Lecar, Single channel currents induced by complement in antibody-coated cell membranes, Proc. Natl. Acad. Sci. USA 78:6421 (1981).
14. M.D.P. Boyle, S.H. Ohanian, and T. Borsos, Studies on the terminal stages of antibody-complement-mediated killing of a tumor cell. I. Evidence for the existence of an intermediate, T*, J. Immunol. 116:1272 (1976).
15. R.P. Rubin, "Calcium and Cellular Secretion," Plenum Press, New York (1982).
16. R.G. Shulman, T.R. Brown, K. Vgurbil, S. Ogawa, S.N. Cohen, and J.A. den Hollander, Cellular applications of ^{31}P and ^{13}C nuclear magnetic resonance, Science 205:160 (1979).
17. M. Barany and T. Glonek, Phosphorus-31 nuclear magnetic resonance of contractile systems. in: "Methods in Enzymology, Vol. 85, Part B," D.W. Frederiksen and L.W. Cunningham, eds., Publisher, City (1982), p. 624.

672

18. V.W. Hu, A.F. Esser, E.R. Podack, and B.J. Wisnieski, The membrane attack mechanism of complement: Photolabeling reveals insertion of terminal proteins into target membrane, J. Immunol. 127:380 (1981).

19. E.A. Podack, A.F. Esser, G. Biesecker and H.J. Müller-Eberhard, Membrane attack complex of complement: A structural analysis of its assembly, J. Exp. Med. 151:301.

20. C.H. Hammer, M.L. Shin, A.S. Abramovitz, and M.M. Mayer, On the mechanism of cell membrane damage by complement: Evidence on insertion of polypeptide chains from C8 and C9 into the lipid bilayer of erythrocytes, J. Immunol. 119:1 (1977).

21. V.W. Hu, (Abstract) Photolabeling provides evidence that C9 forms the major part of a transmembrane complement channel, Immunobiology 164:255 (1983).

22. M.B. Whitlow, L.E. Ramm, and M.M. Mayer, (Abstract) Penetration of the C5b-9 complex across the erythrocyte membrane into the cytoplasmic space, Immunobiology 164:311 (1983).

23. S. Bhakdi, O.J. Bjerrum, B. Bhakdi-Lennen, and J. Tranum-Jensen, Complement lysis: Evidence for an amphiphilic nature of the terminal membrane C5b-9 complex of human complement, J. Immunol. 121:2526 (1978).

24. P.J. Sims and P.K. Lauf, Analysis of solute diffusion across the C5b-9 membrane lesion of complement: Evidence that individual C5b-9 complexes do not function as discrete, uniform pores, J. Immunol. 125:2617 (1980).

25. P.J. Sims, Permeability characteristic of complement-damaged membranes: Evaluation of the membrane leak generated by the complement proteins C5b-9, Proc. Natl. Acad. Sci. USA 78:1838 (1981).

26. E.R. Podack, A.F. Esser, G. Biesecker, and H.J. Müller-Eberhard, Membrane attack complex of complement: A structural analysis of its assembly, J. Exp. Med. 151:301 (1980).

27. M.D.P. Boyle, S.H. Ohanian, and T. Borsos, Lysis of tumor cells by antibody and complement. VII. Complement-dependent ^{86}Rb release -- a nonlethal event? J. Immunol. 117:1346 (1976)

28. A.K. Campbell, R.A. Daw, M.B. Hallet, and J.P. Luzio, Direct measurement of the increase in intracellular free calcium ion concentration in response to the action of complement, Biochem. J. 194:551 (1981).

29. E. Martz, W.L. Parker, M.K. Gately, and C.D. Tsoukas, The role of calcium in the lethal hit of T lymphocyte-mediated cytolysis, in: "Mechanisms of Cell-Mediated Cytotoxicity," W.R. Clark and P. Golstein, eds., Plenum Press, New York, (1981), p. 121.

30. S.J. Burakoff, E. Martz, and B. Benacerraf, Is the primary complement lesion insufficient for lysis? Failure of the cells damaged under osmotic protection to lyse in EDTA or at low temperature after removal of osmotic protection. Clin. Immunol. Immunopathol. 4:108 (1975).

31. G. Berke, Interaction of cytotoxic T lymphocytes and target cells. Prog. Allergy 27:69 (1980).
32. P.B. Garlick, G.K. Radda, and P.J. Seeley, Studies of acidosis in the ischemic heart by phosphorus nuclear magnetic resonance, Biochem. J. 184:547 (1979).
33. K.S. Lee and R.W. Tsien, Mechanism of calcium channel blockade by verapamil, D600, diltiazem and nitrendipine in single dialyzed heart cells. Nature 302:790 (1983).
34. J. Schlessinger, The mechanism and role of hormone-induced clustering of membrane receptors, Trends Biol. Sci. 5:210 (1980).
35. J. Braun and E.R. Unanue, Surface immunoglobulin and the lymphocyte cytoskeleton, Fed. Proc. 42:2446 (1983).

INDEX